Adult Emergency Nursing Procedures

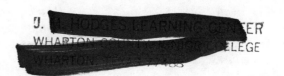

The Jones and Bartlett Series in Nursing

Adult Emergency Nursing Procedures, Proehl

Basic Steps in Planning Nursing Research, *Third Edition*, Brink/Wood

Bone Marrow Transplantation, Whedon

Cancer Chemotherapy: A Nursing Process Approach, Barton Burke et al.

Cancer Nursing: Principles and Practice, *Second Edition*, Groenwald et al.

Chemotherapy Care Plans, Barton Burke

A Clinical Manual for Nursing Assistants, McClelland/Kaspar

Children's Nutrition, Lifshitz/Finch/Lifshitz

Chronic Illness: Impact and Intervention, *Second Edition*, Lubkin

Clinical Nursing Procedures, Belland/Wells

A Comprehensive Curriculum for Trauma Nursing, Bayley/Turcke

Comprehensive Maternity Nursing, *Second Edition*, Auvenshine/Enriquez

Concepts in Oxygenation, Ahrens/Rutherford

Critical Care Review, Wright/Shelton

Emergency Care of Children, Thompson

Essential Medical Terminology, Stanfield

Family Life: Process and Practice, Janosik/Green

Fundamentals of Nursing with Clinical Procedures, *Second Edition*, Sundberg

1991-1992 Handbook of Intravenous Medications, Nentwich

Handbook of Oncology Nursing, Johnson/Gross

Health Assessment in Nursing Practice, *Third Edition*, Grimes/Burns

Health and Wellness, *Fourth Edition*, Edlin/Golanty

Healthy People 2000, U.S. Department of Health & Human Services

Human Development: A Life-Span Approach, *Fourth Edition*, Freiberg

Instruments for Clinical Nursing Research, Oncology Nursing Society

Intravenous Therapy, Nentwich

Introduction to the Health Professions, Stanfield

Introduction to Human Disease, *Third Edition*, Crowley

Journal of Perinatal Education, ASPO

Management and Leadership for Nurse Managers, Swansburg

Management of Spinal Cord Injury, *Second Edition*, Zejdlik

Math for Health Professionals, *Third Edition*, Whisler

Medical Terminology, Stanfield

Memory Bank for Chemotherapy, Preston

Memory Bank for IVs, *Second Edition*, Weinstein

Memory Bank for Medications, *Second Edition*, Kostin/Evans

Mental Health and Psychiatric Nursing: A Caring Approach, Davies/Janosik

The Nation's Health, *Third Edition*, Lee/Estes

Nursing and the Disabled: Across the Lifespan, Fraley

Nursing Assessment: A Multidimensional Approach, *Third Edition*, Bellack/Edlund

Nursing Diagnosis Care Plans for Diagnosis-Related Groups, Neal/Paquette/Mirch

Nursing Management of Children, Servonsky/Opas

Nursing Pharmacology, *Second Edition*, Wallace

Nursing Research: A Quantitative and Qualitative Approach, Roberts/Burke

Nutrition and Diet Therapy: Self-Instructional Modules, *Second Edition*, Stanfield

Pediatric Emergency Nursing Procedures, Bernardo/Bove

Perioperative Nursing Care, Fairchild

Perioperative Patient Care, *Second Edition*, Kneedler/Dodge

A Practical Guide to Breastfeeding, Riordan

Psychiatric Mental Health Nursing, *Second Edition*, Janosik/Davies

Ready Reference of Common Emergency and Prehospital Drugs, Cummings

Ready Reference for Critical Care, Strawn

The Research Process in Nursing, *Third Edition*, Dempsey/Dempsey

Understanding/Responding, *Second Edition*, Long/Prophit

Writing a Succesful Grant Application, *Second Edition*, Reif-Lehrer

Adult Emergency Nursing Procedures

Jean A. Proehl
RN, MN, CEN, CCRN

JONES AND BARTLETT PUBLISHERS
BOSTON LONDON

Editorial, Sales, and Customer Service Offices

Jones and Bartlett Publishers
One Exeter Plaza
Boston, MA 02116

Jones and Bartlett International
PO Box 1498
London W6 7RS England

The selection and dosage of drugs presented in this book are in accord with standards accepted at the time of publication. The authors and publisher have made every effort to provide accurate information. However, research, clinical practice, and government regulations often change the accepted standards in this field. Before administering any drug, the reader is advised to check the manufacturer's product information sheet for the most up-to-date recommendations on dosage, precautions, and contraindications. This is especially important in the case of drugs that are new or seldom used.

Library of Congress Cataloging-in-Publication Data

Adult emergency nursing procedures / editor, Jean A. Proehl.
    p.   cm.
    Includes bibliographical references and index.
    ISBN 0-86720-328-5
    1. Emergency nursing. 2. Emergency medicine.   I. Proehl, Jean A.
    [DNLM: 1. Emergency Nursing — methods — handbooks.   WY 39 A244]
RT120.E4A285   1992
610.73′61 — dc20
DNLM/DLC
for Library of Congress   92-15314
                                   CIP

Printed in the United States of America
97 96 95 94 93   10 9 8 7 6 5 4 3 2 1

For Madeline,
my editor in utero

Contents

Circulation Procedures

Venous Access

Blood Product Administration

Electrical Therapy

Cardiac Pacing

Invasive Monitoring

Preface

Emergency nursing encompasses a vast and varied body of knowledge. The phrase "Jack (or Jane)-of-all-trades" comes to mind when thinking of the numerous procedures an emergency nurse may be required to perform or assist with at a moment's notice. Every effort has been made to make this a comprehensive reference for practicing emergency nurses. Novices will find the basic procedures such as oral airway insertion and peripheral intravenous cannulation a helpful review. Veterans will appreciate information about infrequently performed procedures such as arterial line insertion or open thoracotomy. Managers will be able to replace their "policy and procedure" manuals with "policy only" manuals and refer to this book for information on procedures.

Wherever possible, research findings have been incorporated to provide the most recent, up-to-date information available. The authors have personal, hands-on knowledge of these procedures and you will find helpful hints scattered throughout the book. Every attempt has been made to incorporate regional variations in practice by including authors from around the country and having them review each other's chapters.

Some of these procedures provide a historic glimpse of practices no longer in common use (i.e., theraputic phlebotomy, burr holes). However, anything is possible in the emergency department! I have wished for a book like this many times during my emergency nursing career. The most memorable was the time I helped insert a Sengstaken-Blakemore tube at 4:00 AM during a snowstorm (the gastroenterologist could not reach the hospital). Neither the physician nor myself had ever seen it done, let alone done it ourselves. The instructions on the package insert helped but they did not answer all of my questions. In this book, the emphasis is on providing you with the information that you need to perform the procedure safely, without a lot of extraneous information.

One essential characteristic of a good emergency nurse is the ability to be flexible and change priorities as new situations arise. This book will provide you with some of the information you need to meet the challenges of emergency nursing in the '90s.

Contributors

Marilyn K. Bourn, RN, MSN, CEN, REMTP
Senior EMS Educator
Instructor, Department of Surgery
University of Colorado Health Sciences
Center
Denver, CO

Scott S. Bourn, RN, MSN, CEN
Clinical Nurse, Emergency Department
University Hospital
Denver, CO
President, Scott Bourn Associates
Lafayette, CO

Nancy Carrington, RN, MA, CEN
Director of Nursing, Maternal/Child
Health and Ambulatory Care
St. Francis Medical Center
Trenton, NJ

Michael Cernuska, RRT
Clinical Supervisor, Respiratory Care
Northwest Hospital
Seattle, WA

Mary E. Echternacht, RN, BSN
Emergency Department Charge Nurse
Swedish Medical Center
Englewood, CO

Sharon Gavin Fought, PhD, RN
Faculty, Department of Physiological
Nursing
University of Washington
Seattle, WA

Barbara E. Gamrath, RN, MN, CEN
Clinical Specialist
Physio-Control Corporation
Redmond, WA
Clinical Nurse
Emergency Department
Valley Medical Center
Renton, WA

Ruth Altherr Giebel, MS, RN
Cardiovascular Research Nurse
Community Hospitals Indianapolis
Indianapolis, IN

Manjula D. Gray, RN, BSN, MA, CCRN
Emergency Department Manager
Auburn General Hospital
Auburn, WA

Linell M. Jones, RN, BSN, CEN, CCRN
Assistant Head Nurse
Department of Emergency Services
Valley Medical Center
Renton, WA

Dean M. Kelly, RN, BSN, CEN
Emergency Clinical Supervisor
St. Elizabeth Hospital Medical Center
Lafayette, IN

Stephanie Kitt, RN, MSN
Director of Nursing, Emergency and
Trauma Services
Northwestern Memorial Hospital
Chicago, IL

Margo E. Layman, RNC, BSN, CEN
Unit Supervisor, Medical/Surgical Unit
Clinton County Hospital
Frankfort, IN

Anjula D. Littleton, RN, BSN, CCRN
Staff Nurse
Cardiovascular Consultants
Auburn, WA

Christine A. Miller, RN, MS
Director, Emergency Department
Swedish Medical Center
Englewood, CO

Janet A. Neff, RN, MN, CEN, CCRN
Trauma Coordinator
Stanford University Hospital
Stanford, CA
Formerly: Base Hospital Coordinator

Valerie Novotny-Dinsdale, RN, MSN, CEN
Clinical Nurse Specialist: Emergency
Department
Northwest Hospital
Seattle, WA

Jean A. Proehl, RN, MN, CEN, CCRN
Emergency Clinical Nurse Specialist
Broward General Medical Center
Ft. Lauderdale, FL
Formerly:
Emergency Clinical Nurse Specialist
Swedish Medical Center
Englewood, CO

Wendy R. Reeves, RN, BSN, CCRN
Trauma Nurse Coordinator
Broward General Medical Center
Ft. Lauderdale, FL

Cass Robertson, RN, CRNI
Nurse Manager, IV Therapy
Swedish Medical Center
Englewood, CO

Ruth L. Schaffler, RN, MA, CEN
ER/Trauma Nurse Educator
St. Joseph Hospital and Health Care
Center
Tacoma, WA

Dorothy Schulte, RN, MS
Rural Facilities Manager
St. Anthony Hospital Systems
Frisco, CO

Ruth A. Slabach, MSN, SCN, RN
*Nursing Information Systems
Specialist*
MidWest Medical Center
Indianapolis, IN
Formerly: *Emergency Clinical
Specialist*

Marijane Smallwood, RN, BSN
*Director Emergency/Outpatient
Services*
MidWest Medical Center
Indianapolis, IN

Dawn M. Swimm, RN, CEN
Clinical Instructor, Emergency
Department
General Hospital Medical Center
Everett, WA

Lori D. Taylor, RN, BSN, CEN
Trauma Coordinator
Sacred Heart Medical Center
Spokane, WA

Acknowledgments

I would like to gratefully acknowledge the following people who made many of the illustrations possible: Peter Rosen, MD for generously sharing many of the illustrations from his book, *Atlas of Emergency Medicine*, Chris Schumann, RN for drawing original illustrations, and Robert R. Simon, MD and Earle W. Wilkins, Jr., MD for permission to reproduce numerous figures from their texts.

In my quest for content accuracy, many people provided their expertise and deserve credit: Linda V. Hackley, RN, BSN, CEN for reviewing the entire manuscript for clarity and accuracy, Bradley M. Calhoun, BS, RRT who answered my respiratory therapy questions, and all of the contributing authors for diligently researching their own procedures and reviewing those of their colleagues.

Introduction

This book assumes that the reader possesses basic nursing knowledge. Thus, some information is not included in the procedures because it is assumed to be part of standard nursing practice. These assumed practices include, but are not limited to

- Verifying the patient's identification and introducing yourself
- Obtaining an appropriate history and physical examination
- Placing the patient in a position of comfort when possible
- Explaining the procedure to the patient
- Providing emotional support
- Obtaining verbal and/or written consent as indicated by institutional policy
- Attending to life-threatening emergencies first
- Including the family and significant others in explanations, follow-up teaching, and emotional support
- Teaching the patient about prescribed medications
- Draping the patient to provide privacy and conserve warmth
- Washing your hands and maintaining aseptic technique when indicated
- Protecting yourself with universal barrier precautions
- Documenting your assessment findings, interventions, and the patient's response to them.

This book is intended to be a working manual. Each chapter follows the same format to make information easier to find. Margins are provided to insert institution-specific comments about the procedure (e.g., this tray is kept only in C.S., or we use Technique A in this department). By personalizing the book in this fashion it becomes an even more valuable resource, especially for new or inexperienced staff members.

Nursing practice varies from state to state and from institution to institution. An asterisk (*) has been used throughout the book to indicate portions of the procedure usually performed by a physician. This is not intended to prescribe nursing or medical practice but rather to indicate the usual role delineation in the experience of the authors. The information about physician components will help the nurse anticipate needs and expedite safe care.

1

Universal Barrier Precautions

Janet A. Neff, RN, MN, CEN, CCRN

Universal precautions were designed for use with all patients when the risk of blood exposure is high and the infective status of the patient is unknown. A broader program of protection, referred to as body substance isolation, is designed to prevent exposure to bloodborne pathogens as well as other pathogens. This chapter will consider both.

INDICATIONS

Potential contact with patient fluids, secretions, and drainage which are assumed to be infective in nature. **All patients should be regarded as potential carriers of disease.**

BACKGROUND INFORMATION

1. The Centers for Disease Control (CDC) and the Occupational Safety and Health Administration (OSHA) mandate protection for healthcare workers to prevent occupational exposure to pathogens.
2. OSHA reports that approximately 2,000,000 workers are at risk of exposure in hospitals, with the highest risk areas including the emergency department (ED).
3. Hepatitis B virus (HBV) is a pathogen that can result in serious illness and death. The CDC estimate that there are 18,000 cases in United States healthcare workers each year, of which approximately 200 die from the infection. "One ml of HBsAg positive blood may contain 100 million infectious doses of virus; thus, exposure to extremely small inocula of HBV-positive blood may transmit infection" (Department of Labor, 1989).

    One percent of hospitalized patients are HBV carriers, yet most are asymptomatic and their charts do not reflect this status. HBV can survive for one week in a dried condition on environmental surfaces (Bond, 1981). This supports the need for protective precautions and prophylactic vaccination for high risk personnel.

    Any product approved by the Environmental Protection Agency (EPA) as a high level disinfectant or sterilizing agent will kill HBV, and dilute solutions of household bleach are also effective. The selection and proper use of sterilization and disinfection for medical equipment is complex but rely on prevention of drying and encrusting of organic material on ED equipment (Rutala, 1989).
4. An infection with the human immunodeficiency virus type 1 (HIV-1), which results in AIDS, is fatal. CDC report that of 1,201 healthcare worker exposures to HIV-infected blood, 37% could have been prevented if the recommended infection control precautions had been followed. Documented modes of HIV transmission pertinent to healthcare workers include parenteral, mucous membrane, or nonintact skin contact with HIV-infected blood or blood products.

CONTRAINDICATIONS AND CAUTIONS

1. Staff may initially be less skilled at procedures when wearing protective devices such as gloves.
2. Protective devices are not infallible and can contribute to increased exposure by others if misused (for example, not removing soiled gloves before touching equipment such as telephones).
3. Barrier precautions should not be selectively used based on patient history, nor should action await positive laboratory findings. **All patients should be regarded as potentially infectious.**
4. Latex deteriorates and becomes permeable to microscopic organisms when exposed to petroleum-based products (ointments).

EQUIPMENT AND PROCEDURAL STEPS

1. Gloves should be worn for potential or actual direct contact with blood or body fluids, mucous membranes, nonintact tissues, or contaminated items and surfaces. Gloves not only serve to protect the provider but also to reduce transmission of infectious disease to other patients and providers. However, protection is dependent upon appropriate disposal of gloves after contamination and handwashing after removal. The gloves cannot be effectively washed and reused.

   Studies have shown that sterile gloves are less permeable than nonsterile examination gloves (DeGroot-Kosolcharoen, 1989; Yangco, 1989), and that gloves incorporated within suction kits have poorer performance. The Technical Panel on Infections within Hospitals (1989) rates latex and vinyl equally provided the gloves are intact. A leakage rate of 2.5% is the acceptable quality level established by the American Society for Testing and Materials.

   High risk gloves, for use in settings such as prehospital and emergency services, are thicker and often more form fitting. They also offer improved durability, dexterity, and greater ease in working with materials such as tape.

2. Numerous factors such as cost, flammability, reusability, disposability, and expected exposure level must be considered when selecting aseptic barrier gowns. Cover gowns or over garments that are tightly woven or made of fused material should be worn when exposure to body substances is possible. Fluid-resistant and fluid-proof over garments should also be available when there is high potential for blood exposure or when exposed skin and clothing are likely to be grossly contaminated, such as in gastric lavage, major trauma, and gastrointestinal bleeding. The issue of whether cover gowns such as lab coats or scrub jackets should be left in the department for cleaning or laundering is still debated. The trend toward employee purchase and laundering of scrubs may be questionable in high risk departments.

3. Masks and goggles or combination face shields should be available for situations where splatter can be expected such as during intubation, suctioning, wound cleansing, chest tube insertion, and arterial access. Eye protection should be broad enough to protect against frontal, inferior, or lateral splashing, and designed to avoid distortion and dizziness with head movement. Masks serve to protect employees from respiratory droplet contamination and body fluid splashes. Masks are functional for a limited time due to the accumulation of moisture and handling during use. Most references state that masks should be changed periodically, however, one reference suggests that they may be worn up to eight hours provided they remain dry (American Hospital Association, 1979).

4. Resuscitation devices for patient ventilation should be readily accessible and incorporate double lumen systems and one-way valves to protect the provider. Mouth-to-mouth resuscitation is not necessary in properly prepared emergency settings.

5. Impermeable, containment devices for disposal of sharp instruments must be in close proximity to the area of use, contain an easy entry port, prohibit inappropriate access, and be routinely emptied. Needles should not be recapped but instead dropped directly into a sharps container. The greatest potential for needlestick exposure is during needle recapping or manipulation (Dept. of Labor, 1989). OSHA has revised its needle recapping policy to allow use of mechanical devices for safe recapping, which are particularly useful when handling arterial blood gases and titration of drug doses (OSHA permits, 1990).

6. An institutional guidebook that outlines the means of disposal and cleansing of instruments, room disinfection, containment and management of soiled laundry and waste should be available. The role of emergency nursing staff, ancillary and housekeeping personnel should be clear. The manual should also review infectious diseases including the infective material, room requirements, special considerations, duration of isolation required, and terminal disinfection instructions.

7. Protocols for caregiver exposure to communicable diseases should be formalized and available for quick reference in the emergency department. A plan must be available for exposures occurring at any time. Emergency departments are often involved in following up with prehospital personnel who may have been exposed to an infectious disease. Working in conjunction with the prehospital primary provider and infectious disease/risk management staff, the emergency department can develop an effective system to follow up, refer, and treat prehospital personnel as indicated.

COMPLICATIONS

1. Noncompliance with universal body substance exposure precautions may result in otherwise preventable illness or death of healthcare workers and may result in transmission of disease to other patients.

2. Legal, ethical, and confidentiality issues must be carefully considered.

PATIENT TEACHING

Barrier devices (gown, gloves, etc.) are routinely used when there is any chance of body fluid exposure. These measures help protect healthcare workers and patients from disease transmission.

REFERENCES

American Hospital Association. 1979. *Infection control in the hospital,* 4th ed. Chicago: American Hospital Association.

Bond, W.W., Favero, M.S., & Peterson, N.J. 1981. Survival of hepatitis B virus after drying and storage for one week. *Lancet,* 1:550–551.

DeGroot-Kosolcharoen, J., & Jones, J.M. 1989. Permeability of latex and vinyl gloves to water and blood. *American Journal of Infection Control,* 17, 1:196–201.

Department of Labor. 1989. Occupational exposure to bloodborne pathogens; Proposed rule and notice of hearing. *Federal Register,* 54, 102:23041–23139. (29 CFR Part 1910).

OSHA permits recapping devices, requires free HBV vaccine. 1990. *Hospital Infection Control*, 17, 6:69–72.

Petersen, D. 1988. *Safety management: A human approach*, 2nd ed. New York: Aloray.

Rutala, W.A. 1989. Draft guideline for selection and use of disinfectants. *American Journal of Infection Control*, 17, 1:24A–38A.

Technical Panel on Infections within Hospitals: American Hospital Association. 1989. Management of HIV infection in the hospital. *American Journal of Infection Control*, 17, 4:24A–44A.

Yangco, B.G., & Yangco, N.F. 1989. What is leaky can be risky: A study of the integrity of hospital gloves. *Infection Control and Hospital Epidemiology*, 10, 12:553–556.

SUGGESTED READINGS

Association for the Advancement of Medical Instrumentation. 1988. *Good hospital practice: Steam sterilization and sterility assurance.* Arlington: Association for the Advancement of Medical Instrumentation.

Centers for Disease Control. 1989. Guidelines for prevention of transmission of human immunodeficiency virus and hepatitis B virus to health-care and public-safety workers. *MMWR*, 38, S–6:1–21.

Reed, B. 1990. Infectious diseases. In S. Kitt and J. Kaiser (eds) *Emergency nursing/ A physiologic and clinical perspective.* Philadelphia: Saunders; 667–701.

Technical Panel on Infections within Hospitals: American Hospital Association. 1989. Management of HIV infection in the hospital. *American Journal of Infection Control*, 17, 4:24A–44A.

Primary Survey

Jean A. Proehl, RN, MN, CEN, CCRN

INDICATIONS

To rapidly assess and intervene for life-threatening conditions in critically ill or injured patients.

CONTRAINDICATIONS AND CAUTIONS

1. The presence of an environmental hazard such as fire or noxious fumes which mandates immediate evacuation of the area.
2. Do not proceed to the next assessment step until interventions for life-threatening conditions have been implemented.

EQUIPMENT

Towel rolls or other lateral head
      supports
2–3″ adhesive tape
Stethoscope
Flashlight
Other equipment as indicated for
      resuscitative procedures

PROCEDURAL STEPS

1. Assess airway patency while simultaneously maintaining cervical spine immobilization with manual stabilization. Airway patency is assessed by looking for chest rise and fall, listening and feeling for air movement from the nose and mouth. If the airway is partially or completely obstructed, implement the appropriate intervention. Potential interventions include the following and are described elsewhere in this text:
    Ch. 4: Airway Procedures – Positioning
    Ch. 31: Pharyngeal Suctioning
    Ch. 5: Airway Procedures – Foreign Object Removal
    Ch. 6: Oral Airway Insertion
    Ch. 7: Nasal Airway Insertion
    Ch. 8: Esophageal Obturator Airway and Gastric Tube Airway Insertion
    Ch. 9, 10, 11: Endotracheal Intubation
    Ch. 12: Pharyngeal Tracheal Lumen Airway
    Ch. 13: Cricothyroidotomy
    Ch. 14: Percutaneous Transtracheal Ventilation
    Ch. 15: Tracheostomy
2. If cervical spine injury is a possibility, immobilize the head with towel

rolls or other lateral head supports and wide tape across the forehead. Cervical spine immobilization should be maintained throughout the primary and secondary survey.

3. Assess breathing adequacy by observing respiratory rate, depth, and difficulty. If respiratory compromise is present, breath sounds should be briefly auscultated bilaterally. If respirations are absent or abnormal, implement the appropriate intervention. Potential interventions include the following and are described elsewhere in this text:

   Ch. 16: Positioning the Dyspneic Patient
   Ch. 31, 32, 33, 34: Suctioning
   Ch. 21, 22, 23, 24, 25, 26, 27, 28, 29, 30: Oxygen Therapy
   Ch. 35: Mouth-to-Mask Ventilation
   Ch. 36: Bag-Valve-Mask Ventilation
   Ch. 37: Anesthesia Bag Ventilation
   Ch. 38: Oxygen-Powered Breathing Devices
   Ch. 41: Needle Thoracostomy
   Ch. 42: Chest Tube Insertion
   Flutter valve or occlusive dressing for sucking chest wound

4. Assess circulation by evaluating the radial or carotid pulse for rate and strength. Observe the skin for warmth, color, and moisture. Check for exsanguinating external hemorrhage. If circulation is absent or altered, institute ECG monitoring (see Ch. 57) and implement the appropriate interventions. Potential interventions include the following and are described elsewhere in this text:

   Ch. 55: Positioning the Hypotensive Patient
   Direct pressure for external hemorrhage
   Ch. 60: External Cardiac Massage
   Ch. 62, 63, 64, 65, 66, 67, 68, 69, 70: Intravenous Fluid Administration
   Ch. 71: Pneumatic Antishock Garment
   Ch. 83: Pericardiocentesis
   Ch. 84: Defibrillation
   Ch. 85: Cardioversion
   Ch. 86, 87, 88: Cardiac Pacing
   Ch. 89: Emergency Thoracotomy/Internal Defibrillation

5. Evaluate neurologic status by assessing the patient's best motor, verbal, and eye opening responses using the Glasgow Coma Scale criteria, Table 2.1. Assess pupil size, equality, and reaction to light. Interventions for altered levels of consciousness may include the administration of glucose, naloxone, and thiamine per physician orders.

Table 2.1 Glasgow coma scale.

Best Response	Score
Eye Opening	
Spontaneous	4
To voice	3
To pain	2
None	1
Motor Response	
Obeys commands	6
Localizes pain	5
Withdraws from pain	4
Flexion to pain	3
Extension to pain	2
None	1
Verbal Response	
Oriented	5
Confused	4
Inappropriate	3
Incomprehensible	2
None	1
TOTAL	3 to 15

COMPLICATIONS

1. Failure to recognize and intervene appropriately for life-threatening conditions before progressing to the next assessment step may result in patient deterioration.
2. Intervening for noncritical problems (such as extremity fractures) before correcting life-threatening conditions may result in patient deterioration.

PATIENT TEACHING

Do not move until spinal injury has been ruled out.

SUGGESTED READINGS

American College of Surgeons, Committee on Trauma. 1988. *Advanced trauma life support course: Student manual.* Chicago: American College of Surgeons.

American Heart Association. 1987. *Textbook of advanced cardiac life support.* Dallas: American Heart Association.

Butman, A.M., & Paturas, J.L. (eds). 1986. *Pre-hospital trauma life support.* Akron, OH: Educational Direction.

Rea, R.E. (ed). 1991. *Trauma nursing core course (provider) manual,* 3rd ed. Chicago: Award Printing.

3

Secondary Survey

Jean A. Proehl, RN, MN, CEN, CCRN

INDICATIONS

1. To rapidly and systematically assess injured patients from head-to-toe to identify all injuries.
2. To rapidly and systematically assess critically ill patients in whom the etiology of signs and symptoms is unclear.

CONTRAINDICATIONS AND CAUTIONS

1. Do not begin the secondary survey until the primary survey has been completed and resuscitation procedures initiated as indicated. See Ch. 2: Primary Survey.
2. Continue to monitor airway, breathing, circulatory, and neurological status during the secondary survey and interrupt the secondary survey to initiate interventions as indicated.
3. Prioritize and initiate interventions for injuries or conditions discovered in the secondary survey *after* the entire head-to-toe examination is complete.

EQUIPMENT

Stethoscope
Blood pressure cuff
Clock or watch with a second hand
Thermometer (not immediately
          indicated for all patients)
Sheet or blanket

PROCEDURAL STEPS

1. Maintain cervical spine immobilization for all trauma patients as initiated in the primary survey.
2. Remove all clothing to facilitate a complete patient assessment. Cover the patient to preserve body temperature.
3. Obtain blood pressure, pulse, and respirations. Temperature determination may be deferred but should be performed as quickly as possible in the very old and very young and in patients with potential hypo- or hyperthermia.
4. If the patient is conscious, elicit information about painful areas and in-

struct him/her to report tenderness elicited by palpation. Obtain a brief history of the mechanism of injury and any chronic diseases.

5. Inspect the head and face for wounds, deformities, discolorations, or bloody or serious drainage from the nose or ears. Palpate the entire head and face for wounds, deformities, or tenderness. In the conscious and cooperative patient, evaluate extraocular movements, gross vision, and dental occlusion. Note any unusual odors, for example, gasoline, fruity breath, or ethanol.

6. Inspect the anterior neck for wounds, jugular vein distention, discolorations, or deformities. Gently palpate the posterior neck for wounds, deformities, tenderness, or muscle spasm from the base of the skull to the upper back. Palpate the anterior neck for deformities, crepitus, tenderness, or tracheal deviation (best palpated in the notch above the manubrium).

7. Inspect the anterior and lateral chest for wounds, deformities, discolorations, respiratory expansion, symmetry, and paradoxical movement. Palpate the anterior and lateral chest for deformities, tenderness, or crepitus. Auscultate breath sounds to determine if they are present and equal bilaterally. Auscultate heart sounds to determine if they are clear or muffled.

8. Inspect the abdomen for wounds, discolorations, or distention. Auscultate all quadrants for the presence of bowel sounds. Gently palpate the abdomen for tenderness, guarding, or masses (palpate areas known to be painful last).

9. Inspect pelvic area and genitalia for wounds, deformities, discolorations, or bleeding from the urinary meatus. Palpate for pelvic tenderness, crepitus, or instability by gently pressing in on the anterior superior iliac crests bilaterally and pushing down on the pubic symphysis. Palpate femoral pulses for presence and equality.

10. Inspect all extremities for wounds, deformities, or discolorations. Palpate all extremities for tenderness, deformities, muscle spasm, and distal pulses. In the conscious patient, determine gross motor and sensory function by having the patient wiggle toes and fingers and asking if he/she can feel you touching them.

11. Obtain assistance to maintain cervical spine alignment and support injured extremities while logrolling the patient to the side. In some patients it may be necessary to roll the patient to both sides to adequately assess the posterior surfaces. Inspect the posterior surfaces for wounds, deformities, or discolorations. Palpate all posterior surfaces for tenderness, deformities, or muscle spasm.

12. *Perform a rectal exam to assess sphincter tone and, in male patients, the prostate.

*Indicates portions of the procedure usually performed by a physician.

COMPLICATIONS

1. Failure to recognize and intervene appropriately for life-threatening conditions that develop or worsen during the secondary assessment may result in patient deterioration.

2. Failure to maintain cervical spine immobilization throughout the secondary survey may result in trauma to the spinal cord.

3. Failure to complete the secondary survey and prioritize interventions before instituting interventions may result in patient deterioration.

4. Intervening for noncritical problems (such as extremity fractures) before correcting life-threatening conditions may result in patient deterioration.

PATIENT TEACHING

Do not move until spinal injury has been ruled out.

SUGGESTED READINGS

American College of Surgeons, Committee on Trauma. 1988. *Advanced trauma life support course: Student manual.* Chicago: American College of Surgeons.

Butman, A.M., & Paturas, J.L. (eds). 1986. *Pre-hospital trauma life support.* Akron, OH: Educational Direction.

Rea, R.E. (ed). 1991. *Trauma nursing core course (provider) manual,* 3rd ed. Chicago: Award Printing.

4

Positioning

Mary E. Echternacht, RN, BSN

INDICATIONS

To relieve upper airway obstruction due to displacement of the tongue into the posterior pharynx and/or occlusion by the epiglottis at the level of the larynx.

CONTRAINDICATIONS AND CAUTIONS

1. If the patient has a suspected neck injury, the head and neck should remain in a neutral position – do not hyperextend the neck.
2. Positioning alone may not be sufficient to attain and maintain an open airway. Additional interventions (suctioning, intubation, etc.) may be necessary.

PROCEDURAL STEPS

1. Place patient in supine position.
2. Lift the chin forward to anteriorly displace the mandible while tilting the head back with a hand on the forehead. See Figure 4.1. This maneuver will result in hyperextension of the neck.
3. If head-tilt, chin-lift is unsuccessful, use the jaw thrust maneuver. Grasp the lower jaw and gently bring it forward. See Figure 4.2.

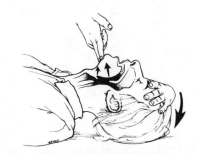

Figure 4.1 Head-tilt, chin-lift. (American Heart Association, 1987: 27. Reprinted by permission.)

COMPLICATIONS

1. If the airway remains obstructed, an oropharyngeal or nasopharyngeal airway should be inserted. See Ch. 6: Oral Airway Insertion; Ch. 7: Nasal Airway Insertion.
2. Injury to the spinal cord may occur if the head and/or neck are moved in patients with cervical spine injuries.

SUGGESTED READINGS

American Heart Association. 1987. *Textbook of advanced cardiac life support.* Dallas: American Heart Association.
Rosen, P., & Sternbach, G.L. 1983. *Atlas of emergency medicine,* 2nd ed. Baltimore: Williams & Wilkins.

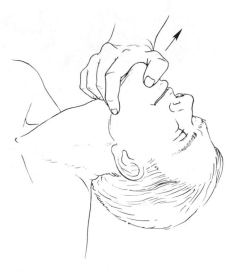

Figure 4.2 Jaw thrust. (Rosen & Sternbach, 1983: 11. Reprinted by permission.)

5

Foreign Object Removal

Mary E. Echternacht, RN, BSN

Foreign object removal is also known as the Heimlich Maneuver, subdiaphragmatic thrust, abdominal thrust, chest thrust.

INDICATIONS

To relieve upper airway obstruction caused by foreign objects and characterized by some or all of the following signs and symptoms:
1. The patient develops sudden inability to speak.
2. The patient exhibits the universal sign for choking—clutching the neck. See Figure 5.1. (Wilkins, 1989)
3. The patient has noisy airflow during inspiration.
4. The patient uses accessory muscles during respiration.
5. The patient has no spontaneous breathing or becomes cyanotic.

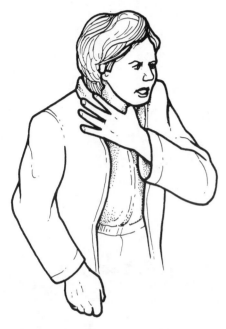

Figure 5.1 Universal sign for choking.
(Baker et al., 1988: 91. Reprinted by permission.)

CONTRAINDICATIONS AND CAUTIONS

1. In the conscious patient, a voluntary cough may serve as the best method to achieve increased airway pressure and relieve the obstruction (Rosen, 1988).
2. Chest thrusts should not be used in the patient who has chest injury, e.g., flail chest, cardiac contusion, or sternal fracture (Simon, 1987).
3. Chest thrusts may be necessary if the abdominal thrust is anatomically impossible due to obesity or advanced pregnancy (White, 1986).
4. Correct hand placement is essential during delivery of abdominal thrusts to avoid injury to underlying organs.
5. It is not recommended that foreign bodies in the upper airway be removed digitally, because this may move the obstruction distally (Wilkins, 1989).

EQUIPMENT

Oral suction (if available)
Magill forceps and laryngoscope
(optional for foreign object
removal that can be
visualized in the upper
airway)

PATIENT PREPARATION

1. The patient may be sitting, standing, or supine.
2. Suction any blood or mucous you can visualize in the patient's mouth.
3. Remove broken or loose fitting dentures.
4. Be prepared to perform more definitive airway management, such as cricothyroidotomy. See Ch. 13: Cricothyroidotomy.

PROCEDURAL STEPS

1. Stand behind the sitting or standing patient and wrap your arms around the abdomen. If the patient is supine, kneel, straddling the patient's thighs.
2. Hand placement is as follows:
   a. **For the standing or sitting patient,** make a fist with one hand and cover the fist with your other hand. Hand placement on the patient's abdomen should be below the xiphoid process and above the navel. See Figure 5.2. (American Heart Association, 1987)

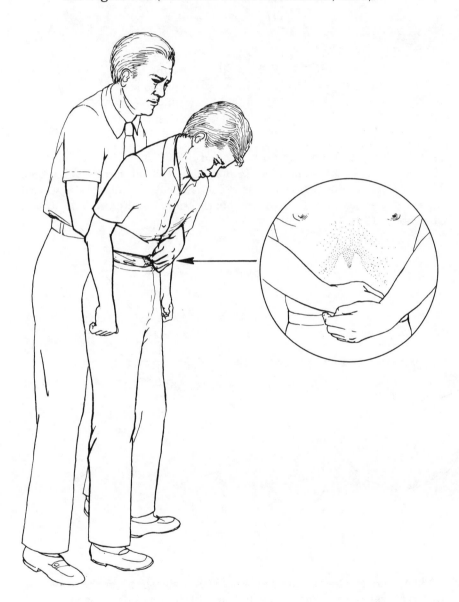

Figure 5.2 Correct hand placement for abdominal thrust for a patient sitting or standing.
(Rosen & Sternbach, 1983: Reprinted by permission.)

   b. **For the supine patient,** place one hand over the other with the heel of the bottom hand against the patient's abdomen below the xiphoid process and above the navel. See Figure 5.3 on page 14. (American Heart Association, 1987)
4. Thrust quickly compressing abdomen inward and upward.
5. Repeat abdominal thrusts several times if necessary to relieve airway obstruction. Assess the airway frequently to determine the success of the maneuver.
6. **For the pregnant or obese patient,** the chest thrust may be performed. The patient may be supine, sitting, or standing. Put one hand directly

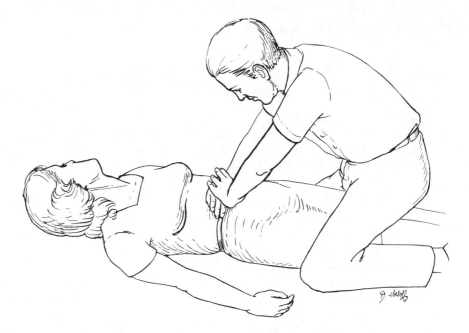

**Figure 5.3   Correct hand placement
for abdominal thrust in the supine
patient.**
(Rosen & Sternbach, 1983: 33. Reprinted by permission.)

over the other and position bottom hand in mid-sternal area above the
xiphoid process (the same position used in external cardiac massage).
Thrust straight down toward the spine. Repeat chest thrusts several
times if necessary to relieve airway obstruction. See Figure 5.4. (Rosen,
Sternbach, 1983)

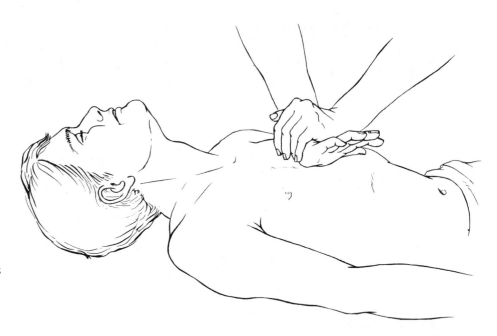

**Figure 5.4   Correct hand placement
for chest thrust.**
(Rosen & Sternbach, 1983: 37. Reprinted by permission.)

*Indicates portions of the procedure
usually performed by a physician.

7.   *When there is direct visualization of the foreign body in the upper airway, removal by forceps may be indicated. Use Magill forceps and laryngoscope to retrieve material seen in the posterior pharynx. This
maneuver, if unsuccessful, may dislodge or further impact the foreign
body with the resultant inability to remove it by the other artificial
cough techniques (Hoffman, 1982).

COMPLICATIONS

1. Abdominal pain, ecchymosis
2. Nausea, vomiting
3. Fractured ribs
4. Injury to underlying abdominal or chest organs

PATIENT TEACHING

Prevention tips
1. Eat slowly.
2. Cut food into small pieces.
3. Chew food thoroughly.
4. Don't laugh or talk while chewing.
5. Make sure dentures fit.
6. Avoid excessive alcohol.
7. Sit down while eating.

REFERENCES

American Heart Association. 1986. *Cardiopulmonary resuscitation,* 3rd ed. Tulsa: CPR Publishers.

Hoffman, J. 1982. Treatment of foreign body obstruction of the upper airway. *Western Journal of Medicine,* 136:11-22.

Baker, F.J., Jr., Strauss, R., & Walter, J.J. 1988. Cardiac arrest, in R. Rosen, F. Baker, R. Barkin, G. Braen, R. Daily, & R. Levy (eds). *Emergency medicine: Concepts and clinical practice,* 2nd ed. St. Louis: Mosby. 91-92.

Rosen, P., & Sternbach, G.L. 1983. *Atlas of emergency medicine,* 2nd ed. Baltimore: Williams & Wilkins.

Simon, R., & Brenner, B. 1987. *Emergency procedures and techniques,* 2nd ed. Baltimore: Williams & Wilkins.

White, R. 1986. Foreign body airway obstruction: Considerations in 1985. *Circulation,* 74:60-62.

Wilkins, E. (ed). 1989. *Emergency medicine: Scientific foundations and current practice,* 3rd ed. Baltimore: Williams & Wilkins.

6

Oral Airway Insertion

Mary E. Echternacht, RN, BSN

INDICATIONS

To maintain airway patency under the following conditions:
1. The unconscious patient with a loss of tonicity to the submandibular muscles resulting in airway obstruction (American Heart Association, 1987).
2. The patient's airway has not been successfully opened by other maneuvers—head-tilt, chin-lift, or jaw thrust.
3. The patient is being ventilated by a bag-valve-mask device. An oral airway elevates the soft tissues of the posterior pharynx making it easier to ventilate the lungs and minimizing gastric insufflation (Rosen & Sternbach, 1983).
4. To prevent an orally intubated patient from biting the endotracheal tube.

CONTRAINDICATIONS AND CAUTIONS

1. Insertion of an oral airway in a conscious or semiconscious patient may stimulate the gag reflex and cause the patient to vomit.
2. Incorrect placement of an oral airway may compress the tongue into the posterior pharynx causing further obstruction.
3. Failure to clear the oropharynx of foreign material before insertion of the airway may result in aspiration (Rosen, 1983).

EQUIPMENT

Oropharyngeal suction equipment
Oropharyngeal airway
Tongue blade

PATIENT PREPARATION

1. Place the patient in a supine position.
2. Suction the patient's oropharynx of blood, secretions, or other foreign material.
3. Select the appropriate oropharyngeal airway size. Align the tube on the side of the patient's face and choose an airway that extends from the tragus to the corner of the mouth. (Grauer, 1987). See Figure 6.1.

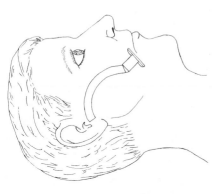

Figure 6.1. Sizing the oropharyngeal airway.

PROCEDURAL STEPS

1. Insert the airway upside down into the mouth. As the tip of the airway reaches the posterior wall of the pharynx, rotate the device 180° into proper position. See Figure 6.2.
2. As an alternative procedure, use a tongue blade to depress and displace the tongue out of the way. Insert the airway right side up into the oropharynx.
3. The distal tip of the airway should lie between the base of the tongue and the back of the throat. The flange of the tube should sit comfortably on the lips. Auscultate the lungs for equal and clear breath sounds during ventilation.

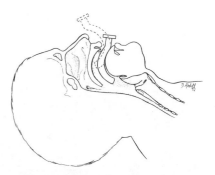

Figure 6.2. Correct placement of oropharyngeal airway. (Rosen & Sternbach, 1983: 7. Reprinted by permission.)

COMPLICATIONS

1. Trauma to lips, tongue, teeth or oral mucosa
2. Aspiration
3. Hypoxia secondary to aspiration or improper placement

REFERENCES

American Heart Association. 1987. *Textbook of advanced cardiac life support,* Dallas: American Heart Association.

Rosen, P., & Sternbach, G.L. 1983. *Atlas of emergency medicine,* 2nd ed. Baltimore: Williams and Wilkins.

Grauer, K., & Cavallaro, D. 1987. *ACLS: Certification preparation and a comprehensive review,* 2nd ed. St. Louis: Mosby.

Nasal Airway Insertion

Mary E. Echternacht, RN, BSN

INDICATIONS

To maintain airway patency under the following conditions:
1. When the use of an oropharyngeal airway is contraindicated—in the conscious or semiconscious patient with a gag reflex.
2. When the patient has severe facial trauma making placement of other airway adjuncts technically difficult.

CONTRAINDICATIONS AND CAUTIONS

1. Insertion of a nasal airway may stimulate the gag reflex causing the patient to vomit.
2. If the tube is too long it may enter the esophagus causing gastric insufflation and hypoventilation (American Heart Association, 1987).
3. Epistaxis may occur leading to aspiration of blood.
4. The nasal airway should not be used in the presence of facial fractures causing nasal obstruction or basal skull fractures involving the cribiform plate creating the risk of intracranial tube placement (Morris, 1988).

EQUIPMENT

Nasopharyngeal suction equipment
Lubricant
Nasopharyngeal airway.
         Recommended sizes
         (American Heart
         Association, 1987) are
         indicated in millimeters for
         outer diameter (o.d.) as
         follows:

Large adult: 11.4-mm o.d. = 34-Fr
Medium adult: 10.0-mm o.d. = 30-FR
Small adult: 8.7-mm o.d. = 26-Fr

PATIENT PREPARATION

1. Place the patient in a supine position.
2. Assess the nasal passages for trauma, foreign body, or septal deviation.
3. Select and lubricate nasal airway. Use the largest airway that will easily pass through the nares.
4. Prepare suction equipment for use if necessary.

PROCEDURAL STEPS

1. Pass the airway along the floor of the nostril with the bevel facing the nasal septum. See Figure 7.1.
2. If resistance is encountered, slight rotation of the tube may facilitate passage as the device reaches the hypopharynx.
3. Maintain anterior displacement of the mandible by chin-lift and/or jaw-thrust when using nasal airway to ensure proper positioning. (American Heart Association, 1987)
4. Auscultate the lungs for equal and clear breath sounds during respirations.

COMPLICATIONS

1. Epistaxis
2. Aspiration
3. Hypoxia secondary to aspiration or improper placement

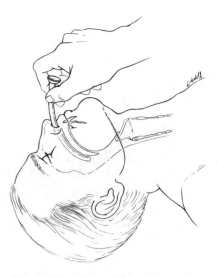

Figure 7.1. Correct placement of nasopharyngeal airway. (Rosen & Sternbach, 1983: 9. Reprinted by permission.)

REFERENCES

American Heart Association. 1987. *Textbook of advanced cardiac life support.* Dallas: American Heart Association.

Rosen, P. & Sternbach, G.L. 1983. *Atlas of emergency medicine,* 2nd ed. Baltimore: Williams and Wilkins.

Morris, I.R. 1988. *Emergency medicine concepts and clinical practice,* 2nd ed. St. Louis: Mosby.

Esophageal Obturator Airway and Gastric Tube Airway Insertion

Scott S. Bourn, RN, MSN, CEN

Esophageal obturator airway and gastric tube airway are also known as EOA (esophageal obturator airway) and EGTA (esophageal gastric tube airway).

The esophageal obturator airway (EOA) and the esophageal gastric tube airway (EGTA) are airway adjuncts that may be used instead of endotracheal tubes. Both airways are rigid, cuffed, plastic airways that are blindly inserted into the esophagus. Placement of the cuffed tube into the esophagus effectively prevents vomiting and aspiration, and insufflation of air into the stomach during ventilation is minimized. Ventilation of the lungs is provided through a mask which is placed over the mouth and nose.

The esophageal obturator airway is a blind tube which is placed into the esophagus. See Figure 8.1. Ventilation is provided through holes near the proximal end of the tube. While this tube effectively seals the esophagus and

Figure 8.1.   A. The esophageal obturator airway (EOA); B. The EOA in place.
(McCabe, 1989: 3. Reprinted by permission.)

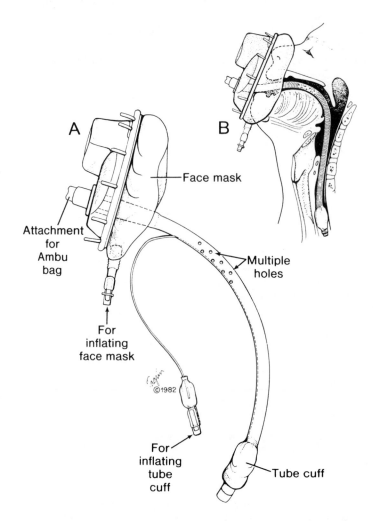

prevents vomiting and aspiration, there is no mechanism to vent or empty the stomach. This limitation has resulted in cases of esophageal perforation and stomach rupture (Pons, 1988).

The esophageal gastric tube airway is an improved version of the EOA. See Figure 8.2. The EGTA is an open tube which incorporates a gastric tube to facilitate venting and evacuation of stomach contents. Ventilation is provided through a separate port in the mask. This modification prevents the high gastric pressures which lead to esophageal perforation and gastric rupture when the EOA is utilized (Pons, 1988).

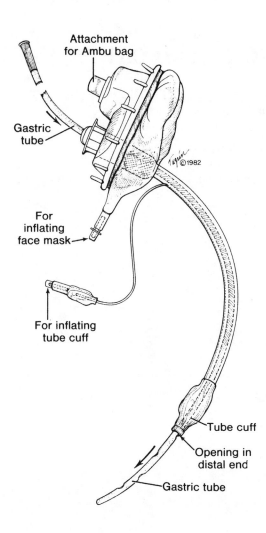

Figure 8.2. The esophageal gastric tube airway (EGTA).
(McCabe, 1989: 4. Reprinted by permission.)

Proponents of the EOA and EGTA airways cite the following advantages of their use:
1. Minimal training is required for insertion.
2. Minimal skill is required for use.
3. Both can be inserted blindly without visualizing the glottis.
4. Insertion requires minimal movement of the cervical spine.

INDICATIONS

To secure the airway in cases of inadequate airway or ventilation in adult patients without a gag reflex. **Note:** Most sources consider endotracheal intubation to be the most effective method of airway protection (Don Michael,

1985; Pons, 1988; Hammargren, 1985). Reports on the effectiveness of ventilation and arterial blood gas analysis of the EOA and EGTA are conflicting. Meislin (1980) reported that the EOA was as effective as endotracheal intubation in maintaining arterial blood gases. A later study (Shea, 1985) found no statistically significant differences in survival and neurological sequellae between patients managed with the EOA or EGTA and those who were intubated. Conflicting with these results are two studies which document inadequate arterial blood gases as compared to intubation (Auerbach & Geehr, 1983) and an inability to successfully oxygenate 69% of patients managed using the EOA (Smith, 1983).

CONTRAINDICATIONS AND CAUTIONS

1. Absolute contraindications for the use of the EOA or EGTA include
   a. Patients under five feet tall
   b. Patients with an intact gag reflex
   c. Patients with known esophageal disease
   d. Patients who have ingested corrosives
2. Facial trauma may make it difficult to achieve an adequate seal with the mask.

EQUIPMENT

EOA or EGTA
Stethoscope for auscultation of
    tube position
Additional supportive equipment:
    Suction, with tonsil tips
    Bag-valve-mask
    Oxygen source and connecting
      tubing
    Pulse oximeter for monitoring
      saturation during tube
      placement and confirming
      tube placement (optional)
    Limb restraints

PATIENT PREPARATION

1. Assess patient's color and ventilatory status prior to attempting placement.
2. Initiate supplemental ventilation and/or oxygenation using a bag-valve-mask if required.
3. Place the patient in a supine position or position indicated by the patient's condition.
4. Place the head in a neutral position, unless contraindicated by a spinal injury or other condition.
5. Restrain patient as indicated to prevent accidental extubation.

1. Inflate the cuff to test for air leaks. Deflate after testing.
2. Attach the mask to the EOA or EGTA tube.
3. Turn on suction and place the tonsil-tip next to the patient's head.
4. Hyperventilate the patient for approximately 3 to 5 minutes (optimal) via bag-valve-mask with 100% oxygen (Dauphinee, 1988).
5. Place the patient in the sniffing position (head extended and neck flexed) unless spinal precautions prohibit it.
6. Provide manual stabilization of the head if cervical spine immobilization is indicated.
7. Grasp the lower jaw and elevate it slightly.
8. Insert the EOA or EGTA into the mouth with the curve of the tube directed toward the feet.
9. Advance the tube until the mask is flush on the face.
10. Inflate the cuff (approximately 35 cc).
11. Maintain the head in the sniffing position and seal the mask on the face.
12. Initiate ventilation using a bag-valve-mask.
13. Check for correct tube placement. See Ch. 9.
14. Secure the tube. See Ch. 9.
15. If using an EGTA, insert the gastric tube through the lumen of the EGTA and attach it to low suction.

COMPLICATIONS

1. Esophageal perforation (Pons, 1988; Kassels, Robinson & O'Bara, 1980)
2. Gastric rupture (this complication may be decreased with the use of the EGTA).
3. Complete airway obstruction caused by kinking of the tube or overinflation of the distal balloon in the esophagus. Obstruction is caused by anterior displacement of the trachea (Low, 1982).
4. Inadvertent, unrecognized endotracheal intubation. (**Note:** Inaccurate placement of any airway device, including the endotracheal tube, has serious consequences. This complication is not limited to the EOA or EGTA).
5. Aspiration of vomitus or blood. This complication is neither caused nor prevented by use of the EOA or EGTA.

REFERENCES

Auerbach, P.S. 1983. Inadequate oxygenation and ventilation using the esophageal gastric tube airway in the prehospital setting. *Journal of the American Medical Association,* 250:3067–3071.

Dauphinee, K. 1988. Orotracheal intubation. *Emergency Medicine Clinics of North America,* 6:699–713.

Don Michael, T.A. 1985. Comparison of the esophageal obturator airway and endotracheal intubation in prehospital ventilation during CPR. *Chest,* 87:814–819.

Hammargren, Y., Clinton, J.E., & Ruiz, E. 1985. A standard comparison of esophageal obturator airway and endotracheal tube ventilation in cardiac arrest. *Annals of Emergency Medicine,* 14:953–958.

Kassels, S.J., Robinson, W.A., & O'Bara, K.J. 1980. Esophageal perforation associated with the esophageal obturator airway. *Critical Care Medicine,* 8:386–389.

Low, R.B., Jensen, R.D., & Cavanaugh, K.J. 1982. Marked anterior displacement of the trachea and larynx from an esophageal obturator airway. *Annals of Emergency Medicine*, 11:670–672.

McCabe, C.J. 1989. Pre-hospital medical care. In E.W. Wilkins (ed.), *Emergency medicine: Scientific principles and current practice*, 3rd ed. Baltimore: Williams & Wilkins.

Meislin, H.W. 1980. The esophageal obturator airway: A study of respiratory effectiveness. *Annals of Emergency Medicine*, 9:54–59.

Pons, P.T. 1988. Esophageal obturator airway. *Emergency Medicine Clinics of North America*, 6:693–698.

Shea, S.R., MacDonald, J.R., & Gruzinski, G. 1985. Prehospital endotracheal tube airway or esophageal gastric tube airway: A critical comparison. *Annals of Emergency Medicine*, 14:102–112.

Smith, J.P., Bodai, B.I., Aubourg, R., & Ward, R.E. 1983. A field evaluation of the esophageal obturator airway. *Journal of Trauma*, 23:317–321.

9

General Principles of Endotracheal Intubation

Scott S. Bourn, RN, MSN, CEN

Endotracheal intubation refers to the procedure of inserting a tube directly into the trachea. The endotracheal tube (ET) may be placed through the nose or mouth. Methods of insertion include visual (using laryngoscopy), blind (through the nose or mouth), or digital (also blind). Details of these procedures are included in Chapters 10 and 11 on oral and nasal intubation.

INDICATIONS

To secure the airway in cases of inadequate ventilatory rate and/or depth. Intubation is the superior means of airway control for the following reasons:
1. The cuffed tube protects the trachea and lungs from gastric contents, saliva, or blood and fluid from the upper airway.
2. Direct access to the lungs provides an easy route for supplemental ventilation.
3. Direct access to the lungs allows suctioning of secretions from the lungs.
4. Direct access to the lungs allows administration of medications for rapid absorption through the pulmonary tree. The mnemonic NAVEL refers to medications commonly administered through an ET: naloxone, atropine, Valium, epinephrine, lidocaine.

CONTRAINDICATIONS AND CAUTIONS

1. There are no absolute contraindications to endotracheal intubation. However, the procedure should be carefully considered when performed in the patient with
   a. An intact gag reflex
   b. Potential or actual cervical spine injury
   c. Head trauma and/or increased intracranial pressure
   d. Epiglottitis
   e. Facial fractures
2. An additional caution involves the need to provide adequate ventilation before, during, and after intubation efforts. Bag-valve-mask ventilation must be provided during preparation for intubation and to sustain ventilation if the initial intubation attempt is unsuccessful. (Jorden, 1988) **This is essential regardless of the method of intubation selected.**
3. Specific precautions exist for each method of endotracheal intubation. These will be discussed in the chapters devoted to nasal and oral intubation, Chapters 10 and 11, respectively.

EQUIPMENT

Endotracheal tubes
  1–5-mm, uncuffed; 6–9-mm,
    cuffed. Should include half
    sizes from 6–9-mm
  Size estimates are made based
    on the size of the patient's
    little finger. For most adult
    males an 8.0-mm tube is
    appropriate, while most
    females will accept a
    7.5-mm tube. Nasal
    intubation generally
    requires a tube 0.5-mm
    smaller than the tube used
    for oral intubation.
Laryngoscope handle
Laryngoscope blades
  Curved (sizes 1–4)
  Straight (sizes 1–4)
Stylets to fit each size endotracheal
    tube
Lighted stylet (optional)
10-cc syringe for inflating cuff
Lubricating or lidocaine jelly for
    nasal intubation
Cetacaine, cocaine, or
    Neosynephrine drops or
    spray for nasal intubation
    (optional)

Airflow detector, such as the Beck
    Airway Airflow Monitor, for
    nasal intubation (optional)
Paralytic or sedative (short acting)
    agent for intubation of
    combative patients
Tube ties or tape
Stethoscope for auscultation of
    tube position
Additional supportive equipment
  Suction, complete with tonsil
    and catheter tips
  Bag-valve-mask or anesthesia
    bag
  Oxygen source and connecting
    tubing
  Extra laryngoscope bulbs and
    batteries
  Carbon dioxide detector for
    tube position confirmation
    (optional) **Note:** disposable,
    single-patient-use units are
    available.
  Pulse oximeter to monitor
    oxygen saturation during
    intubation and to help
    confirm tube placement
    (optional)
  Limb restraints

PATIENT PREPARATION

1. Assess patient's color and ventilatory status prior to intubation attempt.
2. Initiate hyperventilation with 100% oxygen using a bag-valve-mask. See Ch. 36.
3. Administer sedative, paralytic agents, or topical anesthesia as ordered.
4. Restrain patient as indicated to prevent accidental extubation.

PROCEDURAL STEPS

Specific steps of intubation depend upon the method of insertion used. See Chapters 10 and 11 for the specific steps for nasal and oral intubation.

Confirm Tube Placement

A number of methods may be employed to confirm correct endotracheal tube placement. (Bourn, 1989; Birminghan, 1986)
1. Direct visualization of the tube passing through the cords.
2. Chest movement with ventilation.
3. Breath sounds:
   a. Upper lobes, both sides
   b. Lower lobes, both sides
   c. Unilaterally absent or decreased breath sounds (usually the left) sug-

gests that the tube was advanced into a mainstem bronchus. With-draw the tube slightly and reassess until breath sounds are equal bilaterally.

4. Epigastric sounds: the presence of burping sounds over the epigastrium during ventilation suggests esophageal placement. Remove the tube immediately and hyperventilate the patient before attempting intubation again.

5. Bag-valve-mask compliance: Ventilation of the stomach is easier than the lungs; while a tube obstruction, bronchospasm, or tension pneumothorax makes ventilation more difficult.

6. Condensation in the ET tube on exhalation confirms tube position in the trachea.

7. Transillumination of the neck using a lighted stylet: If the neck glows after intubation with the lighted stylet the tube is correctly placed in the trachea.

8. Pulse oximetry: maintenance of an adequate oxygen saturation confirms tube placement. However, oximetry is slow to respond after accidental extubation. (Guggenberger, 1989)

9. End-tidal CO_2 measurement, using a detector or monitor: this is the most accurate method of confirming tube placement. The end-tidal CO_2 detector will respond to accidental extubation within one breath. (Guggenberger, 1989)

10. Presence of gastric contents in endotracheal tube: If food is present in the tube, recheck the position; may indicate esophageal intubation.

11. Chest x-ray documentation of tube location in the trachea just above the carina.

Secure the Endotracheal Tube

To prevent accidental extubation, the endotracheal tube must be carefully secured. While individual departments frequently use different techniques, a number of principles apply

1. A bite block or oral airway should be inserted after oral intubation to prevent the patient from biting the tube and occluding the airway.

2. In order to allow suctioning and mouth care, the mouth must not be occluded by tape, ties, or other devices.

3. The method used should prevent accidental advancement or withdrawal of the tube.

4. When possible, the method used should minimize pressure points on the skin to prevent long-term complications.

5. When tape or ties are used, they should completely encircle the head for maximum security.

6. When possible, the markings on the tube should be noted at the teeth and documented so that movement of the tube can be checked visually.

7. There are two commonly employed methods. See Figure 9.1 on page 28.

   Tape
   a. Tear about 24 inches of 1″ adhesive tape.
   b. Split the tape in half for the last 4 inches of each end.
   c. Slide the tape under the patient's neck, adhesive side up. Center the length of the tape under the middle of the neck.
   d. Bring each end of the tape up the side of the head and wrap the split ends around the tube securely. Split the tape further if necessary.

   Tube ties or umbilical tape
   a. Cut off about 24 inches of umbilical tape.
   b. Place the tape under the patient's neck, centered under the middle of the neck.
   c. Bring the ends up the side of the head and wrap them once around the ET tube. See Figure 9.1a.
   d. Tie a secure overhand knot around the tube, then wrap the ends around the tube again. See Figure 9.1b.

e. Tie another firm overhand knot, then a square knot to complete the procedure. See Figure 9.1c.
8. Whatever method is used, the tube position should be reconfirmed after it has been secured.

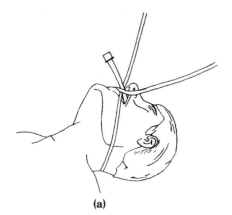 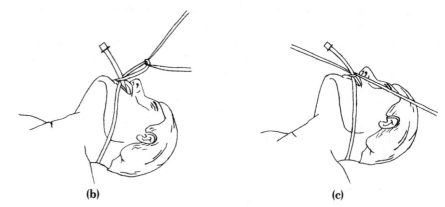

(a) (b) (c)

Figure 9.1. Steps for securing the endotracheal tube using tube ties.

COMPLICATIONS

1. Esophageal intubation. This is a serious complication because the patient's lungs will not be ventilated and gastric distension may occur. Gastric distention increases the risk of vomiting and may decrease the patient's tidal volume.
2. Dislodgement of the tube. Frequent reassessment of tube position, especially after the patient is moved, is necessary.
3. Damage to teeth, nasal mucosa, posterior pharynx, or larynx (depending upon the method of insertion).

PATIENT TEACHING

1. You will not be able to speak while the tube is in place.
2. Swallowing may help diminish gagging.
3. Do not move or manipulate the tube in any way.

REFERENCES

Birmingham, P.K., Cheney, F.W., & Ward, R.J. 1986. Esophageal intubation: A review of detection techniques. *Anesthesia Analgesia,* 65:886–891.

Bourn, S.S. 1989. You can breath easy (methods of confirming endotracheal tube placement). *Journal of Emergency Medical Services,* 14, 5:59–62.

Guggenberger, H., Lenz, G., & Federle, R. 1989. Early detection of inadvertent oesophageal intubation: pulse oximetry vs. capnography. *Acta Anesthesiol Scand,* 33:112–115.

Jorden, R.C. 1988. Airway management. *Emergency Medicine Clinics of North America,* 6, 4:671–686.

SUGGESTED READINGS

Colbert, J. 1987. Succinylcholine: Controlled paralysis for endotracheal intubation. *Emergency Medical Services,* 16, 4:22–23.

Cooper, R., & Bourn, S. 1990. Clearing the way to airway control. *Journal of Emergency Medical Services,* 15, 6:40–53.

Garnett, A.R., Ornato, J.P., Gonzales, E.R., & Johnson, E.B. 1987. End-tidal carbon dioxide monitoring during cardiopulmonary resuscitation. *Journal of the American Medical Association,* 257:512–515.

Orringer, M.B. 1980. Endotracheal intubation and tracheostomy: Indications, techniques, and complications. *Surgical Clinics of North America,* 60:1447–1464.

10

The information in this chapter should be used in conjunction with the information found in Ch. 9.

Oral Endotracheal Intubation

Scott S. Bourn, RN, MSN, CEN

INDICATIONS

To secure an airway in the presence of an inadequate airway or ventilation. Oral intubation is the procedure of choice in unconscious patients, patients without a gag reflex, and patients with no risk of vertebral injury.

CONTRAINDICATIONS AND CAUTIONS

There are no absolute contraindications to oral intubation. However, the procedure should be carefully considered and performed when the patient has

1. An intact gag reflex
2. Potential or actual cervical spine injury. Laryngoscopy is known to cause spinal movement (Aprahamian, 1984). However, retrospective research has shown no increase in spinal cord injury in patients who were orally intubated. The ideal airway technique for potential or actual spinal cord injured patients is not clear (Rhee, 1990; Holley, 1989).

   Several blind methods of oral intubation exist, including digital (tactile) intubation and blind oral intubation using a lighted stylet. Both of these methods produce a minimum of spinal movement, and may be performed even in cases of excessive pharyngeal bleeding, when direct visualization is impossible (Stewart, 1984; Ellis, 1986).
3. Epiglottitis complicates any intubation attempt because of the potential for laryngospasm and complete airway obstruction. Ideally, intubation of the patient with epiglottitis should be done in the operating room where a surgical airway can be inserted quickly should intubation fail.

PATIENT PREPARATION

1. Assess patient's color and ventilatory status prior to intubation attempt.
2. Initiate hyperventilation with 100% oxygen using a bag-valve-mask. See Ch. 36.
3. Administer sedative, paralytic agents, or topical anesthesia as ordered.
4. Restrain patient as indicated to prevent accidental extubation.

PROCEDURAL STEPS

1. Inflate the cuff to test for air leaks. Deflate after testing.
2. Turn on suction and place the tonsil-tip next to the patient's head.
3. Hyperventilate the patient for approximately 3–5 minutes (optimal) via bag-valve-mask with 100% oxygen (Dauphinee, 1988).

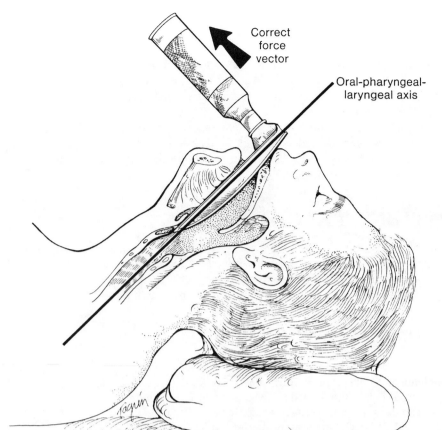

Correct force vector

Oral-pharyngeal-laryngeal axis

Figure 10.1. The laryngoscope is lifted up and away from the intubator to align the airway structures. (Cullen, 1989: 990. Reprinted by permission.)

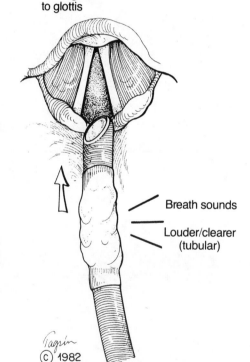

Tube moving closer to glottis

Breath sounds

Louder/clearer (tubular)

© 1982

4. Place the patient in the sniffing position unless spinal precautions prohibit it.
5. Provide manual stabilization of the head if spinal movement is contraindicated.
6. If the patient is too combative to tolerate the procedure, a short-term sedative or paralytic agent may be administered to allow intubation. (Morris, 1988)
7. *Insert the laryngoscope with the left hand. The tongue should be swept to the left side and the laryngoscope inserted and lifted up and away from the intubator. See Figure 10.1. Be careful not to rock the laryngoscope on the patient's teeth!
8. *Visualize the vocal cords and the larynx. See Figure 10.2.
9. If the cords are not visible, downward cricoid pressure (also known as the Sellick maneuver) may move the glottis into view (Dauphinee, 1988). The Sellick maneuver may also serve to prevent aspiration of emesis by occluding the esophagus during intubation (Sellick, 1961).
10. *Place the endotracheal tube through the cords using the right hand. The tube should be advanced until the cuff disappears through the cords.
11. *Remove the laryngoscope, maintaining a grip on the endotracheal tube.
12. Attempt ventilation through the endotracheal tube.
13. Check for correct tube placement. See Chapter 9.
14. If the tube is in the correct position, continue ventilations while inflating the cuff. Instill air until an adequate seal is attained; 10 to 15 ml of air are usually required.
15. Secure the tube. See Chapter 9 for specific methods.
16. Obtain a chest x-ray to confirm correct placement.

Figure 10.2. After the cords are visualized, the tube should be advanced through the cords until the cuff disappears. (Cullen, 1989: 993. Reprinted by permission.)

*Indicates portions of the procedure usually performed by a physician.

COMPLICATIONS

1. Esophageal intubation. This is a serious complication because the patient's lungs will not be ventilated and gastric distention may occur. Gastric distention increases the risk of vomiting and may decrease the patient's tidal volume.
2. Dislodgement of the tube. Frequent reassessment of tube position, especially after the patient is moved, is necessary.
3. Damage to teeth, nasal mucosa, posterior pharynx, or larynx (depending upon the method of insertion).

PATIENT TEACHING

1. You will not be able to speak while the tube is in place.
2. Swallowing may help diminish gagging.
3. Do not move or manipulate the tube in any way.

REFERENCES

Aprahamian, C., Thompson, B.M., Finger, W.A., & Darin, J.C. 1984. Experimental cervical spine injury model: Evaluation of airway management and splinting techniques. *Annals of Emergency Medicine,* 13:584–587.

Cullen, D.J. 1989. Orotracheal intubation. In E. Wilkins (ed). *Emergency medicine: Scientific foundations and current practice,* 3rd ed. Baltimore: Williams & Wilkins.

Dauphinee, K. 1988. Orotracheal intubation. *Emergency Medicine Clinics of North America,* 6:699–713.

Ellis, D.G., Stewart, R.D., Kaplan, R.M., Jakymec, A., Freeman, J.A., & Bleyaert, A. 1986. Success rates of blind orotracheal intubation using a transillumination technique with a lighted stylet. *Annals of Emergency Medicine,* 15:138–142.

Holley, J., & Jorden, R. 1989. Airway management in patients with unstable cervical spine fractures. *Annals of Emergency Medicine,* 18:1237–1239.

Jorden, R.C. 1988. Airway management. *Emergency Medicine Clinics of North America,* 6:671–686.

Morris, I.R. 1988. Pharmacologic aids to intubation and the rapid sequence induction. *Emergency Medicine Clinics of North America,* 6:753–768.

Rhee, K.J., Green, W., Holcroft, J.W., & Mangill, J.A. 1990. Oral intubation in the multiply injured patient: The risk of exacerbating spinal cord damage. *Annals of Emergency Medicine,* 19:511–514.

Sellick, B.A. 1961. Cricoid pressure to control regurgitation of stomach contents during induction of anaesthesia. *Lancet,* 2:404–408.

Stewart, R.D. 1984. Tactile orotracheal intubation. *Annals of Emergency Medicine,* 13:175–178.

11

Nasal Endotracheal Intubation

Scott S. Bourn, RN, MSN, CEN

The information in this chapter should be used in conjunction with the information found in Ch. 9: General Principles of Endotracheal Intubation.

INDICATIONS

To secure an airway in the presence of inadequate airway or ventilation. Nasal intubation is the procedure of choice in conscious patients (Jorden, 1988), patients with a gag reflex (Jorden, 1988), and patients with suspected vertebral injury (Aprahamian, 1984). It can also be used in any patient with trismus from such causes as seizure, posturing, or tetany.

CONTRAINDICATIONS AND CAUTIONS

There are no absolute contraindications to nasal intubation. However, the procedure should be carefully considered and performed in the following situations:
1. *Respiratory arrest.* Because ventilatory sounds are an important component of insertion, apneic patients should usually be intubated using an oral method (Yaron, 1988). However, the procedure is possible in respiratory arrest. The use of a lighted stylet improves the accuracy significantly (Verdile, 1990).
2. *Potential facial and basilar skull fractures.* Many sources cite head trauma as a contraindication of nasal intubation due to concerns that the endotracheal tube will pass through the cribiform plate into the brain (Yaron, 1988). Patients with extensive facial or nasal fractures are poor candidates for nasal intubation (Dauphinee, 1988). However, there is only one documented case of endotracheal tube penetration into the brain (Horellou, 1978). Unless there are significant midface fractures, nasal intubation may be used in head trauma with caution (Iserson, 1985; Jorden, 1988).
3. Coagulopathy or anticoagulant therapy increase the risk of epistaxis (Dauphinee, 1988).
4. Obstructions of the nose or posterior nasopharynx, including trauma, tumor, or foreign body (Dauphinee, 1988).
5. Epiglottitis complicates any intubation attempt because of the potential for laryngospasm and complete airway obstruction. Ideally, intubation of the patient with epiglottitis should be done in the operating room where a surgical airway can be placed quickly should intubation fail.

PATIENT PREPARATION

1. Assess patient's color and ventilatory status prior to intubation attempt.
2. Initiate hyperventilation with 100% oxygen using a bag-valve-mask. See Ch. 36.
3. Administer sedative, paralytic agents, or topical anesthesia as ordered.
4. Restrain patient as indicated to prevent accidental extubation.

33

PROCEDURAL STEPS

1. Inflate the cuff to test for air leaks. Deflate after testing.
2. Turn on suction and place the tonsil-tip suction next to the patient's head.
3. Administer 100% oxygen via bag-valve-mask for at least two minutes to prevent hypoxia during the procedure (Morris, 1988).
4. Prepare the patient and tube. Instill topical vasoconstrictors, and/or anesthetics. Intravenous lidocaine (1.0–1.5 mg/kg) preintubation is also recommended by some sources to prevent increases in intracranial pressure during intubation (Morris, 1988). Lubricate the tube liberally with a water-soluble lubricant.
5. Place the patient in the sniffing position unless spinal precautions prohibit it.
6. Provide manual stabilization of the head if cervical spine immobilization is indicated.
7. If the patient is too combative to tolerate the procedure, a sedative agent such as diazepam (Valium) may be administered.
8. Insert the endotracheal tube through the nostril and advance it along the floor of the nasal passage, directing it toward the bottom of the ear. Resistance will be felt at the posterior pharyngeal wall; gentle pressure should facilitate entry to the posterior oropharynx. The tube is advanced until it reaches the glottis, usually heralded by a cough or gag. Retract the tube slightly. See Figure 11.1.

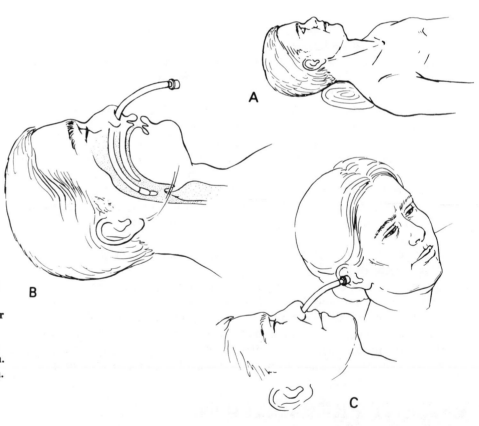

Figure 11.1.
A. Place the patient in the sniffing position.
B. Advance the tube along the floor of the nasal cavity. Continue advancing until the glottis is reached.
C. Listen to the respiratory pattern. The tube is advanced on inspiration.
(Rosen & Sternbach, 1983: 17. Reprinted by permission.)

A number of devices may be used with nasal intubation to improve the accuracy of this blind technique. The Beck Airway Airflow Monitor (Great Plains Ballistics, Inc. Lubbock, Texas) is a whistle device which fits over the proximal end of the endotracheal tube and accentuates breath sounds, making intubation easier (Yaron, 1988). The use of a lighted stylet improves the accuracy of nasal intubation in apneic patients, and may offer an additional method for confirming tube position (Verdile, 1990).

9. Listen to the breath sounds to develop a sense of timing and rhythm. Advance the tube through the glottis on inspiration, stabilizing the larynx with the nondominant hand. This hand may be able to feel a "snap" as the tube passes through the cords (Dauphinee, 1988). Advance the tube an additional 2–4 cm.

10. Continue to listen for breath sounds through the tube. If they sound loud and air movement is felt, hold the tube in position. If breath sounds are absent through the tube and no air movement is felt, the tube has entered the esophagus. Retract the tube to the posterior pharynx and retry.

11. Check for correct tube placement. See Ch. 9: General Principles of Endotracheal Intubation.

12. If the tube is in correct position, maintain ventilations and/or supplemental oxygen while inflating the cuff. Instill air until an adequate seal is attained; 10 to 15 cc of air are usually required.

13. Secure the tube. See Ch. 9: General Principles of Endotracheal Intubation, for specific methods.

14. Obtain a chest x-ray to confirm correct placement.

COMPLICATIONS

1. Esophageal intubation. This is a serious complication because the patient's lungs will not be ventilated and gastric distension may occur. Gastric distension increases the risk of vomiting and may decrease the patient's tidal volume.

2. Dislodgement of the tube. Frequent reassessment of tube position, especially after the patient is moved, is necessary.

3. Damage to nasal mucosa, posterior pharynx, or larynx.

PATIENT TEACHING

1. You will not be able to speak while the tube is in place.
2. Swallowing may help diminish gagging.
3. Do not move or manipulate the tube in any way.

REFERENCES

Aprahamian, C., Thompson, B.M., Finger, W.A., & Darin, J.C. 1984. Experimental cervical spine injury model: Evaluation of airway management and splinting techniques. *Annals of Emergency Medicine*, 13:584–587.

Dauphinee, K. 1988. Nasotracheal intubation. *Emergency Medicine Clinics of North America*, 6:715–723.

Horellou, M.F., Mathe, D., & Feiss, P. 1978. A hazard of naso-tracheal intubation. *Anaesthesia*, 33:73–74.

Iserson, K.V. 1985. Nasotracheal intubation: Myth vs. reality. *Annals of Emergency Medicine*, 14:162.

Jorden, R.C. 1988. Airway management. *Emergency Medicine Clinics of North America*, 6:671–686.

Morris, I.R. 1988. Pharmacologic aids to intubation and the rapid sequence induction. *Emergency Medicine Clinics of North America*, 6:753–768.

Rosen, P., & Sternbach, G.L. 1983. *Atlas of emergency medicine*, 2nd ed. Baltimore: Williams & Wilkins.

Verdile, V.P., Chiang, J., Bedger, R., Stewart, R.D., Kaplan, R., Paris, P.M. 1990. Nasotracheal intubation using a flexible lighted stylet. *Annals of Emergency Medicine,* 19:506–510.

Yaron, M. 1988. Airway management in the resuscitation of trauma patients. *Medical Instrumentation,* 22, 3:129–134.

12

Pharyngeal Tracheal Lumen Airway

Dean M. Kelly, RN, BSN, CEN

The Pharyngeal Tracheal Lumen (PTL) Airway is a product of Respironics Incorporated.

The information in this chapter should be used in conjunction with the information in Ch. 9: General Principles of Endotracheal Intubation.

INDICATIONS

To establish an airway and ventilate a patient in respiratory arrest. The PTL airway should be used when tracheal intubation is unsuccessful, or personnel trained in tracheal intubation are not available. Placement of a PTL airway does not require the use of a laryngoscope.

CONTRAINDICATIONS AND CAUTIONS

1. Children under the age of fourteen
2. Conscious or semiconscious patients
3. Known caustic poisoning cases
4. Known esophageal disease
5. Immediately *remove* the PTL if the gag reflex returns or the patient regains consciousness.
6. If ventilation is inadequate as assessed by chest excursion, breath sounds, etc., remove the PTL and attempt an alternative route for ventilation.
7. Inadequate tightening of neck strap may result in leakage around the oral cuff (Respironics, 1988).

EQUIPMENT

Oxygen source
PTL airway
Suction and catheters

Nasogastric tube
Bag-valve-mask
Water soluble lubricant

PATIENT PREPARATION

1. Place the patient in a supine position with the neck hyperextended, unless cervical spine injury is suspected. If cervical spine injury is suspected, leave the neck in a neutral position.

PROCEDURE

1. Assure that both cuffs are completely deflated. See Figure 12.1.
2. Lubricate tube with a water soluble lubricant.
3. Grasp the tongue and jaw between the thumb and index finger of your nondominant hand and lift straight upward. Remove dentures if present and suction oropharynx if necessary.

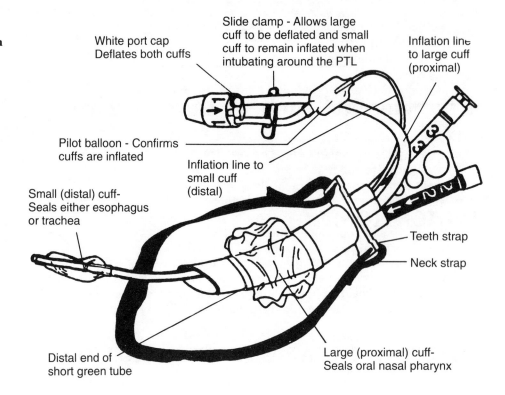

Figure 12.1   PTL Airway.
(Reprinted with permission from
Respironics, Inc.)

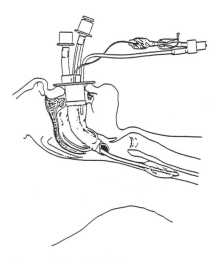

Figure 12.2.   PTL airway inserted
into patient.
(Niemann, & Rosborough, 1984: 8.
Reprinted by permission.)

4. With your dominant hand, insert the PTL into the mouth and advance it behind tongue (the curve of the PTL airway should go with that of the airway) until the teeth strap touches the patient's teeth. See Figure 12.2. You will feel some resistance as the PTL is inserted, but no force should be used. If the tube does not advance with only slight resistance, either redirect it or withdraw and attempt again.

5. Secure the neck strap by slipping it over the head and tighten it firmly with the velcro fasteners.

6. Inflate both cuffs simultaneously by blowing vigorously into #1 inflation valve. (**Note:** Make sure the white cap is closed.)

7. Immediately ventilate with a bag-valve-mask into the #2 green tube while observing for rise and fall of chest, indicating the #3 tube is in the esophagus. Then continue ventilating via the green tube with high flow oxygen and a bag-valve-mask. Lung sounds must also be verified anteriorly and laterally.

8. If chest does not rise upon ventilating into the #2 green tube, the #3 tube may have entered the trachea. Remove the stylet from tube #3 and ventilate with high flow oxygen and a bag-valve-mask while assessing lung sounds and chest rise and fall to confirm that the #3 tube is in the trachea.

9. Once the airway is in place, decompress the stomach by placing a nasogastric tube down the *nonairway* tube, either #2 or #3.

10. If adequate ventilation is verified but you have air leakage, try tightening the head strap or increasing the cuff pressure by blowing forcefully into the #1 inflation valve.

11. To replace the PTL with an endotracheal tube while ventilating through the #2 short green tube:
    a. Decompress the stomach.
    b. Hyperventilate the patient.
    c. Pinch the pilot balloon inflation line with the plastic slide clamp. Next open the white cap on the #1 inflation valve. The large oral cuff

will deflate to atmospheric pressure and may be deflated further by orally sucking air out through the uncapped port of the #1 valve.

   d. Insert laryngoscope and quickly intubate the trachea around the PTL airway.

   e. An alternative is to hyperventilate the patient. Then deflate both cuffs by opening the white cap on the #1 inflation valve. Remove the PTL airway and intubate the patient.

12. If the long, clear #3 tube is in the trachea:

   a. Pass a tube-changing stylet through the #3 tube.

   b. Deflate cuffs and remove the PTL.

   c. Insert the proper endotracheal tube over the stylet to reintubate the patient.

13. If the patient starts to regain the gag reflex, immediately turn the patient to the side, open the white cap on the #1 inflation valve, and remove the PTL airway (Respironics, 1988; Hunt, 1989).

COMPLICATIONS

1. The PTL may not adequately seal the esophagus, therefore, aspiration is always a threat.
2. Inadequate ventilation
3. Assessing tube placement and deciding which lumen to ventilate through can be difficult (Hunt, 1989).

REFERENCES

Hunt, R.C., Clifton, A.S., & Whitley, T.W. 1989. Pharyngeal tracheal lumen airway training: Failure to discriminate between esophageal and endotracheal modes and failure to confirm ventilation. *Annals of Emergency Medicine,* 18:947–952.

Niemann, J.T., Rosborough, J.P., Myers, R., & Scarberry, E.N. 1984. The pharyngeotracheal lumen airway: Preliminary investigation of the new adjunct. *Annals of Emergency Medicine,* 13:591–596.

Respironics, Inc., 1988. Monroeville, PA.

13

Surgical Cricothyroidotomy

Dean M. Kelly, RN, BSN, CEN

Surgical cricothyroidotomy is also known as cricothyrotomy.

INDICATIONS

To establish an airway when endotracheal or nasotracheal intubation is indicated, but not possible, or is contraindicated. Example situations include:

    a. edema of the glottis,
    b. fracture of larynx,
    c. severe facial trauma,
    d. inhalation burns,
    e. foreign body or severe bleeding obstructing the glottic area,
    f. airway compromise in the presence of suspected or proven cervical spine injury.

CONTRAINDICATIONS AND CAUTIONS

1. Any airway impairment that can be corrected by more conservative adjuncts (i.e., endotracheal intubation, etc.)
2. In children under 12 years of age, the cricoid cartilage provides the only circumferential support to the upper trachea, therefore, surgical cricothyroidotomy is *not* recommended (American College of Surgeons, 1988).

EQUIPMENT

Sterile gloves
Masks
Antiseptic solution
Gauze dressings
Sterile drapes
#11 scalpel
Hemostat or tracheal spreader

Local anesthetic (with epinephrine)
5-ml syringe, 18-G needle, 25–27-G
    needle for anesthesia
Tape/ties to secure tube
Tracheostomy or endotracheal tube
    (size #5)

PATIENT PREPARATION

1. Place the patient supine with the neck in a neutral position.
2. Cleanse the anterior neck with antiseptic solution.

PROCEDURAL STEPS

1. *Drape the neck with sterile towels.
2. *Anesthetize the area with a local anesthetic if the patient is conscious.

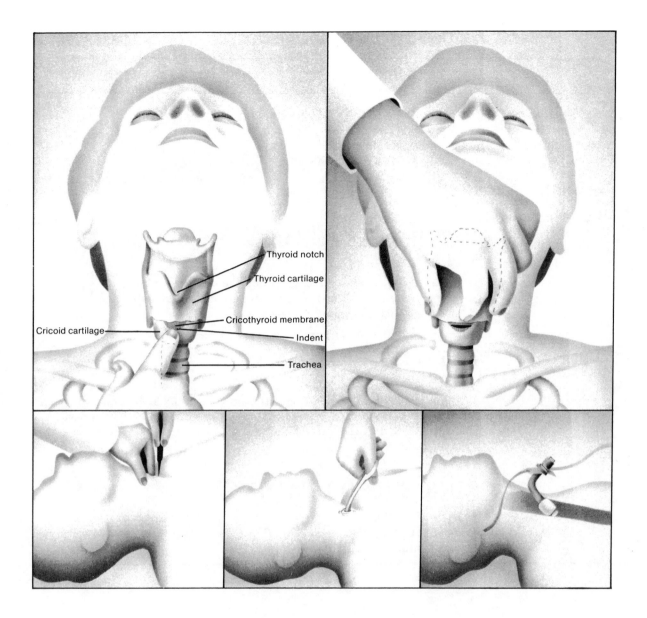

Thyroid notch

Thyroid cartilage

Cricothyroid membrane

Cricoid cartilage

Indent

Trachea

3. *Manually stabilize the thyroid cartilage and incise over the cricothyroid membrane. Then, incise through the cricothyroid membrane. See Figure 13.1.

4. *Open the incision with the scalpel handle, hemostat, or tracheal spreader.

5. *Insert a cuffed endotracheal tube or tracheostomy tube into the trachea. (**Note**: The excess endotracheal tube can be cut off as long as the inflation/deflation lumen for the cuff is not severed.)

6. Inflate the cuff and ventilate the patient.

7. Observe respiratory excursion and auscultate the chest anteriorly and laterally for bilateral breath sounds.

8. Secure the tube with tape or ties and document the centimeter measurement at the skinline.

9. Place a sterile dressing around the incision area.

10. Obtain arterial blood gases. See Chapter 17.

Figure 13.1. Surgical cricothyroidotomy.
(American College of Surgeons, 1988: 44. Reprinted by permission.)

*Indicates portions of the procedure usually performed by a physician.

COMPLICATIONS

1. False passage of the tube into subcutaneous tissues
2. Asphyxia
3. Aspiration
4. Esophageal or tracheal trauma
5. Cellulitis
6. Mediastinal emphysema
7. Hoarseness, vocal cord paralysis after tube removal (Hammond, 1984; American College of Surgeons, 1988).

PATIENT TEACHING

1. You will not be able to speak while the tube is in place.
2. Report any air leak at the incision site or respiratory difficulty.
3. Do not touch the tube or incision site.

REFERENCES

American College of Surgeons, Committee on Trauma. 1988. *Advanced trauma life support course (Student manual)*. Chicago: American College of Surgeons.

Hammond, B., & Lee, G. 1984. *Quick reference to emergency nursing*. Philadelphia: Lippincott.

SUGGESTED READING

Knezevich, B. 1986. *Trauma nursing: Principles and practice*. Norwalk, CT: Appleton-Century-Crofts.

14

Percutaneous Transtracheal Ventilation

Mary E. Echternacht, RN, BSN

Percutaneous transtracheal ventilation (PTV) is also known as needle cricothyrotomy.

INDICATIONS

To rapidly establish an airway under the following conditions:
1. Endotracheal intubation is difficult or contraindicated – massive facial trauma (Toye, 1986).
2. A temporary airway is needed to stabilize the patient until more definitive airway management can be accomplished – until cervical spine injuries have been ruled out (Rosen, 1988).
3. Surgical airway intervention – cricothyrotomy or tracheostomy are contraindicated or not available (Rosen, 1988).

CONTRAINDICATIONS AND CAUTIONS

1. PTV does not provide complete control of the airway and aspiration may occur (Simon, 1987).
2. Ventilation through this device should not exceed 1–2 hours. A tendency toward CO_2 retention has been demonstrated (Simon, 1987).
3. A patent larynx is essential for passive exhalation (Swartzman, 1984).
4. The catheter may easily kink or dislodge after placement into the trachea. Constant monitoring of ventilations is necessary.
5. Unsuccessful catheter insertion on the first attempt may present a problem. Ventilation via a second puncture may result in subcutaneous emphysema or air leak from the original site (Jorden, 1988).
6. Tracheal suctioning cannot be performed through the catheter.
7. There is no standard ventilatory device for PTV. The method described here can be accomplished with commonly available equipment. Other options include the use of intermittent high-pressure oxygen delivery by attaching noncollapsible tubing to an O_2 source on one end and to the catheter at the other. A valve, such as an Elder or Robertshaw valve, or Shrader blow gun is placed in the tubing to allow for intermittent oxygen delivery. See Figure 14.1. The customary frequency of inflation is once every 5 seconds (12 breaths per minute) and the duration 1 second, for this method (Jorden, 1988).
8. The delivery of normal tidal volumes in patients weighing more than 15 kg with bag-valve or continuous flow low-pressure sources via large cannula is unlikely (Yealy, 1989).

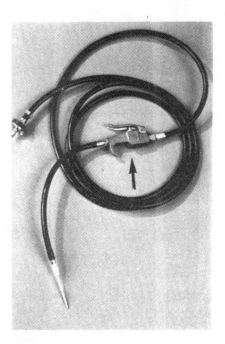

Figure 14.1. A high-pressure oxygen delivery device (Shrader blow gun).
(Jorden, 1988: 749. Reprinted by permission.)

EQUIPMENT

Antiseptic solution
10–14-G over-the-needle catheter
3-ml syringe
Bag-valve-mask

3.0 or 3.5 endotracheal tube tapered
   adaptor
Suction equipment (pharyngeal)
High-flow oxygen source

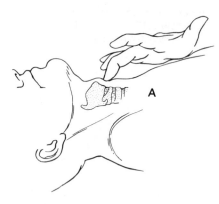

Figure 14.2. Locating the cricothyroid membrane.
(Rosen & Sternbach, 1983: 21. Reprinted by permission.)

*Indicates portions of procedure
usually performed by a physician.

PATIENT PREPARATION

1. Place the patient in a supine position with the neck in neutral alignment.
2. Cleanse the anterior neck with antiseptic solution.
3. Aspiration is a possible complication. Have suction equipment immediately available.
4. Restrain the patient as needed to prevent accidental dislodgement of catheter.
5. Sedate the patient as needed.

PROCEDURAL STEPS

1. *Locate cricothyroid membrane. See Figure 14.2.
2. *Pass over-the-needle catheter (with syringe attached) at 45° angle caudally and cannulate the trachea through the cricothyroid membrane. Air can be aspirated into the syringe when entrance to the trachea has been achieved (Simon, 1987). See Figure 14.3.

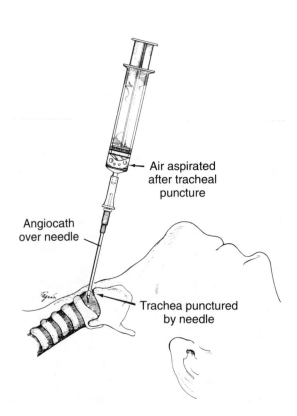

Air aspirated
after tracheal
puncture

Angiocath
over needle

Trachea punctured
by needle

Figure 14.3. Tracheal cannulation.
(Wilkins, 1989: 999. Reprinted by permission.)

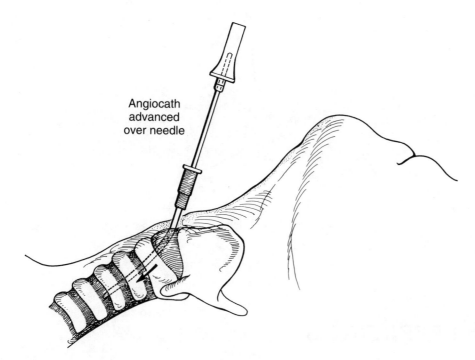

Angiocath
advanced
over needle

Figure 14.4   Catheter placement in
trachea.
(Wilkins, 1989: 1000. Reprinted by
permission.)

3.   *Remove the syringe and needle while manually stabilizing the catheter.
     Advance the catheter as needed. See Figure 14.4.
4.   Attach the catheter to the narrow tip of the endotracheal tube adapter.
     Connect the wider end to a bag-valve-mask and ventilate the patient
     with high-flow oxygen. See Figure 14.5 on page 46.
5.   Secure the catheter by manually holding it at all times (Jorden, 1988).
6.   Auscultate chest to assess ventilation. Visualize chest for rise and fall as
     oxygen is delivered. Exhalation is passive out the glottis and ultimately
     the mouth and nose (Jorden, 1988).

COMPLICATIONS

1.   Subcutaneous and/or mediastinal emphysema (Rosen, 1988)
2.   Hemorrhage at the site of the needle puncture
3.   Posterior tracheal wall puncture
4.   Pneumothorax (rare)
5.   Ventricular ectopy secondary to hypoventilation, hypoxia (Swartzman,
     1984)
6.   Hypotension secondary to inadequate ventilation (Swartzman, 1984)
7.   Inadequate ventilation resulting in hypoxia and hypercapnea

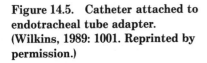

**Figure 14.5. Catheter attached to
endotracheal tube adapter.
(Wilkins, 1989: 1001. Reprinted by
permission.)**

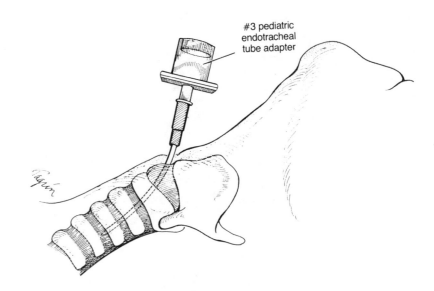

#3 pediatric
endotracheal
tube adapter

REFERENCES

Jorden, R.C. 1988. Percutaneous transtracheal ventilation. *Emergency Medicine
Clinics of North America*, 6: 745–753.

Rosen, P., Baker, F., Barkin, R., Braen, G., Dailey, R., & Levy, R. 1988. *Emergency
medicine: Concepts and clinical practice*, 2nd ed. St. Louis: Mosby.

Rosen, P., & Sternbach, G.L. 1983. *Atlas of emergency medicine*, 2nd ed. Baltimore:
Williams & Wilkins.

Simon, R., Brenner, B. 1987. *Emergency procedures and techniques*, 2nd ed. Baltimore: Williams & Wilkins.

Swartzman, S., Wilson, M., Hoff, B., Bunegin, L., Smith, R., & Sjostrand, U. 1984.
Percutaneous transtracheal jet ventilation for cardiopulmonary resuscitation:
Evaluation of a new jet ventilator. *Journal of Critical Care Medicine*, 12:8–13.

Toye, F., & Weinstein, J. 1986. Clinical experience with percutaneous tracheostomy
and cricothyroidotomy in 100 patients. *The Journal of Trauma*, 26:1034–1040.

Yealy, D.M., Plewa, M.C., & Stewart, R.D. 1989. Pediatric transtracheal ventilation:
An analysis of cannulae and oxygen sources. *Annals of Emergency Medicine*,
18:11–12.

SUGGESTED READING

Cameron, P., & McMichan, J. 1984. Percutaneous transtracheal ventilation simplified. *Journal of Anesthesia and Analgesia,* 63:168–169.

McLellan, I., Gordon, P., Khawaja, S., & Thomas, A. 1988. Percutaneous transtracheal high frequency jet ventilation as an aid to difficult intubation. *Canadian Journal of Anesthesia* 35:404–405.

Wilkins, E. 1989. Emergency Medicine *Scientific Foundations and Current Practice,* 3rd ed. Baltimore: Williams & Wilkins.

15

Tracheostomy

Mary E. Echternacht, RN, BSN

INDICATIONS

To establish an airway under the following conditions:
1. Inability to perform endotracheal intubation or cricothyrotomy.
2. Severe laryngotracheal trauma with loss of anatomical landmarks making endotracheal intubation impossible (Rosen et al., 1988).
3. Tracheal transection in which the distal trachea retracts into the mediastinum (Rosen, et al., 1988).
4. Epiglottitis, neoplasm, space abscess, or foreign body in the pharynx which prevents endotracheal intubation (Rosen, et al., 1988).

CONTRAINDICATIONS AND CAUTIONS

1. Tracheostomy is rarely done in the emergency setting as it is a difficult procedure with multiple associated complications. Definitive airway management can usually be accomplished by other means.
2. Complications in the emergency setting are usually due to haste, inadequate lighting, equipment problems, and managing a patient who is struggling to breathe (Worth, 1982).
3. Skill and experience are needed to perform a tracheostomy. This procedure should be done only by a qualified professional.
4. Patients with suspected neck injuries require strict immobilization. This will prevent optimal positioning for tracheostomy.
5. Tracheostomy is an extremely bloody procedure. Universal precautions need to be employed by all personnel. See Ch. 1.

EQUIPMENT

Sterile gloves
Masks
Protective goggles
Antiseptic solution
Scalpel blade #15, #11
Local anesthetic
Tracheostomy tube with obturator (size #6, 7, or 8 for adults)
Metzenbaum scissors
Mayo scissors
Scissors (sharp and blunt)
Tissue forceps (with and without teeth)
Mosquito forceps (curved)
Needle holder
Tracheal dilator and hook
Kelly clamps (curved)
Retractors (Weitlander, Senn, or Army-Navy)
Adhesive tape
Gauze dressings
Sterile towels and clamps
5-ml syringe with 18-G needle, 27-G needle for anesthesia
Suction equipment, pharyngeal and tracheal
Bag-valve-mask
High-flow oxygen source
3-0, 4-0 silk suture

PATIENT PREPARATION

1. When possible the patient should be ventilated using an endotracheal tube, cricothyrotomy, or other method until tracheostomy is completed.
2. Place patient in supine position with neck in extension and support under shoulders, using a blanket or small pillow. See Figure 15.1.
3. Cleanse the skin from mandible to below the clavicles with antiseptic solution.
4. *Drape the chest and neck.
5. *Infiltrate the skin with a local anesthetic.
6. Restrain patient as needed to prevent accidental extubation.
7. Sedate patient as needed.
8. Hemorrhage is a major complication during exposure of the trachea. Have tracheal and pharyngeal suction equipment immediately available.

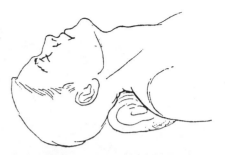

Figure 15.1 Patient positioning for tracheostomy.
(Rosen, & Sternbach, 1983: 7. Reprinted by permission.)

PROCEDURAL STEPS

1. *Make a midline skin incision vertically to expose the strap muscles. See Figure 15.2.
2. *Retract the strap muscles laterally to expose the pretracheal fascia and thyroid isthmus. See Figure 15.3 (Orringer, 1980; Piotrowski, 1988; Price, 1983).

*Indicates portions of the procedure usually performed by a physician.

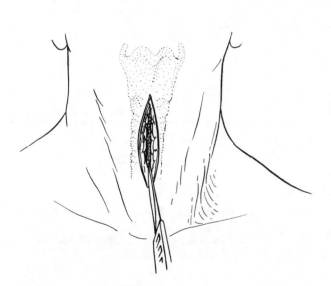

Figure 15.2 Midline incision.
(Rosen & Sternbach, 1983: 25. Reprinted by permission.)

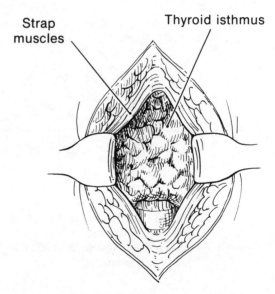

Strap muscles   Thyroid isthmus

Figure 15.3 The Thyroid isthmus exposed.
(Rosen & Sternbach, 1983: 25. Reprinted by permission.)

3. *Clamp the thyroid isthmus and bluntly dissect to divide the isthmus and expose the trachea. See Figure 15.4 on page 50. Have suction available as this step may result in massive hemorrhage (Orringer, 1980; Piotrowski, 1988; Price, 1983).
4. *Incise through the tracheal rings to enter the trachea. See Figure 15.5. Take care to control depth of penetration to minimize risk of injury to posterior trachea and esophagus (Worth, 1982; Orringer, 1980).
5. Suction tracheal secretions.
6. *Insert tracheal tube and obturator. See Figure 15.6. Remove the obturator, inflate the cuff with 5–8 ml of air, and ventilate patient with a bag-valve-mask. Auscultate lungs to assess tube placement and verify tube position with a chest x-ray.

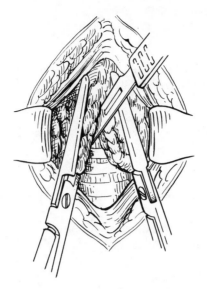

Figure 15.4   The trachea exposed. (Rosen & Sternbach, 1983: 25. Reprinted by permission.)

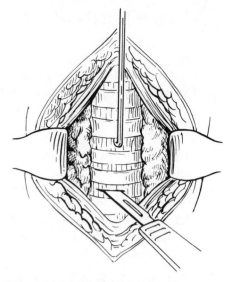

Figure 15.5   Tracheal entry. (Rosen & Sternbach, 1983: 25. Reprinted by permission.)

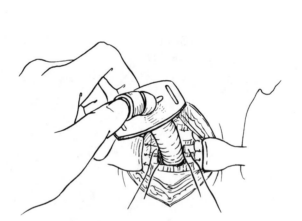

Figure 15.6   Insertion of tracheal tube and obturator. (Rosen & Sternbach, 1983: 27. Reprinted by permission.)

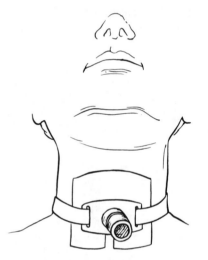

Figure 15.7   Tracheostomy tube tied in place. (Rosen & Sternbach, 1983: 27. Reprinted by permission.)

7. Tie the tracheostomy tube in place with tracheostomy tape around the neck. See Figure 15.7.
8. *Suture the anterior cervical skin loosely to the tracheostomy tube flange (Wilkins, 1989).
9. Cleanse and dress the wound with gauze dressings.
10. Deliver humidified oxygen as soon as possible.

COMPLICATIONS

1. Cardiopulmonary arrest secondary to hypoxia
2. Hemorrhage and injury to the thyroid gland, esophagus, laryngeal nerve, great vessels, or trachea
3. Pneumothorax

4. False passage of the tube into pleura, esophagus, or surrounding vessels
5. Bradycardia, hypotension secondary to hypoxia
6. Subglottic stenosis (late)

PATIENT TEACHING

1. Report respiratory difficulty immediately.
2. You will not be able to speak with the tube in place.

REFERENCES

Piotroski, J.J., & Moore, E.E., 1988. Emergency department tracheostomy. *Emergency Medical Clinics of North America,* 6:737–743.

Orringer, M.B., 1980. Endotracheal intubation and tracheostomy. *Surgical Clinics of North America,* 60:1447–1463.

Price, H.C., & Postma, D.S. 1983. Tracheostomy. *Ear, nose and throat,* 62:44–59.

Rosen, P., Baker, F., Barkin, R., Braen, G., Dailey, R., & Levy, R. 1988. *Emergency medicine: Concepts and clinical practice,* 4. 2nd ed. St. Louis: Mosby.

Rosen, P., & Sternbach, G.L. 1983. *Atlas of emergency medicine,* 2nd ed. Baltimore: Williams & Wilkins.

Worth, M.H., Jr. 1982. *Principles and practice of trauma care.* Baltimore: Williams & Wilkins.

16

Positioning the Dyspneic Patient

This procedure is also known as High-Fowler's position.

Ruth Altherr Giebel, MS, RN

INDICATIONS

To facilitate spontaneous ventilations in the presence of respiratory distress, as can be seen in acute pulmonary edema.

CONTRAINDICATIONS AND CAUTIONS

This position can only be used if the patient is responsive and has a nonobstructed airway.

PROCEDURAL STEPS

1. Raise head of bed to an upright position at a 90° angle.
2. Support patient's feet with footboard if available. Consider use of knee gatch on the hospital bed to maintain position. Knee gatch should only be used for a limited time due to pressure created on the popliteal vessels. See Figure 16.1.
3. An alternative to the High-Fowler's position is the orthopneic position. For this position the patient is positioned along the side of the bed

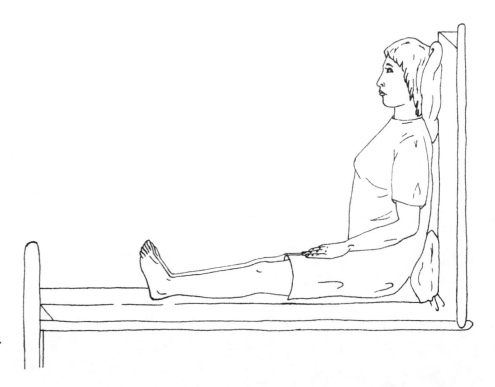

Figure 16.1   High-Fowler's position.

52

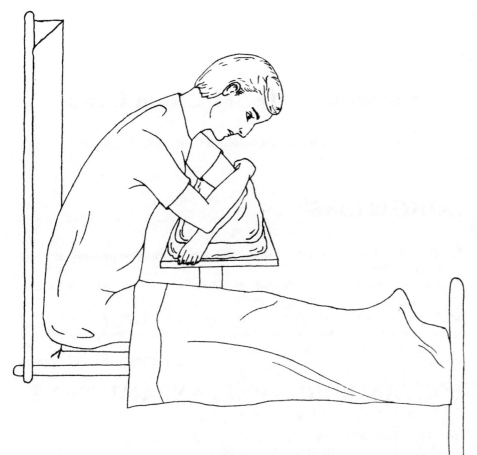

Figure 16.2   Orthopneic position.

with feet dangling or in bed with a overbed table placed across the lap. The table is raised to a comfortable position and padded with a pillow. This is of particular benefit for patients with respiratory distress due to chronic obstructive lung disease (COLD). In addition, the dangling position may help relieve dyspnea due to pulmonary edema (Kozier, 1979). See Figure 16.2.

PATIENT TEACHING

1. Patient comfort is of utmost importance. Allow the patient to assume the position of choice.

REFERENCES

Kosier, B., & Erb, G. 1989. Supporting a client in Fowler's position. In *Techniques in Clinical Nursing*, Redwood City, CA: Addison-Wesley.

17

Drawing Arterial Blood Gases

Ruth A. Slabach, MSN, SCN, RN

Arterial blood gases are also known as ABGs.

INDICATIONS

1. To evaluate acute respiratory distress and assist in determining therapeutic interventions.
2. To document the existence and severity of a problem with oxygenation or carbon dioxide exchange.
3. To analyze acid-base balance.
4. To evaluate the effectiveness of respiratory interventions, e.g., continuous ventilatory assistance or oxygen therapy.

CONTRAINDICATIONS AND CAUTIONS

Relative contraindications:
1. Previous surgery in area (e.g., cutdown)
2. Patients on anticoagulants or with known coagulopathy
3. Skin infection or other damage to skin (e.g., burns) at the puncture site
4. Decreased collateral circulation
5. Patients with severe atherosclerosis
6. Patients with severe injury to the extremity

EQUIPMENT

(Usually available in a prepackaged kit, see Figure 17.1.)
Syringe (3–5-ml size)
20–23-G needle with clear hub (smallest gauge should be used for radial puncture)
Antiseptic pledgets

1–3-ml heparin 1:1000 u/ml (if syringe is not preheparinized)
Stopper (cap) for syringe
Gauze dressings
Ice and container
Local anesthetic (optional)

PATIENT PREPARATION

1. Select the puncture site depending on the clinical situation, how rapidly the sample must be obtained, and the circulatory status of the patient.
2. The preferred site is the radial artery in most patients. The brachial artery may also be used. The femoral artery is most frequently used in critically ill or injured patients but should be avoided whenever possible due to a greater potential for complications, e.g., hematomas and/or hemorrhage, because bleeding is more difficult to control.
3. Patient must be on uninterrupted prescribed oxygen therapy (or room

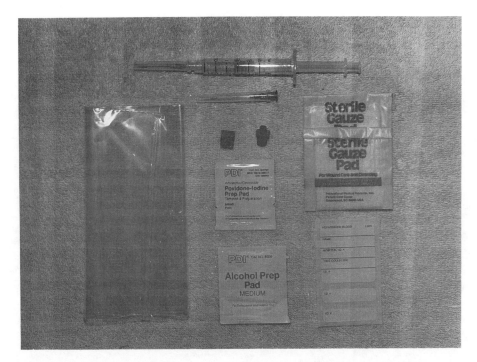

Figure 17.1 Typical equipment found in a prepackaged ABG kit. The syringe is preheparinized.

air) for 15–20 minutes before the arterial blood gas (ABG) is drawn if the test is to reflect any change in the patient's status.

4. If the radial artery is chosen as the puncture site, it is optional to check for patency of collateral circulation to the hand by performing the Allen's test. Some sources dispute the reliability and accuracy of the Allen's test (McGregor, 1987; Stead, 1985; Williams, 1987). If used, it is performed as follows:

   a. Elevate the patient's hand and arm for several seconds. Ask the patient to make a fist. Use your thumbs (or index and middle fingers), apply direct pressure over the radial and ulnar arteries simultaneously. See Figure 17.2. If the patient is unconscious or uncooperative, elevate the hand above the level of the heart and squeeze it until blanching occurs.

   b. While maintaining pressure over the arteries, ask the patient to open the fist and relax the hand. Note the blanched appearance of the palm.

   c. Release pressure from the ulnar artery while maintaining pressure on the radial artery. Observe the hand or palm closely for immediate flushing indicating patency of the ulnar artery. The entire hand should regain color within 5–10 seconds. A flushed hand within 5–10 seconds indicates adequate collateral circulation and the radial artery may be used for arterial puncture (Barker, 1985).

   d. If the hand remains blanched for longer than 10–15 seconds, the radial artery should not be used.

PROCEDURAL STEPS

1. Prepare the syringe (if not preheparanized). Draw up 1–2 ml heparin and rotate the syringe to coat the barrel and fill the dead space of the syringe and needle. Holding the syringe upright, expel the excess heparin and air bubbles from the syringe.

2. Palpate the pulse and determine the point of maximal impulse.

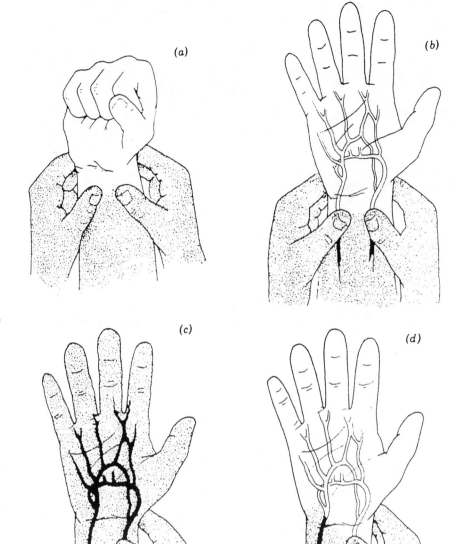

Figure 17.2 Allen's test.

a. Elevate the patient's hand and arm for several seconds. Ask the patient to make a fist. Using your thumbs (or index and middle fingers), apply direct pressure over the radial and ulnar arteries simultaneously.

b. While maintaining pressure over the arteries, ask the patient to open the fist and relax the hand. Note the blanched appearance of the palm.

c. Release pressure from the ulnar artery while maintaining pressure on the radial artery. Observe the hand or palm closely for immediate flushing indicating patency of the ulnar artery. The entire hand should regain color within 5–10 seconds.

d. If the hand remains blanched for longer than 10–15 seconds, the radial artery should not be used.

(May, 1984: 84. Reprinted by permission.)

3. Local anesthesia may be useful in particularly anxious patients. Inject approximately 1 ml of anesthetic into the skin, subcutaneously on either side and above the artery. Aspirate prior to injecting the anesthetic to avoid injecting into the vessel. Wait 3–4 minutes to allow for effective anesthesia.

4. For a radial stick, stabilize the wrist over a small rolled towel or washcloth. The wrist should be dorsiflexed about 30°.

5. For a brachial stick, place a rolled towel under the patient's elbow hyperextending the elbow. Rotate the patient's wrist outward.

6. For a femoral stick, rotate the leg slightly outward. Choose a site near the inguinal fold, approximately 2 cm below the inguinal ligament.

7. Cleanse the overlying skin with an antiseptic solution.

8. Use the index finger of your free hand to palpate the arterial pulse just proximal to the puncture site. See Figure 17.3. An alternative technique is to bracket above and below the arterial pulsation with two fingers of one hand and perform the puncture between the two fingers. See Figure 17.4.

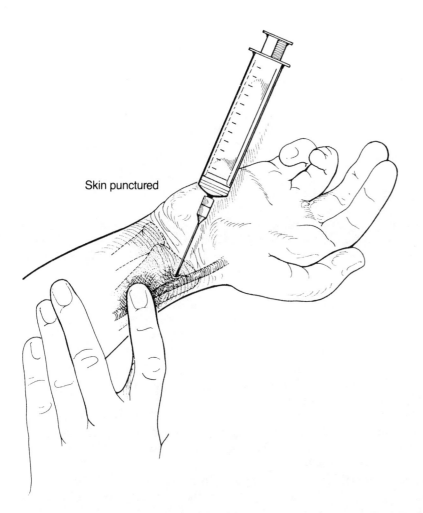

Skin punctured

Figure 17.3 Radial artery puncture.
The index finger of one hand is used
to palpate the arterial pulse just
proximal to the puncture site.
(Wilkins, Jr. 1989: 1013. Reprinted
by permission.)

9. Grasp the syringe as if holding a pencil. Direct the needle, bevel up, and puncture the skin slowly at approximately a 45–60° angle to the radial or brachial artery (90° to the femoral artery). Watch the needle hub constantly for the appearance of blood.
10. When blood appears, stop advancing the needle, and allow the blood to

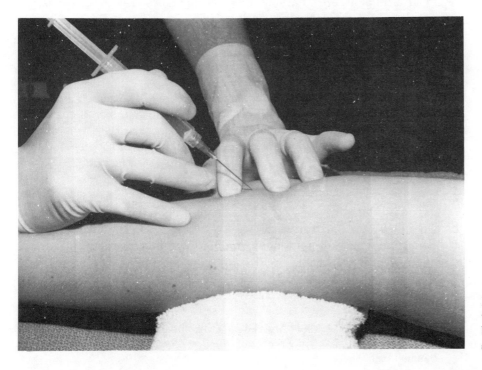

Figure 17.4 Brachial artery puncture. Two fingers of one hand may be used to bracket the artery and stabilize it.

flow freely into the syringe. The blood should fill the syringe without aspiration except in patients with severe hypotension. In these patients, red arterial blood should appear spontaneously in the needle hub. At this time, gentle aspiration may be used to obtain the sample.

11. If the puncture is unsuccessful, both walls of the artery may have been pierced. Withdraw the needle slightly until the tip reenters the artery and blood flows into the syringe. If the needle fails to enter the artery, and a good pulse is still present, withdraw the needle to just above the bevel and redirect it to the point of maximal pulse.

12. The disappearance of a pulse usually indicates arterial spasm or hematoma formation. If this occurs, withdraw the needle immediately, apply direct pressure, and select another site.

13. Obtain a sample of 2–5 ml. Remove the needle from the artery. Immediately apply direct pressure with dry gauze to the puncture site for at least five minutes (longer for patients on anticoagulants or with clotting disorders).

   The next three steps should be performed by an assistant.

14. Prepare the blood sample for the laboratory by immediately expelling all air bubbles. With the syringe upright, finger tap the air bubbles to the top of the syringe and expel them into a gauze dressing or alcohol pledget to catch drops of blood.

15. Stick the needle into a rubber stopper or remove the needle with forceps and cap the syringe with a rubber plug. Gently rotate the syringe between your hands to mix the heparin and blood.

16. Label the syringe. Indicate the concentration of oxygen the patient was receiving and the patient's temperature. An elevated temperature can increase the pO_2 significantly. Place the syringe on ice and take it to the lab for analysis immediately.

17. Place a dry sterile gauze over the puncture site securing it firmly with tape. Check the circulation and pulses of the extremity every 15 minutes for 1 hour.

COMPLICATIONS

1. Compression neuropathies may occur secondary to hematomas caused by arterial punctures. Patients on anticoagulants or with other coagulopathies are at greatest risk (Barker, 1985).

2. If air bubbles are not removed from the sample, the pO_2 can increase yielding inaccurate test results.

3. The blood sample may clot if the heparin and blood are not adequately mixed.

4. Thrombosis may occur with repeated puncture of the same site.

5. Arterial spasm or hematoma formation may cause impaired circulation to the extremity.

6. Nerve injury may occur with inadvertent puncture of the nerve.

PATIENT TEACHING

1. Do not rub the puncture site.
2. Report any pain, numbness, or tingling following the arterial puncture.

REFERENCES

Barker, W.J., &Wyte, S.R. 1985. Arterial puncture and cannulation. In J. Roberts, & J. Hedges. (eds). *Clinical Procedures in Emergency Medicine*. Philadelphia: Saunders; 352–366.

May, H.L., ed. 1984. *Emergency medical procedures.* New York: Wiley.

McCabe, C.J. 1989. Radial arterial puncture. In E.W. Wilkins Jr. (ed). *Emergency Medicine: Scientific Foundations and Current Practice.* Baltimore: Williams & Wilkins; 1013.

McGregor, A.D. 1987. The Allen test – an investigation of its accuracy by fluorescein angiography. *Journal of Hand Surgery* (British). 12-B:82–85.

Stead, S.W., & Stirt, J.A. 1985. Assessment of digital blood flow and palmar collateral circulation. *International Journal of Clinical Monitoring and Computing,* 2:29–34.

Williams, T., & Schenken, J.R. 1987. Radial artery puncture and the Allen test. *Annals of Internal Medicine,* 106, 1:164–165.

Wilkins, E.W., Jr. (ed). 1989. *Emergency medicine: Scientific foundations and current practice.* Baltimore: Williams & Wilkins.

SUGGESTED READINGS

American Heart Association. 1987. *Textbook of advanced cardiac life support.* Dallas: American Heart Association.

Kersten, L.D. 1989. *Comprehensive respiratory nursing.* Philadelphia: Saunders.

Simon, R.R., & Brenner, R.E. 1987. *Emergency procedures and techniques,* 2nd ed. Baltimore: Williams & Wilkins.

18

Pulse Oximetry

Dorothy M. Schulte, RN, MS

Pulse oximetry is also known as pulse ox, ear ox.

INDICATIONS

To quickly and noninvasively monitor oxygen saturation (SpO_2) in patients who are at risk for hypoxemia. Clinical situations may include:
1. Cardiac compromise (CHF, cardiac arrest, chest pain)
2. Pulmonary compromise (SOB, pulmonary emboli, respiratory distress, croup, pneumothorax, asthma)
3. Drug overdose with potential for hypoventilation
4. Hemorrhage/shock
5. High altitude illness/high altitude pulmonary edema
6. Ongoing assessment during minor surgical procedures requiring IV sedation
7. Ongoing assessment during airway management, endotracheal intubation, and suctioning
8. Ongoing assessment during patient transport
9. Ongoing assessment of response to oxygen therapy to titrate the patient's SpO_2 to the desired level

CONTRAINDICATIONS AND CAUTIONS

There are no absolute contraindications for pulse oximetry. However, in the following instances readings may be unobtainable or inaccurate (Szaflarski, 1989).
1. Hemodynamic compromise resulting in a decrease of mean blood pressure to 50mm Hg or less or pulse pressure narrowing.
2. Shock, cardiac arrest, excessive vasoconstriction due to hypothermia, peripheral vascular disease, or other abnormalities which result in poor tissue perfusion.
3. Arterial line or direct arterial compression to extremity to which sensor is applied (blood pressure cuff, tourniquet, PASG).
4. Severe anemia (oximetry requires adequate hemoglobin concentration to function).
5. High carboxyhemoglobin levels (secondary to CO exposure or heavy cigarette smoking) will result in falsely elevated SpO_2.
6. Increased levels of methemoglobin will result in falsely elevated SpO_2.
7. Administration of intravenous dyes (methylene blue, indigo, carmine) will result in falsely low SpO_2.
8. Increased serum bilirubin levels result in falsely low SpO_2.

Table 18.1 Factors determining sensor selection.

Patient size
Available monitoring sites
Adequacy of perfusion
Amount of patient movement
Duration of monitoring time
Requirements for sterility
Shielding from ambient light sources

(Szaflarski & Cohen, 1989)

EQUIPMENT

Pulse oximeter
Appropriate sensor (probe) See Table 18.1 and Figure 18.1.

Cardiac monitor (optional, dependent on type of oximeter available)

QUICK SENSOR APPLICATION REFERENCE

DURASENSOR® DS-100A adult digit oxygen transducer

- For patients who weigh over 40 kg (88 lbs).
- Short-term monitoring only.
- Preferred site is index finger.
- Alternate sites are smaller fingers. *No thumbs or toes!*
- For low-motion environments.
- Accuracy specifications: ± 3 digits (70–100% SaO_2) ± 1 S.D.
- Reusable durable sensor.
- Change sensor site every 4 hours.
- Never tape sensor shut.

OXISENSOR™ R-15 adult nasal oxygen transducer

- For patients who weigh over 50 kg (110 lbs).
- Only site for application is across nasal bridge.
- For no-motion environments.
- Accuracy specifications: ± 3.5 digits (80–100% SaO_2) ± 1 S.D.
- For one time use only—may *not* be reapplied.
- Requires skin preparation prior to sensor application. (Preparation solution enclosed.)

OXISENSOR D-25 adult digit oxygen transducer

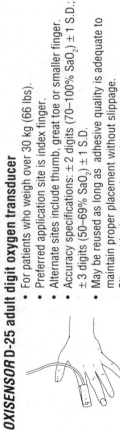

- For patients who weigh over 30 kg (66 lbs).
- Preferred application site is index finger.
- Alternate sites include thumb, great toe or smaller finger.
- Accuracy specifications: ± 2 digits (70–100% SaO_2) ± 1 S.D.; ± 3 digits (50–69% SaO_2) ± 1 S.D.
- May be reused as long as adhesive quality is adequate to maintain proper placement without slippage.
- Site must be inspected every 8 hours.

OXISENSOR D-20 pediatric digit oxygen transducer

- For patients who weigh 10–50 kg (22–110 lbs).
- Preferred application site is index finger.
- Alternate sites include thumb, great toe or smaller digit.
- Accuracy specifications: ± 2 digits (70–100% SaO_2) ± 1 S.D.; ± 3 digits (50–69% SaO_2) ± 1 S.D.
- May be reused as long as adhesive is adequate to maintain proper placement without slippage.
- Site must be inspected every 8 hours.

OXISENSOR I-20 infant digit oxygen transducer

- For patients who weigh 1–20 kg (2.2–44 lbs).
- Preferred application site is great toe.
- Alternate sites include thumb or other digits.
- Use supplied additional tape to secure the I-20 to the patient's foot or hand.
- Accuracy specifications: ± 2 digits (70–100% SaO_2) ± 1 S.D. (in neonatal population); ± 3 digits (70–95% SaO_2) ± 1 S.D.
- Limited reuse with adhesive dots supplied with I-20.
- Site must be inspected every 8 hours.

OXISENSOR N-25 neonatal oxygen transducer

- For patients who weigh under 3 kg (6.6 lbs) or over 40 kg (88 lbs).
- Preferred application site for neonates is around ball of foot.
- Alternate site for neonates is across palm of hand.
- Accuracy specifications in neonatal population: ± 3 digits (70–95% SaO_2) ± 1 S.D.
- Limited reuse with adhesive dots supplied with N-25.
- Site must be inspected every 8 hours.

Warning: Carefully read the Directions for Use provided with each *NELLCOR* sensor for descriptions, complete instructions, warnings, cautions, and specifications.

Figure 18.1 Various sensor types, indications for use, and appropriate placement. (Courtesy of Nellcor Incorporated, Hayward, CA. Reprinted by permission.)

61

PATIENT PREPARATION

1. It is *not* necessary to remove nail polish or wash dirty skin as accuracy of readings is not dependent on these variables (Szaflarski, 1989).

PROCEDURAL STEPS

1. Select the appropriate sensor for patient size and site of placement.
2. Prepare skin with recommended prep solution (if necessary) as specified on sensor instructions.
3. Apply the sensor to site. Accurate readings depend on proper sensor placement. Sensors contain two light sources (red and infrared) and a photodetector. The saturation is determined by the ratio of red to infrared as sensed by the photo detector. Therefore, it is important to place the two light sources directly opposite of the photodetector to assure accuracy of readings.

*Most oximeters will give some indication as to why readings are not obtainable.

4. *If unable to obtain readings assess:
   a. Circulation in extremity through capillary refill, color, and temperature.
   b. Sensor position. Both light sources must pass through the pulsating arterial bed and reach the photosensor.
   c. Presence of ambient light sources in room (surgical lamps, fiber optic lights, fluorescent lights, infrared heating lamps, direct sunlight) as the photodetector cannot differentiate bright external lights from those transmitted from the sensor light source.
   d. Dirt or blood on sensor at light source or photodetector site.
   e. Patient movement.
6. Trouble shooting options:
   a. Massage the extremity to increase circulation or apply isopropyl alcohol topically to cause vasodilation.
   b. Change the site and/or the type of sensor.
   c. Reposition the sensor to assure light sources are opposite of photosensor.
   d. Decrease ambient light by turning off external light sources, shutting blinds, or placing tape over the sensor.
   e. Clean the probe with alcohol.
   f. If the oximeter has the ability to synchronize data processing to the ECG and if the patient has poor tissue perfusion or increased movement, interface the oximeter with cardiac monitor.
7. If the oximetry reading does not correlate with patient's clinical presentation, assess pulse rate apically or radially and compare with the oximeter's pulse reading. If the readings differ, repeat Steps 6a.–f. or obtain an arterial blood gas reading.
8. Document oximeter reading and concomitant oxygen therapy.
   Note: Notation of SpO_2 indicates measurement of arterial oxygen saturation by pulse oximetry rather than by arterial blood gas analysis and is used because blood analysis and oximetry readings may differ due to machine capabilities and patient status.

COMPLICATIONS

False high or false low readings (See Contraindications and Cautions.)

Hold the extremity where the sensor is placed as still as possible to prevent inaccurate or unobtainable readings.

REFERENCES

Szaflarski, N. & Cohen, N. 1989. Use of pulse oximetry in critically ill adults. *Heart and Lung,* 18:444–453.

SUGGESTED READINGS

Gilroy, N., & McGaffigan, P. 1989. Noninvasive monitoring of oxygenation with pulse oximetry. *Journal of Emergency Nursing,* 15:26–31.
Schroeder, C.H. 1988. Pulse oximetry: A nursing care plan. *Critical Care Nurse,* 8:50–67.

19

Assessing Pulsus Paradoxus

Manjula D. Gray, RN, BSN, MA, CCRN

Manjula D. Gray, RN, BSN, MA, CCRN

Pulsus paradoxus is also known as paradoxical pulse.

INDICATIONS

To assess hemodynamic status in conditions that may cause a greater than normal decline in left ventricular outflow during inspiration. These conditions include: cardiac tamponade, constrictive pericarditis, asthma, COPD, severe congestive heart failure, tension pneumothorax, and superior vena cava syndrome.

CONTRAINDICATIONS AND CAUTIONS

1. Surgical procedures or disease processes that prevent performing blood pressures in both of the upper extremities (e.g., amputation, mastectomy, extra anatomical bypass, and dialysis fistula).
2. Severe dysrythmias will prevent accurate measurement of pulsus paradoxus.

EQUIPMENT

BP cuff (cuff sphygmomanometer)
Stethoscope

PROCEDURAL STEPS

1. Assess the patient for any irregular cardiac rhythms.
2. Instruct patient to breath normally.
3. Obtain the patient's blood pressure and note the systolic finding. Deflate the cuff.
4. Reinflate the blood pressure cuff, slightly above the patient's previous systolic reading.
5. Deflate the cuff slowly, 2 mm Hg at a time, and listen for the first systolic Korotkoff sound. Watch the patient's respiratory pattern. This sound will be heard only during expiration. Note this systolic reading.
6. Continue to deflate the cuff 2 mm Hg at a time and listen to the Korotkoff sound while watching the patient's respiratory cycle, until the Korotkoff sound is heard both during inspiration and expiration. Note the systolic reading.
7. The difference in mm of Hg between the first Korotkoff sound heard only during expiration and the first Korotkoff sound heard both during expiration and inspiration is the measurement of the paradoxical pulse. For example, if the first Korotkoff sound on expiration was heard at 150 mm Hg and the first Korotkoff sound during inspiration and expiration

was heard at 130 mm Hg, then the paradoxical pulse is said to be 20 mm Hg.

8. A difference of 10 mm Hg or less is considered normal (King, 1982).

REFERENCE

King, D.E. 1982. Assessment and evaluation of the paradoxical pulse. *Dimensions of Critical Care Nursing*, 1:266–274.

20

Peak expiratory flow measurement is also known as peak flow.

Peak Expiratory Flow Measurement

Manjula D. Gray, RN, BSN, MA, CCRN

INDICATIONS

To assess peak expiratory flow rate in obstructive airway diseases (especially asthma) and evaluate response to bronchodialator therapy.

EQUIPMENT

Peak flowmeter (Assess, Flo Scope, Wright, etc.)
Disposable mouthpiece

PATIENT PREPARATION

If possible, place the patient in a sitting position with legs dangling to maximize diaphragmatic excursion.

PROCEDURAL STEPS

1. Insert the mouthpiece into the flowmeter. See Figure 20.1.
2. Make sure that the indicator is at the bottom of the scale (zero).
3. Instruct the patient:
   a. to hold the flow meter vertically or horizontally according to the manufacturer's directions;
   b. to not block the openings;
   c. to inhale deeply;
   d. while holding his/her breath, to place the mouth firmly around the mouthpiece, sealing the circumference with the lips;
   e. to exhale as forcefully as possible.
4. The position of the indicator is the peak expiratory flow measurement.
5. Have the patient repeat the procedure twice more.
6. Document the highest value of the three.
7. The normal range for adults is between 350 to 750 liters per minute, based on age and height of the person. See Figure 20.2. A peak flow less than 100 L/min (< 60% predicted) indicates a severe exacerbation (Corre, 1985).

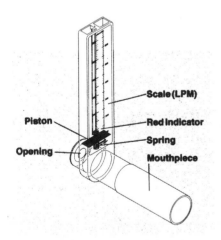

Scale (LPM)
Piston
Red Indicator
Spring
Opening
Mouthpiece

Figure 20.1 Assess peak flowmeter. (Reproduced by permission from Healthscan Products Inc.)

COMPLICATIONS

Bronchospasm and increased dyspnea.

PATIENT TEACHING

Report any increase in shortness of breath, faintness, or dizziness.

PREDICTED AVERAGE PEAK EXPIRATORY FLOW (liters per minute)

NORMAL MALES*

Age (Years)	Height				
	60″	65″	70″	75″	80″
20	554	602	649	693	740
25	543	590	636	679	725
30	532	577	622	664	710
35	521	565	609	651	695
40	509	552	596	636	680
45	498	540	583	622	665
50	486	527	569	607	649
55	475	515	556	593	634
60	463	502	542	578	618
65	452	490	529	564	603
70	440	477	515	550	587

NORMAL FEMALES*

Age (Years)	Height				
	55″	60″	65″	70″	75″
20	390	423	460	496	529
25	385	418	454	490	523
30	380	413	448	483	516
35	375	408	442	476	509
40	370	402	436	470	502
45	365	397	430	464	495
50	360	391	424	457	488
55	355	386	418	451	482
60	350	380	412	445	475
65	345	375	406	439	468
70	340	369	400	432	461

NORMAL CHILDREN AND ADOLESCENTS†

Height (Inches)	Males & Females	Height (Inches)	Males & Females
43	147	55	307
44	160	56	320
45	173	57	334
46	187	58	347
47	200	59	360
48	214	60	373
49	227	61	387
50	240	62	400
51	254	63	413
52	267	64	427
53	280	65	440
54	293	66	454

* Leiner GC, *et al*: Expiratory peak flow rate. Standard values for normal subjects. Use as a clinical test of ventilatory function. *Am Rev Resp Dis 88*: 644, 1963.
† Polgar G, Promadhat V: *Pulmonary function testing in children: Techniques and standards*. Philadelphia, W.B. Saunders Company, 1971.
NOTE: All tables are averages and are based on tests with a large number of people. The peak flow of an individual can vary widely.

Figure 20.2   Peak expiratory flow measurement chart.
(Reproduced by permission from Healthscan Products Inc.)

REFERENCE

Corre, K.A. & Rothstein, R.J. 1985. Assessing severity of adult asthma and need for hospitalization. *Annals of Emergency Medicine,* 14:45–52.

SUGGESTED READING

Roberts, R.R., & Hedges, J.R. 1985. *Clinical procedures in emergency medicine.* Philadelphia: Saunders.

21

General Principles of Oxygen Therapy

Ruth A. Slabach, MSN, SCN, RN

INDICATIONS

To provide supplemental oxygen to patients with adequate spontaneous respirations.

CONTRAINDICATIONS AND CAUTIONS

1. The primary physical hazard of oxygen therapy is fire. Oxygen supports combustion. Smoking should not be permitted in the room and spark producing appliances should be removed from the immediate vicinity.
2. Oxygen induced hypoventilation must always be considered as a possible hazard with patients who are known or suspected to have a chronic lung disease with chronic carbon dioxide retention.
3. Oxygen masks are contraindicated in patients with facial burns or patients needing frequent access to the facial area for nursing care. Nasogastric tubes may interfere with a tight seal of the mask.
4. Aspiration is a potential hazard with a mask in place. Special caution must be used with unconscious or comatose patients. Elevating the head of the bed may decrease the risk.

EQUIPMENT

Prescribed oxygen delivery device
Flowmeter (regulator must be used
        for cylinder systems)
Nut and tailpiece ("Christmas tree")
Oxygen source
No-smoking signs

PATIENT PREPARATION

Explain no-smoking instructions to patient and post no-smoking signs.

PROCEDURAL STEPS

1. Attach the flowmeter to the oxygen source.
2. Attach the nut and tailpiece to the flowmeter.
3. Attach the flared vinyl tip of the oxygen tubing to the tailpiece.

4. Adjust oxygen to the flow rate prescribed by the physician or protocol. The float ball in the flowmeter should be positioned so that the flow rate line is in the middle of the ball.
5. Place mask on patient's face or insert cannula prongs into nostril.
6. Mold the malleable metal nose strip (on oxygen masks) to the patient's nose.
7. Pad straps with gauze or cotton as needed to prevent discomfort or irritation.

COMPLICATIONS

1. Excessive drying of nasal mucosa. Standard humidification equipment delivers a very limited amount of humidity to the patient (Darin, 1982).
2. Mask or cannula may be easily dislodged.
3. Masks are of standard sizes and may not comfortably and snugly fit all patients.
4. Facial irritation may result from the mask being too tight or plastic rubbing the face.
5. Some patients may complain of a feeling of suffocation with a mask covering both the mouth and nose.
6. The mask must be removed for the patient to eat, drink, expectorate, or blow their nose. Patient may be placed on nasal cannula of corresponding oxygen concentration while eating.
7. Patients may complain of the mask being hot.

PATIENT TEACHING

1. No smoking while oxygen is in the room.
2. Remove mask only to eat, to clear nasal passages, to expectorate, or when vomiting occurs. Replace the mask immediately. The mask may be replaced with a nasal cannula of comparable oxygen concentration while the patient is eating.
3. Explain proper position of mask and importance of snug fit.

REFERENCES

Darin, J., Broadwell, J., & MacDonell, R. 1982. An evaluation of water-vapor output from four brands of unheated prefilled bubble humidifiers. *Respiratory Care,* 27:41–50.

SUGGESTED READINGS

American Heart Association. 1987. *Textbook of advanced cardiac life support.* Dallas: American Heart Association.
Kersten, L.D. 1989. *Comprehensive respiratory nursing.* Philadelphia: Saunders.
Morrissey, W.L., & Smith, M.H. 1985. Inhalation techniques and oxygen delivery. In J. Roberts, & J. Hedges. (eds). *Clinical procedures in emergency medicine.* Philadelphia: Saunders, 30–45.
Rarey, K.P., & Youtsey, J.W. 1981. *Respiratory patient care.* Englewood Cliffs, NJ: Prentice Hall.
Simon, R.R., & Brenner, R.E. 1987. *Emergency procedures and techniques,* 2nd ed. Baltimore: Williams & Wilkins.

22

Application and Removal of Oxygen Tank Regulators

Ruth A. Slabach, MSN, SCN, RN

The oxygen tank is also known as C cylinder, D cylinder, E cylinder, G cylinder, etc.

The regulator is also known as: adjustable regulator, regulator/flowmeter, control valve (a regulator reduces the cylinder pressure to a working pressure before the oxygen enters the flowmeter) (the flowmeter controls and measures liter flow of oxygen to the patient) See Figure 22.1.

The sealing washer is also known as O ring, gasket.

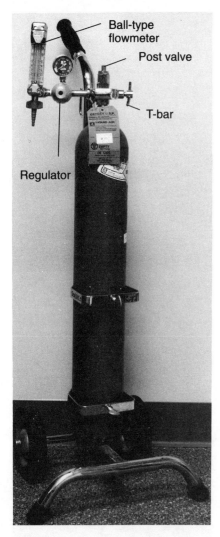

Figure 22.1 An E cylinder in a portable stand with regulator and flowmeter attached.

INDICATIONS

Oxygen cylinders are used to provide oxygen
1. while transporting patients,
2. where no piped oxygen source is available.

CONTRAINDICATIONS AND CAUTIONS

1. Secure oxygen cylinders in support stands to avoid damage during transport and storage. The pressurized oxygen may turn the cylinder into a "torpedo" if damage occurs to the regulator.
2. Cylinders are heavy and cumbersome to handle.
3. To prevent fire, never permit oil, grease, or other highly flammable materials to come in contact with oxygen cylinders, valves, regulators, or fittings.
4. Check the cylinder for an adequate amount of oxygen before transport. A full E cylinder will last approximately 2 hours at a flow rate of 5 liters per minute.
5. To prevent accidental readjustment of oxygen flow, never drape anything over the cylinder or regulator.
6. Use only the proper wrench or key to open and close the post valve. See Figure 22.1.
7. If a support stand is not available, carefully lay cylinder on floor away from personnel.

EQUIPMENT

Cylinder of oxygen (E cylinder is most commonly used size inhospital; see Figure 22.1)
Regulator (Pin-Index Safety System compatible with oxygen cylinder; see Figure 22.2)
Wrench or key (some cylinder posts may have a knob, and do not require a wrench)

PROCEDURAL STEPS

Application of regulator

1. Secure the cylinder in a support stand or cart.
2. Remove the protective seal from the post valve.
3. Turn post valve outlet away from any personnel. Turn the post valve on

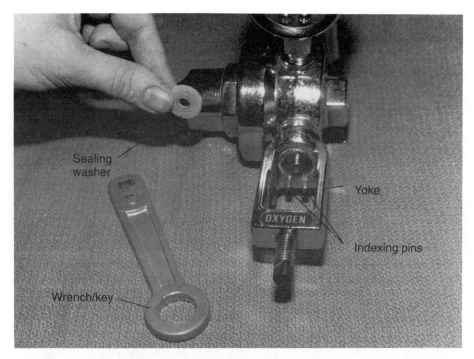

Figure 22.2 A sealing washer is usually provided with the dust cover. Note the two indexing pins that indicate the appropriate regulator for an E cylinder. Do not force regulator connectors onto cylinders or alter the indexing.

(counter-clockwise) and off quickly with the key (a loud "whooshing" sound will be heard). This clears (cracks) the valve and eliminates any dust or foreign materials. If you have difficulty remembering which direction to turn the key, the saying "righty-tighty, lefty-loosey" may help.

4. Place the yoke on the cylinder, making sure the fittings are compatible, ensuring that any necessary gasket or sealing washer is in place. See Figure 22.2.
5. Tighten the yoke by turning the "t-bar" clockwise. See Figure 22.3.
6. Turn the flowmeter off.
7. Slowly open the post valve until the pressure gauge reaches cylinder pressure. The pressure gauge on a full E cylinder reads 2200 psi.
8. Check the pressure gauge to ascertain adequate cylinder pressure for a

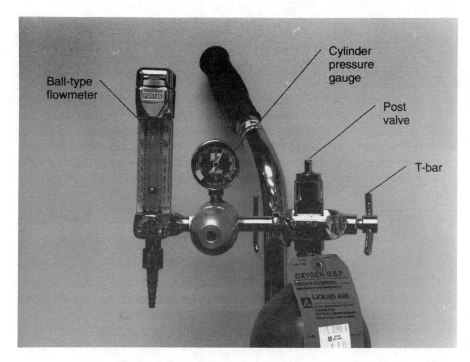

Figure 22.3 Close up view of regulator and "needle gauge" flowmeter on E cylinder.

reasonable supply of gas. Do not use the cylinder for transporting a patient if the pressure gauge reads below 500 psi.

9. Connect the desired form of patient oxygen delivery device. See Ch. 23–30.
10. Open the flowmeter so that flow rate prescribed by the physician or protocol registers on the flowmeter. If using the "ball-type" flowmeter the middle of the ball should be on the desired level. See Figure 22.4.
11. Secure the tank in an appropriate carrier.
12. When the cylinder is not in use, turn the post valve off and bleed the system by turning the flowmeter on until the pressure gauge reads zero.

Removal of regulator

1. Secure the cylinder in an upright position.
2. Turn the post valve off with appropriate key or wrench.
3. Open flowmeter to bleed the system until the pressure gauge reads zero.
4. Loosen yoke and remove regulator.
5. Label tank "empty" or "in use" and store in rack.

COMPLICATIONS

1. The "ball-type" flowmeters are constructed to be used in an upright position. See Figure 22.4. Laying them on their side affects the accuracy of their reading, but not the accuracy of the actual flow. The "needle gauge" flowmeters may be used in any position without affecting the accuracy of their reading. See Figure 22.3.
2. Removing the regulator before bleeding the system may damage the sealing washers.
3. A cylinder containing less than 500 psi should not be used for transporting patients.

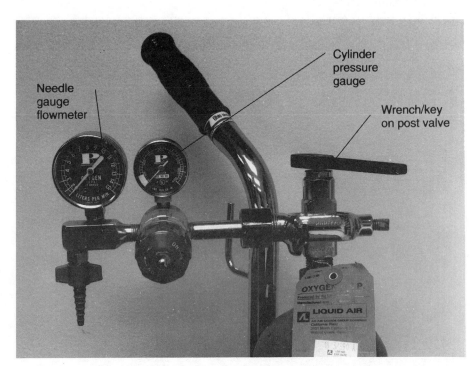

Figure 22.4 Close up view of regulator and "ball type" flowmeter on E cylinder.

SUGGESTED READINGS

Kersten, L.D. 1989. *Comprehensive respiratory nursing.* Philadelphia: Saunders.

Morrissey, W.L., & Smith, M.H. 1985. Inhalation techniques and oxygen delivery. In J. Roberts, & J. Hedges, (eds). *Clinical procedures in emergency medicine.* Philadelphia: Saunders, 30–45.

23

Nasal Cannula

Ruth A. Slabach, MSN, SCN, RN

Nasal Cannula is also known as cannula, O₂ prongs, nasal prongs.
   Note: The information in this chapter should be used in conjunction with the information in Ch. 21: General Principles of Oxygen Therapy.

INDICATIONS

To provide 22–45% supplemental oxygen to patients with adequate spontaneous ventilations.

CONTRAINDICATIONS AND CAUTIONS

1. The concentration of oxygen delivered is unpredictable. At any given flow rate, the concentration may vary depending on the ratio of mouth-to-nose breathing and respiratory pattern of the patient.
2. Flows greater than 6 liters per minute should not be used because such high flow rates are very uncomfortable to the patient when delivered by nasal cannula.
3. Patients with partially obstructed nasal cavities will receive less oxygen.

EQUIPMENT

Nasal cannula   Oxygen source

PROCEDURAL STEPS

1. Insert cannula prongs into nostrils, making sure the curves of the prongs follow the contour of the nasal passage.
2. Pass cannula tubing over patient's ears, and adjust the plastic slide up tubing toward neck for a comfortable fit under the chin. See Figure 23.1.
3. If nasal cannula has an elastic band, place the band around the back of patient's head and adjust for a comfortable fit. See Figure 23.2.

COMPLICATIONS

1. Cannula may be dislodged easily.
2. Cannula may become plugged with nasal secretions.
3. To fit an individual patient's nares more comfortably, the tips of the nasal prongs may be trimmed with a scissors.

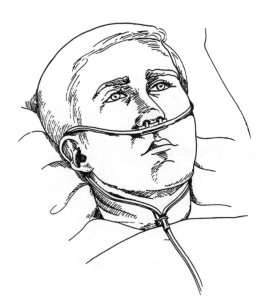

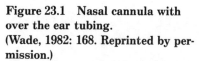

Figure 23.1   Nasal cannula with over the ear tubing.
(Wade, 1982: 168. Reprinted by permission.)

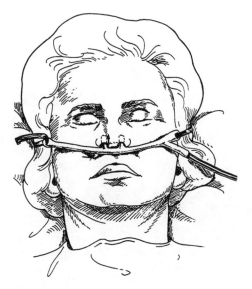

Figure 23.2   Nasal cannula with adjustable elastic band.
(Wade, 1982: 168. Reprinted by permission.)

SUGGESTED READINGS

American Heart Association. 1987. *Textbook of advanced cardiac life support.* Dallas: American Heart Association.

Kersten, L.D. 1989. *Comprehensive respiratory nursing.* Philadelphia: Saunders.

Morrissey, W.L., & Smith, M.H. 1985. Inhalation techniques and oxygen delivery. In J. Roberts & J. Hedges, (eds). *Clinical procedures in emergency medicine.* Philadelphia: Saunders, 30–45.

Rarey, K.P., & Youtsey, J.W. 1981. *Respiratory patient care.* Englewood Cliffs, NJ: Prentice Hall.

Rea, R.E. (ed). 1991. *Trauma nursing core course (provider) manual,* 3rd ed. Chicago: Award Printing Corporation.

Simon, R.R., & Brenner, R.E. 1987. *Emergency procedures and techniques,* 2nd ed. Baltimore: Williams & Wilkins.

Wade, J.F. 1982. *Comprehensive respiratory care,* 3rd ed. St. Louis: Mosby.

24

Simple Face Mask

Ruth A. Slabach, MSN, SCN, RN

The simple face mask is also known as simple oxygen mask, face mask, simple mask.

Note: The information in this chapter should be used in conjunction with the information in Ch. 21: General Principles of Oxygen Therapy.

INDICATIONS

To provide 40–60% supplemental oxygen to patients with spontaneous respirations.

CONTRAINDICATIONS AND CAUTIONS

1. The concentration of oxygen delivered is variable and depends on flow rate, ventilatory pattern, and anatomic dead space.
2. Flow rates less than 5 liters per minute should never be used. Flow rates of 5 liters and above are necessary to prevent the rebreathing of carbon dioxide.
3. Improper mask fit may allow room air to dilute the oxygen concentration excessively.

EQUIPMENT

Simple oxygen mask   Oxygen source

PROCEDURAL STEPS

1. Place mask on patient's face.
2. Slip the elastic retaining strap over the head. Strap may be placed below or above the ears depending on the patient's comfort and mask fit. See Figure 24.1.

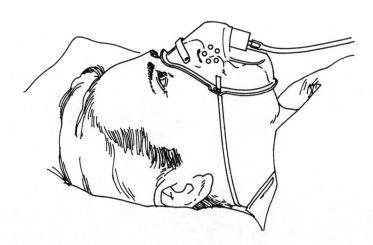

Figure 24.1 Simple face mask. (Rarey & Youtsey, 1981: 22. Reprinted by permission.)

SUGGESTED READINGS

American Heart Association. 1987. *Textbook of advanced cardiac life support.* Dallas: American Heart Association.

Kersten, L.D. 1989. *Comprehensive respiratory nursing.* Philadelphia: Saunders.

Morrissey, W.L., & Smith, M.H. 1985. Inhalation techniques and oxygen delivery. In J. Roberts, & J. Hedges, (eds). *Clinical procedures in emergency medicine.* Philadelphia: Saunders, 30–45.

Rarey, K.P., & Youtsey, J.W. 1981. *Respiratory patient care.* Englewood Cliffs, NJ: Prentice Hall.

Rea, R.E. (ed). 1991. *Trauma nursing core course (provider) manual,* 3rd ed. Chicago: Award Printing Corporation.

Simon, R.R., & Brenner, R.E. 1987. *Emergency procedures and techniques,* 2nd ed. Baltimore: Williams & Wilkins.

25

Partial Rebreather Mask

Ruth A. Slabach, MSN, SCN, RN

The partial rebreather mask is also known as partial rebreathing mask, reservoir mask.

Note: The information in this chapter should be used in conjunction with the information in Ch. 21: General Principles of Oxygen Therapy.

INDICATIONS

To provide 50–80% supplemental oxygen to patients with adequate spontaneous respirations.

CONTRAINDICATIONS AND CAUTIONS

1. The concentration of oxygen delivered is variable and depends on flow rate, ventilatory pattern, and anatomic dead space.
2. Improper mask fit may allow room air to dilute the oxygen concentration excessively.

EQUIPMENT

Partial rebreather mask (similar to a simple face mask, with the addition of a reservoir bag, allowing the patient to inhale oxygen-rich air from the reservoir bag)

Oxygen source

PATIENT PREPARATION

1. Explain the importance of keeping the reservoir bag from kinking and obstructing the flow of oxygen.

PROCEDURAL STEPS

1. Turn the oxygen to the prescribe flow rate (usually 8–12 liters per minute).
2. Occlude the outlet from the reservoir bag to the mask until the reservoir bag inflates.
3. Place mask on patient's face and slip the elastic retaining strap over the patient's head. Strap may be placed either above or below the ears depending on patient's comfort and mask fit. See Figure 25.1.
4. Adjust the flow rate of the oxygen so that the reservoir bag remains inflated during both maximal inspiration and expiration. The bag should never completely collapse.

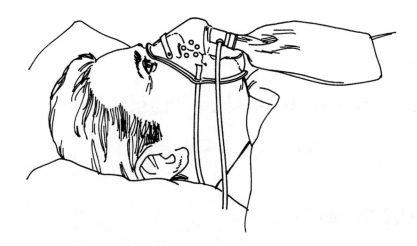

**Figure 25.1 Partial rebreather
mask.
(Rarey & Youtsey, 1981: 23.)**

COMPLICATIONS

1. Pinching of the reservoir bag blocks the flow of oxygen to be inhaled
    from it. This reduces the delivered oxygen concentration in comparison
    to that of a simple mask.
2. If the prescribed flow rate is insufficient to maintain bag inflation, in-
    crease the flow rate and notify the physician.

PATIENT TEACHING

Position your head so that reservoir bag does not kink.

SUGGESTED READINGS

American Heart Association. 1987. *Textbook of advanced cardiac life support.* Dal-
    las: American Heart Association.
Kersten, L.D. 1989. *Comprehensive respiratory nursing.* Philadelphia: Saunders.
Morrissey, W.L., & Smith, M.H. 1985. Inhalation techniques and oxygen delivery. In
    J. Roberts, & J. Hedges. (eds). *Clinical procedures in emergency medicine.* Phila-
    delphia: Saunders, 30–45.
Rarey, K.P., & Youtsey, J.W. 1981. *Respiratory patient care.* Englewood Cliffs, NJ:
    Prentice Hall.
Rea, R.E. (ed). 1991. *Trauma nursing core course (provider) manual,* 3rd ed. Chicago:
    Award Printing Corporation.
Simon, R.R., & Brenner, R.E. 1987. *Emergency procedures and techniques,* 2nd ed.
    Baltimore: Williams & Wilkins.

26

Nonrebreather Mask

Ruth A. Slabach, MSN, SCN, RN

The nonrebreather mask is also known as 100% mask, nonrebreathing mask.

Note: The information in this chapter should be used in conjunction with the information in Ch. 21: General Principles of Oxygen Therapy.

INDICATIONS

To deliver 85–100% supplemental oxygen to patients with adequate spontaneous respirations.

CONTRAINDICATIONS AND CAUTIONS

1. The concentration of oxygen delivered is varied and depends on flow rate, patient's ventilatory pattern, and differences in design among various brands of masks.
2. Improper mask fit or removal of the one-way valves from the side exhalation ports allows room air to dilute the oxygen concentration excessively.

EQUIPMENT

Nonrebreather mask (similar to a partial rebreather mask except for two features: (1) a one-way valve lies between the mask and reservoir bag preventing exhaled gas from entering the bag, and (2) one-way valves on the side exhalation ports allow gas to leave the mask during exhalation and prevent room air from entering during inspiration)

Oxygen source

PATIENT PREPARATION

1. Explain importance of not allowing the reservoir bag to kink, thereby obstructing the flow of oxygen.

PROCEDURAL STEPS

1. Turn the oxygen to the prescribed flow rate (usually 12–15 liters per minute).
2. Occlude the outlet from the reservoir bag to the mask until the reservoir bag inflates.
3. Slip the elastic retaining strap over the patient's head. Strap may be placed either above or below the ears depending on patient's comfort and mask fit. See Figure 26.1.
4. Adjust the flow rate of the oxygen so that the reservoir bag remains inflated during both maximal inspiration and expiration. The bag should never completely collapse.

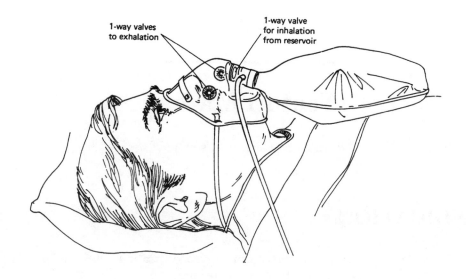

1-way valves to exhalation

1-way valve for inhalation from reservoir

Figure 26.1 Nonrebreather mask. (Rarey & Youtsey, 1981: 24.)

COMPLICATIONS

1. Carbon dioxide will accumulate and be rebreathed by the patient if the bag is pinched off or the inhalation valve is obstructed. Some brands have a safety relief valve that allows the patient to inhale room air in this instance.
2. If the prescribed flow rate in insufficient to maintain bag inflation, check for bag or valve obstruction. If no obstruction exists, increase the flow rate and notify the physician.

PATIENT TEACHING

1. Proper mask position and snug fit are important for accurate oxygen delivery.
2. Position your head so that the reservoir bag is not kinked.

SUGGESTED READINGS

American Heart Association. 1987. *Textbook of advanced cardiac life support.* Dallas: American Heart Association.

Kersten, L.D. 1989. *Comprehensive respiratory nursing.* Philadelphia: Saunders.

Morrissey, W.L., & Smith, M.H. 1985. Inhalation techniques and oxygen delivery. In J. Roberts, & J. Hedges (eds). *Clinical procedures in emergency medicine.* Philadelphia: Saunders, 30–45.

Rarey, K.P., & Youtsey, J.W. 1981. *Respiratory patient care.* Englewood Cliffs, NJ: Prentice Hall.

Rea, R.E. (ed.) 1991. *Trauma nursing core course (provider) manual,* 3rd ed. Chicago: Award Printing Corporation.

Simon, R.R., & Brenner, R.E. 1987. *Emergency procedures and techniques,* 2nd ed. Baltimore: Williams & Wilkins.

27

Venturi Mask

Ruth A. Slabach, MSN, SCN, RN

The venturi mask is also known as Ventimask, air entrainment mask.
  Note: The information in this chapter should be used in conjunction with the information in Ch. 21: General Principles of Oxygen Therapy.

INDICATIONS

1. To provide supplemental oxygen at precise concentrations from 24–50% to patients with adequate spontaneous respirations.
2. Major advantages: (a) allows inhalation of a constant oxygen concentration regardless of the rate or depth of respiration, (b) an accidental increase in flow rate does not alter oxygen concentration.

CONTRAINDICATIONS AND CAUTIONS

1. Not useful for oxygen concentrations greater than 50%.
2. The mask must fit snugly so that room air cannot be inhaled around the mask.
3. Air entrainment ports on the mask must never be blocked. See Figure 27.1. If this occurs, the venturi mask functions as a simple mask with varying oxygen concentrations delivered to the patient.

EQUIPMENT

Venturi mask
Oxygen source

Color-coded adaptors (oxygen diluters) for various oxygen concentrations

PROCEDURAL STEPS

1. Attach the appropriate adaptor to the venturi mask to deliver the prescribed oxygen concentration.
2. For multi-vent barrels, select the prescribed oxygen concentration by setting the indicator on the diluter to the appropriate percentage on the barrel. Firmly slide the locking ring into position over the diluter.
3. Turn oxygen to the flow rate prescribed to deliver the necessary oxygen concentration. See Table 27.1.
4. Place the mask on patient's face.
5. Slip the elastic retaining strap over the patient's head. Strap may be placed below or above the patient's ears depending on the patient's comfort and mask fit.

COMPLICATIONS

1. Increased oxygen concentrations will result if the air entrainment ports become obstructed.

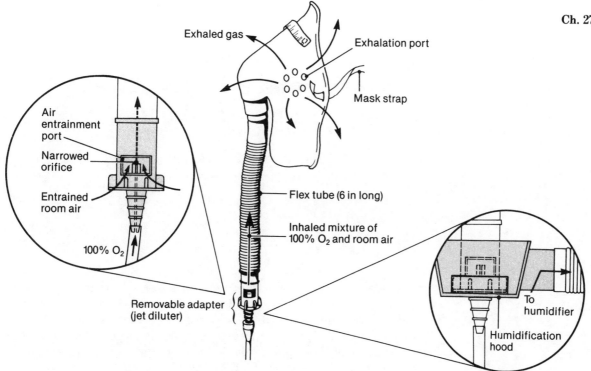

Figure 27.1 Venturi mask. The arrows indicate the movement of gas during respiration. A humidification hood may be added to protect air entrainment ports and to provide humidification.
(Kersten, 1989: 611. Reprinted by permission.)

Table 27.1 Recommended oxygen liter flow (Hudson Multi-Vent air entrainment mask product insert). Note: these are recommended flow rates only. Other brands may use different flow rates. (Courtesy of Hudson RCI, Temecula, CA.)

O_2 concentration	Recommended O_2 liter flow (liters per minute)
24%	3
26%	3
28%	6
30%	6
35%	9
40%	12
50%	15

SUGGESTED READINGS

American Heart Association. 1987. *Textbook of advanced cardiac life support.* Dallas: American Heart Association.

Kersten, L.D. 1989. *Comprehensive respiratory nursing.* Philadelphia: W.B. Saunders.

Morrissey, W.L., & Smith, M.H. 1985. Inhalation techniques and oxygen delivery. In J. Roberts, & J. Hedges, (eds.). *Clinical procedures in emergency medicine.* Philadelphia: W.B. Saunders, 30–45.

Rarey, K.P., & Youtsey, J.W. 1981. *Respiratory patient care.* Englewood Cliffs, NJ: Prentice Hall.

Simon, R.R., & Brenner, R.E. 1987. *Emergency procedures and techniques,* 2nd ed. Baltimore: Williams & Wilkins.

28

Continuous Positive Airway Pressure Mask

Valerie Novotny-Dinsdale, RN, MSN, CEN
Michael Cernuska, RRT

The continuous positive airway pressure mask is also known as CPAP mask, positive end expiratory pressure (PEEP) during spontaneous respirations.

INDICATIONS

1. To provide positive end expiratory pressure to a spontaneously breathing patient. This technique provides positive end expiratory pressure at the end of each inhalation which helps prevent alveolar collapse on exhalation. Usually, the patient has a diffuse pulmonary infiltrate on chest x-ray accompanied by hypoxemia that is refractory to supplemental oxygen (Luce et al., 1988). Use of a CPAP mask has also been shown to decrease the need for intubation and mechanical ventilation in patients with acute pulmonary edema (Bernsten et al. 1991).
2. To maintain positive pressure throughout the entire breathing cycle (as in those at risk for adult respiratory distress syndrome).
3. To restore or maintain oxygenation by increasing end expiratory lung volume above normal during regular tidal breathing. This usually applies when the PaO_2 is < 60 mm Hg on an FiO_2 > 0.5 (Sunderrajan, 1989).

CONTRAINDICATIONS AND CAUTIONS

Absolute

1. Inadequate cardiac output. CPAP increases intrathoracic pressure thereby diminishing venous return to the right side of the heart (Morrison, 1979).
2. Diminished or absent respiratory drive.
3. Untreated pneumothorax (when the intrapleural pressure is equal to atmospheric pressure).
4. Obtundation or the use of physical restraints. The patient must be alert and strong enough to pull off the mask in case of nausea or vomiting, to protect the airway.

Relative

1. Hypovolemia. As noted earlier, CPAP decreases ventricular filling. A patient that is concurrently hypovolemic and requiring CPAP should be monitored closely.
2. Unilateral or focal infiltrate evident on chest x-ray rather than a homogenous infiltrate. CPAP goes to the point of least resistance causing overdistention of the alveoli of the unaffected lung (Luce, 1988).

EQUIPMENT

Pole-mounted humidifier.
Blender, flow generator, or high
flow oxygen and air
flowmeters (1 each)
$^1/_4''$ I.D. (inner diameter) tubing ("Y"
if flowmeters are used
instead of a blender)
One-way valve assembly to act as a
safety breathing valve
+15 cm H_2O PEEP valve to act as
an overpressure relief valve

3-liter anesthesia bag as a pressure
reservoir (bag tail must be
closed)
Fittings needed to assemble unit.
See Figure 28.1.
Pressure alarm and tubing
Tight fitting mask with appropriate
size PEEP valve
Ventilator "Y" with flex tube and
swivel adapter (for CPAP
intubated patients)

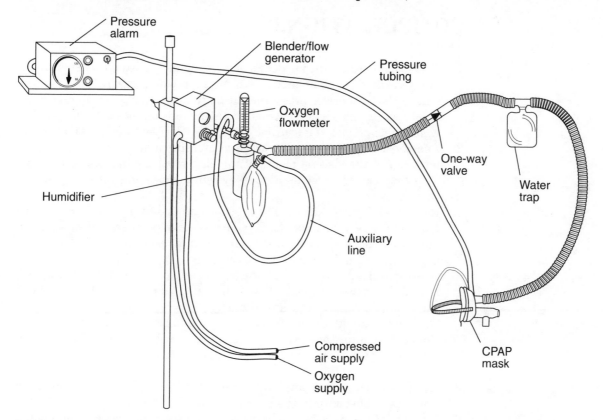

Figure 28.1 Continuous positive airway pressure (CPAP) mask set-up.

PATIENT PREPARATION

Insert a gastric tube (see Ch. 98), if ordered, to help prevent gastric distention.

PROCEDURAL STEPS

1. Assemble as shown in Figure 28.1 and according to method used (mask or artificial airway).
2. Adjust blender or flowmeters to deliver required FiO_2.
3. Evaluate readings on oxygen analyzer to determine FiO_2.

4. Attach apparatus to patient. If a mask is used, evaluate for comfortable fit and leaks (particularly around the eyes).
5. Adjust gas flow so that reservoir bag remains distended throughout the respiratory cycle.
6. Adjust alarm 2–3 cm below baseline CPAP (to sound if circuit pressure is lost).
7. Check the following CPAP setup components for proper functioning at least every two hours: manometer for proper level of ordered CPAP; proper FiO_2 setting; that the mask is still secure; drain tubing of collected water; and that the disconnect alarm is on and functioning.
8. Assess and document the patient's spontaneous respiratory rate and tidal volume. Consider use of an oximeter to continuously monitor oxygen saturation (see Ch. 18, Pulse Oximetry).

COMPLICATIONS

1. Decreased cardiac output demonstrated by decreased blood pressure or bradycardia due to the increase in intrathoracic pressure and lung volume. As intrathoracic pressure returns to atmospheric pressure, the venous return and right ventricular output are increased while the left ventricular preload and cardiac output are decreased (Morrison, 1979).
2. Pneumothorax. A rise in intrapleural pressure may cause a break in the integrity of the visceral pleura of the lung resulting in a pneumothorax. This tear can also act as a one-way valve creating a tension pneumothorax.
3. Decreased urinary output. The positive end expiratory pressure overdistends the alveoli against the capillary walls and causes a drop in blood pressure. Antidiuretic hormone is released in response to this "perceived hypovolemia" and leads to decreased urine output (Sunderrajan, 1989).
4. Air-trapping after removal of positive airway pressure. When the alveoli have been opened with CPAP and the CPAP is removed, the alveoli can clamp shut resulting in trapped air.

   Note: Should the above complications occur, immediately remove the patient from the system and if necessary, be prepared to manually ventilate the patient. Suction and resuscitation equipment must be immediately accessible.
5. Damage to the membranes of the eyes if the mask is too loose and high flow gas is blown up to the eyes.
6. Damage to the eyes from a harness that is too tight resulting in poking into the eye sockets.

PATIENT TEACHING

1. Report symptoms of nausea and/or vomiting immediately. CPAP can cause overinflation of the stomach in patients who do not have a nasogastric tube in place.
2. Report decreased tolerance for the procedure immediately. Symptoms include a feeling of claustrophobia or anxiety. This can be a result of increased intrathoracic pressure, as noted in complications, or restriction of the diaphragm due to an overinflated stomach.

REFERENCES

Bernsten, A., Holt, A., Vedig, A., Skowronski, G., & Baggoley, C. 1991. Treatment of severe cardiogenic pulmonary edema with continuous positive airway pressure delivered by face mask. *New England Journal of Medicine*, 325, 26:1825–1830.

Morrison, M. 1979. Respiratory intensive care nursing, 2nd ed. Boston: Little, Brown.

Luce, J., Tyler, M., & Pierson, D. 1988. Intensive respiratory care. Philadelphia: Saunders.

Sunderrajan, E.V. 1989. Mechanical ventilation and weaning. In S.R. Braun, (ed), Concise textbook of pulmonary medicine. New York: Elsevier: 393–396.

SUGGESTED READINGS

Kacmarek, R.M., Dimas, S., & Reynolds, J., 1982. Technical aspects of positive end expiratory pressure. *Respiratory Care,* 27:270–273.

Luce, J. 1984. The cardiovascular effects of mechanical ventilation and positive end expiratory pressure. *JAMA,* 252:807.

29

T-Piece

Valerie Novotny-Dinsdale, RN, MSN, CEN
Michael Cernuska, RRT

The T-piece is also known as T-piece aerosol nebulizer set-up, tee piece, or Briggs adaptor.

INDICATIONS

To provide humidification and oxygen to patients with artificial airways and spontaneous breathing patterns that meet the following parameters (Kacmarek, 1988):

VC (vital capacity) > 15 ml/kg

IE (inspiratory effort) > −25 mm Hg @ FRC (functional residual capacity)

Vt (tidal volume) > 7–10 ml/kg

Ve (Minute Exhalatory Volume) < 10 L/min

CONTRAINDICATIONS AND CAUTIONS

1. Patients who are obtunded without spontaneous respirations or who do not meet minimum spontaneous parameters will require mechanical ventilation.
2. The temperature at the patient end of the circuit should be at body temperature (optional for normothermic patients requiring short term use).
3. Tubing must be checked and drained often for excess water. A water trap may be included in the circuit and is recommended if extended use is anticipated. The water trap is placed in the lowest portion of the aerosol tubing.

EQUIPMENT

Heated aerosol (optional)   T-piece set up (see Figure 29.1)
Oxygen analyzer   Flowmeters (air or O_2)

PROCEDURE

1. Assemble the aerosol nebulizer, add 1000 ml of sterile water if the unit is not prefilled.
2. Plug the heating element into an electrical outlet (if used).
3. Connect flowmeter to the oxygen source and attach nebulizer.
4. Set the FiO_2 with the Venturi on the nebulizer.
5. Turn the primary flowmeter to 14 liters per minute of oxygen. Analyze the FiO_2 with an oxygen analyzer and label the flowmeters with the proper L/min settings. To maintain adequate flow, Table 29.1 can be used. Always run the flowmeter powering the nebulizer at 14 L/min or greater and/or adjust bleed in until desired FiO_2 is obtained.

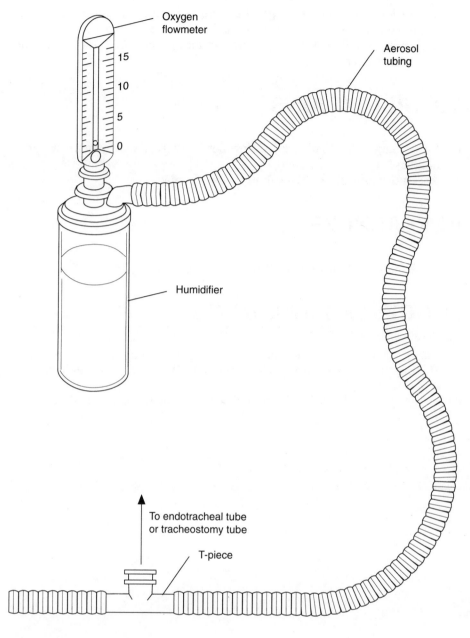

Figure 29.1   T-piece setup (bleed-in flowmeter and heater not shown).

Table 29.1

FiO$_2$	Nebulizer powered flow required	Bleed in desired
.21	air flowmeter	not used
.22–.27	air flowmeter	O$_2$ flowmeter
.28–.45	O$_2$ flowmeter	not used
.45–.80	O$_2$ flowmeter	O$_2$ flowmeter

6. Check to see that mist is visible at the T-piece. If it is not visible, the unit may be faulty or the flow rate not high enough. Attach the T-piece to the endotracheal or tracheostomy tube.

7. It is important to maintain a "high flow" system. If the patient inspira-

tory flow rate exceeds the output from the nebulizer, the resultant flow deficit will result in "room air" entrainment and a decreased FiO_2. To assure a high flow system, the Venturi should never be turned higher than the 40% setting. Any FiO_2 greater than .40 must be achieved by bleeding in additional flow to the system. This assures the patient of at least 40 L/min total flow. Be sure to analyze for proper FiO_2 after set up and equipment changes.

COMPLICATIONS

1. FiO_2 changes due to unsecured flowmeter controls and entrainment port handles.
2. Aspiration of water if the tubing is not drained.

REFERENCES

Kacmarek, R.M., & Stoller, J.K. 1988. *Current respiratory care.* Toronto: Decker, 271.

SUGGESTED READINGS

Bowser, M. 1980. Techniques of ventilator weaning. In G. Burton, G.N. Gee, & J.E. Hodgkin, (eds). *Respiratory Care: A Guide to Clinical Practice.* Philadelphia: Lippincott, 664–671.

Pierson, D., & Luce, J. 1988. *Critical care medicine.* Philadelphia: Saunders.

30

Tracheal Collar

Sharon Gavin Fought, PHD, RN
Jean A. Proehl, RN, MN, CEN, CCRN

The tracheal collar is also known as Puritan collar, tracheostomy collar.
Note: The information in this chapter should be used in conjunction with the information in Ch. 21: General Principles of Oxygen Therapy.

INDICATIONS

To facilitate the delivery of oxygen, warmed air, humidification, and medications to patients with tracheostomies or laryngectomies (Moorehouse, 1982).

CONTRAINDICATIONS AND CAUTIONS

Do not use a tracheal collar if the patient is unable to protect his own airway (i.e., vomiting and unable to turn or cough to prevent aspiration via the stoma).

EQUIPMENT

Humidification system with
heating element (optional)
Oxygen or medical air source
Oxygen delivery system (tubing,
connectors)

Gauze dressings
Tracheal collar

PROCEDURAL STEPS

1. Assemble the equipment:
   a. fill the humidification/warming system container with sterile water;
   b. attach the tubing to the humidifier;
   c. connect the humidifier system to the oxygen source.
2. Clean and dry the area around the stoma as needed.
3. Turn on the oxygen at the source to determine if the system is intact and functioning; a stream of humidified air/oxygen should be observed flowing from the connecting tube.
4. Set the oxygen flow rate (and temperature setting, if appropriate) as prescribed.
5. Attach the connecting tubing to the tracheal collar.
6. Place the tracheal collar over the patient's stoma, being careful not to occlude the stoma.
7. Secure the collar in place by snapping together the two ends of the elastic band. The band should be secure enough to prevent movement of the collar, but loose enough that one finger can easily fit under the elastic. The collar should be comfortable for the patient. See Figure 30.1.
8. Empty pooled water from the oxygen delivery tubing as it accumulates. This collected water can serve as a potential source of contaminants and

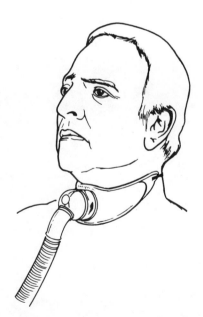

Figure 30.1 Tracheal collar in place.
(Blodgett, 1987: 23.)

can inadvertently be "dumped" into the patient's trachea when the tubing is repositioned. This may also be prevented by placing a water trap/collection bag in the aerosol tubing.

9. Use gauze dressings to remove water and secretions that accumulate around the stoma. The patient may also begin to feel "cold" as water evaporates from his skin. Provide extra sheets or blankets as needed.

COMPLICATIONS

1. Respiratory infection
2. Inadvertent aspiration of water collected in tubing
3. If the patient is to be transported, a humidified oxygen source may be needed during transport.
4. Decreased FiO_2 if excessive water accumulates in the tubing.

PATIENT TEACHING

1. Leave the collar in place.
2. Immediately report any shortness of breath.
3. Do not cover the inhalation port with bed linens or tissues, etc.

REFERENCES

Blodgett, D. 1987. *Manual of respiratory care procedures,* 2nd ed. Philadelphia: Lippincott.

Moorehouse, M.F., Geissler, A.C., & Doenges, M.E. 1982. *Critical care plans.* Philadelphia: F.A. David.

SUGGESTED READINGS

Swearingen, P. (ed). 1984. *The Addison-Wesley photo atlas of nursing procedures.* Menlo Park, CA: Addison-Wesley.

Luce, J.M., Tyler, M.L., & Pierson, D.J. 1984. *Intensive respiratory care.* Philadelphia: Saunders.

31

Pharyngeal Suctioning

Marijane Smallwood, RN, BSN

Pharyngeal suctioning is also known as oropharyngeal suctioning, Yankauer suctioning, nasopharyngeal suctioning, tonsillar suctioning.

INDICATIONS

1. To assure airway clearance for patients incapable of clearing their own oropharynx. Pharyngeal suctioning may be used with conscious or unconscious, intubated or nonintubated patients.
2. To maintain airway patency and maximize oxygenation of the patient by clearing the oropharynx.
3. To improve ventilation of the oropharynx during procedures such as insertion of posterior nasal packing.
4. To stimulate coughing and deeper breathing in the nonintubated patient.

CONTRAINDICATIONS AND CAUTIONS

1. Oropharyngeal secretions may be thick (e.g., blood or vomitus). Use a large bore suction catheter, tonsillar/pharyngeal suction tip device (Yankauer), or the suction connecting tubing alone for more effective airway clearance.
2. Excessive suctioning may traumatize the pharyngeal tissue, create bleeding, swelling, or localized inflammation. Use of a beveled tip and limiting suctioning to 10–15 seconds per attempt helps decrease the amount of trauma.
3. Hypoxemia may result from prolonged suctioning.
4. Suctioning may cause coughing and/or gagging, which should be avoided in patients with head injuries. Coughing creates increased intracranial pressure and decreases the cerebral blood flow (American Heart Association, 1987). If gagging leads to vomiting, further airway compromise may occur.
5. Suctioning may stimulate the vagal response leading to bradycardia and hypotension.
6. If possible, use the less traumatic oropharyngeal route rather than the nasopharyngeal approach.

EQUIPMENT

Portable or wall-continuous suction unit with regulator
Suction cannister
Suction connecting tubing
Tonsillar or pharyngeal suction tip (see Figure 31.1) or large bulb syringe (Asepto, similar to a turkey baster)
Large bore suction catheter or #14–18 French whistle tip with a vent port or Y connector
30–60 ml of tap water to clear the connecting tubing
Container to hold water (an emesis basin works well)
Water-soluble lubricant for catheter inserted via nasopharyngeal route
Emesis basin
Tissues

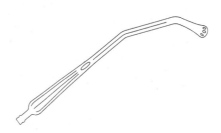

Figure 31.1 Tonsillor or pharyngeal suction catheter (Yankauer). (Rarey & Youtsey, 1981: 199. Reprinted by permission.)

93

PATIENT PREPARATION

1. For optimal airway alignment, place patient in semi-Fowler's position. However, pharyngeal suctioning may be performed in any position.
2. The patient may feel breathless during the 10–15 second procedure. A high-flow oxygen mask may be set up for use in between suctioning. Instruct the patient to use the oxygen mask and take deep breaths until he/she feels comfortable.
3. Warn the patient that the suctioning procedure may stimulate the gag or cough reflex. Provide an emesis basin and tissues.
4. Prior to using the nasopharyngeal route, assess for nasal patency by inspecting each nare for any obstruction such as polyps, structural deformity, or trauma. Occlude each nare and ask the patient to inhale to determine which side is most patent. Use the most patent nare for suctioning.

PROCEDURAL STEPS

1. Assemble suction cannister and attach to suction unit.
2. Attach connecting tubing to the suction cannister.
3. Select an appropriate catheter or suction device. To prevent hypoxia and trauma, the suction catheter for nasopharyngeal route should not be greater than one-half the size of the nare.
4. Set the suction gauge between 120–200 mm Hg. Full suction assists in rapid removal of large amounts of fluid or debris present in the oropharynx. Occlude the suction tubing to test the level of suction as measured by the suction gauge.

Oropharyngeal route

1. Attach the catheter or pharyngeal suction tip to the connecting tubing.
2. Insert the catheter or pharyngeal suction tip into the back of the mouth without applying suction. If using a Yankauer tip, gently sweep the posterior pharynx area while applying suction for 10–15 seconds.
3. If using a catheter, insert into the area on either side of the glottis. Apply suction intermittently for 10–15 seconds, gently rotating as you withdraw the catheter.
4. Flush the catheter by aspirating water through the connecting tubing.

Large bulb syringe

1. Depress large bulb syringe and gently advance to area of pooled secretions and debris in the oropharynx. Release the large bulb to aspirate secretions and debris.
2. Depress large bulb syringe into a basin to dispose of secretions and debris.
3. Flush the large bulb syringe by aspirating and expelling water until clear.
4. Repeat above steps until the airway is clear.

Nasopharyngeal route

1. Nasopharyngeal suctioning is used when the oral route is not accessible (e.g., clenched teeth or oral trauma).

2. Examine both nares, choose the more patent one. Avoid using a nare partially blocked by polyps or a deviated nasal septum.
3. Attach a suction catheter to the connecting tubing. Apply a small amount of water soluble lubricant to the catheter.
4. Without applying suction, gently insert the catheter medially into the nare. If coughing is stimulated, pull back on the catheter slightly.
5. Apply suction intermittently and rotate slightly while withdrawing the catheter.
6. Flush the catheter and connecting tubing by aspirating water through the tubing.
7. If repeated suctioning is required, a nasopharyngeal airway may be inserted to prevent additional mucosal trauma and to act as a guide for the catheter. See Ch. 7: Nasopharyngeal Airway Insertion.

COMPLICATIONS

Infection is a potential complication if the correct technique is not used. A new catheter must be used each time for nasopharyngeal suctioning, because contamination of the tracheobronchial area is possible. Repeated passage of the catheter past the upper respiratory tract promotes bacterial colonization in the lungs, which may lead to pneumonia (Kersten, 1989). However, a catheter or pharyngeal suction tip for the oropharynx may be used repeatedly for the same patient unless it is grossly contaminated or becomes clogged with large debris.

PATIENT TEACHING

1. Cough when possible to assist in clearing the airway.
2. Report any respiratory difficulty.
3. For a conscious patient with excessive oral secretions, a tonsil suction tip may be set up and the patient instructed how to suction himself/herself.

REFERENCES

American Heart Association 1987. *Textbook of advanced cardiac life support.* Dallas: American Heart Association.
Kersten, L. 1989. *Comprehensive respiratory nursing.* Philadelphia: Saunders.

SUGGESTED READINGS

Belland, K., & Wells, M. 1986. *Clinical nursing procedures.* Boston: Jones and Bartlett.
Petty, T. 1982. *Intensive and rehabilitative respiratory care.* Philadelphia: Lea & Febiger.
Rarey, K., & Youtsey, J., 1981. *Respiratory patient care.* Englewood Cliffs, NJ: Prentice Hall.

32

Nasotracheal Suctioning

Marijane Smallwood, RN, BSN

INDICATIONS

1. To maintain airway patency, maximize oxygenation, and reduce lower airway resistance in the nonintubated patient through removal of secretions.
2. To stimulate coughing in the weak or debilitated patient unable to clear secretions without assistance.
3. To obtain a sputum specimen when the patient is unable to do so without assistance.

CONTRAINDICATIONS AND CAUTIONS

1. To prevent hypoxia and tissue trauma, select a suction catheter no more than one-half the diameter of the nare to be suctioned.
2. Suctioning may exacerbate increased intracranial pressure or severe hypertension and should be performed with caution in these patients (Kersten, 1989).
3. Hypoxia may occur during suctioning particularly in patients with a history of pulmonary or cardiac disease.
4. Continuous suction may cause trauma to mucosa. Suction should be applied no longer than 10–15 seconds.
5. The nasotracheal route should not be used for patients with severe facial or head trauma to prevent penetration of the cranial vault with the suction catheter (Rea, 1991).

EQUIPMENT

Portable or wall-continuous suction unit with regulator
Suction cannister
Suction connecting tubing
Water-soluble lubricant
Sterile suction catheter (14 French is the standard size for adults)
Sterile water or 0.9% saline solution to flush tubing

Sterile container for flush solution
Sterile gloves
Oxygen source with oxygen mask or nasal cannula
Towels
Emesis basin and tissues
(Commercially prepared suction catheter kits are also available.)

PATIENT PREPARATION

1. For optimum airway alignment, place the patient in semi-Fowler's position. In the supine position, place the head in a neutral position.

2. Have the patient blow the nose to clear the nasal passages.
3. Provide an oxygen source prior to and following the suctioning. If a nasal cannula is being used, the prongs may be adjusted so that one nare continues to receive oxygen.
4. Inform the patient that a brief feeling of breathlessness is normal during the procedure. Encourage the patient to continue breathing rather than holding his/her breath.
5. Inform the patient that the procedure may stimulate the gag or cough reflex. Provide an emesis basin and tissues. Encourage the patient to expectorate any mucous produced.
6. Drape towels over the patient's chest to protect the patient from contamination by secretions.

PROCEDURAL STEPS

1. Assemble the suction cannister and attach to wall or portable suction unit. Attach connecting tubing to the suction cannister.
2. Set the suction gauge between 80–100 mm Hg. Full suction is no longer recommended. Pressures over 100 mm Hg increase trauma to the area and are no more effective in removing secretions (Kersten, 1989). Occlude the suction tubing to test the level of suction being delivered as measured by the suction gauge.
3. Examine both nares and choose a patent one. Avoid using a nare partially blocked by polyps, hemorrhaging, or a deviated nasal septum. Select a sterile suction catheter. To prevent hypoxia and trauma, the suction catheter for the nasotracheal route should not be greater than one-half the internal diameter of the nare.
4. Preoxygenate the respiratory compromised patient with high flow oxygen for two minutes prior to suctioning or place the prong of a nasal cannula in the opposite nare or have an assistant hold an oxygen mask with high-flow oxygen to the mouth (Kersten, 1989). Patients may be asked to take slow, deep breaths through their mouth during the procedure. Preoxygenation is a key method to prevent a decrease in the patient's PaO_2 baseline (Riegel & Forshee, 1985).
5. Dispense a small amount of water-soluble lubricant onto a sterile field such as the inside of the catheter package.
6. Put on sterile gloves.
7. Attach sterile suction catheter to connecting tubing.
8. Hold the suction catheter in your dominant hand, which must remain sterile. Your other hand controls the suction control vent and is considered clean.
9. Apply water-soluble lubricant to suction catheter.
10. Gently advance catheter through the nasal passage in a medial, downward direction.
11. Have the patient open mouth and extend tongue to prevent retraction of the tongue when gagging is stimulated.
12. Have the patient take slow deep breaths or cough gently. Coughing assists in opening the glottis which permits insertion of the catheter into the trachea.
13. When the patient coughs, advance the suction catheter until resistance is met or spontaneous coughing is noted.
14. When resistance is met, withdraw the catheter 2 or 3 centimeters and apply suction intermittently for 10 seconds. Gently rotate while withdrawing it.
15. Withdraw the suction catheter to the epiglottis area or until spontaneous coughing or gagging is absent. When secretions are excessive necessitating repeat suctioning, do not withdraw the catheter beyond the epiglottis. This prevents having to traverse the nasal passages again.

Discontinuation of suctioning is heavily dependent on the patient's tolerance of the procedure.

16. Reoxygenate the patient with high flow oxygen for 2 minutes or longer before repeating the procedure.
17. Flush the catheter by aspirating sterile water or saline solution through the tubing.

Alternative method

1. Pass an unconnected suction catheter through the nare to the point of the epiglottis. Listen at the end of the suction catheter for breath sounds. Advance catheter 1–2 centimeters until coughing is stimulated, then quickly advance the catheter into the trachea. Attach to connecting tubing and proceed to suction.

or

2. Advance catheter until no breath sounds are heard. Withdraw catheter 1–2 centimeters. Ask the patient to cough and pass the catheter into the tracheal area. Listen for breath sounds or watch for condensation in the catheter to verify tracheal entry. Proceed with suctioning (Kersten, 1989).

COMPLICATIONS

1. Infection of the lower respiratory tract is a potential complication because the catheter is contaminated when passed through the nasopharyngeal area.
2. The patient may refuse to allow the procedure to be repeated.
3. Prolonged suctioning may deplete the residual volume of the lung leading to alveolar collapse/atelectasis and hypoxia. Hypoxia can be decreased by providing adequate pre- and postoxygenation and limiting suctioning to 10–15 seconds per attempt.
4. Suctioning may stimulate a vagal response resulting in hypotension or bradycardia.
5. Forcing the suction catheter or repeated insertions may result in mucosal damage or local inflammation of the nasopharynx or trachea. Passing the catheter during inspiration is essential to avoid mucosal damage.

PATIENT TEACHING

1. Cough and deep breathe to assist in clearing the airway.
2. Increase fluid intake as allowed to loosen and thin secretions by adequate hydration.
3. Good oral hygiene decreases the chance for infection or bacterial colonization.

REFERENCES

Kersten, L. 1989. *Comprehensive respiratory nursing.* Philadelphia: Saunders.
Rea, R.E. 1991. *Trauma nursing core course (provider) manual*, 3rd ed. Chicago: Award Printing.
Riegel, B., & Forshee, T. 1985. A review and critique of the literature on preoxygenation for endotracheal suctioning. *Heart & Lung*, 14:507–518.

SUGGESTED READINGS

Miller, S., Sampson, L., & Soukoup, M. 1985. *AACN procedure manual for critical care.* Philadelphia: Saunders.

Petty, T. 1982. *Intensive and rehabilitative respiratory care.* Philadelphia: Lea & Febiger.

33

Endotracheal Suctioning

Marijane Smallwood, RN, BSN

Marijane Smallwood, RN, BSN

Endotracheal suctioning is also known as ET suctioning.

INDICATIONS

1. To remove secretions via an endotracheal tube, which may obstruct the airways and cause hypoxia.
2. To obtain a sputum specimen for laboratory analysis.

CONTRAINDICATIONS AND CAUTIONS

1. Do not deflate the endotracheal tube cuff prior to suctioning. The inflated cuff assists in preventing aspiration of any contents into the lungs if the gag reflex is stimulated and vomiting occurs.
2. Suctioning may exacerbate increased intracranial pressure or severe hypertension (Kersten, 1989).
3. Suctioning should not exceed 10–15 seconds per attempt to prevent hypoxia (Kersten, 1989).
4. For patients receiving mechanical ventilation with positive end expiratory pressure (PEEP), a PEEP adaptor may be added to the bag-valve-mask device to prevent interruption of maximum oxygenation. PEEP adaptor usage remains controversial as compared to delivering 100% oxygen without PEEP (Douglas, 1985).

EQUIPMENT

Portable or wall-continuous suction unit with regulator
Suction cannister
Suction connecting tubing
Sterile suction catheter, 14–18 French for adults, with intermittent suction control vent
Sterile gloves
Sterile container
Sterile water or saline solution
Bag-valve-mask (BVM) or anesthesia bag connected to a high-flow oxygen source
Towel
(Commercially prepared, disposable suction catheter kits are also available.)

PATIENT PREPARATION

1. While endotracheal suctioning can be accomplished in any position, Fowler's position with neutral head alignment is optimum. If the patient is conscious or semiconscious, restraining the patient may assist in decreasing excessive movement during the procedure.
2. Drape a towel over the patient's chest to protect the patient from contamination by secretions.

3. Warn the patient that suctioning may stimulate uncontrolled coughing or brief periods of breathlessness.
4. The benefit of using a 3–10 ml saline bolus to thin or loosen tenacious secretions is controversial. Research indicates this practice has little to no value for thinning, mobilizing, or removing dried secretions (Ackerman, 1985). Approximately 10–20% of the saline is recovered by suctioning after instillation and distribution of the saline to the lung periphery is limited.

PROCEDURAL STEPS

1. Obtain assistance if possible.
2. Assemble the suction cannister and attach to wall or portable suction unit. Attach connecting tubing to the suction cannister.
3. Set the suction gauge between 80–100 mm Hg. Full suction is no longer recommended. Pressures over 100 mm Hg increase trauma to the area and are no more effective in removing secretions (Kersten, 1989). Occlude the suction tubing to test the level of suction being delivered as measured by the suction gauge.
4. Select a suction catheter that is no larger than one-half the diameter of the endotracheal tube. A 14 French is usually appropriate for an adult.
5. Attach suction catheter to the connecting tubing. Hold the suction catheter in your dominant hand, which must remain sterile. Use your other hand to control the suction vent. This hand is considered clean.
6. Have your assistant remove the patient from the ventilator or T-piece and preoxygenate the patient with high-flow oxygen (100% concentration) via a BVM or anesthesia bag for one minute or 6–8 hyperinflations (Goodnough, 1985).
7. Immerse the tip of the catheter into the saline and aspirate a small amount to lubricate the catheter.
8. Have your assistant stabilize the endotracheal tube to prevent excessive movement or tube displacement.
9. Gently insert the catheter through the endotracheal tube and advance until resistance is met. Pull the catheter back 1–2 centimeters. Do not apply suction during introduction of the catheter.
10. Withdraw the catheter slowly while applying intermittent suction and rotating the catheter. Suction should be applied no longer than 10–15 seconds per attempt (Kersten, 1989).
11. Have your assistant hyperventilate the patient with 100% oxygen concentration. Postoxygenation is required for 2 minutes or until the oriented patient signals recovery (Goodnough, 1985).
12. Reconnect the patient to the ventilator or T-piece.
13. Rinse the catheter and connecting tubing by aspirating sterile water or saline through the tubing.
14. Steps 8–11 may be repeated if excessive secretions exist. Allow the patient at least 1 minute to recover before repeating the procedure.
15. If necessary, suction the nares or oropharynx before disposing of the catheter and gloves.

Alternative technique: Closed suction system

1. The closed suctioning system device is placed between the endotracheal tube and the ventilator or T-piece to permit suctioning without interrupting ventilation (Birdsall, 1986). The attached sheathed suction catheter passes through a seal into the endotracheal tube. See Figure 33.1.
2. The traditional endotracheal suctioning technique is followed.
3. The irrigation port is used to instill saline or water to rinse the catheter

and connecting tubing. A self-sealing system prevents the fluid from entering the endotracheal tube.

Note: The closed suctioning system cannot be used with an endotracheal tube smaller than a #7. The 14 French catheter in the prepackaged suction kit will leave half the airway open in a #7 endotracheal tube to not interrupt ventilation during the suction procedure (Birdsall, 1986). The closed suction system is more common in the intensive care setting, but is available for ED use.

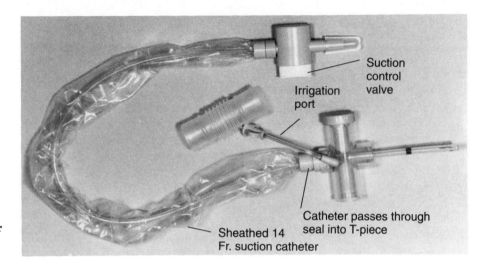

Figure 33.1   Closed suction catheter system. (Photo courtesy of Ballard Medical.)

COMPLICATIONS

1. Prolonged suctioning may cause hypoxia or atelectasis.
2. Hypoxia and hypercarbia produced during endotracheal suctioning increases the cerebral blood volume and increases the intracranial pressure (ICP) (McGinnis, 1988). Caution should be used when providing respiratory care to the patient with a head injury by limiting suctioning to 10–15 seconds per attempt. Administering prophylactic medication such as intravenous Lidocaine 50–100 mg two minutes prior to suctioning may prevent an increase in the ICP, but is still being studied (McGinnis, 1988).
3. The procedure may create a feeling of suffocation and lead to excessive anxiety for the patient.
4. Improper suctioning technique may cause traumatization of the tracheal mucosa.
5. The patient may develop a respiratory tract infection due to colonization of the airway with bacteria.
6. Aspiration of vomitus may occur particularly if the endotracheal cuff is faulty or with an incompetent glottis in the unconscious patient. Postintubation aspiration has been reduced with the advent of the low pressure, high volume cuffs.
7. Suctioning may stimulate a vagal response resulting in hypotension or bradycardia.
8. Patients receiving anticoagulants or thrombolytics may have blood-tinged secretions. Suctioning should be limited for these patients.

PATIENT TEACHING

1. Avoid touching or moving the endotracheal tube to decrease the incidence of mucosal damage at the point of entry (mouth or nose) and at the tracheal entry area.
2. Report any respiratory distress immediately.

REFERENCES

Ackerman, M. 1985. The use of bolus normal saline instillations in artificial airways: Is it useful or necessary? *Heart & Lung,* 14:505–506.

Birdsall, C. 1986. How do you use a closed suction adapter? *American Journal of Nursing,* 86:1222–1223.

Douglas, S., & Larson, E. 1985. The effect of a positive end-expiratory pressure adapter on oxygenation during endotracheal suctioning. *Heart & Lung,* 14:396–400.

Goodnough, S. 1985. The effects of oxygen and hyperinflation on arterial oxygen tension after endotracheal suctioning. *Heart & Lung,* 14:11–17.

Kersten, L. 1989. *Comprehensive respiratory nursing.* Philadelphia: Saunders.

McGinnis, G. 1988. Central nervous system I: Head injuries. In V. Cardona, P. Hurn, P. Mason, A. Scanlon-Schilpp, & S. Veise-Berry, (eds). *Trauma Nursing: From resuscitation through rehabilitation.* Philadelphia: Saunders, 365–418.

SUGGESTED READINGS

Barnes, C., & Kirchhoff, K. 1986. Minimizing hypoxemia due to endotracheal suctioning: a review of the literature. *Heart & Lung,* 15:164–175.

Millar, S., Sampson, L., & Soukup, M. 1985. *AACN procedure manual for critical care.* Philadelphia: Saunders.

34

Tracheostomy Suctioning

Marijane Smallwood, RN, BSN

INDICATIONS

1. To remove secretions via a tracheostomy tube, which may obstruct the airways and cause hypoxia.
2. To obtain a sputum specimen for laboratory analysis.

CONTRAINDICATIONS AND CAUTIONS

1. Suctioning may exacerbate increased intracranial pressure or severe hypertension (Kersten, 1989).
2. Suctioning should not exceed 10–15 seconds per attempt to prevent hypoxia (Kersten, 1989).
3. Always use sterile technique for tracheostomy suctioning to prevent contamination and bacterial colonization of the airway.
4. Do not deflate the tracheostomy cuff prior to suctioning. The inflated cuff assists in preventing aspiration if the gag reflex is stimulated and vomiting occurs.
5. For patients receiving mechanical ventilation with positive end expiratory pressure (PEEP), a PEEP adaptor may be added to the bag-valve-mask device to prevent interruption of maximum oxygenation. The advantage of the PEEP adaptor remains controversial as compared to delivering 100% oxygen without PEEP (Douglas & Larson, 1985).
6. Instillation of 2–5 ml of sterile saline into the tracheostomy (tracheal lavage) to thin or loosen tenacious secretions is controversial. Research indicates this practice has little to no value in thinning, mobilizing, or removing dried secretions (Ackerman, 1985). Approximately 10–20% of the saline is recovered by suctioning after instillation and distribution of the saline to the lung periphery is limited.

EQUIPMENT

Portable or wall-continuous suction unit with regulator.
Suction cannister
Suction connecting tubing
Sterile suction catheter, 14–18 French for adults, with intermittent suction control vent
Sterile gloves
Sterile container
Sterile water or saline solution
Bag-valve-mask (BVM) or anesthesia bag connected to a high-flow oxygen source
Towel
(Commercially prepared, disposable suction catheter kits are also available.)

PATIENT PREPARATION

1. While tracheostomy suctioning can be accomplished in any position, Fowler's position with the head in neutral position is optimum.
2. Drape a towel over the patient's chest to protect the patient from contamination by secretions.
3. Warn the patient that suctioning may stimulate uncontrolled coughing or brief periods of breathlessness.
4. If the patient is conscious or semiconscious, restraining the patient may assist in decreasing excessive movement during the procedure.

PROCEDURAL STEPS

1. Obtain assistance if possible.
2. Assemble the suction cannister and attach to wall or portable suction unit. Attach connecting tubing to the suction cannister.
3. Set the suction gauge between 80–100 mm Hg. Full suction is no longer recommended. Pressures over 100 mm Hg increase trauma to the area and are no more effective in removing secretions (Kersten, 1989). Occlude the suction tubing to test the level of suction being delivered as measured by the suction gauge.
4. Select a suction catheter that is no larger than one-half the diameter of the endotracheal tube. A 14 French is usually appropriate for an adult.
5. Attach the suction catheter to the connecting tubing. Hold the suction catheter in your dominant hand which must remain sterile. Use your other hand to control the suction vent. This hand is considered clean.
6. If the patient has a double-walled tracheostomy, remove the inner cannula and place in saline filled basin during the procedure. The inner cannula may be cleaned with hydrogen peroxide and a pipe cleaner. Rinse it in saline before reinserting. See Figure 34.1.

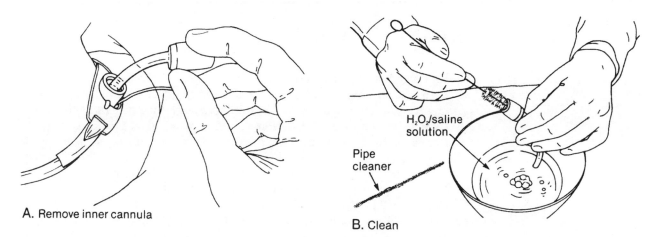

A. Remove inner cannula

H₂O₂/saline solution

Pipe cleaner

B. Clean

7. Have your assistant remove the patient from the ventilator or T-piece if necessary, and preoxygenate the patient via BVM or anesthesia bag with high-flow oxygen (100% concentration) for one minute or 6–8 hyperinflations (Goodnough, 1985).
8. Immerse the tip of the catheter into the saline and aspirate a small amount to lubricate the catheter.
9. Gently insert the catheter through the tracheostomy tube and advance it until resistance is met. Pull back 1–2 centimeters. Do not apply suction during introduction of the catheter.

Figure 34.1 A. Remove inner cannula. B. Clean inner cannula. (Kersten, 1989: 677. Reprinted by permission.)

10. Withdraw the catheter slowly applying intermittent suction and using a rotating motion. Suction should be applied for no longer than 10–15 seconds (Kersten, 1989).
11. Have your assistant hyperventilate the patient with 100% oxygen. Post-oxygenation is required for up to 2 minutes or until the oriented patient signals recovery (Goodnough, 1985).
12. Replace the clean inner cannula. See Figure 34.2.

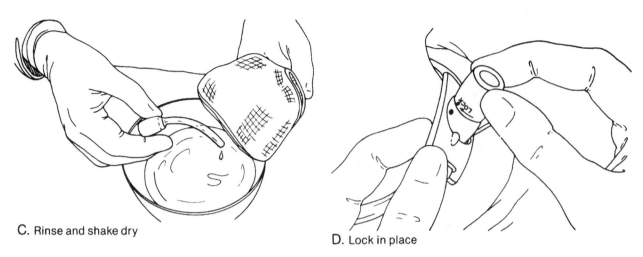

C. Rinse and shake dry

D. Lock in place

Figure 34.2   C. Rinse inner cannula, shake dry. D. Reinsert cannula and turn clockwise to lock in place. (Kersten, 1989: 677. Reprinted by permission.)

13. Reconnect the patient to the ventilator or T-piece, if necessary.
14. Rinse the catheter and connecting tubing by aspirating sterile water or saline through the tubing.
15. Steps 9–11 may be repeated if excessive secretions exist. Allow the patient at least 1 minute to recover before repeating the procedure.
16. If necessary, suction the nares or oropharynx before disposing of the catheter and gloves.

Alternative technique: Closed suction system
   See Ch. 33, Endotracheal Suctioning.

COMPLICATIONS

1. Prolonged suctioning may cause hypoxia or atelectasis.
2. Hypoxia and hypercarbia produced during endotracheal suctioning increases the cerebral blood volume and increases the intracranial pressure (ICP) (McGinnis, 1988). Caution should be used when providing respiratory care to the patient with a head injury by limiting suctioning to 10–15 seconds per attempt. Administering prophylactic medication such as intravenous lidocaine 50–100 mg two minutes prior to suctioning may prevent an increase in the ICP, but is still being studied (McGinnis, 1988).
3. The procedure may create a feeling of suffocation and lead to excessive anxiety for the patient.
4. Improper suctioning technique may cause traumatization of the tracheal mucosa.
5. The patient may develop a respiratory tract infection due to colonization of the airway with bacteria.
6. Aspiration of vomitus may occur particularly if the tracheal cuff is faulty or with an incompetent glottis in the unconscious patient.
7. Suctioning may stimulate a vagal response resulting in hypotension or bradycardia.
8. Patients receiving anticoagulants or thrombolytics may have blood-tinged secretions. Suctioning should be limited for these patients.

PATIENT TEACHING

1. Avoid moving during suctioning to help prevent tube displacement.
2. Report any respiratory distress immediately.

REFERENCES

Ackerman, M. 1985. The use of bolus normal saline instillations in artificial airways: Is it useful or necessary? *Heart & Lung,* 14:505–506.

Douglas, S., & Larson, E. 1985. The effect of a positive end-expiratory pressure adapter on oxygenation during endotracheal suctioning. *Heart & Lung,* 14:396–400.

Goodnough, S. 1985. The effects of oxygen and hyperinflation on arterial oxygen tension after endotracheal suctioning. *Heart & Lung,* 14:11–17.

Kersten, L. 1989. *Comprehensive respiratory nursing.* Philadelphia: Saunders.

McGinnis, G. 1988. Central nervous system I: Head injuries. In V. Cardona, P. Hurn, P. Mason, A. Scanlon-Schilpp, & S. Veise-Berry (eds). *Trauma nursing from resuscitation through rehabilitation.* Philadelphia: Saunders, 365–418.

SUGGESTED READINGS

Barnes, C., & Kirchhoff, K. 1986. Minimizing hypoxemia due to endotracheal suctioning: a review of the literature. *Heart & Lung,* 15:164–175.

Millar, S., Sampson, L., & Soukup, M. 1985. *AACN procedure manual for critical care.* Philadelphia: Saunders.

35

Mouth-to-Mask Ventilation

Ruth L. Schaffler, RN, MA, CEN

Mouth-to-mask ventilation is also known as face mask and face shield ventilation.

INDICATIONS

1. To ventilate a patient with ineffective or absent spontaneous respirations and protect the rescuer from direct contact with the patient's mouth or secretions.

   Note: Mouth-to-mask ventilation may provide a greater tidal volume than ventilation with a bag-valve-mask, especially if the rescuer is not highly skilled in the use of the bag-valve-mask (American Heart Association, 1987).

CONTRAINDICATIONS AND CAUTIONS

1. Clear any airway obstruction before ventilating the patient.
2. Both hands of a rescuer are needed to provide an adequate seal around the mask and to maintain an open airway. If cardiopulmonary resuscitation (CPR) is indicated, two rescuers are preferred because it is very difficult for one person to quickly open the airway and reestablish the mask's seal with each return to the head after doing chest compressions. A face shield lays over the patient's face and CPR can be administered by one rescuer.
3. The concentration of oxygen delivered in exhaled air is approximately 16%, but delivery can be enriched by adding supplemental oxygen.
4. Use of a face mask may not be appropriate for patients who have severe facial trauma, trismus, excessive oral bleeding, or vomitus.
5. Face masks are not used for patients who have a stoma following a laryngectomy.

EQUIPMENT

Pocket mask (collapsible, see Figure 35.1)
or
Face mask with or without:
    6″ flexible tubing (see Figure 35.2)
    one-way valve
    mouthpiece
or
Face shield (see Figure 35.3)
Oropharyngeal or nasopharyngeal airway (if needed)

Suction equipment (if needed)
Oxygen tubing and source (optional, but preferred)
    Note: Desirable characteristics for a face mask or shield include transparent material, capability of providing a tight-fitting seal, one-way valves, durability and ease of cleaning if reusable.

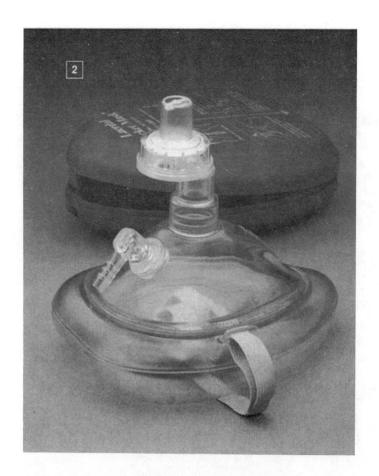

Figure 35.1 Example of a pocket mask.
(Laerdal Medical Corporation product information. Copyright 1989 by Laerdal Medical Corporation. Reprinted by permission.)

PATIENT PREPARATION

1. Place the patient in a supine position on a firm surface when possible. (**Note:** If necessary, ventilations can be delivered to persons who are seated or who are floating in water).
2. Open the airway using the head-tilt, chin-lift or jaw-thrust. See Ch. 4, Airway Positioning.
3. An oral or nasal airway may be needed. See Ch. 6, Oral Airway Insertion or Ch. 7, Nasal Airway Insertion.
4. Assess breathing status.

PROCEDURAL STEPS

Mouth-to-mask

1. Kneel at the top of the patient's head.
2. Place the mask over the patient's nose and mouth with the narrow end of the mask over the nose.
   (**Note:** A properly sized mask should extend from the bridge of the nose to the space between the lower lip and the chin and should provide an airtight seal on the patient's face.)
3. Apply pressure to the sides of the mask using the thenar aspects of the palm of both hands to seal the air cuff tightly against the patient's face.
4. Lift upward on the patient's mandible using the index, middle, and ring fingers of both hands to maintain a head tilt. See Figure 35.4.
5. Blow into the opening of the mask until you observe the patient's chest rise.

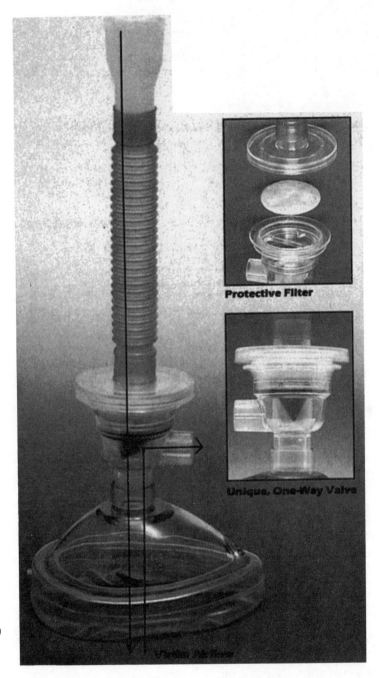

Protective Filter

Unique, One-Way Valve

Victim Airflow

Figure 35.2 Example of a face mask with one-way valve, 6″ flexible tubing, and attached mouthpiece. (Armstrong Medical Industries Inc. product information. Copyright 1989 by Armstrong Medical Industries Inc. Reprinted by permission.)

6. Remove your mouth from the opening to allow for passive exhalation by the patient.
7. Ventilate the patient 12 times per minute until the patient has spontaneous respirations or an alternative method of ventilation is established.
8. Connect oxygen tubing to the mask as soon as possible, if an inlet is present, and adjust the flow rate to a minimum of 10 L/min.

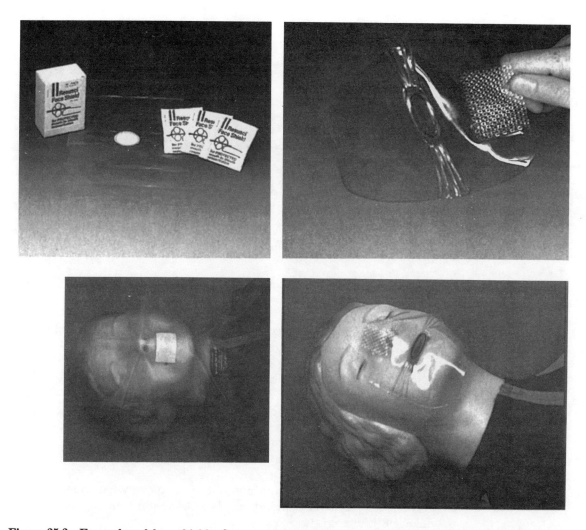

Figure 35.3 Examples of face shields. Some models provide one-way valves, others only filters. (Armstrong Medical Industries Inc. product information. Copyright 1989 by Armstrong Medical Industries Inc. Reprinted by permission.)

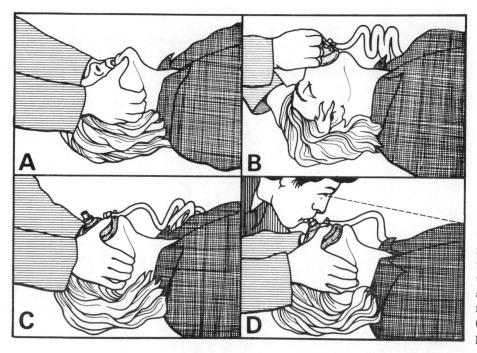

Figure 35.4 Mouth-to-mask ventilation. A. Open the airway. B. Place mask over mouth and nose. C. Maintain a tight seal against the face using both hands. D. Observe rise and fall of the chest during the respiratory cycle. (Campbell, 1988:67.) Reprinted by permission.

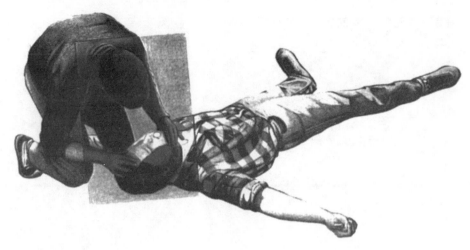

Figure 35.5   Mouth-to-shield ventilation. The filter is positioned over the mouth to form a barrier between the patient and the rescuer.
(From product information by Armstrong Medical Industries Inc. Copyright 1989 by Armstrong Medical Industries Inc. Reprinted by permission.)

Face shield

1. Place the shield on the patient's face with the filter or one-way valve over the mouth. See Figure 35.5.
2. Position yourself at the side of the patient's head.
3. Administer ventilations according to the guidelines established by the American Heart Association (1986):
   a. Pinch the patient's nose using the thumb and index finger of the hand maintaining the head-tilt.
   b. Take a deep breath and blow through the one-way valve on the face shield while watching for the patient's chest to rise (adequate tidal volume is 800–1200 ml).
   c. Allow the patient to exhale passively.
   d. Rescue breathing should be performed 12 times a minute or every 5 seconds.
   e. Reassess the need for continued ventilation every few minutes.
4. Oxygen delivery to the patient may be enhanced by putting a nasal cannula at 6 L/min on the *rescuer*.

COMPLICATIONS

1. Loss of oxygen and tidal volume due to an ineffective seal around the mask.
2. Insufficient airway patency as a result of improper chin-lift or head-tilt position.
3. Failure to recognize obstruction from excessive secretions or bleeding in the upper airway.
4. Gastric distension from excessive ventilatory pressures, which may lead to regurgitation and aspiration.
5. Improper assembly of one-way valves does not permit air to enter the patient's lungs.

REFERENCES

American Heart Association. 1986. Standards and guidelines for cardiopulmonary resuscitation and emergency cardiac care. *Journal of the American Medical Association,* 255:2841–3044.

American Heart Association. 1987. *Textbook of advanced life support.* Dallas: American Heart Association.

Campbell, J.E. (ed). 1988. *Basic trauma life support: Advanced prehospital care.* 2nd ed. Englewood Cliffs, NJ: Prentice-Hall.

SUGGESTED READINGS

American Academy of Orthopedic Surgeons 1987. *Emergency care and transportation of the sick and injured,* 4th ed. Chicago: American Academy of Orthopedic Surgeons.

Harrison, R., et al. 1982. Mouth-to-mask ventilation: A superior method of rescue breathing. *Annals of Emergency Medicine,* 11:74–75.

Nickalls, R.W.D., & Thomson, C.W. 1986. Mouth-to-mask respiration. *British Medical Journal,* 292:1350.

Simon, R.R. & Brenner, B.E. 1987. *Emergency procedures and techniques,* 2nd ed. Baltimore: Williams & Wilkins.

36

Bag-Valve-Mask Ventilation

Dawn M. Swimm, RN, CEN

Dawn M. Swimm, RN, CEN

Bag valve mask is also known as manual resucitator, Ambu bag, self-inflating bag.

INDICATIONS

To manually provide positive pressure ventilatory support in the presence of inadequate respirations or apnea.

CONTRAINDICATIONS AND CAUTIONS

1. Avoid excessive airway pressure or tidal volumes which can cause gastric distension and pneumothoraces.
2. Care should be taken to properly fit mask and provide a good seal. Frequently two people are required for adequate ventilation of a nonintubated patient: one to maintain the airway and the mask seal and the other to squeeze the bag (Jesudian, 1985).

EQUIPMENT

Oral airway (for nonintubated
    patient)
Pharyngeal suctioning equipment

Bag-valve-mask with oxygen
    reservoir
Oxygen connecting tubing

PATIENT PREPARATION

1. Open and secure the airway.
   Ch. 4: Airway Positioning
   Ch. 5: Foreign Object Removal
   Ch. 6: Oral Airway Insertion
   Ch. 7: Nasal Airway Insertion
   Ch. 8: Esophageal Obturator/Gastric Tube Airway
   Ch. 9, 10, 11, 12: Endotracheal Intubation
   Ch. 13: Cricothyroidotomy
   Ch. 14: Percutaneous Transtracheal Ventilation
   Ch. 15: Tracheostomy
2. Suction the airway of any obvious debris. See Ch. 31: Pharyngeal Suctioning.

PROCEDURAL STEPS

1. Connect oxygen tubing to oxygen flow meter and set at desired liter flow. **Note:** If utilizing an oxygen reservoir, 90–100% oxygen can be administered when using a 10–15 liter/minute flow. Without the reservoir, oxygen concentrations will drop to 40–60% (Burton, 1984).

2. Attach the oxygen tubing to the oxygen inlet on the bag-valve-mask.
3. a. For the nonintubated patient, choose the appropriate size of mask and secure to bag. See Figure 36.1.

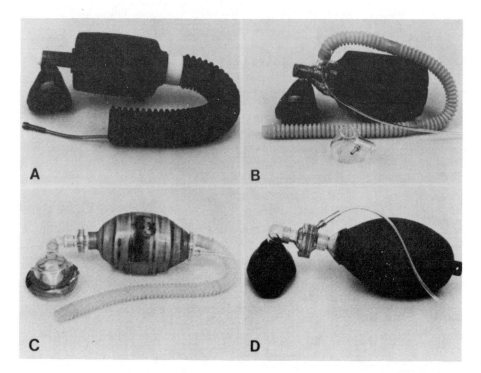

Figure 36.1 Various types of bag-valve-mask ventilators.
(Burton, 1984: 915. Reprinted by permission.)

   b. Assure equipment function by placing the mask against your hand and noting gas flow through the mask.
   c. Stand behind the patient's head. Seat the mask on the face covering the nose, mouth, and tip of the chin. The narrow end of the mask goes over the patient's nose.
   d. Hold the mask firmly with your thumb over the patient's nose and your fingers grasping the bony edge of the mandible. See Figure 36.2.
   e. Two-person technique may be used with one maintaining the airway and mask seal, while the other squeezes the bag. See Figure 36.3.
4. For the intubated patient, attach the bag to the adaptor of the endotracheal tube.

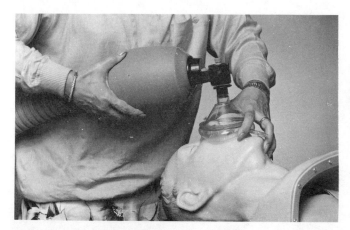

Figure 36.2 Application of a bag-valve-mask by a single rescuer.
(Jesudian et al., 1985: 122. Reprinted by permission.)

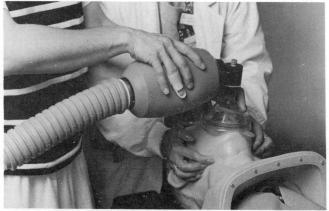

Figure 36.3 Application of a bag-valve mask by two rescuers.
(Jesudian et al., 1985: 122. Reprinted by permission.)

5. With your free hand, squeeze the bag to force air into the lungs. Squeezing the bag against your thigh or the stretcher will assist in generating an adequate tidal volume.
6. The gentle symmetrical rise and fall of the chest signals an adequate tidal volume and mask seal (American Heart Association, 1987).

COMPLICATIONS

1. Excessive tidal volumes may cause gastric distension, leading to vomiting and aspiration.
2. Excessive airway pressures can result in pneumothoraces.
3. Inadequate tidal volumes or mask seal will result in inadequate ventilation.
4. Ophthalmic damage can occur if the mask is too large and pressure is exerted on the eyes during ventilation.

REFERENCES

American Heart Association. 1987. *Textbook of advanced cardiac life support.* Dallas: American Heart Association.

Burton, G.G., & Hodgkin, J.E. 1984. *Respiratory care,* 2nd ed. Philadelphia: Lippincott.

Jesudian, M.C., Harrison, R.R., Keenan, R.L., & Maull. K.I. 1985. Bag-valve-mask ventilation: two rescuers are better than one: preliminary report. *Critical Care Medicine,* 13, 2:122–123.

SUGGESTED READINGS

American Association of Critical-Care Nurses. 1984. *Core curriculum for critical care nursing,* 3rd ed. Philadelphia: Saunders.

Cummins, R.O. 1985. Ventilation skills of emergency medical technicians: A teaching challenge for emergency medicine. *Annals of Emergency Medicine,* 15, 1187–1192.

McPherson, S.P., & Spearman, C.B. 1985. *Respiratory therapy equipment.* 3rd ed. St. Louis: Mosby.

Wade, J.F. 1982. *Comprehensive respiratory care,* 3rd ed. St. Louis: Mosby.

37

Anesthesia Bag

Dawn M. Swimm, RN, CEN

Anesthesia bag is also known as: flow inflating bag, bellows, manual resucitator, balloon bag.

INDICATIONS

1. To manually provide ventilations in the event of apnea.
2. To assist respirations in the event of ineffective respiratory pattern.
3. If desired, high concentrations of oxygen may be delivered via this system.

CONTRAINDICATIONS AND CAUTIONS

1. Overinflation may result in gastric distension or pneumothoraces.
2. Care should be taken to establish proper mask size and seal to ensure adequate ventilation in the nonintubated patient.
3. Frequently two people are needed to effectively ventilate the nonintubated patient via an anesthesia bag.

EQUIPMENT

Anesthesia bag
Oxygen flow meter
Oxygen connecting tubing
Suction equipment (as indicated)
Airway adjuncts (as indicated)

Mask (if patient is not intubated)
(**Note:** If the anesthesia bag has a pressure gauge port, you will need a pressure gauge.)

PATIENT PREPARATION

1. Secure an open airway. See
   Ch. 4: Airway Positioning:
   Ch. 5: Foreign Object Removal
   Ch. 6: Oral Airway Insertion
   Ch. 7: Nasal Airway Insertion
   Ch. 8: Esophageal Obturator/Gastric Tube Airway
   Chs. 9, 10, 11, 12: Endotracheal Intubation
   Ch. 13: Cricothyroidotomy
   Ch. 14: Percutaneous Transtracheal Ventilation
   Ch. 15: Tracheostomy
2. Suction the airway of any obvious debris. See Ch. 31: Pharyngeal Suctioning.

PROCEDURAL STEPS

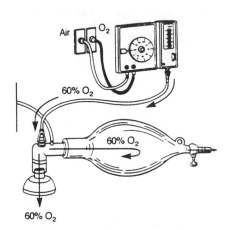

Figure 37.1 Anesthesia bag attached to oxygen blender.
(American Heart Association, 1987b: 3A, 14. Reprinted by permission.)

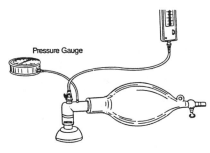

Figure 37.2 Anesthesia bag/mask system with pressure gauge attached.
(American Heart Association, 1987a: 3A, 12. Reprinted by permission.)

1. Connect oxygen tubing to oxygen flow meter and to gas inlet on the anesthesia bag. (**Note:** If less than 100% oxygen is indicated, an air/oxygen blender will be needed. See Figure 37.1)
2. Turn on oxygen flow meter to allow the bag to fill to half. Adjust flow control valve to maintain the bag at approximately half full. (**Note:** This allows for ease in compression of the bag and will usually deliver adequate tidal volumes. For the adult bag this is 10–12 liters/minute.)
3. If the patient is not intubated, choose a mask which covers the patient's nose, mouth, and tip of the chin.
4. Attach mask or endotracheal tube to the anesthesia bag.
5. Pressure gauges are optional. If there is a pressure port, attach pressure gauge to bag. (**Note:** Pressure measurement is not a primary concern with the adult patient, but the gauge must be attached for the bag to properly inflate.) See Figure 37.2.
6. Test the unit by placing the mask against your hand and squeezing the bag to feel the flow and observe reinflation of the bag.
7. If using a mask, stand behind the patient's head, seat the mask on the face covering the nose, mouth, and tip of the chin. Hold the mask firmly in place using your thumb and forefinger of one hand and allow your remaining fingers to grasp the bony edge of the mandible.
8. For the intubation patient, attach the bag to the adaptor of the endotracheal tube.
9. With your free hand, squeeze the bag, forcing air into the lungs. (**Note:** If the anesthesia bag does not have a flow control valve, you will need to occlude the distal opening of the bag as you squeeze. If you have two people available for airway management, one can maintain the airway and mask seal while the other ventilates. See Ch. 36: Bag-Valve-Mask Ventilation.)
10. Symmetrical rise and fall of the chest signals adequate tidal volume and mask seal.

COMPLICATIONS

Via bag- mask

1. Overinflation can cause gastric distension which may lead to vomiting and aspiration.
2. Inadequate pressure can result in inadequate ventilation.
3. Inadequate seal of the face mask can result in inadequate ventilation.
4. Damage to the eyes can occur if mask is too large and pressure is exerted during bag-mask ventilation.

Via bag-endotracheal tube

1. Excessive airway pressures can cause pneumothoraces.
2. Inadequate pressure can result in inadequate ventilation.
3. Overinflation of the lungs can cause gastric distension.

REFERENCES

American Heart Association. 1987a. *Textbook of neonatal resuscitation.* Dallas: American Heart Association.

American Heart Association. 1987b. *Textbook of advanced cardiac life support.* Dallas: American Heart Association.

SUGGESTED READINGS

American Association of Critical-Care Nurses. 1984. *Core Curriculum for Critical Care Nursing,* 3rd ed. Philadelphia: Saunders.

McPherson, S. P., & Spearman, C.B. 1985. *Respiratory Therapy Equipment,* 3rd ed. St. Louis: Mosby.

Wade, J.F. 1982. *Comprehensive Respiratory Care,* 3rd ed. St. Louis: Mosby.

38

Oxygen-Powered Breathing Devices

Scott S. Bourn, RN, MSN, CEN

Oxygen-powered breathing devices are also known as demand valve, Robertshaw, or Elder valve.

Oxygen-powered breathing devices are ventilators that utilize oxygen to deliver positive pressure ventilation. Most are manually triggered, although there are some units which can be programmed for specific rates and volumes, thus freeing the operator to perform other tasks. Guidelines for which rates and volumes to use with these units can be found in Ch. 39: Mechanical Ventilation.

INDICATIONS

To provide positive pressure ventilation to intubated and nonintubated patients in the presence of

1. Respiratory arrest
2. Hypoventilation of any cause
3. Hypoxemia
4. Significant acidosis
5. Inadequate chest wall function, caused by severe chest trauma, CNS dysfunction, or neuromuscular disease
6. Severe shock, ARDS, pulmonary contusion
7. Conditions requiring hypocapnia (i.e., increased intracranial pressure)

CONTRAINDICATIONS AND CAUTIONS

There are no absolute contraindications to the use of mechanical ventilation. However, a number of circumstances require care.

1. The conscious patient may resist assisted ventilation. This "bucking the ventilator" increases intracranial pressure and decreases the efficacy of ventilation. It may be necessary to sedate and/or paralyze the patient to deliver adequate ventilations.
2. Caution must be taken to avoid overinflation which may cause pulmonary barotrauma and lead to pneumothorax, tension pneumothorax, or pneumomediastinum. With a nonintubated patient, overinflation may also lead to gastric distension, vomiting, aspiration, and gastric rupture.
3. Careful maintenance of equipment is essential. Oxygen-powered ventilators have a pressure "pop-off" valve which should terminate ventilations. The typical setting for this valve is 50 cm H_2O for adults and 30 cm H_2O for infants and children (Safar, 1986). Periodic testing and maintenance is necessary to ensure that the pop-off valve is functioning correctly.
4. Special care must be exercised when using positive pressure ventilation equipment on children and infants because of the potential for barotrauma and gastric distension. Some sources (American Heart Association, 1988) do not recommend the use of these devices on children.

EQUIPMENT

Oxygen-powered ventilator   Oxygen source
Suction

PATIENT PREPARATION

1. *If possible, intubate the patient (see Ch. 9).
2. Have suction assembled and turned on at the patient's head throughout the procedure.
3. Initiate assisted ventilations via bag/valve/mask (see Ch. 36) or mouth-to-mask (see Ch. 35) unless the oxygen-powered ventilator is ready for immediate use.

*Indicates portions of the procedures usually performed by a physician

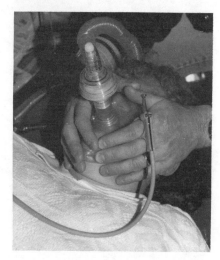

Figure 38.1   Sealing the mask to the patient's face is most effective using two hands.

PROCEDURAL STEPS

1. Attach the oxygen-powered ventilator to an oxygen source.
2. If the patient is not intubated, position the head in a neutral, slightly hyperextended position to open the airway. Utilize the jaw-lift method in cases when manipulation of the head is not desired. See Ch. 4: Airway Positioning.
3. If the patient is not intubated, seal the mask tightly to the patient's face. A two-handed seal is preferred over one hand. See Figure 38.1.
4. Attach the ventilator to the mask or endotracheal tube.
5. Initiate ventilation by triggering the ventilator. If the patient is breathing spontaneously, inspiration will trigger the ventilator.
6. Watch the chest rise. Stop insufflation of air when the chest stops rising. Overinflation leads to gastric distension and/or pulmonary barotrauma. If the patient is breathing spontaneously, patient resistance and exhalation will stop air insufflation automatically. Assess breath sounds bilaterally.
7. Continue ventilations at the desired rate and depth.
8. Consider insertion of a nasogastric tube to prevent gastric distension, especially in the nonintubated patient.
9. Assess arterial blood gases 15 to 30 minutes after initiation of ventilation. Readjust ventilatory rate and depth as indicated.

COMPLICATIONS

1. Increased intrathoracic pressure may cause
   a. decreased venous return to the heart and hypotension;
   b. increased intracranial pressure.
2. Increased airway pressure may cause
   a. barotrauma to airways which occurs in 10–20% of patients receiving mechanical ventilation (Chadwick, 1983);
   b. barotrauma may cause pneumothorax, pneumomediastinum, pneumopericardium, subcutaneous emphysema, or air embolism;
   c. gastric distension and/or rupture in nonintubated patients. Mortality from gastric rupture is 80–90% (Smith, 1980).
3. Ventilator-induced respiratory alkalosis.

REFERENCES

American Heart Association. 1988. *Textbook of Pediatric Advanced Life Support.* Dallas: American Heart Association.

Chadwick, W. 1983. Airway and ventilator management. *Emergency Medicine Clinics of North America,* 1, 241–260.

Safar, P. 1986. Cardiopulmonary cerebral resuscitation: Basic and advanced life support. In G.R. Schwartz, P. Safar, J.H. Stone, P.B. Storey, D.K. Wagner, (eds). *Principles and Practice of Emergency Medicine,* 2nd ed. Philadelphia: Saunders; 233–234.

Smith, L.B., & Gainey, M.D. 1980. Gastric rupture secondary to resuscitation with a positive pressure breathing apparatus: A report of two fatal cases. *Emergency Medical Services,* May–June, 39–41.

SUGGESTED READINGS

Peterson, G.W., & Baier, H. 1983. Incidence of pulmonary barotrauma in a medical ICU. *Critical Care Medicine,* 11, 2:67–69.

Safar, P., & Caroline, N. 1986. Respiratory care techniques and strategies. In G.R. Schwartz, P. Safar, J.H. Stone, P.B. Storey, D.K. Wagner, (eds). *Principles and Practice of Emergency Medicine,* 2nd ed. Philadelphia: Saunders; 346–405.

Shapiro, B.A., Harrison, R.A., & Trout, C.A. 1975. *Clinical Application of Respiratory Care.* Chicago: Year Book Medical Publishers.

39

Mechanical Ventilators

Scott S. Bourn, RN, MSN, CEN

Mechanical ventilators are also known as ventilator, vent, or by specific brand name (Bird, Bennett, MA-1, etc.)

INDICATIONS

To provide supplemental ventilation for a prolonged period of time in the presence of
1. Respiratory arrest
2. Hypoventilation of any cause
3. Hypoxemia
4. Significant acidosis
5. Inadequate chest wall function, caused by severe chest trauma, CNS dysfunction, or neuromuscular disease
6. Severe shock, ARDS, pulmonary contusion
7. Conditions requiring hypocapnia (i.e., increased intracranial pressure)

CONTRAINDICATIONS AND CAUTIONS

1. The conscious patient may resist mechanical ventilation. This "bucking the ventilator" increases intracranial pressure and decreases the efficacy of ventilation. In this case, it may be necessary to sedate and/or paralyze the patient to deliver adequate ventilations.
2. It is essential that the rate, tidal volume, and airway pressure be appropriate for the patient. Incorrect ventilator settings may deliver inadequate minute ventilation, cause acid/base abnormalities or create barotrauma to the airways. Guidelines for setting the ventilator follow.
3. Patients with pneumothorax should be monitored carefully to ensure that the pneumothorax does not become larger or develop into a tension pneumothorax because of increased airway pressures. In some cases, prophylactic chest tubes may be inserted to prevent the development of tension pneumothorax.

EQUIPMENT

Endotracheal tube
Bag-valve-mask with oxygen
    reservoir
Suction

Mechanical ventilator (See
    following discussion.)
Oxygen source (at least 2 outlets)

Two basic types of ventilators exist: *Pressure-cycled ventilators* terminate the inspiratory phase when a preset airway pressure is met. This is a simple, cost-effective ventilator. A disadvantage is that a patient who is fighting the ventilator will raise the airway pressure and terminate ventilation. This may cause inadequate ventilation. *Volume-cycled ventilators* terminate the inspiratory phase when a preset volume of air has been delivered.

124
Ch. 39 Mechanical Ventilators

The ventilator varies the inspiratory time until the proper volume is delivered. To prevent damage from high airway pressures, a maximum pressure limit is set; ventilation is terminated if the pressure setting is exceeded.

Ventilators also vary in the degree of respiratory assist. *Controlled mechanical ventilation,* or CMV provides total respiratory support. Both respiratory volume and rate are controlled by the ventilator. This mode requires no ventilatory effort by the patient. *Assist-control ventilation* augments the patient's own respiratory efforts, delivering a predetermined volume of air when triggered by the patient's own inspiration. In this mode, the patient controls that rate and the ventilator controls the volume. Unfortunately, if the patient's rate slows, the minute ventilation may become inadequate. *Intermittent mandatory ventilation,* or IMV, is a combination of controlled mandatory and assist-control ventilation. IMV allows the patient to breathe spontaneously, and supplements the patient's ventilations with a preset number of "ventilator breaths." This mechanism assures adequate ventilation while allowing the patient to maintain independent respiration as much as possible.

While IMV is optimal for long-term ventilatory assist, most cases in the emergency department are managed with controlled mechanical ventilation.

PATIENT PREPARATION

*Indicates portions of the procedures usually performed by a physician.

1. *Intubate the patient. (See Ch. 9: General Principles of Intubation.)
2. Initiate assisted ventilation using a bag-valve-mask and supplemental oxygen.
3. Have suction assembled and turned on at the patient's head throughout the procedure.

Figure 39.1 Control panel of a common ventilator, the Bennett MA-1. (A) on-off switch, (B) sensitivity setting for assisted ventilation, (C) peak flow in liters per minute, (D) rate, (E) volume control, (F) normal pressure limit, (G) sigh pressure limit, (H) sigh volume limit, (I) sigh interval, (J) control button for manual breaths or sighs, (K) oxygen percentage, (L) expiratory resistance control, (M) nebulizer for medication administration, (N) pressure gauge, (O) alarm light for patient initiated breaths, (P) alarm light for high pressure, (Q) ratio alarm, activated when I:E ratio is less than 1:1, (R) sigh light, (S) oxygen light: lights green if FiO₂ greater than 21% has been selected, lights red if oxygen has not been connected to the ventilator and a value greater than 21% has been selected on the oxygen control knob (K).
(Burton & Hodgkin, 1984: 597. Reprinted by permission.)

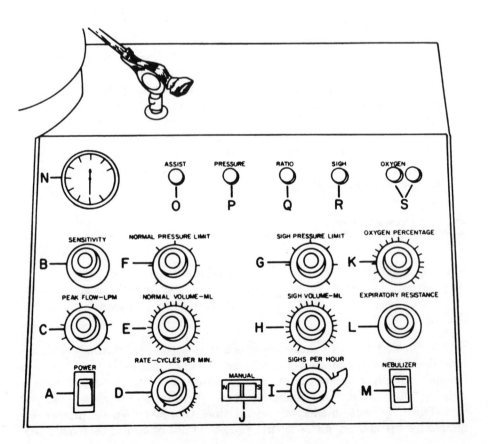

1. Plug the ventilator in and attach to the oxygen source. Turn the unit on. See Figure 39.1.
2. Set the inspired oxygen concentration (FiO_2). In most cases, 100% should be the initial setting. It is safest to begin at 100%, and decrease it as indicated by PaO_2 or oxygen saturation (Otto, 1986).
3. Set the tidal volume. A good guideline is 12–15 ml/kg (Otto, 1986).
4. Set the respiratory rate. For most patients, 8–12 breaths per minute (at 12–15 ml/kg) will produce adequate ventilation (Otto, 1986).
5. Set the ventilator mode (control, assist-control, or IMV).
6. Adjust positive end expiratory pressure (PEEP) if desired. If PEEP is used, it is best to start with 5 cm H_2O or less.
7. Attach the patient to the ventilator after settings have been established.
8. Set the maximum airway pressure. This is usually 6–10 cm H_2O above the peak airway pressures as read on the pressure monitor of the ventilator.
9. Assess arterial blood gases 15 to 30 minutes after initiation of ventilation. Readjust ventilator settings as indicated.
10. Further discussion of ventilator settings is beyond the scope of this text. Please refer to Dettenmeier & Johnson (1991) for more information.

COMPLICATIONS

1. Increased intrathoracic pressure may cause
   a. decreased venous return to the heart and hypotension;
   b. increased intracranial pressure.
2. Increased airway pressure may cause
   a. barotrauma to airways (occurs in 10–20% of patients receiving mechanical ventilation (Chadwick, 1983);
   b. barotrauma may cause pneumothorax, pneumomediastinum, pneumopericardium, subcutaneous emphysema, or air embolism.
3. Ventilator-induced respiratory alkalosis.

REFERENCES

Burton, G.G., & Hodgkin, J.E. 1984. *Respiratory care: A guide to clinical practice*, 2nd ed. Philadelphia: Lippincott.

Chadwick, W. 1983. Airway and ventilator management. *Emergency Medicine Clinics of North America*, 1, 2:241–260.

Dettenmeier, P., & Johnson, T. 1991. The art and science of mechanical ventilator adjustments. *Critical Care Nursing Clinics of North America*, 3:575–583.

Otto, C.W. 1986. Ventilatory management in the critically ill. *Emergency Medicine Clinics of North America*, 4, 4:635–654.

SUGGESTED READINGS

Peterson, G.W., & Baier, H. 1983. Incidence of pulmonary barotrauma in a medical ICU. *Critical Care Medicine*, 11, 2:67–69.

Safar, P., & Caroline, N. 1986. Respiratory care techniques and strategies. In G.R. Schwartz, P. Safar, J.H. Stone, P.B. Storey, D.K. Wagner, (eds). *Principles and Practice of Emergency Medicine*, 2nd ed. Philadelphia: Saunders; Chapter 20.

Shapiro, B.A., Harrison, R.A., & Trout, C.A. 1975. *Clinical Application of Respiratory Care*. Chicago: Year Book Medical Publishers.

40

Nebulizer Therapy

Scott S. Bourn, RN, MSN, CEN

Nebulizer therapy is also known as neb, updraft, SVN (small volume nebulizer), and acorn neb

INDICATIONS

To deliver medications to the respiratory tree for the treatment of
1. acute bronchospasm
2. excessive mucous buildup
3. croup or epiglottitis.

Advantages of nebulized medications are that the medication is delivered directly to the site of action (the lungs), therefore, a lower dose may be used; the reduced dose decreases systemic absorption and side effects; delivery of nebulized medications to the lungs is very rapid, so the onset of action is faster than with subcutaneous or oral routes; the delivery of nebulized medications humidifies inspired air which helps loosen bronchial secretions.

CONTRAINDICATIONS AND CAUTIONS

1. With an unconscious or confused patient, who cannot cooperate with the procedure, a mask may be used, but it is significantly less effective.
2. Absent or severely diminished breath sounds, unless the nebulized medication is to be delivered through an endotracheal tube utilizing positive pressure. A patient with decreased air exchange may not be able to adequately move the medication into the respiratory tract.
3. Use with caution in patients with cardiac irritability. Inhaled catecholamines increase cardiac rate and may precipitate dysrhythmias.
4. Nebulized medications are no longer administered via Intermittent Positive Pressure Breathing (IPPB), because it is irritating and increases bronchospasm. The only patients who should receive nebulized medications via positive pressure are those whose underlying condition mandates assisted ventilation.

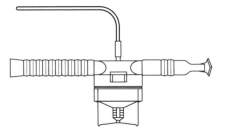

Figure 40.1 The assembled nebulizer. The corrugated tubing in this illustration acts as a reservoir. The corrugated tubing may also be placed between the nebulizer and the mouthpiece to allow large droplets to "rain out."

EQUIPMENT

Nebulizer and connecting tubing
    See Figure 40.1.
Short, corrugated tubing
Oxygen cannula

Compressed gas source (oxygen or air)
Medication to be administered See Table 40.1.

PATIENT PREPARATION

1. Place the patient in a position that allows for deep ventilation and maximal diaphragmatic movement. Sitting up is ideal. (See Ch. 16: Positioning the Dyspneic Patient.)
2. Assess the breath sounds, pulse rate, respiratory status, and spirometry

Table 40.1

127

Ch. 40 Nebulizer Therapy

Type of Medication	Name	Typical Adult Dose
Bronchodilator	Isoetharine (Bronkosol)	0.25–1.0 mg
	Metaproterenol (Alupent)	0.25 ml
	Albuterol (Ventolin, Proventil)	0.25 ml
	Terbutaline (Brethine)	0.25 mg
	Atropine	0.025–0.075 mg/kg
	Isoproterenol (Isuprel)	0.30 ml
Decongestants	Racemic Epinephrine (Vaponephrine)	10–15 drops
Mucolytics (break up mucous)	N-acetylcysteine (Mucomyst)	1–2 ml of 20% solution
Steroids	Beclomethasone (Vanceril)	84 mcg

Dosages are from "Respiratory Pharmacology" by M.R. Anderson, 1989, *Emergency Care Quarterly*, 5(1), 23–36.

or peak flow (See Ch. 20: Peak Expiratory Flow Measurement) prior to administration of the medication.

3. Teach the patient the correct procedure:
   a. Complete exhalation;
   b. Slow inhalation through the mouth, inhaling the medication through the mouthpiece;
   c. Brief pause after inspiration is complete;
   d. Slow exhalation;
   e. Several resting breaths after inhalation of the medication to prevent tingling and carpopedal spasm caused by repeated deep ventilations.

PROCEDURAL STEPS

1. Place the patient on supplemental oxygen, with the flow rate determined by patient condition, pulse oximetry, or arterial blood gases. Inhalation of catecholamines alters pulmonary ventilation/perfusion ratios and will *exacerbate hypoxemia* for a short period (Anderson, 1989).
2. Place the correct dose of the medication into the nebulizer.
3. Add the ordered amount of sterile normal saline to the nebulizer, 2.5 ml is a common amount of diluent.
4. Attach the nebulizer to a source of compressed gas. Oxygen is preferred because of the hypoxemia discussed in Step 1.
5. Attach the corrugated tubing to the nebulizer. Some authorities place the tubing between the nebulizer and the mouthpiece, to allow large droplets to "rain out" in the tubing; this decreases deposition of these droplets on the tongue and may reduce side effects. Other sources place the tubing on the opposite side of the nebulizer to serve as a reservoir.
6. Increase the flow rate of the compressed gas until the nebulized medication lightly mists out of the nebulizer mouthpiece. If too forceful a stream is created, much of the medication will be wasted.
7. Hold the nebulizer and control administration of the medication until the patient has demonstrated good technique.
8. When administering nebulized medication to children too young to follow the procedure, replace the mouthpiece with a mask and seal the mask over the nose and mouth.
9. Continue the treatment until the medication is gone or unacceptable side effects, such as severe tachycardia, occur.
10. Reassess and document breath sounds, pulse rate, respiratory status, and pulmonary function tests after the treatment is completed.

COMPLICATIONS

1. Tremor
2. Nausea
3. Headache
4. Tachycardia
5. Circumoral paresthesia or carpopedal spasm secondary to hyperventilation

(Note: The first four complications are usually medication-related.)

PATIENT TEACHING

The patient should be reminded of the importance of proper technique prior to discharge from the emergency department. Additional instruction with return demonstration may be appropriate. The patient should also be instructed to return to the emergency department if respiratory distress recurs.

REFERENCES

Anderson, M.R. 1989. The pharmacology of intervention for respiratory emergencies. *Emergency Care Quarterly, 5,* 1:23–26.

SUGGESTED READINGS

Hawkins, J., Hakala, K., Heller, M.B., Kaplan, R.M., Schneider, S., & Stewart, R.D. 1986. Metered-dose aerosolized bronchodilators in prehospital care: A feasibility study. *The Journal of Emergency Medicine,* 4:273–277.

Shapiro, B.A., Harrison, R.A., & Trout, C.A. 1975. *Clinical Application of Respiratory Care.* Chicago, Year Book Medical Publishers.

41

Needle Thoracostomy

Lori D. Taylor, RN, BSN, CEN

INDICATIONS

To provide immediate decompression of a tension pneumothorax with respiratory and/or cardiovascular compromise. Tension pneumothorax is suspected in the presence of the following: (a) shortness of breath, (b) tracheal deviation, (c) jugular venous distention, (d) hypotension, (e) hyperresonance, and (f) signs of hypoxemia. Performance of a needle thoracostomy converts a tension pneumothorax to a simple pneumothorax.

CONTRAINDICATIONS AND CAUTIONS

1. If this procedure is used in the absence of a tension pneumothorax, there is a 10% to 20% chance of producing a pneumothorax and/or causing damage to the lung (American College of Surgeons, 1989).
2. Needle thoracostomy is frequently done as an interim procedure until tube thoracostomy (chest tube placement) can be carried out. Anticipate this as a follow-up procedure.
3. Initial presentation of a traumatic ruptured diaphragm with evisceration of abdominal contents into a hemithorax can mimic a tension pneumothorax. Placement of a needle in this instance can result in bacterial contamination of the pleural cavity. Suspect a ruptured diaphragm with a history of the application of sudden, compressive forces to the abdomen.
4. Due to the emergent nature of a tension pneumothorax, consideration should be given to the training of nursing and ancillary personnel in this procedure in areas lacking immediate accessibility to a physician. The patient may arrest quickly without immediate intervention.

EQUIPMENT

Razor (optional)
Antiseptic solution
Local anesthetic
5–10-ml syringe, 18-G needle,
    25–27-G needle for
    anesthesia

14–18-G (3–6-cm long)
    over-the-needle catheter
35-ml syringe for aspiration
Adhesive tape

PATIENT PREPARATION

1. Chest x-rays may be deferred initially, depending on the patient's presentation. Consider doing films prior to needle thoracostomy if a ruptured diaphragm is suspected.

2. If time allows, shave and cleanse the chest with antiseptic solution on the side of the tension pneumothorax (the trachea deviates away from the side of pathology). The usual site for needle insertion is the second intercostal space, midclavicular line. See Figure 41.1.

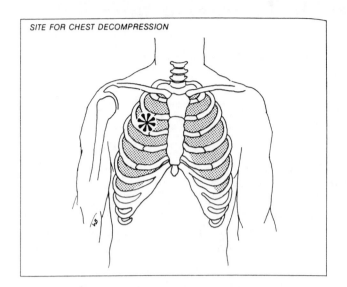

SITE FOR CHEST DECOMPRESSION

Figure 41.1 The usual site for needle thoracostomy.
(Caroline, 1983: 226. Reprinted by permission.)

3. Place the patient in an upright position if cervical spine pathology has been ruled out and patient's condition permits (American College of Surgeons, 1989).

PROCEDURAL STEPS

1. *Infiltrate the area with local anesthetic if the patient is conscious and the patient's condition permits.
2. *Attach the over-the-needle catheter to the 35-ml syringe.
3. *Insert the needle through the skin and direct it toward the top of the second rib. The needle is then directed over the top of the rib (intercostal nerves and arteries run inferior to the rib) and into the pleural space.
4. *Aspiration of air confirms the diagnosis of tension pneumothorax. Further air can be removed manually by gentle aspiration. If no air is aspirated, or if signs and symptoms do not improve, consider the presence of pericardial tamponade, myocardial contusion, or air embolism (Dalbec & Krome, 1986).
5. *Remove the needle and syringe, leaving the catheter in place. The catheter may be secured with tape and left open to air. (A simple pneumothorax now exists.)
6. Assemble equipment and prepare for subsequent chest tube placement. If there will be a delay until a chest tube can be placed (for example, transport nurses and medics operating outside of the hospital setting), a flutter valve can be placed over the hub of the catheter. A simple form of flutter valve utilizes either a 1/4-inch sterile rubber drain or a finger of a sterile glove with the tip removed. The flutter valve can then be secured to the hub of the catheter with tape or suture. See Figure 41.2.

   Another option is to connect an intravenous extension tubing to the catheter and place the free end of the tubing in a container of sterile water. Thus, establishing water-seal chest drainage.
7. After chest tube placement is carried out, the catheter is removed. A thin layer of antibiotic ointment and a sterile dressing is then applied over the puncture site.
8. Obtain chest x-rays post-procedure.

*Indicates portions of the procedure usually performed by a physician.

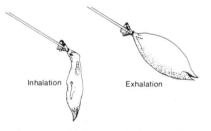

Inhalation   Exhalation

Figure 41.2 Flutter valve made from the finger of a rubber glove.
(Caroline, 1983: 226. Reprinted by permission.)

COMPLICATIONS

1. Infection of puncture site (late)
2. Creation of a pneumothorax if a tension pneumothorax did not exist prior to procedure
3. Hematoma at insertion site
4. Perforation of abdominal viscera if ruptured diaphragm and herniation of abdominal contents is present
5. Pleural infection, empyema (American College of Surgeons, 1989)
6. Use of a steel needle or teflon catheter may lacerate the lung and produce a significant pulmonary injury or hemothorax (American Heart Association, 1987).
7. Placement of the needle too medial (toward the sternum) may result in laceration of the internal mammary artery with significant blood loss and resultant hemothorax.

REFERENCES

American College of Surgeons, Committee on Trauma. 1988. *Advanced trauma life support course: Student manual.* Chicago: American College of Surgeons.

American Heart Association. 1987. *Textbook of advanced cardiac life support.* Dallas: American Heart Association.

Dalbec, D.L., & Krome, R.L. 1986. *Emergency Medical Clinics of North America,* 4:441–457.

SUGGESTED READINGS

Caroline, N.L 1983. *Emergency care in the streets,* 2nd ed. Boston: Little, Brown.

Strange, J.M. 1987. *Shock Trauma Care Plans.* Springhouse, PA: Springhouse Corporation.

Chest Tube Insertion

Lori D. Taylor, RN, BSN, CEN

INDICATIONS

1. To remove air and/or blood from the pleural cavity in the presence of pneumothorax (free air in pleural space), hemothorax (free blood in pleural space), or hemopneumothorax (combination of air and blood).
2. To remove fluid from the pleural cavity in the presence of a large pleural effusion, empyema, or chylothorax. Iatrogenic pleural collections are most commonly seen following central venous access procedures and may require chest tube placement.
3. To provide prophylactic chest drainage in patients with severe blunt chest trauma (flail chest/pulmonary contusions) who will require positive-pressure ventilatory support. Prophylactic chest tubes are also inserted in patients with penetrating thoracic injuries, even without evidence of pneumothorax (Yeston, 1989).

CONTRAINDICATIONS AND CAUTIONS

1. A patient's hemodynamic status may deteriorate rapidly following the evacuation of a massive hemothorax (over 1500–2000 cc). Initiate fluid resuscitation prior to chest decompression and anticipate the need for high volume resuscitation. Autotransfusion may be indicated if available. A large left hemothorax may signal an aortic or great vessel injury.
2. The use of trocar chest tubes is controversial, as trocar use has been associated with damage to thoracic structures.
3. The only absolute contraindication to chest tube placement is the need for open thoracotomy (Dalbec, 1986).
4. A patient with a previous thoracotomy may have scar tissue and adhesions, making chest tube placement difficult.
5. Consideration should be given to decompression of pneumothoraces prior to air transport, as the size of the pneumothorax may increase with increased altitude.

EQUIPMENT

Razor (optional)
Antiseptic solution
Local anesthetic
#10 scalpel
5-ml syringe, 18-G needle, 22–25-G needle for anesthesia
Large curved hemostat
Suture scissors

Needle holder
Sterile towels
Chest tube of appropriate size (Larger sizes, 36–40, are recommended for use for blood or other viscous fluid and small sizes, 18–22, are indicated for air only.)

Selection must also include choosing a tube with or without a trocar.

Large silk suture (0-0 to 2-0)

3-inch adhesive tape

Antibiotic ointment and/or occlusive dressing (petroleum jelly impregnated gauze)

Gauze dressings

Closed chest drainage device

Autotransfusion equipment if indicated/available

Suction connecting tubing (if required by drainage system)

(Note: Prepackaged kits containing much of this equipment are also available.)

PATIENT PREPARATION

1. Obtain x-rays unless the patient's condition mandates immediate chest tube placement.
2. If the time allows, shave and cleanse the chest with antiseptic solution on the side of the injury. The usual site for chest tube placement is the 4th or 5th intercostal space in the anterior or mid-axillary line. See Figure 42.1.

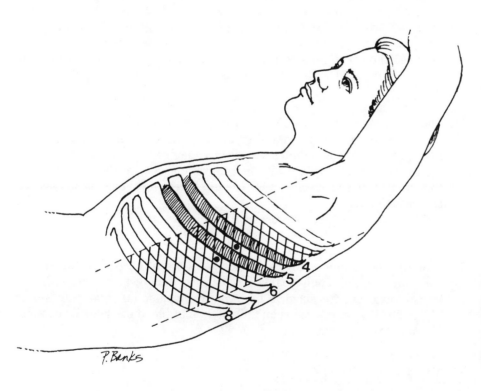

Figure 42.1 Acceptable and preferred locations for chest tube placement.
(Dalbec & Krome, 1986: 449. Reprinted by permission.)

Alternatively, the level of the nipple line can be used as a marker, especially in the unstable patient requiring immediate placement of the tube. Placement lower than this runs the risk if inserting the tube through the diaphragm, possibly into the liver or spleen (Trunkey, 1986).

3. Place the patient in a supine position with the arm on the involved side up over the head. If the patient's injuries permit, elevate the trunk to a 45° angle (Dalbec, 1986).
4. Set up the chest drainage device. See Ch. 43 through 53: Chest Drainage Devices.
5. Set up autotransfusion equipment if indicated. See Ch. 77 through 80: Autotransfusion.

PROCEDURAL STEPS

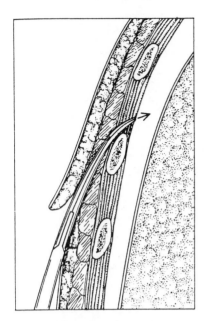

Figure 42.2   The pleural space is then entered using a Kelly clamp. (Civetta et al., 1989: 249. Reprinted by permission.)

*Indicates portions of the procedure usually performed by a physician.

1. *Drape the chest with sterile towels.
2. *Infiltrate the area with local anesthetic if the patient is conscious and if the patient's condition permits.
3. *Using the chest tube, measure the distance from the insertion site to the apex of the lung and note distance on the tube.
4. *Make a 2–3-cm incision through the chest wall, parallel to the ribs. The incision is made one interspace below the desired interspace. This creates a tunnel which allows later removal of the tube without an air leak (Dalbec, 1986).
5. *Bluntly dissect over the superior surface of the rib with the curved hemostat (nerves and arteries run inferior to the ribs). Enter the pleural cavity with the hemostat. The patient will experience pain as the pleural cavity is entered. See Figure 42.2
6. *Widen the pleural opening and skin incision by pulling the opened hemostat back out of the chest wall.
7. *With a gloved finger, palpate through the incision made to verify entry into the pleural space and to check for adhesions of the pleura and for intrathoracic or intrabdominal organs. See Figure 42.3.
8. *Direct the chest tube (with or without trocar) upward through the incision. When using a tube without a trocar, use the hemostat to introduce the tube. Advance the tube to the premeasured distance. The immediate return of blood and/or air confirms appropriate placement.
9. Connect the chest tube to the chest drainage device. This connection should be secured with adhesive tape to prevent accidental disconnection.
10. *Suture the chest tube in place with silk suture.
11. Place a thick layer of antibiotic ointment or an occlusive dressing (such as petroleum jelly impregnated gauze) around the incision site.
12. Place gauze dressings under the chest tube near the insertion site and then cover the site with additional dressings. Secure the dressing and tube in place with adhesive tape. The final dressing should entirely cover the insertion site.
13. *Obtain x-rays to confirm correct tube placement (the last hole on tube should be inside the pleural space) and to assess the status of the pneumothorax or hemothorax.
14. Monitor the drainage device for the presence of large, continuous air leaks (may signal esophageal or large airway damage) or excessive blood loss. Indications for surgical intervention include (a) 1000–1500 ml of blood initially, (b) greater than 200–300 ml of blood per hour, or (c) massive air leaks (Trunkey, 1986).

COMPLICATIONS

1. A malpositioned, nonfunctioning tube (last hole in tube outside of the pleural space with air leak or tube malpositioned in subcutaneous space).
2. Bleeding from the skin incision, intercostal arteries/veins, or from a pulmonary artery/vein (risk increased if chest tube with trocar used).
3. Organ injury (diaphragm, liver, spleen, stomach, or colon).
4. Occlusion or kinking of tube (which may result in the formation of a tension pneumothorax).
5. Pain with re-expansion of the lung.
6. Local hematoma.
7. Local cellulitis (late).

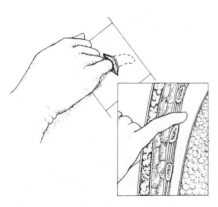

Figure 42.3   A gloved finger is placed into the pleural space confirming thoracic penetration. (Civetta et al., 1989: 249. Reprinted by permission.)

8. Atelectasis/pneumonia due to splinting by patient.
9. Reoccurrence of pathology after removal of the tube.

REFERENCES

American College of Surgeons, Committee on Trauma. 1988. *Advanced trauma life support course: Student manual.* Chicago: American College of Surgeons.

Dalbec, D., & Krome, R. 1986. Thoracostomy. *Emergency Medical Clinics of North America,* 4:441–457.

Trunkey, D., & Lewis, F. 1986. *Current therapy of trauma-2.* Philadelphia: B.C. Decker.

Yeston, N., & Niehoff, J. 1989. Important procedures in the intensive care unit. In R. Civetta, R. Taylor, & R. Kirby (eds). *Critical care,* Philadelphia: Lippincott; 243–271.

SUGGESTED READINGS

Roberts, R., Lange, D., Robin, A., & Barrett, J. 1987. Chest trauma: Emergency diagnosis and management of airway problems and intrathoracic injuries. *Topics in Emergency Medicine,* 9, 3:53–70.

Simon, R. R., & Brenner, R. E. 1987. *Emergency procedures and techniques,* 2nd ed. Baltimore: Williams & Wilkins.

Strange, J. M. 1987. *Shock trauma care plans.* Springhouse, PA: Springhouse.

Williams, S. M. 1990. *Decision making in critical care nursing.* Philadelphia: B. C. Decker.

43

Management of Chest Drainage Systems

Manjula D. Gray, RN, BSN, MA, CCRN

GENERAL PRINCIPLES

1. Do not clamp the tube unless absolutely necessary (to change the water-seal bottle or to check for air leaks), because a tension pneumothorax may develop.
2. Do not raise the bottle above the patient's chest level, as it can cause fluid to reenter the chest and increase the probability of infection (applies to water-seal systems only).
3. Do not allow tubing to coil below the cap of the bottle or lie on the floor because dependent fluid filled loops require increased intrathoracic pressure to continue emptying of the pleural space (Roberts, 1985).
4. The fluid level in the water-seal tube should rise with inspiration and fall with expiration. If the fluctuations are not present, the lung is either fully reexpanded or there is an obstruction. Check the tubing for kinks or occlusion. (The most common cause is the patient lying on the tubing.)
5. The water in the water-seal bottle or chamber should bubble during expiration. If it bubbles constantly, check for an air leak.
   a. Clamp the chest tube near the insertion site. If the bubbling stops, the leak is either at the insertion site or from the patient's lung.
   b. Reinforce the occlusive dressing over the chest tube insertion site. If the bubbling continues, notify the physician, because the air leak is from the patient's lung. This should be brought to the physician's attention immediately if it is a new finding.
   c. If the bubbling continues after clamping at the insertion site, then the air leak is either in the tubing or the equipment. Clamp the tube at short intervals for a few seconds to find the leak. The bubbling will subside if the leak is in the tubing. If not, check the equipment for a crack in the unit or a loose cap.
6. If the tubing becomes disconnected from the patient, or a bottle breaks, place the end of the drainage tubing (approximately 2.5 cm) in a container of sterile water until another chest drainage device can be assembled.
7. If the chest tube is dislodged or the patient pulls it out, have the patient cough or exhale forcibly and apply an occlusive dressing to the area. Notify the physician immediately. Monitor the patient closely for development of a tension pneumothorax until another chest tube can be inserted (Mims, 1985).
8. Milking or stripping chest tubes can cause more than 400 cm water of negative pressure within the pleural space (Erickson, 1989). This negative pressure may damage lung tissue and thus, stripping chest tubes should not routinely be performed. Stripping is necessary when a clot is suspected of obstructing the tube as is the case when the flow of sanguinous drainage suddenly slows or stops.

REFERENCES

Erickson, R.S. 1989. Mastering the ins and outs of chest drainage: Part 2. *Nursing,* 19, 6:46–49.

Mims, B.C. 1985. You can manage chest tubes confidently. *RN,* 48, 1:39–44.

Roberts, R.R., & Hedges, J.R. 1985. *Clinical Procedures in Emergency Medicine.* Philadelphia: Saunders.

44

One-Way Valve

Sharon Gavin Fought, PHD, RN
Jean Proehl, RN, MN, CEN, CCRN

One-way valve is also known as Heimlich valve, flap valve.

INDICATIONS

To allow air and fluid to drain from the pleural cavity while preventing air reentry into the pleural space. A flap valve allows active ambulation and/or discharge from the hospital of patients with chronic pneumothorax or pleural effusion because no other chest drainage device is required. The valve is also useful during interhospital transport.

CONTRAINDICATIONS AND CAUTIONS

It may be necessary to replace the valve with a regular chest drainage device, especially if large amounts of fluid drain from the chest tube.

EQUIPMENT

One-way valve
Adhesive tape
Padded hemostat
Urinary catheter drainage collection
     bag, or

Sterile glove (if necessary for fluid
     collection)

PATIENT PREPARATION

*Indicates those portions of the procedure usually performed by a physician.

1. *Insert a chest tube. See Ch. 42: Chest Tube Insertion.
2. Instruct the patient to lie quietly during the procedure and report any pain or shortness of breath.
3. Whenever possible, have the patient sit upright at a 45–90-degree angle.
4. Assess and document breath sounds and respiratory status.

PROCEDURAL STEPS

1. Untape the connection between the chest tube and the tubing from the chest drainage device.
2. If no collecting device is attached to the valve, securely tape a sterile glove to the distal end of the flap valve. Place the glove and tape so as not to disrupt the integrity of the flap valve. A urinary catheter collecting bag can be used if drainage of large volumes of fluid is anticipated (Finke, 1986).

3. Clamp the chest tube securely with the padded hemostat. The tube should be clamped only briefly and not until you are ready to proceed to the next step.
4. Connect the one-way valve to the chest tube. The "collapsed end" of the valve should be placed distally to allow fluid/air to drain out of the pleural space.
5. Remove the clamp from the chest tube. Ask the patient to cough or to exhale slowly and forcefully as the clamp is removed.
6. Tape the connections securely and anchor the chest tube and valve to the patient's chest. See Figure 44.1.
7. *Obtain a chest x-ray to determine if air has reentered the pleural cavity.
8. Assess and document breath sounds and respiratory status.

COMPLICATIONS

1. Infection related to break in sterile technique.
2. Pneumothorax or tension pneumothorax from air reentering the pleural cavity.
3. Occlusion of tube may result in tension pneumothorax.
4. If the valve becomes disconnected, immediately submerge the end of the chest tube in a glass of water or reconnect the valve and notify the physician.
5. If the chest tube is accidently dislodged from its insertion site, apply an occlusive 3-sided dressing to the site as the patient coughs or exhales forcefully. Notify the physician immediately.

PATIENT TEACHING

1. Report any chest pain, shortness of breath, or system disconnections immediately.
2. Do not attempt to reposition the chest tube or valve.

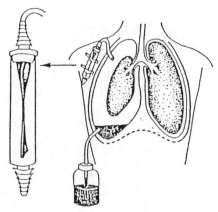

Figure 44.1 The one-way flap or Heimlich valve at the right upper chest can be used alone to manage a pneumothorax during transport. The flap valve can also be used to manage the pneumothorax while concurrently a lower chest tube, for example, is used to treat an existing hemothorax with closed, underwater drainage.
(American College of Surgeons, Committee on Trauma, 1982: 124. Reprinted by permission.)

REFERENCES

American College of Surgeons, Committee on Trauma. 1982. *Early Care of the Injured Patient*, 3rd ed. Philadelphia: Saunders.
Finke, M., & Lanros, N.E. 1986. *Emergency Nursing*. Rockville, MD: Aspen Publishers.

SUGGESTED READINGS

Luce, J.M., Tyler, M.L., & Pierson, J.J. 1984. *Intensive Respiratory Care*. Philadelphia: Saunders.
Persons, C.B. 1987. *Critical Care Procedures and Protocols*. Philadelphia: Lippincott.
Swyer, P.R., & Perlman, M. 1987. Respiratory disturbances in the newborn other than the respiratory distress syndrome. In W.C. Shoemaker, S. Ayers, A. Genvik, P.R. Holbrook, W.L. Thompson, (eds). *Textbook of Critical Care Medicine*, 2nd ed. Philadelphia: Saunders.

45

Chest Drainage Devices: One-Bottle System – Gravity Drainage

Manjula D. Gray, RN, BSN, MA, CCRN

Note: The information in this chapter should be used in conjunction with the information in Ch. 43: Management of Chest Drainage Systems.

INDICATIONS

To remove air and/or fluid from the pleural cavity in conjunction with a chest tube.

CONTRAINDICATIONS AND CAUTIONS

1. The one-bottle system can be used for removing fluid, however, a two- or three-bottle system is preferred, because it reduces the need for frequent readjustment of the water-seal tube so that it is appropriately submerged (the same bottle is used for both water seal and collection chamber).
2. The bottle system is rarely used, because most facilities now use the prefabricated, disposable chest drainage systems. The prefabricated systems have the flexibility of being used either as gravity or suction drainage systems, they are easier to set up and maintain, and they are not as fragile as glass bottles.

EQUIPMENT

*Indicates portions of the procedure usually performed by a physician.

Sterile water-seal/collection bottle
    See Figure 45.1.
Holder for bottle
3–4 ft of sterile tubing
Tubing connectors, 1/4-inch internal
    diameter

Sterile water or saline
Tape
Padded hemostat

PATIENT PREPARATION

*Insert a chest tube. See Ch. 42: Chest Tube Insertion.

PROCEDURAL STEPS

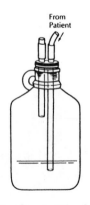

From Patient

Figure 45.1   One-bottle chest drainage system.
(King & Wieck, 1981: 775. Reprinted by permission.)

140

1. Add sterile water to the bottle until the end of the water-seal tube that will be connected to the tubing from the patient is submerged in 1–2 cm of water. This provides the water seal necessary to prevent back flow. The short, stiff tube is the vent tube. See Figure 45.1.
2. Connect the chest tube to the drainage tubing with a connector.

3. Connect the drainage tubing to the water-seal tube.
4. Tape all tube connections securely with adhesive tape (Brunner, 1978).

COMPLICATIONS

1. Tension pneumothorax secondary to obstruction in the system.
2. Open pneumothorax secondary to tubing disconnection, chest tube dislodgement, bottle breakage, or loss of water seal if the water-seal tube is not kept submerged.

PATIENT TEACHING

1. Instruct the patient in deep breathing and coughing.
2. Ask for assistance to get out of bed.
3. Report any chest pain, shortness of breath, or tubing disconnections immediately.
4. Do not lie on the tubing or allow it to kink. The bottle must be kept upright at all times.

REFERENCES

Brunner, L.S., & Suddarth, D.S. 1978. *Lippincott manual of nursing practices,* 2nd ed. Philadelphia: Lippincott.
King, E.M., Weick, L., & Dryer, M. 1981. *Illustrated manual of nursing techniques,* 2nd ed. Philadelphia: Lippincott.

SUGGESTED READING

Mims, B.C. 1985. You can manage chest tubes confidently. RN, 48, 1:39–44.

46

Chest Drainage Devices: Two-Bottle System – Gravity Drainage

Manjula D. Gray, RN, BSN, MA, CCRN

Note: The information in this chapter should be used in conjunction with the information in Ch. 43: Management of Chest Drainage Systems.

INDICATIONS

To remove air and/or fluid from the pleural cavity in conjunction with a chest tube.

CONTRAINDICATIONS AND CAUTIONS

The bottle system is rarely used, because most facilities now use the prefabricated, disposable chest drainage systems. The prefabricated systems have the flexibility of being used either as gravity or suction drainage systems, they are easier to set up and maintain, and they are not as fragile as glass bottles.

EQUIPMENT

*Indicates portions of the procedure usually performed by a physician.

Sterile collection and water-seal bottles (See Figure 46.1.)
Holder for bottles
3–4 ft of sterile tubing

Tubing connectors, 1/4-inch internal diameter
Sterile water or saline
Tape

PATIENT PREPARATION

*Insert a chest tube. See Ch. 42: Chest Tube Insertion.

PROCEDURAL STEPS

1. Add sterile water/saline to the water-seal bottle until the end of the water-seal tube is submerged in 1–2 cm of water. This provides the water seal necessary to prevent back flow. The short, stiff tube is the vent tube.
2. Connect the collection bottle to the water-seal bottle with a short length of sterile tubing attached to the water-seal tube.
3. Connect the chest tube to the drainage tubing with a connector.
4. Connect the drainage tubing to the other short stiff tube of the collection bottle. See Figure 46.1.
5. Tape all tube connections securely with adhesive tape (Brunner 1978).

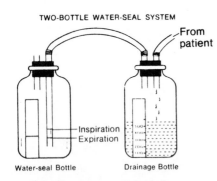

Figure 46.1 Two-bottle gravity drainage system.
(Brunner & Suddarth, 1974: 151. Reprinted by permission.)

COMPLICATIONS

1. Tension pneumothorax secondary to obstruction in the system.
2. Open pneumothorax secondary to tubing disconnection, chest tube dislodgement, bottle breakage, or loss of water seal if the water-seal tube is not kept submerged.

PATIENT TEACHING

1. Instruct the patient in deep breathing and coughing.
2. Ask for assistance to get out of bed.
3. Report any chest pain, shortness of breath, or tubing disconnections immediately.
4. Do not lie on the tubing or allow it to kink. The bottles must be kept upright at all times.

REFERENCES

Brunner, L.S., & Suddarth, D.S. 1978. *Lippincott manual of nursing practices*, 2nd ed. Philadelphia: Lippincott.

SUGGESTED READING

Mims, B.C. 1985. You can manage chest tubes confidently. *RN*, 48, 1: 39–44.

47

Chest Drainage Devices: Two-Bottle System – Suction Drainage

Manjula D. Gray, RN, BSN, MA, CCRN

Note: The information in this chapter should be used in conjunction with the information in Ch. 43: Management of Chest Drainage Systems.

INDICATIONS

To remove air and/or fluid from the pleural cavity in conjunction with a chest tube.

CONTRAINDICATIONS AND CAUTIONS

The bottle system is rarely used, because most facilities now use the prefabricated, disposable chest drainage systems. The prefabricated systems have the flexibility of being used either as gravity drainage or suction drainage systems, they are easier to set up and maintain, and they are not as fragile as glass bottles.

EQUIPMENT

Sterile water-seal/collection and suction bottles (See Figure 47.1.)
Holder for bottles
3–4 ft of sterile tubing
Tubing connectors, 1/4-inch internal diameter

Sterile water or saline
Tape
Wall or portable suction (continuous)

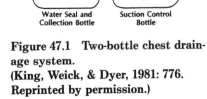

From Patient

To Suction

Water Seal and Collection Bottle   Suction Control Bottle

Figure 47.1   Two-bottle chest drainage system.
(King, Weick, & Dyer, 1981: 776. Reprinted by permission.)

PATIENT PREPARATION

*Insert a chest tube. See Ch. 42: Chest Tube Insertion.

*Indicates portions of the procedure usually performed by a physician.

PROCEDURAL STEPS

1. Add sterile water/saline to the water-seal/collection bottle until the end of the water seal tube is submerged in 1–2 cm of water. This provides the water seal necessary to prevent back flow.
2. The suction control bottle has three openings in the cap. The long stiff tube in the center works as the manometer tube. Fill the suction control bottle with enough sterile water/saline so the manometer tube is submerged in about 10 cm of water. Connect the suction control bottle to the water-seal/collection bottle with a short length of sterile tubing. Connect the other short stiff tube in the suction control bottle to continuous

suction. The depth the manometer tube is submerged in water determines the amount of suction that is applied, not the suction regulator device. One cm of manometer tube submerged in sterile water/saline = 1 cm of water pressure (Brunner, 1988).

3. Connect the chest tube to the drainage tubing with a connector.
4. Connect the drainage tubing to the water-seal tube of the collection bottle. See Figure 47.1.
5. Tape all tube connections securely with adhesive tape (Brunner, 1978).

COMPLICATIONS

1. Tension pneumothorax secondary to obstruction in the system.
2. Open pneumothorax secondary to tubing disconnection, chest tube dislodgement, bottle breakage, or loss of water seal if the water seal is not kept submerged.

PATIENT TEACHING

1. Instruct the patient in deep breathing and coughing.
2. Ask for assistance to get out of bed.
3. Report any chest pain, shortness of breath, or tubing disconnections immediately.
4. Do not lie on the tubing or allow it to kink. The bottles must be kept upright at all times.

REFERENCES

Brunner, L.S., & Suddarth, D.S. 1978. *Lippincott manual of nursing practices,* 2nd ed. Philadelphia: Lippincott.
Brunner, L.S., & Suddarth, D.S. 1988. *Textbook of medical-surgical nursing,* 6th ed. Philadelphia: Lippincott.

SUGGESTED READING

Mims, B.C. 1985. You can manage chest tubes confidently. *RN,* 48, 1: 39–44.

48

Chest Drainage Devices: Two-Bottle System — Emerson Pump

Manjula D. Gray, RN, BSN, MA, CCRN

Note: The information in this chapter should be used in conjunction with the information in Ch. 43: Management of Chest Drainage Systems.

INDICATIONS

To remove air and/or fluid from the pleural cavity in conjunction with a chest tube.

CONTRAINDICATIONS AND CAUTIONS

The Emerson pump is a high-pressure, high-flow system, capable of generating pressures up to −60 cm of water. It is used infrequently because most facilities now use the low-pressure prefabricated, disposable chest drainage systems. The prefabricated systems have the flexibility of being used either as gravity drainage or suction drainage systems.

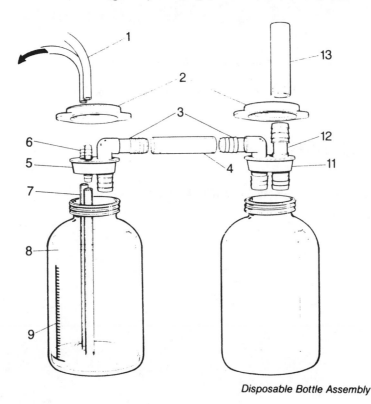

1	Drainage tubes, 4 feet, pair
	Drainage tubes, 6 feet, pair
	Drainage tubes, 8 feet, pair
2	Threaded ring
3	Elbow
4	Tube (short)
5	Stopper for primary bottle
6	Connector
7	Bottle tubes, pair
8	Trap bottle with scale (case of **6**)
9	Scale
10	Trap bottle, secondary (case of **6**)
11	Stopper for secondary bottle
12	Connector
13	Tube (long)
	Primary cap assembly
	1 @ 555-0022
	2 @ 556-00**11**
	1 @ 510-1101
	1 @ 555-0044
	Secondary cap assembly
	1 @ 555-0023
	1 @ 510-1101
	1 @ 510-1102
	1 @ 555-0044

Disposable Bottle Assembly

Figure 48.1 Glass bottle assembly for the Emerson pump. (Reproduced with permission from J.H. Emerson Co., Cambridge, MA.)

EQUIPMENT

Emerson Pump Set (includes connectors, drainage tubes, bottles, bottlecap assemblies, bottle tubes, large tubing, pump, and the mobile stand with its triangular tray) See Figure 48.1.

or

Disposable Emerson pump unit (Figure 48.2)

Sterile water or saline

Tape

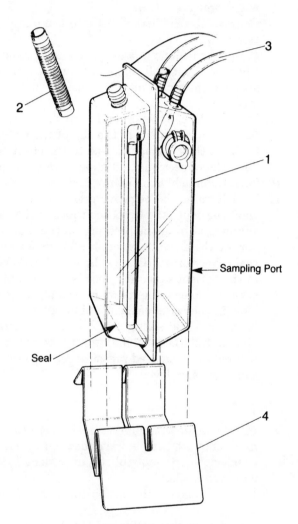

1 Disposable drainage set*
2 Flex-tube (included in drainage set)
3 Drainage tubes (included in drainage set)
4 Bottle stand
* See literature for other models of disposable drainage sets.

Figure 48.2 Disposable Emerson pump unit.
(Reproduced with permission from J.H. Emerson, Co., Cambridge, MA.)

PATIENT PREPARATION

*Insert a chest tube. See Ch. 42: Chest Tube Insertion.

*Indicates portions of the procedure usually performed by a physician.

PROCEDURAL STEPS

Bottle system

1. Add sterile water/saline to the water-seal/collection bottle to the water line. Mark it with time and date. Connect the two, short, stiff narrow tubes to the underside of the cap with three connectors. These tubes should be submerged in 1–2 cm of sterile water in the bottle. This provides the water seal necessary to prevent back flow.
2. If the patient has only one chest tube, cover one of the openings in the bottle cap with the plastic adapter.
3. Connect the water-seal bottle to the fluid-trap bottle with the short, wide connection tube.
4. Connect the fluid-trap bottle to the pump with the large, wide connection tube.
5. Plug the machine in and make sure the red indicator light goes on.
6. Plug the two, small connectors on the primary bottle cap and adjust the speed of the motor until the desired suction is attained (20–30 cm of water).
7. Remove the cap or caps and connect the long tube or tubes (if the patient has two chest tubes) to the cap of the water-seal/collection bottle.
8. Connect the drainage tube(s) to the chest tube(s).
9. Tape all connections and make sure the caps are tight.
10. Turn the machine on and adjust the pressure to the prescribed level.
11. To determine the negative pressure in the patient's pleural space, subtract the depth the tip of the tubes in the water-seal/collection bottle are submerged from the pressure on the machine. For example, if the pressure on the machine is set at -30 cm of water and the tubes in the water-seal/collection bottle are submerged to 20 cm of water, then the pressure in the patient's pleural space is -10 cm of water. Therefore, it is necessary to increase the pressure setting on the machine as fluid accumulates in the water-seal/collection bottle in order to maintain the desired pressure. Fluid should not be allowed to fill the bottle more than one-quarter full (the machine capacity is -60 cm of water; higher fluid levels will require increased pressure settings on the machine to maintain the same pressure level).

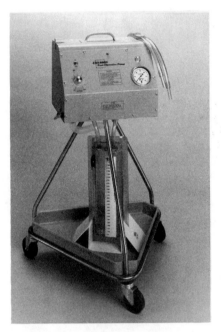

Figure 48.3 Emerson pump. (Reproduced with permission from J.H. Emerson Co., Cambridge, MA.)

Disposable system

1. Fill the disposable unit's underwater seal chamber up to the water-seal mark through the pump connection port.
2. Connect the patient tube(s) to patient fittings on the disposable unit. See Figure 48.2.
3. Place the disposable unit on the stand in the triangular tray. See Figure 48.3.
4. Connect the disposable unit to the pump with the flex tube.
5. The level of accumulated fluid in the disposable unit does not effect the vacuum level applied to the patient, because there is no underwater seal in the primary collecting compartment (Emerson Co).

COMPLICATIONS

1. Tension pneumothorax secondary to obstruction in the system.
2. Open pneumothorax secondary to tubing disconnection, chest tube dislodgement, bottle breakage, or loss of water seal if the water-seal tube is not kept submerged.

3. If there is a loss of electrical power or the Emerson pump malfunctions, disconnect the water-seal bottle from the fluid-trap bottle. This will prevent buildup of back pressure by providing an air vent.

PATIENT TEACHING

1. Instruct the patient in deep breathing and coughing.
2. Ask for assistance to get out of bed.
3. Report any chest pain, shortness of breath, or tubing disconnections immediately.
4. Do not lie on the tubing or allow it to kink. The bottles must be kept upright at all times.

REFERENCES

Brunner, L.S., & Suddarth, D.S. 1978. *Lippincott manual of nursing practices,* 2nd ed. Philadelphia: Lippincott.

SUGGESTED READING

Mims, B.C. 1985. You can manage chest tubes confidently. *RN,* 48, 1:39–44.
Pfister, S., & Bullas, J.B. 1985. Caring for a patient with a chest tube connected to the Emerson pump. *Critical Care Nurse,* 5, 2:26–32.

49

Chest Drainage Devices: Three-Bottle System

Manjula D. Gray, RN, BSN, MA, CCRN

Note: The information in this chapter should be used in conjunction with the information in Ch. 43: Management of Chest Drainage Systems.

INDICATIONS

To remove air and/or fluid from the pleural cavity in conjunction with a chest tube.

CONTRAINDICATIONS AND CAUTIONS

The bottle system is rarely used, because most facilities now use the prefabricated, disposable chest drainage systems. The prefabricated systems have the flexibility of being used either as gravity or suction drainage systems, they are easier to set up and maintain, and they are not as fragile as glass bottles.

EQUIPMENT

Sterile collection, suction, and
    water-seal/overflow bottles
    (Figure 49.1)
Holder for bottles
4–5 ft of sterile tubing
Tubing connectors, 1/4-inch internal
    diameter

Sterile water or saline
Tape
Wall or portable suction
    (continuous)

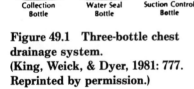

Figure 49.1 Three-bottle chest drainage system. (King, Weick, & Dyer, 1981: 777. Reprinted by permission.)

*Indicates portions of the procedure usually performed by a physician.

PATIENT PREPARATION

*Insert a chest tube. See Ch. 42: Chest Tube Insertion.

PROCEDURAL STEPS

1. Add sterile water/saline to one of the bottles with two openings in the cap, until the end of the long, stiff tube is submerged in 1–2 cm of water. This provides the water seal necessary to prevent back flow. This is the water-seal/collection overflow bottle.
2. The other bottle with two openings in the cap is the collection bottle. One short, stiff tube is connected to the drainage tubing and the other short, stiff tube is connected to the water-seal tube with a short length of sterile tubing.
3. The suction bottle has three openings in the cap. The long, stiff tube in

the center is the manometer tube. Fill the suction bottle with enough sterile water so the manometer tube is submerged in about 10 cm of water. Connect one of the short, stiff tubes of the suction bottle to the water-seal bottle with a short length of sterile tubing. Connect the other short, stiff tube in the suction bottle to the suction. It is the depth the manometer tube is submerged in water that determines the amount of suction that is applied, not the suction regulator devices. For example, 1 cm of manometer tube submerged in sterile water/saline = 1 cm of water pressure (Brunner, 1988).

4. Connect the chest tube to the drainage tubing with a connector.
5. Connect the drainage tubing to the other short, stiff tube of the collection bottle (Figure 49.1).
6. Tape all tube connections securely with adhesive tape (Brunner, 1978).

COMPLICATIONS

1. Tension pneumothorax secondary to obstruction in the system.
2. Open pneumothorax secondary to tubing disconnections, chest tube dislodgement, bottle breakage, or loss of water seal if the water-seal tube is not kept submerged.
3. When the suction source is functioning, there is continuous bubbling from the manometer tube in the suction bottle. If the bubbling stops check the suction source. If it is a malfunctioning suction source, disconnect the tubing to the suction at the bottle to provide an air vent for gravity drainage.

PATIENT TEACHING

1. Instruct the patient in deep breathing and coughing.
2. Ask for assistance to get out of bed.
3. Report any chest pain, shortness of breath, or tubing disconnections immediately.
4. Do not lie on the tubing or allow it to kink. The bottles must be kept upright at all times.

REFERENCES

Brunner, L.S., & Suddarth, D.S. 1978. *Lippincott manual of nursing practices,* 2nd ed. Philadelphia: Lippincott.
Brunner, L.S., & Suddarth, D.S. 1988. *Textbook of medical-surgical nursing,* 6th ed. Philadelphia: Lippincott.
King, E.M., Wieck, L., & Dyer, M. 1981. *Illustrated manual of nursing techniques,* 2nd ed. Philadelphia: Lippincott.

SUGGESTED READING

Mims, B.C. 1985. You can manage chest tubes confidently. *RN,* 48, 1:39–44.

50

Chest Drainage Devices: Pleur-evac

Janet A. Neff, RN, MN, CEN, CCRN

Pleur-evac is also known as A-8000 series chest drainage unit; newer version of A-4005 equivalent.

Note: The information in this chapter should be used in conjunction with the information in Ch. 43: Management of Chest Drainage Systems.

INDICATIONS

1. To collect and monitor the amount and type of pleural fluid drainage and to detect a pleural air leak via a chest tube.
2. To maintain a safe and effective level of intrapleural pressure by regulating the amount of air flow and suction generated, and manipulating any excess negative or positive pressure within the drainage unit.
3. To assist in the assessment of a patient's pulmonary status.

CONTRAINDICATIONS AND CAUTIONS

1. Although these devices are less likely to break than glass bottle systems, they may crack or internal parts may malfunction.
2. The unit must be kept upright when in use.
3. If autotransfusion (ATS) is necessary, a unit with a preattached ATS unit (A-7050 [A-5000]) or with an option to attach ATS (A-7000 [A-5005]) should be initially selected. The A-8000 has no ATS option.

EQUIPMENT

Note: Unitized chest drainage units integrate the functions of a 3-bottle glass system into a plastic disposable unit. See Figure 50.1.

Sterile water
1- or 2-inch tape
Disposable gloves
Pleur-evac A-8000 adult/pediatric single use chest drainage unit (CDU) with preattached funnel. See Figure 50.2.

High flow, continuous suction apparatus with regulator such as wall suction or Emerson pump
Some portable suction pumps can not generate sufficient air flow capacity (20 L/min desired).

PATIENT PREPARATION

*Indicates portions of the procedure usually performed by a physician.

*Insert a chest tube. See Ch. 42: Chest Tube Insertion.

PROCEDURAL STEPS

1. Attach funnel to suction tubing connector and fill to 2-cm water level FILL TO HERE mark with approximately 70 mL sterile water (sterile saline is not as desirable, because with evaporation, salt crystals may form). The water seal is necessary to maintain a closed system.
2. The water will turn blue for greater visibility. Disconnect funnel. The unit can be attached to patient now if necessary.

3. Suction (optional): Remove atmospheric vent cover (muffler) and fill the suction control chamber with sterile water to dotted line (-20 cm H_2O or as ordered:

Suction pressure	Water volume
-15 cm H_2O	280 ml
-20 cm H_2O	415 ml
-25 cm H_2O	540 ml

4. Replace the muffler – do not occlude the atmospheric vent.
5. Attach the long latex tube from the collection chamber to the patient's chest tube and tape securely. Maintain the unit in an upright position and below the level of the patient's chest; secure it with attached hooks or the locking floor stand.
6. Attach the tubing on suction control chamber to a suction source. The connector can be cut to allow maximal size in relation to the chest tube size. A large internal diameter is important (Besson, 1983).
7. Adjust the suction until gentle, continuous bubbling occurs.

   Higher suction pressures are used for large air leaks. Adding suction to the system improves evacuation of gas from the pleural space by creating a lower pressure within the unit than within the patient. The amount of bubbling does not indicate greater pressure against the pleura, but rather increased air flow capacity – excessive bubbling is not desirable because it increases evaporation and noise.
8. The Pleur-evac A-6000 series has been designed with a dry suction control system. The water-seal chamber must be filled first as usual, but no water is necessary for suction control. Suction pressure is regulated by a control dial (to the left of unit), which is rotated until the orange/red fluorescent stripe is in line with the level of suction desired. Settings range from -10-cm H_2O to -40-cm H_2O. An indicator window contains a fluorescent float that is visible when the dialed suction level is being maintained. If the float is not visible, the suction source may be too low or the unit may be broken. See Figure 50.3.

   The A-6000 suction regulator automatically deals with fluctuations due to changes in the suction source or the patient's air leak, thereby maintaining the desired level of H_2O) suction pressure without manipulation.
9. The collection chambers hold up to 2500 mL and are calibrated for easy measurement. Recognize that the calibration of mL is varied as the volume increases, so each collection column is not equivalent in volume. Assess and record the type and volume of drainage. If blood in large quantities is rapidly evacuated, change to an ATS system. (See Ch. 78: Pleur-evac Autotransfusion System.)

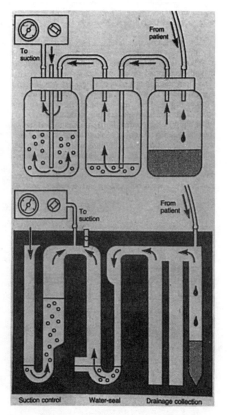

Figure 50.1 Comparison of principles of a three-bottle system to a Pleur-evac chest drainage unit. (Luce et al., 1984: 166. Reprinted with permission.)

Figure 50.2 Pleur-evac A-8000 chest drainage unit.
   S-1: Atmospheric vent, used to fill suction control chamber.
   S-2: Self-sealing diaphragm
   S-3: Suction control pressure scale
   S-4: Suction tubing
   W-1: Water-seal pressure scale
   W-2: Positive pressure relief valve
   W-3: High negativity float valve
   W-4: Filtered high negativity relief valve
   W-5: Self-sealing diaphragm
   C-1: Collection chamber
   C-2: Self-sealing diaphragm
(From *Pleur-evac-Instructions for Use.* Deknatel, 1989, Fall River, MA: Pfizer Hospital Products Group. Copyright 1989 by Pfizer Hospital Products Group. Reprinted by permission.)

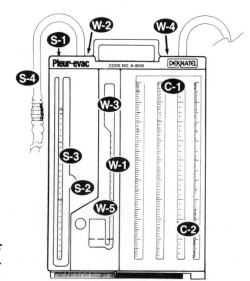

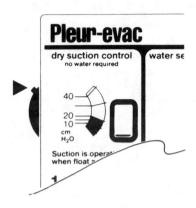

Figure 50.3 Pleur-evac A-6000 dry suction control regulation system with fluorescent float.
(From *Pleur-evac-Instructions for use.* Deknatel, 1989, Fall River, MA: Pfizer Hospital Products Group. Copyright 1989 by Pfizer Hospital Products Group. Reprinted by permission.)

10. Avoid dependent loops in patient tubing because this generates the same effect as a higher water-seal level, requiring more effort to evacuate fluid and air.

11. Fluid in the water-seal chamber is expected to oscillate or "tidal" with respirations. Fluid will rise with spontaneous inspiration (more negative) and fall (more positive) with expiration, although the opposite occurs with positive pressure ventilation and the oscillation is less evident when suction is applied. Tidaling decreases or stops if the patient tubing is kinked or obstructed or the lung has reexpanded.

12. An air leak is detected by viewing the water-seal chamber for bubbling. Some Pleur-evac units have an air flow meter with a Lo to Hi display. Air leaks do not always occur with each breath, so careful observation is necessary. Normal air evacuation would be seen on exhalation; if it occurs on inspiration as well (constant bubbling), a significant pulmonary air leak may be present or a leak within the system exists.

    Bubbling in the water seal without bubbling in the suction chambers means that the suction must be increased.

13. Negativity within the system arises from the suction-control setting (cm H_2O), from maneuvers to clear the drainage tubing (milking, stripping), and from within the patient, such as during increased inspiratory effort. The degree of negativity is reflected in the water-seal chamber which is calibrated in units of cm H_2O. On gravity drainage, the negativity is measured solely from the water seal chamber; on suction, the negativity is calculated by adding the cm H_2O pressure in water-seal and suction-control chambers. Evaporation will lower the water level over time and the chamber should be refilled with the suction off to ensure an accurate level.

14. Excess negativity can be manually relieved by depressing the high negativity relief valve on the top of the unit and should be done while suction is on.

15. Excess positive pressure ($> +2$ cm H_2O) is automatically relieved.

16. Fluid samples should not be taken from the latex tubing since it is not self-sealing, however, a special port is provided.

COMPLICATIONS

1. Enlarging pneumo/hemothorax evolving into a tension status if there is inadvertent compression of the patient tubing, biologic obstruction, or insufficient suction.

2. Incomplete drainage of fluid may result in fibrothorax.

3. Capillary damage and entrapment of lung tissue may occur if excessive negative pressure is generated by maneuvers such as stripping or milking chest tubes (Duncan, 1982).

4. Tipping of the unit will result in loss of the water seal until the unit is repositioned upright. A water-seal float valve prevents permanent loss of water from the water-seal chamber.

PATIENT TEACHING

1. Report any shortness of breath, chest pain, or system disconnections immediately.

2. Do not lie on the tubing or allow it to be kinked. Keep the unit upright at all times.

REFERENCES

Besson, A., & Saegesser, F. 1983. *Color atlas of chest trauma and associated injuries,* volume one. Oradell, NJ: Medical Economics.

Duncan, C., & Erickson, R. 1982. Pressures associated with chest tube stripping. *Heart & Lung,* 11, 2:166–171.

SUGGESTED READINGS

Hamilton, H.K. (ed). 1984. *Nurse's clinical library: Respiratory disorders.* Springhouse, PA: Springhouse.

Luce, J.M., Tyler, M.L., & Pierson, D.J. 1984. *Intensive respiratory care.* Philadelphia: Saunders.

51

Chest Drainage Devices: Thora-Klex

Janet A. Neff, RN, MN, CEN, CCRN

Thora-Klex® is also known as 7700 chest drainage system. Thora-Klex is produced by Davol, Inc., a subsidiary of C.R. Bard Inc.

Note: The information in this chapter should be used in conjunction with the information in Ch. 43: Management of Chest Drainage Systems.

INDICATIONS

1. To collect and monitor the amount and type of pleural fluid drainage and to detect a pleural air leak via a chest tube.
2. To maintain a safe and effective level of intrapleural pressure by regulating the amount of air flow and suction generated, and manipulating any excess negative or positive pressure within the drainage unit.
3. To assist in the assessment of a patient's pulmonary status.
4. To ensure maintenance of water seal regardless of position of chest drainage unit in relation to the patient, i.e., in instances where tipping or horizontal placement is likely, e.g., air transport, rapid transfer to OR/CT, etc.

CONTRAINDICATIONS AND CAUTIONS

1. Although these devices are less likely to break than glass bottle systems, they may crack or internal parts may malfunction.
2. In patients with significant change in air leak or with an inconsistent suction source, the unit requires frequent manual adjustments.

EQUIPMENT

Thora-Klex 7700 chest drainage unit (CDU) See Figure 51.1.
Sterile water
Syringe and needle (18-gauge or smaller bore)
1- or 2-inch tape
Disposable gloves

High flow, continuous suction apparatus with regulator such as wall suction or Emerson pump. Some portable suction pumps can not generate sufficient air flow capacity (20 L/min desired).

PATIENT PREPARATION

*Indicates portions of the procedure usually performed by a physician.

*Insert a chest tube. See Ch. 42: Chest Tube Insertion.

PROCEDURAL STEPS

The unit is ready for use on a patient immediately after removal from package. Instructions are readily available on the front of the unit on a pull-out card.

1. Attach the long latex tube from the collection chamber to the patient's chest tube and tape securely. The connector can be cut to allow maximal size in relation to the chest tube size. A large internal diameter is important (Besson, 1983).

2. Place the unit approximately 30 cm below the level of the patient's chest (Elliot, 1990). Secure it with attached hooks or the floor stand.

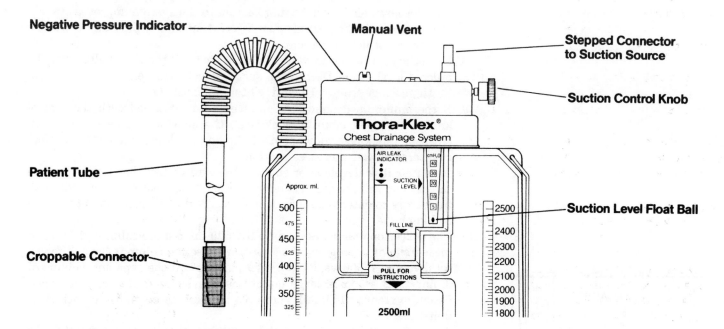

Figure 51.1   Thora-Klex 7700 chest drainage unit.

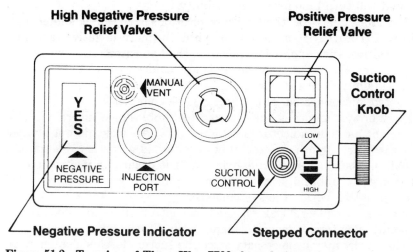

Figure 51.2   Top view of Thora-Klex 7700 chest drainage unit.

Figures 51.1, 51.2, and 51.3 are from *Thora-Klex 2500/4000 mL chest drainage system: Quick reference guide.* Davol, 1990, Cranston, RI. Copyright 1989 by Davol, Inc. Reprinted by permission.

3. There is no true water seal in the Thora-Klex device, because it is a dry system. A seal is maintained by a one-way vacuum seal valve which is preset at 1.5–2.0 cm H_2O. The one-way valve maintains a closed system and allows air to flow in only one direction, away from the patient. The effective seal is not lost when the unit is tipped in any position.

4. Push and turn the suction control dial counterclockwise until it is fully open in order to maximize air flow. See Figure 51.2. **Note:** Do not use the manual vent when on gravity drainage.

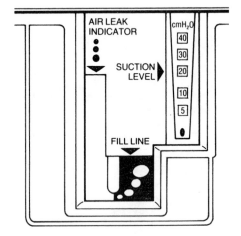

Figure 51.3 Thora-Klex 7700 chest drainage unit air leak indicator and suction level chambers.

5. The Thora-Klex is a dry suction system. Attach tubing from suction source to suction connector on top of the control module. See Figure 51.2.

6. Adjust suction control on CDU by pushing and turning the suction control knob clockwise until closed.

7. Adjust suction pressure on suction source: −80 to −120 mm Hg wall suction; −40 to −60 cm H₂O portable suction pump. Higher vacuum is used for large air leaks. Adding suction to the system improves evacuation of gas from the pleural space by creating a lower pressure within the unit than within the patient.

8. Push the suction control knob in and turn until the float ball sits at the ordered level of cm H₂O in the suction-level chamber. See Figure 51.3. Settings range from −10 cm H₂O to −40 cm H₂O.

9. If the minimum desired suction level is not obtained with the control knob fully open (counterclockwise), the suction source must be increased. Clockwise movement of the control knob decreases suction; counterclockwise increases suction.

10. As an air leak develops or suction pressure varies; the suction level to the patient will change. Therefore, observe the position of the float ball frequently to detect changes, which require manual resetting of the control knob.

11. The collection chambers hold up to 2500 ml and are calibrated for easy measurement. Recognize that the two collection columns have different total volumes (500 vs 2000). Assess and record the type and volume of drainage. If blood in large quantities is evacuated, add an autotransfusion system (ATS). All Thora-Klex units are compatible with ATS units. See Ch. 79.

12. Avoid dependent loops in patient tubing, because this generates the same effect as a higher water-seal level, requiring more effort to evacuate fluid and air.

13. Inject 15 ml sterile water into the air leak indicator via the injection port on the top of the unit to create a fluid filled chamber to detect air leaks. The fluid will turn blue for easier visibility.

14. Fluid will rock gently or "tidal" with respirations in the air leak indicator. Fluid will rise with spontaneous inspiration (more negative) and fall (more positive) with expiration, however, the opposite occurs with positive pressure ventilation. Oscillation is less evident when suction is applied. Tidaling decreases or stops if the patient tubing is kinked, obstructed, disconnected, or the lung has reexpanded.

15. A pleural or system air leak is detected by bubbles passing from left to right in the air leak indicator. See Figure 51.3. Air leaks do not always occur with each breath, so careful observation is necessary. Pleural air evacuation would be seen on exhalation, if it occurs on inspiration as well (constant bubbling), a significant pulmonary air leak may be present or a leak within the system exists.

16. If there is a large pleural leak, the suction control knob should be turned maximally counterclockwise to increase air flow capacity, however, a physician order may be necessary since the suction level is changing, as in the suction chamber in water-seal systems.

17. The presence of negativity within the unit is displayed on the top of the unit by a YES indicator. In gravity systems, the YES will display intermittently with the respiratory pattern; but on suction, the YES should be constant. The unit must remain negative in order to continue to evacuate fluid and air from the chest.

18. Negativity within the system arises from the suction level setting (cm H₂O), from maneuvers to clear the drainage tubing (milking, stripping), and from within the patient during increased inspiratory efforts. The de-

gree of negativity is reflected by the suction level float ball with a range of 0 to −40 cm H$_2$O.

19. Excess negativity (> −50 cm H$_2$O) is automatically reduced to a relatively safe level of approximately −35 cm H$_2$O by a high negative pressure relief valve. See Figure 51.2. The manual vent on top of the unit will lower the negative pressure further in order to return to the ordered level.

The manual vent is activated by use of a coin or pen; it cannot be accidentally adjusted. To confirm that suction control is restored to the desired level after decreasing negativity within the system (i.e., after stripping the chest tube), and after any change from a higher to lower suction setting, adjust the suction control (float ball) to desired setting and depress the manual vent until a bubble is seen passing from left to right, then release.

If system negativity exceeds that of the suction control, fluid will rise up the left side of the air leak indicator and bubbling may occur from right to left. The manual vent procedure should be followed. A similar phenomenon will occur when the lung reexpands, but there will be concurrent lack of tidaling, and no bubbling.

20. Excess positive pressure (> +2 cm H$_2$O) is automatically relieved.

21. Fluid samples are optimally taken from the self-sealing latex tubing, although a port is available on the back of the first collection chamber.

COMPLICATIONS

1. Enlarging pneumo/hemothorax evolving into a tension status if there is inadvertent compression of the patient tubing, biologic obstruction, or insufficient suction.

2. Incomplete drainage of fluid may result in fibrothorax.

3. Capillary damage and entrapment of lung tissue may occur if excessive negative pressure is generated by maneuvers such as stripping or milking chest tubes (Duncan, 1982) or undetected excess negativity.

PATIENT TEACHING

1. Report any shortness of breath, chest pain, or system disconnections immediately.

2. Do not lie on the tubing or allow it to be kinked.

REFERENCES

Besson, A., & Saegesser, F. 1983. *Color atlas of chest trauma and associated injuries,* volume one. Oradell, NJ: Medical Economics.

Duncan, C., & Erickson, R. 1982. Pressures associated with chest tube stripping. *Heart & Lung,* 11, 2:166–171.

Elliott, D. 1990. *Why waterless chest drainage?* (Report No. 118910M). Cranston, RI: Davol.

Pfizer Hospital Products Group. 1990. *A comparison of Davol's Thora-Klex® and Deknatel's Pleur-evac® A-6000 dry suction chest drainage units* (Research report No. 356). Fall River, MA: Pfizer.

SUGGESTED READINGS

Ames, S.W., & Kneisl, C.R. 1988. *Essentials of Adult Health Nursing* (Ch. 14: The nursing process for clients with respiratory dysfunction). Menlo Park, CA: Addison-Wesley.

Hamilton, H.K. (ed). 1984. *Nurse's clinical library: Respiratory disorders* Springhouse, PA: Springhouse.

Luce, J.M., Tyler, M.L., & Pierson, D.J. 1984. *Intensive respiratory care.* Philadelphia: Saunders.

Traver, G. 1982. *Respiratory nursing: The science and the art.* New York: Wiley.

52

Chest Drainage Devices: Argyle Double Seal

Janet A. Neff, RN, MN, CEN, CCRN

The Argyle® Double Seal, Thora Seal®, and Sentinel Seal® are produced by Sherwood Medical.

Note: The information in this chapter should be used in conjunction with the information in Ch. 43: Management of Chest Drainage Systems.

INDICATIONS

1. To collect and monitor the amount and type of pleural fluid drainage and to detect a pleural air leak via a chest tube.
2. To maintain a safe and effective level of intrapleural pressure by regulating the amount of air flow and suction generated, and manipulating any excess negative or positive pressure within the drainage unit.
3. To assist in the assessment of a patient's pulmonary status. The actual negative pressure reaching the patient is easily seen in the assessment chamber.

CONTRAINDICATIONS AND CAUTIONS

1. Although these devices are less likely to break than glass bottle systems, they may crack or internal parts may malfunction.
2. The unit must be kept upright when in use.
3. The Argyle Double Seal chest drainage unit (CDU) has no autotransfusion (ATS) option. If ATS is indicated, an Argyle Thora Seal or Sentinel Seal CDU with ATS attachment should be used.

EQUIPMENT

Note: This unitized chest drainage unit integrates the functions of a 4-bottle glass system into a plastic disposable unit See Figure 52.1.
Argyle Double Seal CDU with four chambers; underwater seal, suction control, collection, and patient assessment See Figure 52.2.
Sterile water
1- or 2-inch tape

Disposable gloves
High flow, continuous suction apparatus with regulator such as wall suction (100–160 mm Hg) or Emerson pump (> 45 cm H_2O, Some portable suction pumps can not generate sufficient air flow capacity (20 L/min desired).

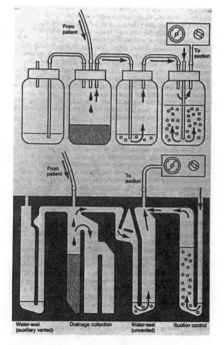

Figure 52.1 Comparison of principles of a four-bottle system to an Argyle chest drainage unit. (Luce et al., 1984: 167. Reprinted by permission.)

PATIENT PREPARATION

*Insert a chest tube. See Ch. 42: Chest Tube Insertion.

*Indicates portions of the procedure usually performed by a physician.

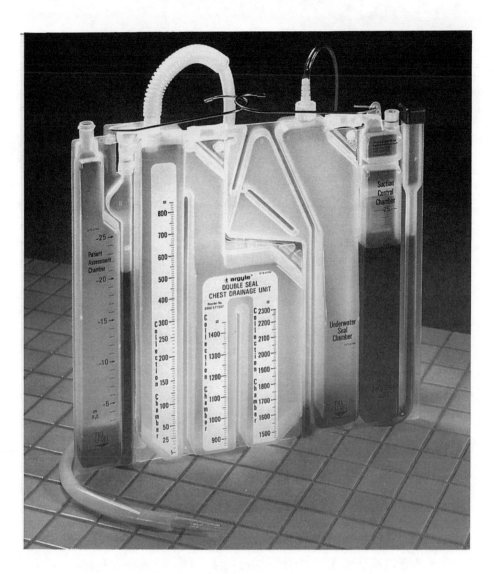

**Figure 52.2 Argyle Double Seal
chest drainage unit.
(Sherwood Medical, 1989: 5. Reprinted by permission.)**

PROCEDURAL STEPS

1. Remove connector with tubing attached inside the water-seal chamber and fill to 2-cm water level FILL LEVEL mark (dark line below arrow, not the dashed line) with approximately 55 ml sterile water (sterile saline is not as desirable, because with evaporation, salt crystals may form). The water seal is necessary to maintain a closed system.

   No funnel is provided. It may help to use a 50-ml piston syringe with the plunger removed. After filling chamber, screw the tapered connector with attached tubing, approximately 10 inches, and 5-in-1 connector onto the water-seal chamber.

2. The water will turn blue for easier visibility.

3. The assessment chamber contains an auxiliary underwater seal and a manometer which must be filled to FILL LEVEL with approximately 55 ml sterile water. This fluid will also turn blue. The unit can be attached to patient now.

4. Suction (optional): Remove vented green cap (muffler) and fill the suction control chamber with sterile water to dashed line (-20 cm H_2O) or as ordered. Fluid will turn blue.

5. Replace the muffler since this unit is noisy.

6. Attach the long latex tube from the collection chamber to the patient's chest tube and tape securely. Maintain the unit in an upright position and below the level of the patient's chest; secure it with attached hooks.

7. Connect the tubing from the suction source to the 5-in-1 connector which is attached to the tubing at the top of water-seal chamber.

8. Adjust the suction until gentle, continuous bubbling occurs in the suction control chamber.

   Higher suction source pressures are used for large air leaks. Adding suction to the system improves evacuation of gas from the pleural space by creating a lower pressure within the unit than within the patient. The amount of bubbling does not indicate greater pressure against the pleura, but rather increased air flow capacity — excessive bubbling is not desirable because it increases evaporation and noise.

   Bubbling in the suction chamber indicates only that the patient is receiving no less than the indicated pressure. However, more negative pressure (vacuum) may be in effect and can be easily detected in the assessment chamber.

9. The narrow column attached to the assessment chamber will reflect the actual negative pressure reaching the patient. If this column shows higher negative pressure (read at level of float ball) than the ordered level, the suction source must be adjusted.

10. The Argyle Thora Seal has been designed with a nonbubbling suction control system with a manometer and precision suction regulator. This system is much quieter and more compact. The Argyle Thora Seal suction regulator automatically deals with fluctuations due to changes in the suction source or the patient's air leak, thereby maintaining the desired suction pressure.

11. The collection chambers hold up to 2300 ml and are calibrated for easy measurement. Recognize that the calibration of ml is varied as the volume increases, so each collection column is not equivalent in volume. Assess and record the type and volume of drainage.

12. Avoid dependent loops in patient tubing because this generates the same effect as a higher water-seal level, requiring more effort to evacuate fluid and air.

13. Fluid is expected to oscillate or "tidal" approximately 2–5 cm H_2O with respirations: on gravity, the water seal will oscillate; on suction, the tidaling will be seen in the assessment chamber. Fluid will rise with spontaneous inspiration (more negative) and fall (more positive) with expiration, although the opposite occurs with positive pressure ventilation and the oscillation is less evident when suction is applied. Tidaling decreases or stops if the patient tubing is kinked or obstructed or the lung has reexpanded.

14. Air leaks do not always occur with each breath, so careful observation is necessary. An air leak is detected by viewing the water-seal chamber for bubbling. On gravity drainage, bubbling may be seen in either or both water-seal and assessment chambers since the air takes the path of least resistance. On suction, bubbling in the water seal reflects an air leak. If bubbling is noted in the assessment chamber, something is wrong and the patient has additional positive pressure to be relieved. Check the patient, suction source, and all tubings for obstructions. Normal air evacuation would be seen on exhalation, if it occurs on inspiration as well (constant bubbling), a significant pulmonary air leak may be present or a leak within the system exists.

   Bubbling in the water seal without bubbling in the suction chamber means that the suction source must be increased.

15. Negativity within the system arises from the suction control setting (cm H_2O), from maneuvers to clear the drainage tubing (milking, stripping), and from within the patient during increased inspiratory efforts. The degree of negativity is reflected in the assessment chamber which is calibrated in units of cm H_2O. On gravity drainage, the fluid level in the water-seal column will rise and the patient assessment column will de-

crease to equalize; on suction, the negativity is measured from the assessment chamber (narrow column attached).

Evaporation will lower the water levels over time and the chambers should be refilled with the suction off to ensure an accurate level. If overfilled, fluid removal is difficult because no access ports are available. A catheter would have to be inserted from the top and placed to suction.

16. Tipping the unit will rarely result in loss of the water seal unless the unit is almost totally inverted. Water from the underwater seal and suction chambers may mix if the unit is tipped and would need adjustment.

17. Excess negativity is automatically vented at approximately -60 cm H_2O pressure and returned to the original setting.

18. Excess positive pressure ($> +2$ cm H_2O) is automatically relieved from a vent on top of the suction control chamber and the assessment chamber is also open to air, allowing another site for excess positive pressure release.

19. Fluid samples are taken from the self-sealing latex tubing.

COMPLICATIONS

1. Enlarging pneumo/hemothorax evolving into a tension status if there is inadvertent compression of the patient tubing, biologic obstruction, or insufficient suction.
2. Incomplete drainage of fluid may result in fibrothorax.
3. Capillary damage and entrapment of lung tissue may occur if excessive negative pressure is generated by maneuvers such as stripping or milking chest tubes (Duncan, 1982).
4. Tipping of the unit will result in mixing of fluid from some chambers (see 16 above).
5. Suction regulators on portable pumps may be inaccurate. Ensure that they are properly calibrated.

PATIENT TEACHING

1. Report any shortness of breath, chest pain, or system disconnections immediately.
2. Do not lie on the tubing or allow it to be kinked. Keep the unit upright at all times.

REFERENCES

Duncan, C., & Erickson, R. 1982. Pressures associated with chest tube stripping. *Heart & Lung,* 11 2:166–171.

SUGGESTED READINGS

Besson, A., & Saegesser, F. 1983. *Color atlas of chest trauma and associated injuries,* volume one. Oradell, NJ: Medical Economics.

Hamilton, H.K. ed. 1984. *Nurse's clinical library: Respiratory disorders.* Springhouse, PA: Springhouse.

Luce, J.M., Tyler, M.L., & Pierson, D.J. 1984. *Intensive respiratory care.* Philadelphia: Saunders.

Sherwood Medical. 1979. *Clinical aspects of chest drainage: Argyle® Double Seal chest drainage unit.* St. Louis: Sherwood Medical.

53

Chest Drainage Devices: Atrium

Valerie Novotny-Dinsdale, RN, MSN, CEN

The Atrium unit is also known as 2002 single collection water-seal chest drainage unit.

Note: The information in this chapter should be used in conjunction with the information in Ch. 43: Management of Chest Drainage Systems.

INDICATIONS

1. To evacuate air and fluid from the pleural space and reexpand the lung by restoring negative intrapleural pressure.

CONTRAINDICATIONS AND CAUTIONS

1. The unit must be kept in the upright position and below the patient's chest to maximize drainage efficiency.
2. Water-seal and suction-control chambers must be filled to prescribed levels for best results (Atrium, 1989).

EQUIPMENT

Atrium 2002 single collection unit
Tape
2 rubber tipped clamps (to diagnose airleaks and to clamp the tube in 2 places should the unit become full)

500 ml of water (sterile water is needed for blood recovery procedures)

PATIENT PREPARATION

*Insert a chest tube. See Ch. 42: Chest Tube Insertion.

*Indicates those portions of the procedure usually performed by a physician.

PROCEDURAL STEPS

1. To fill the water-seal chamber, remove tape holding the funnel assembly.
2. Hold the preattached funnel, level with the unit and add 25 ml of water.
3. Raise the funnel, turn the suction control stopcock to the on position, and fill the chamber. Once the water has passed to the chamber, the suction control stopcock must be returned to the off position prior to connecting it to the unregulated suction. See Figure 53.1 on page 166.
4. Discard the funnel after use or use it to fill the suction control chamber. See Step 5 below.
5. To fill the suction control chamber, remove the suction control vent plug and pour the amount of sterile water into the chamber needed for the desired suction pressure.

Suction Pressure	Water Volume Needed
-20 cm H_2O	320 cc
-15 cm H_2O	180 cc
-10 cm H_2O	80 cc
-5 cm H_2O	38 cc

(Atrium 2002 single collection water seal chest drainage unit instructions, 1989)

5. Replace the suction control vent plug.
6. Remove the cap from the patient tube connector and connect it to the patient's chest tube.
7. Lower the unit below the patient's chest level and keep it in the upright position by either using the bed attachment hooks or the floor stand.

Figure 53.1   Atrium water-seal chest drainage unit.
(Atrium Medical Corporation, 1989. Reprinted by permission.)

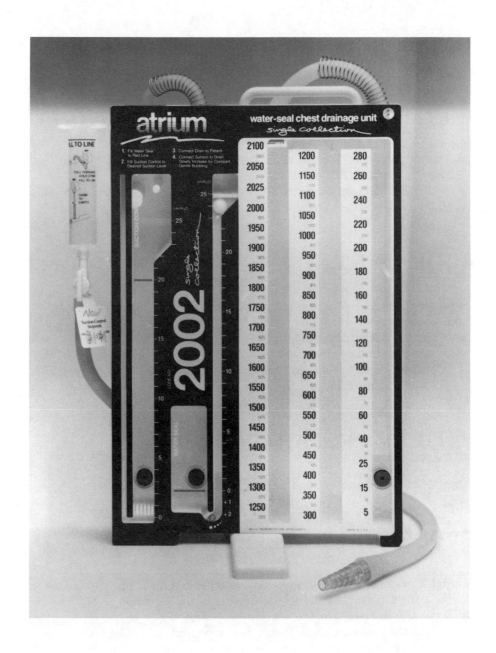

8. Connect the suction source to the suction control stopcock. Tape all connections to prevent accidental disconnections.
9. Slowly increase the suction pressure until constant gentle bubbling occurs.
10. To increase or decrease suction pressure, turn off the suction source and adjust the water level to the desired amount. A syringe and 18-G needle can be used to access the front face grommet.
11. Observe the water seal for air leaks and changes in pressure. No bubbling with the float ball above the air leak zone indicates that there is not an air leak. Constant or intermittent bubbling with the float ball in the air leak zone indicates a leak in either the patient connection or the thoracic cavity. See Figure 53.2.

    To determine the source of the leak, pinch or clamp the patient's tube with rubber tipped hemostats below the catheter connection. If bubbling stops, the air leak is external to the system and may indicate a patient air leak. The patient's chest dressing should be peeled back to see if the chest tube eyelets are visible. If so, this should be treated as a chest tube dislodgement and the physician must be notified immediately. If the bubbling continues, it indicates a leak in the drainage system. All connections should be checked and the unit observed for cracks.
12. Changes in patient pressure can be detected by observing the float ball in the calibrated water-seal column. When connected to suction, the patient's pressure will be equal to the suction-control setting plus the float ball level. Accumulated positive pressure is automatically released by the in-line positive pressure valve.

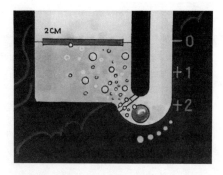

Figure 53.2 Atrium water-seal with float ball in the air leak zone. (Atrium Medical Corporation, 1989. Reprinted by permission.)

COMPLICATIONS

1. Poor drainage due to tubing hanging below the collection chamber.
2. Poor drainage or development of a tension pneumothorax due to kinked or occluded tubing.
3. Accidental disconnection resulting in respiratory distress.
4. Accidental dislodgement of the chest tube.
5. Loss of water seal if the unit is tipped.

PATIENT TEACHING

1. A constant bubbling sound in the unit is normal.
2. Report any respiratory difficulty immediately.
3. Do not lie on the tubing or allow it to be kinked. Keep the unit upright at all times.
4. Report any disconnections immediately and request assistance when changing positions to prevent accidental dislodgements or disconnections.

REFERENCES

Atrium 2002 single collection water seal drainage unit instruction sheet. 1989. Hollis, NH: Atrium Medical Corporation.

54

Thoracentesis

Manjula D. Gray, RN, BSN, MA, CCRN
Anjula D. Littleton, RN, BSN, CCRN

INDICATIONS

1. To diagnose or remove fluid from the pleural cavity (pleural effusion).
2. To remove air from the pleural cavity in tension pneumothorax as a temporizing measure. However, needle thoracostomy and/or placement of a chest tube are the treatments of choice.

CONTRAINDICATIONS AND CAUTIONS

There are no contraindications, however caution should be used in the presence of
1. Compromised respiratory status (i.e., ventilator dependent patient, ruptured diaphgram, and emphysema), because of higher incidence of pneumothorax secondary to lung perforation.
2. Bleeding dyscrasias may cause hemothorax. (R.N. Dewan, MD., personal communication; October 18, 1990).
3. Pleural adhesions may cause perforation of the visceral pleura and/or the lung (Roberts, 1985).
4. The through-the-needle catheter technique should be used for supine patients.

EQUIPMENT

Sterile gloves
Antiseptic solution
Sterile towels
Local anesthetic
5-ml syringe with 25–27-gauge needle for anesthesia
22-gauge 1 1/2-inch needle
50-ml syringe for aspiration
Two 15–18-gauge 2-inch needles or a 14-gauge through-the-needle catheter and a 15-gauge 2-inch needle

Two curved hemostats
Three-way stopcock
Collection tubing (intravenous tubing without drip chamber or back check valve)
500–1000-ml vacuum bottles
Gauze dressings
Tape
Note: Preassembled kits containing some of this equipment are also available.

PATIENT PREPARATION

1. Place the patient in a sitting position, leaning forward on a bedside table with arms crossed. If unable to tolerate sitting position, place the patient in a supine position.

2. Cleanse the site with antiseptic solution. For the patient in supine position drape the area with a sterile towel. For a pneumothorax, the insertion site is the second intercostal space in the midclavicular line. For the removal of pleural fluid, the insertion site is the midscapular line or the posterior axillary line at a level below the top of the fluid (Roberts, 1985).

3. Encourage the patient to refrain from coughing during the procedure to prevent trauma to the lung.

PROCEDURAL STEPS

Rigid Needle Technique

1. *Infiltrate the area with local anesthetic directly inferior to the selected site.
2. *Change to the 22-gauge needle and continue anesthetic infiltration through the intercostal space until the pleura is entered.
3. *Aspirate fluid and clamp the curved hemostat to the needle at the skin surface.
4. *Remove the needle from the chest with the hemostat still clamped to the needle.
5. *Attach the 50-ml syringe and the 15–18-gauge needle to the three-way stopcock.
6. *Attach one end of the collection tubing to the stopcock and attach the other end of the tubing to a 15-gauge needle.
7. *Turn the stopcock off to the collection tubing.
8. *Attach the second hemostat to the needle on the stopcock at the same distance as the hemostat on the anesthetic needle.
9. *Enter the pleural space by inserting the needle to the depth of the hemostat and aspirate fluid. See Figure 54.1 on page 170.
10. *Clamp the tubing with the first hemostat and insert the needle on the connecting tubing into the vacuum bottle.
11. *Turn the stopcock off to the syringe and unclamp the tubing.
12. *Withdraw the desired amount of fluid. Turn the stopcock off to the tubing and withdraw the needle from the patient.
13. Apply sterile dressing and obtain a chest x-ray (Roberts, 1985).
14. Fluid from the syringe or the bottle may be sent to the laboratory for analysis. Commonly performed analyses include Gram's stain, culture and sensitivity, acid-fast staining and culture, differential cell count, cytology, pH, specific gravity, total protein, and lactic dehydrogenase.

Through-the-Needle Catheter Technique

1. *Follow preceding Steps 1 through 4.
2. *Insert the 14-gauge through-the-needle catheter the same distance as the anesthetic needle. See preceding Steps 8 and 9.
3. *Guide the catheter, within the plastic sleeve, through the needle into the pleural space. Discard the plastic sleeve. See Figure 54.2 on page 171.
4. *Withdraw the needle, leaving the catheter in the pleural space.
5. *Attach the catheter to a three-way stopcock and a 50-ml syringe (Wilkins, 1989).
6. *Follow preceding Steps 6 through 14.

COMPLICATIONS

1. Pneumothorax as a result of lung perforation.
2. Pulmonary edema from removing a large quantity of fluid. Do not remove more than 1 liter of fluid at one time, as this may lead to a sudden shift in mediastinal contents.

*Indicates portions of the procedure usually performed by a physician.

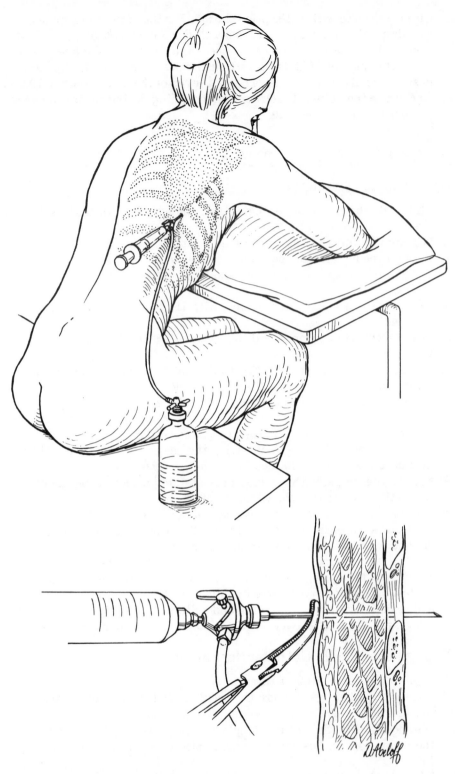

Figure 54.1   Needle thoracentesis.
(Rosen, & Sternbach, 1983: 63. Reprinted by permission.)

3.   Infection.
4.   Shearing of plastic catheter, if catheter is withdrawn through the needle.
5.   Hypoxia in patients with underlying respiratory pathology.
6.   Hemothorax from laceration of the lung, diaphragm, intercostal vessels, or internal mammary vessels (Roberts, 1985).

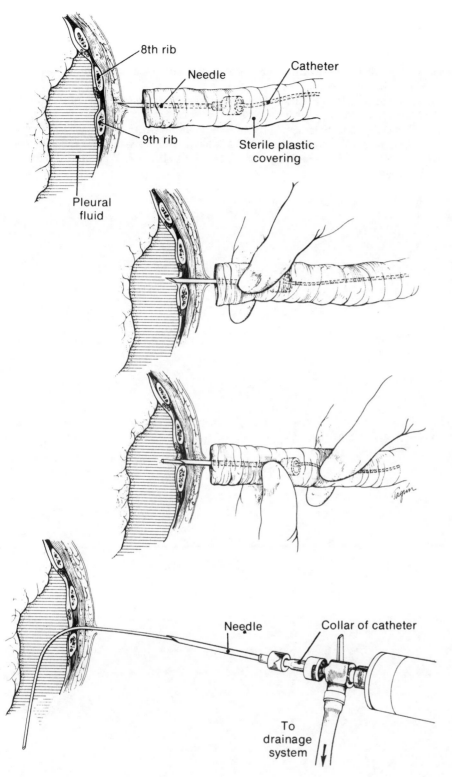

Figure 54.2   Thoracentesis with a through-the-needle catheter. (Wilkins, 1989: 1022. Reprinted by permission.)

PATIENT TEACHING

1. Immediately report any shortness of breath, faintness, bloody sputum, or chest pain.
2. Remain in position of comfort for one hour.

REFERENCES

Roberts, R.R., & Hedges, J.R. 1985. *Clinical procedures in emergency medicine.* Philadelphia: Saunders.

Rosen, P., & Sternbach, G.L. 1983. *Atlas of emergency medicine,* 2nd ed. Baltimore: Williams & Wilkins.

Wilkins, E.W., Jr. 1989. Thoracentesis. In E.W. Wilkins, Jr., J.J. Dineen, P.L. Gross, C.J. McCabe, A.C. Moncure, & P.J. O'Malley (eds). *Emergency medicine: Scientific foundations and current practice,* 3rd ed. Baltimore: Williams & Wilkins; 1021–1022.

55

Positioning the Hypotensive Patient

This position is also known as modified Trendelenberg.

Ruth Altherr Giebel, MS, RN

INDICATIONS

1. Symptomatic hypotension due to hypovolemia, vasovagal reaction, or medications.

CONTRAINDICATIONS AND CAUTIONS

1. Care should be taken to avoid the use of modified Trendelenburg in the case of potential head or brain injuries. This may include stroke, head trauma, brain surgery, and respiratory or cardiac arrests. The appropriate position for a hypotensive patient with possible neurologic impairment is supine and flat (Rollheiser, 1986).
2. In the case of other types of shock, the best position to promote cerebral and cardiac circulation is the flat, supine position (Rollheiser, 1986).

PROCEDURAL STEPS

1. Place patient supine.
2. Raise lower extremities to a maximum elevation of 20–30 degrees. See Figure 55.1.
3. Do not lower the patient's head below the level of the body.

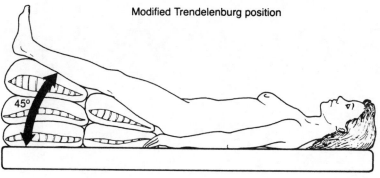

Modified Trendelenburg position

45°

Lower extremities elevated   Patient flat

Figure 55.1   Modified Trendelenberg position.
(Kitt & Kaiser, 1990: 295. Reprinted by permission.)

PATIENT TEACHING

1. Explain that the position is temporary.

REFERENCES

Springhouse Corp. 1986. *Cardiovascular Care Handbook.* Springhouse, PA:
    Springhouse Corp.
Kitt, S., & Kaiser, J. 1990. *Emergency nursing: A physiologic and clinical perspec-
    tive.* Philadelphia: Saunders.
Rollheiser, E.E. 1986. Shock and the Trendelberg position. *AARN Newsletter,* 42,
    8:17–8.

SUGGESTED READINGS

Carey, K.W. (ed). 1984. *Shock.* Springhouse, PA: Springhouse Corp.
Wilcox, S., & Vandam, L.D. 1988. Alas, poor Trendelenberg and his position! *Anesth
    Analg,* 67:574–8.

56

Doppler Ultrasound for Assessment of Blood Pressure and Peripheral Pulses

Ruth Altherr Giebel, MS, RN

INDICATIONS

1. To amplify the blood pressure and/or pulse when auscultation by stethoscope is unsuccessful (i.e., in the presence of hypotension or a noisy environment).
2. To assess peripheral blood flow when circulatory impairment or vascular trauma is suspected.

CONTRAINDICATIONS AND CAUTIONS

1. Avoid using the probe near the eyes as damage to the nerve tissue may result. (Durbin, 1983)
2. Improper probe placement may result in erroneous interpretations. Care should be taken to verify that the signal heard is coming from the vessel intended and not a collateral vessel. This can be done by assessing the quality of the sound as described in the Complications section of this chapter.
3. Excess pressure on the probe may abolish the signal.
4. Verify sensitivity when signals are absent at a position where they would normally be expected. Sensitivity may be verified by checking one's own pulses with the Doppler device.
5. Presence of a signal does not always indicate that circulation and perfusion are adequate to maintain viable tissue. Absence of a signal does not always indicate that there is no blood flow through the vessel.
6. Doppler devices are only able to detect blood velocities that are at least 6-cm/sec (Stair, 1985).
7. Tissue penetration will vary between different types of Dopplers. The higher frequency sound waves yield better resolution for superficial vessels, and the lower frequency sound waves allow penetration of deeper tissues with less scatter. Most Doppler instruments are supplied with a fixed frequency. The frequency required for assessment of blood pressure and peripheral blood flow superficially is 5–10MHz (Stair, 1985).

EQUIPMENT

Doppler probe with a frequency of 5–10 MHz and amplifier. See Figure 56.1.

Ultrasonic transmission gel
Blood pressure cuff
Wet towel or tissue

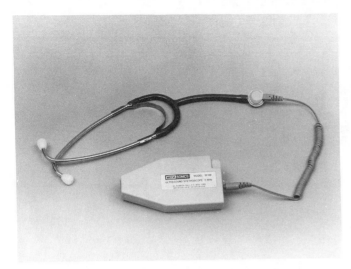

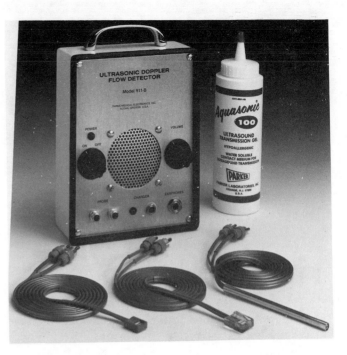

Figure 56.1 Examples of 2 commercially available Doppler probes.
(A. Courtesy of Medasonics, Inc., Mountain View, CA;
b. Courtesy of Parks Medical Electronics, Inc., Aloha, OR.)

PROCEDURAL STEPS

Blood pressure measurement

1. Apply transmission gel to the detector surface of the probe.
2. Turn on the Doppler instrument and insert stethoscope earpieces, if applicable.
3. Adjust the volume control as necessary.
4. Identify the brachial pulse with the Doppler instrument.
5. Obtain the blood pressure in the usual manner substituting the Doppler probe for a stethoscope. Position probe over the brachial artery and tilt it so that it is at a 45-degree angle to the vessel.
   a. Inflate the blood pressure cuff until arterial sounds are no longer audible.
   b. Deflate the cuff slowly, listening for the first sound which is the systolic pressure.
6. Clean the gel from the patient's skin with a wet towel or tissue.
7. Clean the face of the Doppler probe detector with a damp towel or tissue. Do not use alcohol or other organic solvents to clean the probe detector. The probe may be gas sterilized, but should not be autoclaved or immersed in liquid.

Assessment of peripheral blood flow

1. Apply transmission gel to the detector surface of the probe.
2. Turn on the Doppler instrument and insert the stethoscope earpieces, if applicable.
3. Place the probe over the vessel to be assessed and tilt probe so that it is at a 45-degree angle to the vessel. Standard arterial locations include brachial, radial, femoral, popliteal, dorsalis pedis, and posterior tibial.
4. Adjust volume control as necessary.
5. Mark pulse location with a waterproof marker. Compare blood flow bilaterally. Begin assessing the extremity in the most distal aspect. If you do not find a pulse with the Doppler instrument, move to a more proximal site. Continue to move more proximally until you are able to identify blood flow. The findings may then be recorded by describing the pulses at each location assessed as being *absent, present,* or *diminished* (Hudson, 1983).

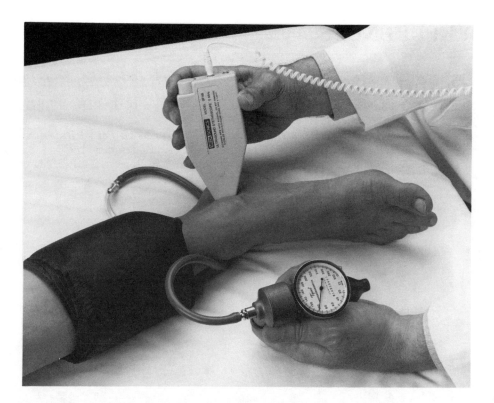

Figure 56.2 Measurement of the systolic blood pressure in the leg.
(*Courtesy of Medasonics, Inc., Mountain View, CA.*)

6. If directed to do so you may obtain a systolic blood pressure on a patient's leg by following these steps:
   a. Place a blood pressure cuff around the patient's ankle, leaving enough room to place the Doppler detector over the artery with the strongest pulse. See Figure 56.2.
   b. Inflate the blood pressure cuff until arterial sounds are no longer audible.
   c. Deflate the cuff slowly. Record the pressure reading at which you hear the first sound. This is the systolic pressure and is the only one attainable by this method.

COMPLICATIONS

1. Absence of a Doppler signal may be due to any of the following:
   a. blood flow at a speed less than the Doppler instrument can detect (6cm/sec) (Stair, 1985);
   b. excess pressure on the probe causing occlusion of the vessel;
   c. volume setting is too low;
   d. insufficient transmission gel;
   e. dead battery;
   f. damaged equipment.
2. Misinterpretation of the signal source. Arterial sounds are loud, high-pitched sounds with one or more softer, lower-pitched diastolic sounds repeated with each cardiac cycle. Venous sounds are normally cyclic, occur with respirations, and produce a high-pitch sound on expiration which resembles a windstorm.
3. Although the output of ultrasonic signals from diagnostic Doppler applications is very low, prolonged unnecessary exposure to ultrasonic signals should be avoided to prevent tissue damage. (*Instructions*, 1985)

REFERENCES

Durbin, N. 1983. The application of Doppler techniques in critical care. *Focus on Critical Care,* 10, 3:45–46.

Hudson, B. 1983. Sharpen your vascular assessment skills with the Doppler Ultrasound Stethoscope. *Nursing,* 13, 5:54–57.

Instructions: A Doppler instrument for the detection of blood flow, Ultrasound Stethoscope Model BF4A. 1985. Mountain View, CA: Medasonics, Inc.

Stair, T. 1985. The clinical use of Doppler ultrasound. In J.R. Roberts & J.R. Hedges (eds). *Clinical Procedures for Emergency Medicine.* Philadelphia: Saunders.

57

Electrocardiographic Monitoring

Ruth Altherr Giebel, MS, RN

INDICATIONS

To monitor cardiac rhythm and rate.

CONTRAINDICATIONS AND CAUTIONS

All equipment should be well-grounded to prevent electrical shock and electrical interference on the ECG tracing.

EQUIPMENT

ECG monitor
ECG Cable (3- or 5-lead system)
Pregelled disposable electrodes (3 to 5)

Razor (optional)
Alcohol sponges (optional)
Gauze dressings (optional)

PROCEDURAL STEPS

1. Turn on the monitor.
2. Select the desired lead. See Figures 57.1–57.5 on page 180.
3. Connect the electrodes to the lead wires and place electrodes on the skin at the appropriate sites, per Figures 57.1, 57.2, 57.3, 57.4, or 57.5. Avoid placing the electrodes over large muscle masses and bony structures.
4. Observe the ECG tracing. Ideally the tracing should be free of excessive artifact with an adequate R wave to allow for accurate heartrate determinations.
5. Set heartrate alarm rates and turn the alarms on.

TROUBLESHOOTING ECG TECHNICAL PROBLEMS

1. AC Interference (Also known as 60-cycle interference). See Figure 57.6 on page 181.

   Possible causes
   a. Nearby electrical equipment, power cords, electrical wiring in room walls and floors.
   b. Improper grounding of electrical equipment in the area.
   c. Unshielded lead wires or patient cable.
   d. Loose connections in the system (i.e., electrodes, lead wires, cable).
   e. Inadequate skin prep.
   f. Dry electrodes.

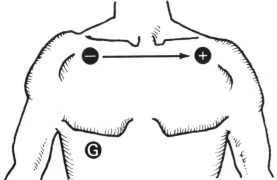

Figure 57.1   Lead II.
(American Heart Association, 1987: 52. Reprinted by permission.)

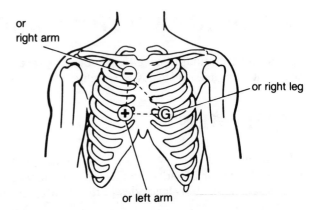

Figure 57.2   Marriott's MCL1, aides in QRS morphology differentiation.
(Persons, 1987: 11. Reprinted by permission.)

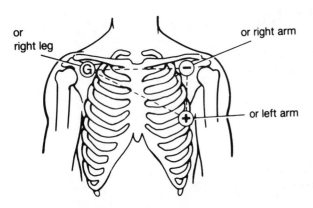

Figure 57.3   Marriott's MCL6, aides in QRS morphology differentiation.
(Persons, 1987: 11. Reprinted by permission.)

Figure 57.4   Lewis lead, aides in locating P waves.
(Persons, 1987: 11. Reprinted by permission.)

Figure 57.5   Five-lead system. (From AACN Procedure Manual for Critical Care(2nd ed.) by S. Millar, L.K. Sampson and S.M. Soukup, 1985, p. 21. Copyright 1985 by W.B. Saunders Company. Reprinted by permission.)

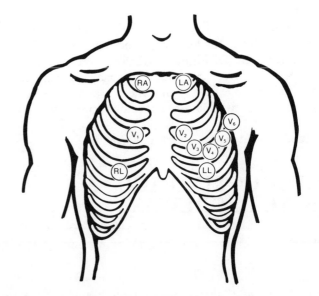

Solutions
a. Properly ground equipment in patient area.
b. Verify electrode, lead, and cable connections.
c. Prep skin using the following procedure and apply new electrodes.
   – Shave area as necessary
   – Cleanse the skin with an alcohol swab.
   – Abrade the skin with dry gauze pad.

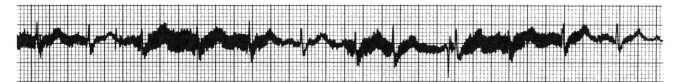

2. Low Voltage See Figure 57.7

Figure 57.6   Common ECG problem patterns: AC electrical interference (60 cycles per second).

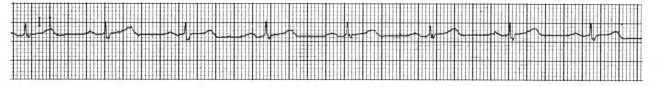

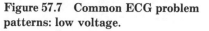

Figure 57.7   Common ECG problem patterns: low voltage.

Possible causes

a. Low gain setting on the ECG monitor.
b. Poor electrode contact or disconnected electrode.
c. Broken or disconnected lead wire.
d. Loose cable connection.
e. Patient position change causing low amplitude of QRS signal.

Solutions

a. Increase gain on monitor.
b. Verify that all connections are intact.
c. Change electrodes.
d. Select another lead to monitor.

3. Excessive Artifact See Figure 57.8.

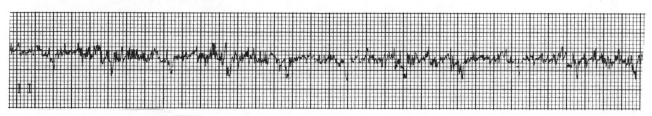

Possible Causes

a. Patient movement.
b. Loose electrode, lead or cable connections.
c. Intermittent electrical interference.

Figure 57.8   Common ECG problem patterns: excessive artifact.

Solutions

a. Verify electrode placement or move electrode to a new location where there is less skeletal muscle.
b. Replace electrode if loose.
c. Verify connections.
d. Support lead wires and cable to prevent tension on the cable-lead system with patient movement.

4. Wandering Baseline See Figure 57.9.

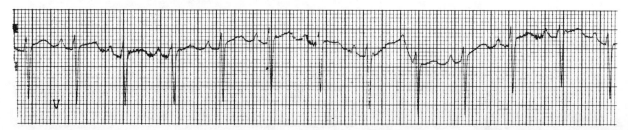

Figure 57.9   Common ECG problem patterns: wandering baseline.

Possible causes

a. Cable movement with respirations or patient movement.

b. Poor electrode contact or location.

c. Excess tension on cable-lead system.

Solutions

a. Reposition cable where it will be exposed to less movement.

b. Change electrodes and select a new location if necessary.

c. Secure cable-lead system to reduce tension.

PATIENT TEACHING

1. Report any chest pain, palpitations, shortness of breath, or related symptoms immediately.
2. Report any disconnections in the system.

REFERENCES

American Heart Association. 1987. *Textbook of advanced cardiac life support.* Dallas: Am. Heart Assoc.

Mock, N. 1985. Lead systems. In S. Millar, L.K. Sampson, & S.M. Soukup (eds). *AACN Procedure Manual for Critical Care.* Philadelphia: Saunders, 16–24.

Persons, C.B. 1987. Hard-wire monitoring. In C.B. Persons (ed). *Critical Care Procedures and Protocols: A Nursing Process Approach.* Philadelphia: Lippincott; 10–16.

SUGGESTED READINGS

Conover, M.B. 1980. *Understanding electrocardiography: Physiological and interpretative.* St. Louis: Mosby.

Suazo, N.L. 1983. Is there a best lead system? *Critical Care Update,* August, 24–26.

58

12-Lead Electrocardiogram

Ruth Altherr Giebel, MS, RN

12-Lead ECG is also known as 12-Lead EKG.

INDICATIONS

1. To aid in the diagnosis of acute myocardial ischemia, injury, and infarction.
2. To diagnose and differentiate cardiac dysrhythmias and conduction defects.

CONTRAINDICATIONS AND CAUTIONS

1. All electrical equipment including the 12-lead ECG machine should be well-grounded to prevent electrical shock and electrical interference on the ECG tracing.
2. Do not touch ECG machine, patient cable, or patient during defibrillation.

EQUIPMENT

12-Lead ECG machine
ECG cable and leads
Electrodes (plates, suction cups, or
     pregelled disposable
     electrodes)

Electrical conductive gel or cream
Damp towels
Tissues

PATIENT PREPARATION

1. Center the patient on the bed so that no parts of the body touch the side rails, the head, or the foot of the bed.

PROCEDURAL STEPS

1. Connect the power cord into a grounded electrical outlet and turn the ECG machine on.
2. Place a small amount of the conductive media on the metal plate of the limb leads and attach to the inner aspect of each forearm and the medial aspect of each leg with rubber straps or tape or apply disposable electrodes to the same site.
3. Determine the location for precordial leads. Lead V1 is located in the 4th intercostal space (ICS) along the right sternal border. Lead V2 is located in the 4th ICS along the left sternal border. Lead V4 is located in the 5th ICS at the midclavicular line. Lead V3 is located midway between V2

and V4 in the 5th ICS. Lead V6 is located in the 5th ICS at the midaxillary line. Lead V5 is located midway between Lead V4 and Lead V6 in the 5th ICS. See Figure 58.1.

Note: Precordial lead sites may be marked with a waterproof marker to allow consistent placement from test to test.

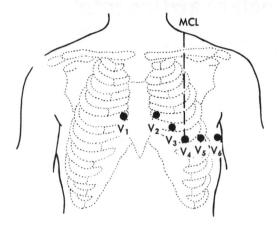

Figure 58.1 Standard precordial chest lead placement.
(Andreoli et. al., 1987: 91. Reprinted by permission.)

4. Apply electrode conductive gel or paste to the precordial sites if nondisposable electrodes are to be used.
5. Connect the patient leads/electrodes to the appropriate extremity and precordial location as indicated on each lead. Limb leads are color coded as follows:
   a. Right arm—white
   b. Left arm—black
   c. Right leg—green
   d. Left leg—red
6. Press the calibration button to verify the standardization of the signal. The calibration pulse should be at least 10 mm for a standard 12-lead ECG. The gain may be decreased in the presence of excessively tall ECG complexes and should be noted as such on the tracing.
7. Set paper speed at 25 mm/sec. The paper speed may be at 50 mm/sec to allow for better visualization of the ECG complexes and should be so noted on the tracing.
8. For a multichannel recording:
   a. connect all leads prior to obtaining the ECG;
   b. depress the auto-run button after inserting paper;
   c. if additional rhythm strips of specific leads are required, you may run them manually by selecting the appropriate lead button.
9. For a single channel ECG machine:
   a. connect the limb leads;
   b. select lead I and place in the run position to record at least 6 seconds;
   c. record leads II, III, aVR, aVF, aVL in the same manner. When changing leads turn the power switch to the on position.
   d. Record each chest lead VI–V6 by moving the precordial electrode between recordings to the next precordial lead location as marked. Turn switch to the on position while moving the electrode.
10. Depress the marker button to identify each lead while running the ECG. The standard code for labeling leads is as follows:

Lead I   _____

Lead II   _____ _____

Lead III   _____ _____ _____

Lead aVR   _____

Lead aVL   _____ _____

Lead aVF   _____ _____ _____

Lead V1   _____ ____

Lead V2   _____ ____ ____

Lead V3   _____ ____ ____ ____

Lead V4   _____ ____ ____ ____ ____

Lead V5   _____ ____ ____ ____ ____ ____

Lead V6   _____ ____ ____ ____ ____ ____ ____

11. After recording all twelve leads turn the recorder off, remove electrodes, and cleanse the sites with tissue or damp towels as needed.

COMPLICATIONS

1. Equipment malfunction
2. Electromicroshock

TROUBLESHOOTING ECG TECHNICAL PROBLEMS

1. AC Interference. See Ch. 57: ECG Monitoring.
2. Wandering Baseline. See Ch. 57: ECG Monitoring.
3. Tremor

   Possible causes
   a. Patient is tense or uncomfortable.
   b. If electrode plates are used, the straps may be too tight.

   Solution
   a. Assist patient into a comfortable position and encourage relaxation.
   b. Loosen electrode straps.
4. Intermittent or Jittery Waveforms

   Possible Causes
   a. Loose connections
   b. Broken lead wires
   c. Poor skin preparation
   d. Contaminated conductive gel or cream
   e. Patient movement and tension

   Solutions
   a. Check all connections.
   b. Test lead wires for breaks by wiggling them and watching for the effect on the recording.
   c. Reapply the electrodes with proper skin preparation technique and with fresh electrode conductive gel or cream.

PATIENT TEACHING

1. You must lie still and not talk during the recording.

REFERENCES

Andreoli, K.A., Lipes, D.P., Wallace, A.K., Kinney, M.R., & Fowkes, V.K. 1987. *Comprehensive cardiac care,* 6th ed. St. Louis: Mosby.

Hill, N.E., & Goodman, J.S. 1987. Importance of accurate placement of precordial leads in the 12-lead electrocardiogram. *Heart and Lung,* 16:561–566.

Mock, N. 1985. 12-Lead ECG. In S. Millar, L.K. Sampson, & S.M. Soukoup (eds). *AACN Procedure Manual for Critical Care,* 2nd ed. Philadelphia: Saunders. 8–15.

SUGGESTED READINGS

Operating and self-training guide for the EKG technician. 1981. Andover, MA: Saunders.

Sumner, S.M. 1985. Guidelines for running a 12-lead E.K.G. *Nursing,* December, 30–33.

59

Measuring Postural Vital Signs

Dorothy M. Schulte, RN, MS

Postural vital signs are also known as orthostatic vital signs, tilt test.

INDICATIONS

1. To safely and noninvasively evaluate a patient's fluid status.
2. To evaluate a patient with a history of significant vomiting, diarrhea, diaphoresis, blunt abdominal or chest trauma, history of acute or chronic internal bleeding, abdominal pain, unexplained syncope, weakness or dizziness, obvious and significant external bleeding, and unexplained hypotension or tachycardia of greater than 120 beats/minute (Wells, 1979).

CONTRAINDICATIONS AND CAUTIONS

1. An assistant may be necessary because a patient with hypovolemia may experience dizziness, light-headedness, or syncope when moving from a lying to a standing position for postural vital sign measurement. Do not leave the patient alone during this procedure.
2. Orthostatic readings taken when a person moves from a lying to a sitting position are less accurate than standing measurements and may result in false negative readings because there are smaller decreases in stroke volume and cardiac output and smaller increases in heart rate when compared to standing (Stenberg, 1967). Studies also indicate that lying to sitting vital sign measurements are not reliable in discriminating between no blood loss and losses of 500–1000 ml (Knopp, 1980).
3. Postural vital sign measurement may not be valid in assessing the presence of hypovolemia in pediatric patients (Bergman, 1983).
4. Postural vital sign measurements may be falsely positive as studies indicate that 20% of all persons greater than 65 and 30–50% of persons over 75 will have postural hypotension associated with age (Robbins, 1984). Another study found 43% of presumed euvolemic patients (no recent history of blood or fluid loss) had positive postural vital signs (Koziol-McLain, 1991).
5. Orthostatic hypotension can be seen in patients on ganglion blockers, sympatholytic drugs, oral diuretics, phenothiazines, antihistamines, cyclic antidepressants, barbiturates, and anticholinergic medications, which could result in postural vital sign changes in the absence of hypovolemia (Caird, 1973).
6. Alcohol abuse may result in orthostatic hypotension in the absence of hypovolemia due to catecholamine disturbance and vasodilating effects (Schatz, 1984).

EQUIPMENT

Sphygmomanometer with blood pressure cuff*

Stethoscope
Stretcher

*An automated blood pressure machine may be used if available.

PATIENT PREPARATION

Have the patient lie in a supine position for 2–5 minutes prior to taking the initial measurements.

PROCEDURAL STEPS

1. Take blood pressure and heart rate measurements while the patient is in the supine position.
2. Have patient move from supine to sitting position (if three measurements are to be taken) or from supine to standing position.
3. Question the patient about weakness, dizziness, or visual dimming associated with position change. Note any pallor or diaphoresis.
4. Within 30 seconds to two minutes take the standing or sitting blood pressure and heart rate measurements. Support the forearm at heart level when taking the blood pressure to prevent an inaccurate measurement.
5. If an intermediate sitting measurement was taken, have the patient move into the standing position and repeat Steps 3 and 4.
6. Return the patient to supine or sitting position.
7. Note on the patient record all measurements taken and if they were taken in lying, sitting, or standing positions. Positive findings are considered to be heart rate increases of greater than 20 beats/minute and systolic blood pressure decreases of greater than 10 mm Hg.
8. Return the patient to supine or sitting position.

COMPLICATIONS

1. Weakness, dizziness, and syncope

REFERENCES

Bergman, G., Reisner, F., & Anwar, R. 1983. Orthostatic changes in normovolemic children: An analysis of the tilt test. *Journal of Emergency Medicine* 1:137–141.

Caird, F.I., Andrews, G.R., & Kennedy, R.D. 1973. Effect of posture on blood pressure in the elderly. *British Heart Journal*, 35:527–530.

Knopp, R., Claypool, R., & Leonardi, D. 1980. Use of the tilt test in measuring acute blood loss. *Annals of Emergency Medicine* 9:29–32.

Koziol-McLain, J., Lowenstein, S.R., & Fuller, B. 1991. Orthostatic vital signs in emergency department patients. *Annals of Emergency Medicine*, 20:606–610.

Robbins, A., & Rubenstein, L. 1984. Postural hypotension in the elderly. *Journal of the American Geriatrics Society*, 32:769–774.

Schatz, I. 1984. Orthostatic hypotension: Clinical diagnosis, testing and treatment. *Archives of Internal Medicine*, 144:1037–1041.

Stenberg, J., Astrand, P., Ekblom, B. Royces, J., & Saltim, B. 1967. Hemodynamic response to work with different muscle groups, sitting and supine. *Journal of Applied Physiology*, 22, 1:61–70.

Wells, J.J. 1979. Clinical assessment and priority setting. *Emergency Nursing Update Series*, 1:2–7.

60

External Cardiac Massage

Ruth Altherr Giebel, MS, RN

External cardiac massage is also
known as external chest
compressions, cardiopulmonary
resuscitation (CPR).

INDICATIONS

To circulate blood in the pulseless patient.

CONTRAINDICATIONS AND CAUTIONS

1. Proper assessment of the patient is necessary to ensure that external cardiac massage is not performed on an adult patient with a pulse. (Standards for CPR & ECC, 1986)
2. Cardiac massage is useless if inadequate ventilatory support is provided.

PATIENT PREPARATION

1. Establish unresponsiveness by shaking or tapping the patient and asking, "Are you OK?".
2. Place the patient in a supine position.
3. Call for help.
4. Establish a patent airway and assess for spontaneous respirations. See Ch. 4: Airway Positioning.
5. If respirations are absent, ventilate the patient with one of the following techniques:
   a. mouth-to-mouth
   b. mouth-to-mask See Ch. 35: Mouth-to-Mask Ventilation.
   c. bag-valve-mask See Ch. 36: Bag-Valve-Mask Ventilation.
6. Place a firm support under the chest.

PROCEDURAL STEPS

1. Give two full breaths.
2. Watch for chest rise and fall to verify adequate ventilation. Assess the carotid pulse. Gently palpate the pulse for 5 to 10 seconds. See Figure 60.1 on page 190.
3. If the patient is pulseless, initiate external chest compressions.
4. Kneel or stand at the victim's side near the chest.
5. Locate proper hand position. See Figure 60.2, left on page 190.
   a. With the middle and index fingers of the hand nearest the legs, find the edge of the rib cage and follow it up to the notch where the ribs meet the sternum at the center of the chest (above the xiphoid process).
   b. Place the middle finger on the notch with the index finger next to it.

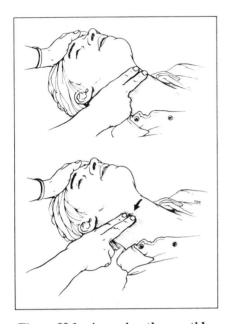

Figure 60.1 Assessing the carotid pulse.
(American Heart Association, 1986: 2919. Reprinted by permission.)

c. Place the heel of the opposite hand on the lower half of the sternum next to your index finger. The long axis of the heel of the hand should be placed along the long axis of the sternum to allow the main force of the compression to be directed onto the sternum.

d. Place the first hand on top of the hand on the sternum so that the hands are parallel.

e. Extend or interlock the fingers so they do not touch the chest wall.

6. Begin chest compressions using the following guidelines for optimum effectiveness. See Figure 60.2, right.

a. With the elbows locked, arms straight, and the shoulders directly over your hands, deliver the thrust of each compression straight down onto the sternum.

b. Depress the sternum 1.5 to 2 inches (for a normal-sized adult) with each compression.

c. Release each compression completely to allow blood flow into the heart prior to the next compression. The release time should equal the time required for the compression.

d. Chest compression should be performed at a minimum rate of 80 per minute, and up to a rate of 100 per minute if possible. For one-rescuer CPR the ratio of compressions to ventilations is 15:2. For two-rescuer CPR the ratio of compressions to ventilations is 5:1.

7. Ventilate the patient during a brief pause in compressions; see Ch. 36: Bag-Valve-Mask Ventilation. If the patient is intubated, no pause in compressions is necessary for ventilation (American Heart Association, 1986).

8. Assessment during external cardiac massage.

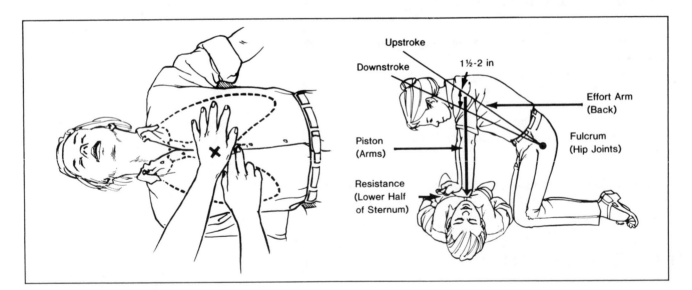

Figure 60.2 External chest compression. Left, locating the correct hand position on the lower half of the body; right, Proper position of the rescuer, with shoulders directly over the victim's sternum and elbows locked.
(American Heart Association, 1986: 2920. Reprinted by permission.)

a. The pulse is reassessed after the first four cycles of compressions and ventilations and every few minutes thereafter.

b. Assess the carotid pulse for 5 seconds. If it is absent, chest compressions are reinstituted after 2 full ventilations are given.

c. If a pulse is present, check for breathing. If both are present, continue to monitor the patient closely. If breathing is absent, continue to ventilate the patient 12 times per minute and closely monitor the pulse.

d. Never interrupt resuscitation efforts for more than 7 seconds except in special circumstances (i.e., during placement of a central intravenous line or transvenous pacemaker).

e. During a 2-person resuce, the ventilator is responsible for monitoring the effectiveness of the pulse produced by chest compressions.
f. Continue cardiac compressions and ventilations until advanced life support personnel and equipment are available, resuscitation is turned over to another equally qualified rescuer, the rescuer(s) is(are) exhausted, or the patient is pronounced dead (American Heart Association, 1986).

COMPLICATIONS

1. Death due to inadequate circulation. This can occur even if chest compressions are correctly applied.
2. Rib fractures.
3. Fracture of the sternum.
4. Rib separation from sternum.
5. Pneumothorax
6. Hemothorax
7. Lung contusions
8. Lacerations of liver and spleen
9. Fat emboli

PATIENT EDUCATION

Chest soreness is common following compressions.

REFERENCES

American Heart Association. 1986. Standards for cardiopulmonary resuscitation (CPR) and emergency cardiac care (ECC), *Journal of the American Medical Association*, 255:2915–2932.

SUGGESTED READING

Kozier, B., & Erb. G. 1989. Administering external CPR to an adult. In *Techniques in Clinical Nursing*. Redwood City, CA: Addison-Wesley.

61

Phlebotomy for Laboratory Specimens

Linell M. Jones, RN, BSN, CEN, CCRN

Phlebotomy for laboratory specimens is also known as blood draw, blood collection, blood tests, venipuncture.

INDICATIONS

To obtain blood for laboratory studies.

CONTRAINDICATIONS AND CAUTIONS

1. Patients undergoing thrombolytic therapy should have very limited punctures. If venipuncture is absolutely necessary, use the smallest possible needle (i.e., 23G).
2. Patients should have initial blood specimens drawn at the time IVs are started whenever possible to limit the number of punctures.
3. Blood should never be drawn proximal to a running IV line. It is preferable to draw from the other arm, but if this is not possible turn off the line for 2 minutes then draw from a site distal to the line.
4. Never do a venipuncture on a standing patient.
5. Avoid venipunctures in an arm containing an arteriovenous shunt or fistula or on the same side as a radical mastectomy.
6. Label all tubes immediately after blood collection. Do not allow unlabeled tubes to leave the patient's bedside or the possession of the person drawing the blood.
7. Patients who are extremely difficult to draw or those who should not have large volumes of blood drawn, such as those on hemodialysis or with blood dyscrasias, may benefit from using neonatal or pediatric blood sample tubes.
8. Use of a tight tourniquet on elderly patients with friable veins may cause the vein to rupture when punctured. Use a loose tourniquet or no tourniquet.
9. Informed consent may be required prior to Human Immunodeficiency Virus (HIV) testing. Refer to your institution's policy.

EQUIPMENT

Tourniquet or blood pressure cuff
Antiseptic solution or prep pads
Needles (21 G or 23 G) and syringe
Vacutainer type holder and needle
    See Figure 61.1.
All necessary evacuated tubes.
    Check with your laboratory.
    Common color codes are
      purple top for hematology;
      red or speckled top for
      chemistry;
      blue top for coagulation;
      yellow for blood culture.
Cotton balls or 2-×-2-inch gauze
    dressings
Tape
Patient labels
Gloves

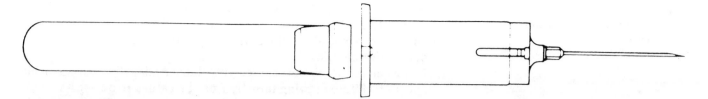

PATIENT PREPARATION

Figure 61.1 Vacutainer blood collection set.
(Used with permission of Becton Dickinson Vacutainer Systems, Rutherford, NJ.)

1. Positively identify the patient.
2. Check for restrictions such as IVs, shunts, thrombolytic therapy, uncooperative patient.
3. Position patient: sitting with arm extended and supported comfortably or lying down with arm extended at side.
4. To prevent aspiration in the event of syncope, be sure patient does not have anything in his or her mouth.
5. Assemble equipment (with extra tubes, needles, syringes) within easy reach.
6. Select site. The most common sites are the veins in the antecubital fossa, the cephalic, basilic, and median cubital (also known as the median basilic). See Figure 66.2. Any vein may be used.
7. Apply the tourniquet or cuff 3–4 inches proximal to the puncture site.
8. Have the patient make a fist and hold it.
9. Palpate for a vein. Palpation is necessary even if the vein is visible to confirm location, direction, and suitability. Vessels that pulsate are arteries. Veins feel like an elastic tube. Thrombosed veins are hard or rigid and roll. Tendons may feel like veins. If in doubt, release the tourniquet while palpating and the fullness should disappear if the structure is a vein.
10. Find the best vein, but do not leave tourniquet on for more than 2 minutes because it may alter some laboratory values (M. Gilbert, personal communication; February 28, 1990).
11. If you are having difficulty finding a vein, be sure the arm is in a dependent position, try the other arm, gently massage the arm from wrist to elbow, tap over the vein site with your finger, apply a warm compress, or switch to a blood pressure cuff instead of a tourniquet.
12. Perform the venipuncture with the bevel of the needle up and inserted at approximately a 15-degree angle in line with the vein. The needle may be inserted directly over the vein or off to the side and then directed into the vein.
13. Withdraw blood.
    a. *Using a syringe.* Gently pull the plunger with one hand while stabilizing the syringe and needle with the other hand. Aspirating too forcefully may collapse the vein or hemolyze the specimen. This method is often used with smaller veins such as in the hand, in the elderly, or in the chronically ill, because the evacuated tube may provide too much suction.
    b. *Evacuated tube method.* The first tube may be placed in the holder and pushed to the line without loss of vacuum prior to the venipuncture. One hand stabilizes the holder while the other presses the tube onto the needle. The tube will fill and automatically stop when the vacuum is exhausted. If multiple samples are drawn, keep the holder and needle stable as the tubes are exchanged. Be sure to use a multiple sample needle to prevent blood from leaking while changing tubes. If no blood enters the tube and the needle is thought to be in the vein, change tubes before withdrawing the needle to verify that the tube does have a vacuum.

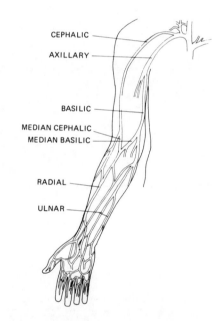

Figure 61.2 Anatomy of veins of upper extremity.
(American Heart Association, 1987: 143. Reprinted by permission.)

193

c. *Butterfly method.* A winged collection set with either luer adapter or tube holder adapters may be used with difficult veins. This method allows you to withdraw blood with very little manipulation of the needle within the vein.

d. Intravenous catheter/evacuated tube holder adapters also are available to facilitate drawing directly from IV catheters during IV start.

14. Gently invert the collection tubes 5–8 times as soon as filled to properly mix samples.

15. The tourniquet may be released as soon as blood enters the collection system or may be left on throughout the procedure.

16. Blood samples should be collected in the following order:
   a. Sterile sample, for culture,
   b. Tubes without additives,
   c. Tubes for coagulation studies, (**Note:** Tubes for coagulation studies must be allowed to fill completely for accurate test results.)
   d. Tubes with additives (Package insert, Becton Dickinson, 1991).

17. Upon completion of blood collection, have the patient relax the hand.

18. Release the tourniquet (if not previously released).

19. Apply a gauze dressing over the site and gently withdraw needle. Apply pressure until bleeding has stopped.

20. Tape the gauze dressing firmly in place.

21. Label blood samples per institutional policy. **Note:** If blood was drawn using syringe it is preferable to remove the stopper from the tube, gently expel the blood into the tube, replace the stopper, and invert the tube 5–8 times. This helps prevent hemolysis.

SPECIAL SITUATIONS

Blood Cultures

Cultures are done in an effort to evaluate bacteremia. Bacteremia may be intermittent, transient, or continuous. It is ideal to obtain cultures one hour prior to the onset of fever or chills, because there is usually a delay between the influx of bacteria and fever spike or chill. However, this is rarely a possibility in the emergency department setting. Two blood cultures from two separate sites may be obtained prior to initiating antimicrobial therapy. Multiple bottles from the same site should be considered a single sample. For confirmation of bacteremia and to rule out contamination or a break in skin cleaning technique, both cultures need to be positive (Reller, 1982).

PROCEDURE

1. Clean the skin and bottle tops with 70% isopropyl alcohol and then swab both with iodine or povidone-iodine. Allow both to air dry.

2. Perform the venipuncture. Sterile gloves may be worn to avoid contaminating the prepared skin.

3. If a syringe was used, replace the needle with a sterile one prior to inoculating the culture bottle.

4. Note the time, site, and any prior administration of antibiotics on the lab slip.

COMPLICATIONS

1. Vasovagal syncope.

2. Failure to obtain blood, usually due to incorrect needle positioning or tube without vacuum.

3. Hematoma formation at puncture site.
4. Hemolysis of sample, usually due to rough handling or forceful aspiration through a small needle.
5. Clotted sample, sample was not mixed properly when drawn.
6. Local reaction to skin cleansing agent.

PATIENT TEACHING

1. Report any increasing soreness at venipuncture site or continued bleeding.

REFERENCES

Reller, L.B., Murray, P.R. & MacLowry, J.D. 1982. *Cumatech 1A, Blood Cultures II.* J.A. Washington II (ed). Washington, DC: American Society for Microbiology.

SUGGESTED READING

Sheehy, S.B. 1985. Laboratory tests in trauma. *Journal of Emergency Nursing,* 11, 2:99–104.

62

Peripheral Intravenous Cannulation

Margo E. Layman, RNC, BSN, CEN

Peripheral intravenous (IV) cannulation is also known as peripheral IV start.

INDICATIONS

To establish venous access for the administration of fluids, electrolytes, medications, blood and blood components, or total parenteral nutrition.

CONTRAINDICATIONS AND CAUTIONS

1. If the patient has a coagulation disorder, care should be taken to prevent bleeding from unsuccessfully attempted sites.
2. Inadequate cleansing of the skin at the cannulation site may result in the introduction of bacteria into the vein.
3. On cannulation, there should be adequate blood return to demonstrate appropriate placement of cannula.
4. A hematoma may form if the needle punctures both the anterior and posterior walls of the vein.
5. Avoid placing IVs over joints because the movement of the joint may cause infiltration.
6. Rotate IV sites every 72 hours to help prevent the development of phlebitis and infection (West, 1983).
7. IV catheters should be promptly removed upon evidence of edema, redness, phlebitis, pain, or subcutaneous infiltration.
8. Shaving the site for intravenous cannulation may promote bacterial growth (West, 1983).
9. Never withdraw the catheter back over the needle, this could shear the catheter off inside the vein.

EQUIPMENT

IV pole
Intravenous solution as ordered
IV tubing (in appropriate sizes)
or
Heparin lock, heparin and saline flush
Local anesthetic or saline, TB syringe (optional)
Tourniquet
Gauze dressings

Adhesive tape
Antiseptic solution or prep pads
Over-the-needle intravenous catheter
Transparent dressing (optional)
Armboard (optional)
Note: Preassembled IV start kits are available.

PATIENT PREPARATION

Assemble IV tubing, spike solution bag, and prime the tubing.

PROCEDURAL STEPS

1. Apply a tourniquet above intended site of cannulation.
2. Identify a vein. If the vein is not distended and easily palpable, lightly pat the area, have the patient open and close the fist, lower the extremity below level of the heart, or apply a warm pack to help distend a vein. Start in the distal extremity to preserve proximal sites for future venipunctures if needed. Bifurcations are good for venipuncture because they are more stable and less prone to rolling.
3. Inject a wheal of local anesthetic or saline intradermally (optional). Some hospitals require a physician order for this.
4. Cleanse the skin with an antiseptic solution using a firm circular swabbing motion from the center of the site outward.
5. Insert the needle through the skin at a 45-degree angle with the bevel up, in line with and alongside the vein. Alternatively, insert the needle directly over the vein (there is an increased risk of posterior wall puncture with this technique). See Figure 62.1.

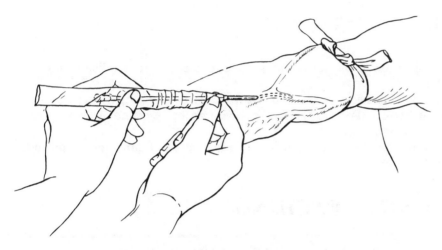

Figure 62.1   Insert the needle through the skin at a 45° angle.
(Rosen & Sternbach, 1983: 73. Reprinted by permission.)

6. Puncture the vein, a flash of blood will appear in the hub of the catheter.
7. Advance the catheter over the needle and into the vein. If any resistance is met on advancement of the catheter, stop immediately, remove the needle and catheter, and apply pressure to the site.
8. Release the tourniquet.
9. Connect the IV tubing and open the roller clamp or attach the heparin lock.
10. Apply 1/4″ tape across the hub of the catheter to secure it, do not place tape over the insertion site or junction of the needle and tubing. Alternatively, apply a transparent dressing over the site and needle hub.
11. If a transparent dressing is not used, apply antimicrobial ointment (optional) to the insertion site and cover with a 2×2 gauze dressing folded in half and taped securely.
12. Tape the IV tubing or heparin lock securely. See Figure 62.2.
13. Label the intravenous site tape with the date, time, size of catheter, and your initials.
14. Adjust the drip rate as ordered or flush heparin lock per institutional policy.

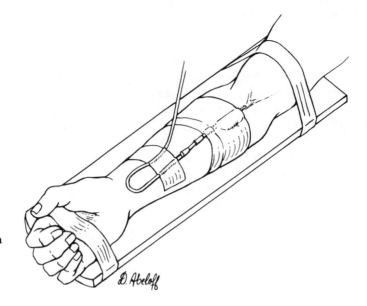

**Figure 62.2   Tape the IV securely in
place.**
(Rosen & Sternbach, 1983: 73. Reprinted by permission.)

COMPLICATIONS

1. Infiltration of the surrounding tissue can occur from a displaced catheter.
2. Embolisms occur rarely from intravenous sites of patients with poor venous return. (Feet and ankle are poor sites for IV cannulation because of
   poor venous return.)
3. Rotate IV sites every 72 hours to help prevent infection or phlebitis
   (West, 1983).

PATIENT TEACHING

1. Do not adjust the flow rate, bend, or pinch the tubing.
2. Report any sensations of swelling, heat, burning, pain, or drainage at the
   puncture site.

REFERENCES

Fincke, M.K., & Lanros, N.E. 1986. *Emergency nursing: A comprehensive review.*
   Rockville, MD: Aspen Publications.
King, E.M. 1981. *Illustrated manual of nursing techniques.* Philadelphia: Lippin-
   cott.
Kozier, B., & Erb, G. 1983. *Fundamentals of nursing: Concepts and procedures.* Los
   Angeles: Addison-Wesley.
Rosen, P., & Sternbach, G. 1983. *Atlas of emergency medicine,* 2nd ed., Baltimore:
   Williams & Wilkins.
West, R.S. 1983. *Managing IV therapy.* Springhouse, PA: Sringhouse Corp.

63

External Jugular Venous Access

Lori D. Taylor, RN, BSN, CEN

INDICATIONS

To obtain peripheral venous access when other peripheral sites (hand, forearm, antecubital fossa) are unavailable or inaccessible due to injury.

Note: The external jugular vein is considered to be a peripheral intravenous site (American Heart Association, 1987). Therefore, its use by nursing and prehospital personnel should be addressed by local policy.

CONTRAINDICATIONS AND CAUTIONS

1. Manipulation of the head and neck is contraindicated in the trauma patient with suspected cervical spine injury.
2. Accessing the external jugular vein during a cardiopulmonary arrest may result in the interruption of resuscitation efforts, making this site less desirable during resuscitation efforts.
3. Use of the external jugular vein is contraindicated with penetrating trauma to the neck, and should be avoided with significant blunt trauma and soft tissue injury to the neck.
4. Securing an intravenous line in the neck area is difficult, with frequent accidental dislodgement. Additionally, accessory equipment such as cervical collars cannot easily be utilized with intravenous access in the neck.

EQUIPMENT

Antiseptic solution
Intravenous (IV) solution and
    tubing
IV needle and catheter (Size and
    length are dependent upon
    the need for the line:
    large bore catheters, such
    as 14–16-G, are indicated
    when large volumes of
    fluids are needed, and small
    catheters, such as 18–20-G,
    will suffice to keep the vein
    open for maintenance
    fluids.) Three choices of IV
    needles are available, and
    include (American Heart
    Association, 1987):
Hollow needles (butterfly-type
    needles)

Indwelling plastic
    over-the-needle catheters
    (preferred in emergent
    situations)
Plastic catheters inserted
    through needles or over
    guidewires with the
    Seldinger technique
Transparent dressing (optional)
Antibiotic ointment
Gauze dressings
5-ml syringe, 18-G and 25–27-G
    needles for local anesthesia
Local anesthetic agent
20–30-ml syringe for obtaining
    blood specimens
Assorted blood collection tubes
Adhesive tape

PATIENT PREPARATION

1. Prepare the IV solution and tubing. Placing extension tubing in-line will facilitate future tubing changes.
2. Place the patient in a supine, head-down position with the head turned away from the side to be utilized for access (contraindicated in trauma patients with possible cervical spine injury).
3. Cleanse the area overlying external jugular vein with antiseptic solution. The external jugular vein runs downward and backward obliquely behind the angle of the mandible and across the sternomastoid muscle. It then courses deeply into the neck just above the midclavicular area. The external jugular vein then enters the subclavian vein. See Figure 63.1.

PROCEDURAL STEPS

*Indicates portions of the procedure usually performed by a physician.

1. *Infiltrate the area of the venipuncture with an intradermal wheal of local anesthetic if the patient is conscious and/or if the patient's condition permits.
2. *Align the IV needle with the vein with the needle tip directed toward the ipsilateral shoulder.
3. *Lightly "tourniquet" the distal end of the vein (just above the clavicle) with the opposite index finger. The opposite thumb can also be used on proximal portion of the vein to assist in anchoring it for puncture. See Figure 63.2.

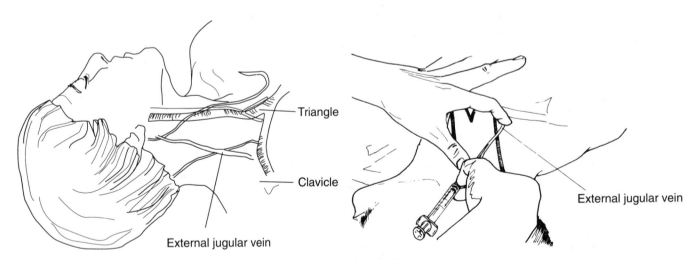

Figure 63.1 Anatomy of the external jugular vein. (American Heart Association, 1987: 144.)

Figure 63.2 External jugular venipuncture. (American Heart Association, 1987: 145. Reprinted by permission.)

4. *Perform the venipuncture midway between the angle of the jaw and the clavicle.
5. *When blood return is noted, advance the catheter off of the needle to the hub. If using a through-the-needle catheter, advance the catheter through the needle. In order to avoid the introduction of air into the venous system, a gloved finger should be placed over the needle hub. Alter-

natively, the patient may be instructed to perform a Valsalva maneuver (strain or cough).

6. *Remove the needle and attach the 20–30-ml syringe if lab specimens are to be obtained. Withdraw blood for lab specimens.
7. Connect the IV tubing and assess flow of the fluid. Monitor closely for swelling indicative of infiltration.
8. Apply antibiotic ointment and a sterile dressing over the puncture site.
9. Secure the needle and tubing with adhesive tape.

COMPLICATIONS

1. Local complications related to external jugular cannulation may include
   a. Infection of puncture site (late)
   b. Hematoma formation at the insertion site (immediate)
   c. Inadvertent arterial puncture
   d. Phlebitis/thrombosis of vein (late)
2. Systemic complications may include
   a. Catheter shear with fragment embolization (high risk when through-the-needle catheters are pulled back through the needle)
   b. Air embolism
   c. Sepsis (late)

REFERENCES

American Heart Association. 1987. *Textbook of advanced cardiac life support.* Dallas: American Heart Association.

SUGGESTED READINGS

American College of Surgeons, Committee on Trauma. 1988. *Advanced trauma life support course: Student manual.* Chicago: American College of Surgeons.

Caroline, N.L. 1983. *Emergency care in the streets,* 2nd ed. Boston: Little, Brown.

Daily, R. 1988. Venous access. In American College of Emergency Physicians, *Emergency medicine: A comprehensive study guide.* New York: McGraw-Hill, 10–25.

Kaye, W., & Dubin, H. Vascular cannulation. In J. Civetta, R. Taylor, & R. Kirby, (eds). *Critical care.* Philadelphia: Lippincott, 211–225.

64

Subclavian Venous Access

Lori D. Taylor, RN, BSN, CEN

INDICATIONS

1. To secure central venous access via the subclavian vein when peripheral access is unobtainable, such as in a full arrest or profound shock with peripheral vasoconstriction.
2. To monitor central venous pressure or other hemodynamic parameters, central access is necessary in order to allow passage of catheters into the heart or pulmonary circulation.
3. To administer certain hypertonic solutions and pharymocologic agents into the central circulation.

CONTRAINDICATIONS AND CAUTIONS

1. Central venous cannulation is associated with much greater risk and higher complication rates than peripheral vascular cannulation. Therefore, the risks versus benefits for this procedure must be weighed carefully.
2. Cardiopulmonary resuscitation may need to be interrupted for a brief period to allow subclavian venipuncture. Therefore, this is not the first choice of access points for intravenous line placement during a cardiopulmonary arrest.
3. Central line access constitutes a relatively strong contraindication to thrombolytic therapy (American Heart Association, 1987).
4. The right subclavian vein is slightly preferred over the left side, because the lung apex is slightly lower on the right, there is a straighter relationship between the right subclavian and superior vena cava, and the thoracic duct is protected from injury (Dailey, 1988).
5. Subclavian access should be utilized as a last resort in children due to anatomical difficulties and high risk of complications. (Chameides, 1988).
6. In the case of chest trauma, the injured side should be considered for subclavian access to avoid inducing a pneumothorax or other pathology on the uninjured side. However, if a clavicle fracture is suspected, utilize the side opposite the fracture.
7. A failed attempt on one side should be followed by repeat attempts on the same side in order to avoid iatrogenic pathology on both sides of the chest (Dailey, 1988).

EQUIPMENT

Antiseptic solution
Razor (optional)

5-ml syringe, 18-G and 27-G needles
for local anesthesia

Local anesthetic
10–20 ml syringe for aspiration of
    blood
Selected intravenous (IV)
    needle/catheter
    (Usually, a
    through-the-needle catheter
    is utilized for this
    procedure. The needle
    length is usually longer
    than those used with
    peripheral cannulation,
    because the vein may be
    several centimeters from the
    puncture site. The catheter
    length for subclavian lines
    should be 15–20 cm. If the
    catheter is to be inserted
    through-the-needle, the
    needle must be a 14-G. If
    the Seldinger technique is

employed, a thin-walled
18-G needle will accept a
standard guidewire
(American Heart
Association, 1987)).
IV solution and tubing
Silk suture (2-0 to 3-0)
Sterile towels
Suture scissors
Needle holder
Transparent dressing (optional)
Antibiotic ointment
Gauze dressings
Adhesive tape
Various blood collection tubes
(Note: Pre-packaged kits
    containing much of this
    equipment and a variety of
    central venous catheters are
    also available).

PATIENT PREPARATION

1. Prepare the IV solutions and tubing.
2. Place the patient in a supine, 15°, head-down position with the head turned away from the side of insertion. This will aid in distending the veins and preventing air embolism (American College of Surgeons, 1989).
3. Placing the shoulders back by putting a rolled towel under the high thoracic spine area will help prevent pneumothorax (Dailey, 1988).
4. Cleanse the area overlying the subclavian area with antiseptic solution and shave if indicated. The subclavian vein arises as a continuation of the axillary vein, with its origin near the lateral portion of the first rib. The vein then runs medially, passing under the middle third of the clavicle and unites with the internal jugular vein near the sternum to form the innominate vein. See Figure 64.1

PROCEDURAL STEPS

1. *Infiltrate the area of the venipuncture with local anesthetic if the patient is conscious and/or if the patient's condition permits.
2. *Determine the depth of catheter placement by measuring from the point of insertion to the desired surface marker on the chest wall (American College of Surgeons, 1989). Note the desired distance on the catheter. See Figure 64.2.
   a. Sternoclavicular joint approximates the subclavian vein.
   b. Middle of the manubrium of the sternum approximates the brachycephalic vein.
   c. Junction of the manubrium and midsternum approximates the superior vena cava.
   d. 5cm below the manubrial-sternal junctions approximates the right atrium.
3. *Attach the 10–20-ml syringe to the selected needle.
4. *Perform the venipuncture inferior to the junction of the middle and medial thirds of the clavicle.

*Indicates portions of the procedure performed by a physician.

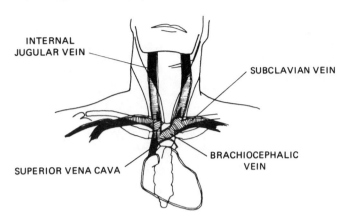

Figure 64.1 Anatomy of the subclavian vein. (American Heart Association, 1987: 147. Reprinted by permission.)

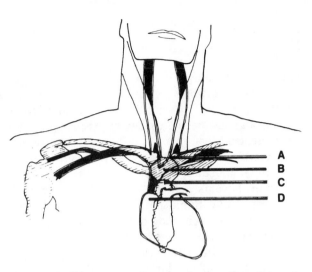

Figure 64.2 Surface markers on chest wall to determine depth of catheter placement. See text for explanation. (American Heart Association, 1987: 148. Reprinted by permission.)

5. *Place the index finger of the opposite hand into the suprasternal notch.
6. *With the syringe and needle parallel to the frontal plane, advance the needle behind the clavicle, in a medial and slightly cephalad direction toward the fingertip in the suprasternal notch. See Figure 64.3.

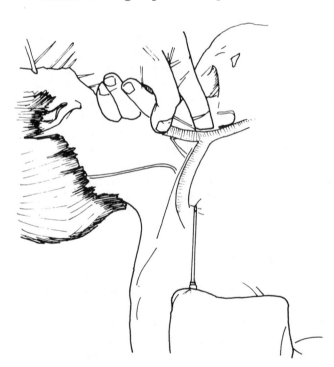

Figure 64.3 Infraclavicular subclavian venipuncture. (American Heart Association, 1987: 151. Reprinted by permission.)

7. *Maintain steady negative pressure on the plunger of the syringe as the needle is advanced. The free flow of blood into the syringe signals entry into the subclavian vein. The appearance of bright red arterial blood may indicate inadvertent entry into the subclavian artery, which runs posterior to the vein.
8. *When blood return is noted, remove the syringe from the needle. In order to avoid introduction of air into the venous system, a gloved finger should be placed over the needle hub. Alternatively, the patient can be instructed to perform a Valsalva maneuver (strain or cough).
9. *If a through-the-needle catheter is to be used, advance it through the needle to the premeasured depth. The needle is then removed. If the

Seldinger technique is to be used, a guidewire (with a J-tip) is advanced through the needle. The needle is then removed, taking care not to dislodge the guidewire. Finally, the catheter is advanced over the guidewire, and the wire removed.

10. *Obtain desired lab specimens.
11. Attach IV tubing and adjust rate of flow of the infusion.
12. *Suture the catheter in place, taking care not to occlude the catheter with the suture.
13. Apply an antibiotic ointment to the puncture site and cover the area with a dressing.
14. Secure the tubing and dressing in place with adhesive tape.
15. *Central venous access should always be followed by a chest x-ray. The chest film is used both to confirm line placement and to rule out postprocedural complications (i.e., pneumothorax).

COMPLICATIONS

1. Local complications from subclavian cannulation may include
   a. Local hematoma formation
   b. Inadvertent arterial puncture
   c. Local cellulitis (late)
   d. Injury to adjacent nerves, lymphatics, or other structures
   e. Malpositioned catheters
   f. Infiltration of IV fluid into the mediastinum or pleural space
2. Systemic complications may include
   a. Pneumothorax is commonly seen following subclavian venous access. The incidence, even with elective lines, is 5–10% and is even higher in emergency situations (Trunkey, 1986).
   b. Hemothorax (bleeding from subclavian vein or other sources)
   c. Hemopneumothorax
   d. Air embolism
   e. Sepsis (late)
   f. Catheter shear with embolization (high risk when a through-the-needle catheter is withdrawn back through the needle)
   g. Ventricular ectopy may be noted during the placement of catheters into the heart or pulmonary circulation.

REFERENCES

American College of Surgeons, Committee on Trauma. 1988. *Advanced trauma life support course: Student manual.* Chicago: American College of Surgeons.

American Heart Association. 1987. *Textbook of advanced cardiac life support.* Dallas: American Heart Association.

Chameides, L. 1988. *Textbook of Pediatric Advanced Life Support.* Dallas: American Heart Association.

Dailey, R. 1988. Venous access. In American College of Emergency Physicians, *Emergency medicine: A comprehensive study guide.* New York: McGraw-Hill, 10–25.

Trunkey, D., & Lewis F. 1986. *Current therapy of trauma-2,* Philadelphia, PA: Decker.

SUGGESTED READINGS

Caroline, N.L. 1983. *Emergency care in the streets,* 2nd ed. Boston: Little, Brown.

Kaye, W., & Dubin, H. Vascular cannulation. In J. Civetta, R. Taylor, & R. Kirby, (eds). *Critical care.* Philadelphia: Lippincott, 211–225.

65

Internal Jugular Venous Access

Lori D. Taylor, RN, BSN, CEN

INDICATIONS

1. To secure control venous access via the internal jugular (IJ) when peripheral access is unobtainable, such as in a full arrest or profound shock with peripheral vasoconstriction.
2. To monitor central venous pressure or other hemodynamic parameters.
3. To administer certain hypertonic solutions and pharmacologic agents into the central circulation.

CONTRAINDICATIONS AND CAUTIONS

1. Central venous cannulation is associated with much greater risk and higher complication rates than peripheral vascular cannulation. Therefore, the risks versus benefits for this procedure must be weighed carefully.
2. Cardiopulmonary resuscitation may need to be interrupted for a brief period to obtain IJ access. Therefore, IJ access is not indicated as an initial intravenous (IV) attempt in a full arrest situation.
3. With suspected cervical spine injury, the manipulation of the head and neck necessary for this procedure is contraindicated.
4. Central line access constitutes a relatively strong contraindication to thrombolytic therapy (American Heart Association, 1987).
5. A failed attempt on one side of the neck should be followed by repeat attempts on the same side. Hematoma formation on both sides of the neck could result in respiratory compromise (American Heart Association, 1987).

EQUIPMENT

Antiseptic solution
Razor (optional)
5-ml syringe, 18-G and 27-G needles for local anesthesia
Local anesthetic
10–20-ml syringe for aspiration of blood
Selected intravenous (IV) needle/catheter (Usually, a through-the-needle catheter is utilized for this procedure, and the needle is longer than that used with peripheral IV access, because the vein may be several centimeters from the puncture site. The catheter length should be sufficient to reach the desired location within the chest).
Sterile towels
IV solution and tubing
Silk suture (2-0 to 3-0)
Suture scissors
Needle holder
Transparent dressing (optional)
Antibiotic ointment

Gauze dressings
Adhesive tape
Various blood collection tubes
(Note: Commercially prepared,
disposable kits for central

venous access are available
and contain many of these
items, as well as various
catheters and needles).

PATIENT PREPARATION

1. Prepare the IV solution and tubing. Placing an extension set in-line will facilitate future tubing changes.
2. Place the patient in a supine, 15°, head-down position with the head turned away from the side of insertion. The right side is preferred for insertion, because the lung dome is lower on the right, there is a straighter angle into the superior vena cava, and the large thoracic duct is protected from injury (Dailey, 1988).
3. Cleanse the area overlying the neck area with antiseptic solution and shave if indicated. The internal jugular vein runs posteriorly and laterally to the internal and common carotid artery (American Heart Association, 1987). As the vein nears the thoracic area, it becomes more lateral and anterior to the common carotid artery. Another landmark utilized in accessing the IJ vein is the sternocleidomastoid muscle. The IJ vein runs medial to this muscle in its upper part and then passes posterior to the two inferior heads of the muscle in its midportion. See Figure 65.1

PROCEDURAL STEPS

Three approaches to the IJ vein are utilized in practice and include a posterior, central, and anterior approach. The central approach is the most commonly used and will be the one outlined in this procedure.

1. *Infiltrate the area of the venipuncture with local anesthetic if the patient is conscious and/or if the patient's condition permits.
2. *Determine the length of catheter placement by measuring from the point of insertion to the desired surface marker on the chest wall (American College of Surgeons, 1989). Note the desired distance on the catheter. See Figure 65.2.
   a. Sternoclavicular joint approximates the subclavian vein.
   b. Middle of the manubrium of the sternum approximates the brachycephalic vein.
   c. Junction of the manubrium and midsternum approximates the superior vena cava.
   d. 5cm below the manubrial-sternal junction approximates the right atrium.
3. *Attach the 10–20 ml syringe to the selected needle.
4. *Insert the needle into the center of the apex of the triangle formed by the two heads of the sternocleidomastoid muscle and the clavicle.
5. *While maintaining negative pressure to the plunger of the syringe, direct the needle toward the ipsilateral nipple at a 30–45° angle to the frontal plane. See Figure 65.3
6. *The free flow of the blood into the syringe signals entry into the IJ vein. See Figure 65.4. The vein is very superficial here, and blood return should be obtained within three centimeters of the puncture site (Dailey, 1988). If not, slowly withdraw the needle, maintaining negative pressure. If the vein is still not entered, redirect the needle 10° laterally (avoid directing the needle more medial, as the carotid artery may be punctured inadvertently).
7. *When blood return is noted, the syringe is removed from the needle. In

*Indicates portion of the procedure usually performed by a physician.

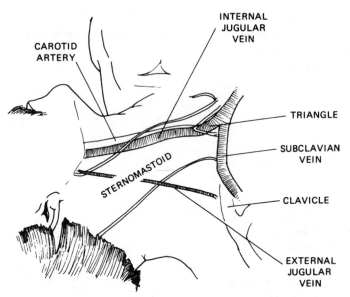

Figure 65.1 Anatomy of the internal jugular vein. (American Heart Association, 1987: 147. Reprinted by permission.)

CAROTID ARTERY

INTERNAL JUGULAR VEIN

TRIANGLE

SUBCLAVIAN VEIN

CLAVICLE

STERNOMASTOID

EXTERNAL JUGULAR VEIN

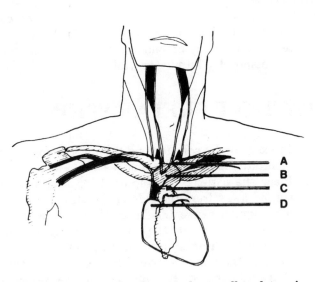

Figure 65.2 Surface markers on chest wall to determine depth of catheter placement. (American Heart Association, 1987: 148. Reprinted by permission.)

A
B
C
D

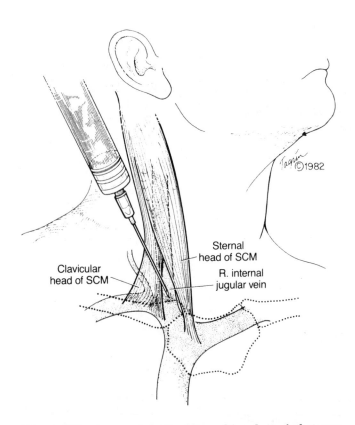

Sternal head of SCM

Clavicular head of SCM

R. internal jugular vein

Figure 65.3 Approach to the internal jugular vein between the sternal and clavicular heads of the sternocleidomastoid muscle. (Wilkins, 1989: 1005. Reprinted by permission.)

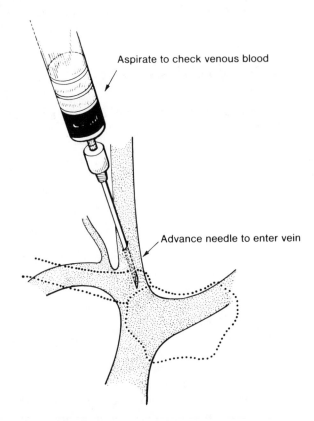

Aspirate to check venous blood

Advance needle to enter vein

Figure 65.4 Entry into vein is signaled by the free flow of blood into syringe. (Wilkins, 1989: 1006. Reprinted by permission.)

order to avoid accidental introduction of air into the needle, a gloved finger should be placed over the needle hub. Alternatively, the patient can be instructed to perform a Valsalva maneuver by straining or coughing.

8. *If a through-the-needle catheter is to be used, it is advanced through the needle to the premeasured distance. The needle is then removed. If

the Seldinger technique is to be used, a guidewire with a J-tip is advanced through the needle. The needle is then removed and the catheter is advanced over the wire. Remove the guidewire after catheter placement. See Figure 65.5.

9. *Obtain desired lab specimens.
10. Attach IV tubing and adjust rate of flow of the infusion. Monitor for signs of extravasation.
11. *The catheter frequently will be sutured in place to prevent accidental dislodgement.
12. Apply a thin layer of antibacterial ointment to the puncture site and cover the area with a dressing.
13. Secure the tubing and dressing in place with adhesive tape.
14. *Central venous access should always be followed by a chest x-ray. The chest film is used both to confirm line placement and to rule out postprocedural complications.

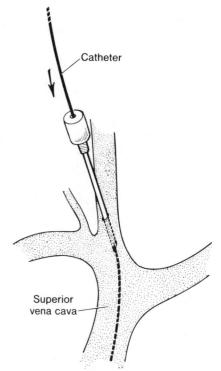

Figure 65.5 Insertion of through-the-needle catheter through the internal jugular vein and into the superior vena cava.
(Wilkins, 1989: 1006. Reprinted by permission.)

COMPLICATIONS

1. Local complications from IJ access may include
   a. Local hematoma formation
   b. Inadvertent arterial puncture
   c. Local cellulitis (late)
   d. Injury to adjacent structures
   e. Malpositioned catheters
   f. Infiltration of infusate into the subcutaneous tissues and/or mediastinum
2. Systemic complications may include
   a. Pneumothorax—the incidence is less with IJ cannulation performed correctly than with subclavian cannulation (Dailey, R., 1988).
   b. Hemothorax
   c. Air embolism
   d. Sepsis (late)
   e. Catheter shear with fragment embolization (higher risk if through-the-needle catheter is used)

REFERENCES

American Heart Association. 1987. *Textbook of advanced cardiac life support.* Dallas: American Heart Association.
Dailey, R. 1988. Venous access. In American College of Emergency Physicians, *Emergency medicine: A comprehensive study guide.* New York: McGraw-Hill; 10–25.
Wilkins, E.W. (ed). 1989. *Emergency medicine: Scientific foundations and current practice,* 3rd ed. Baltimore: Williams & Wilkins.

SUGGESTED READINGS

American College of Surgeons, Committee on Trauma. (1988). *Advanced trauma life support course: Student manual.* Chicago: American College of Surgeons.
Caroline, N.L. 1983. *Emergency care in the streets,* 2nd ed. Boston: Little, Brown.
Kaye, W., & Dubin, H. Vascular cannulation. In J. Civetta, R. Taylor, & R. Kirby, (eds). *Critical care.* Philadelphia: Lippincott, 211–225.

66

Femoral Venous Access

Dean M. Kelly, RN, BSN, CEN

INDICATIONS

1. To place large (i.e., 8.5-French) intravenous catheters for rapid fluid replacement in hypovolemic shock. The femoral vein can be entered even when the peripheral circulation has collapsed (American Heart Association, 1987).
2. To allow central venous access for medications and fluids without interrupting CPR or causing additional congestion at the head and neck of a patient during resuscitation.
3. To insert a pulmonary artery pressure catheter through the right side of heart into the pulmonary artery.
4. To place a temporary cardiac pacemaker in the right ventricle.
5. To obtain venous access for hemodialysis.
6. To place a central venous catheter to obtain central venous pressure (CVP) measurements See Ch. 90: Central Venous Pressure Measurement.
7. To obtain a venous blood sample when peripheral attempts have failed.

CONTRAINDICATIONS AND CAUTIONS

1. Excessive bleeding may occur if the patient is receiving anticoagulant or thrombolytic therapy. Caution should be exercised with such patients.
2. Infection of tissue overlying the puncture site.

EQUIPMENT

IV catheter, as indicated by patient's needs
  (Seldinger type/wire guided catheter is best for percutaneous approach.)
  4- or 5-inch, 8-French catheters are excellent for fluid replacement
  14-G–16-G catheters, which are long enough (24″) to extend above the diaphragm, are used for CVP measurements.
10-ml syringe
Suture (2-0 silk/nylon)
Needle holder
Suture scissors

Scalpel
Antiseptic solution
Gauze dressings
Transparent dressing (optional)
Antibiotic ointment (optional)
Tape
IV solution and administration set as indicated
Local anesthetic (lidocaine, etc.)
5-ml syringe with 27-G and 18-G needles
Blood collection tubes, as indicated
Note: Prepackaged kits containing an IV catheter and many of the other items are also available.

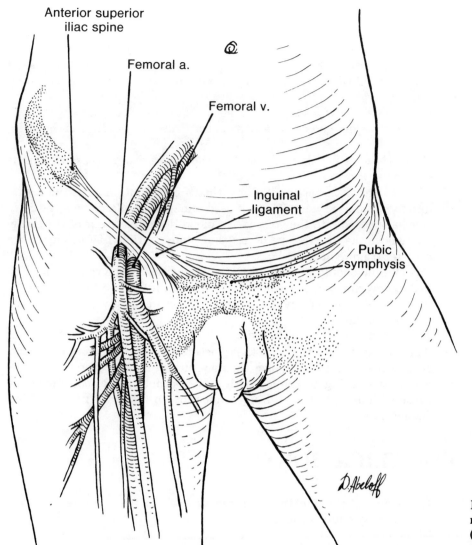

Anterior superior
iliac spine

Femoral a.

Femoral v.

Inguinal
ligament

Pubic
symphysis

D.Abeloff

Figure 66.1 Anatomy of the femoral vein.
(Rosen & Sternbach, 1983: 83. Reprinted by permission.)

PATIENT PREPARATION

1. Place the patient in the supine position with the legs fully extended.
2. Shave or clip hair around the insertion site and cleanse the area well with antiseptic solution. See Figure 66.1 for insertion site.

PROCEDURAL STEPS

1. *Locate the femoral artery by palpating the pulsation just below the inguinal ligament which runs from the anterior superior iliac spine to the pubis bone. The femoral vein usually lies 1–2cm medial to the artery. **Note:** In a pulseless patient with CPR in progress, the femoral vein will also pulsate and may be easier to locate than the femoral artery due to low arterial flow (American Heart Association, 1987).
2. *If the patient is conscious, infiltrate the skin overlying the femoral vein 1–2cm below the inguinal ligament with local anesthetic. **Note:** A venipuncture more than 2cm below the inguinal ligament may pass inadvertently through the superficial femoral artery (Grossman, 1986).
3. *Insert a 10ml syringe with a needle larger than the J-wire into the skin above the artery at a 45° angle cephalad. Insert the needle gently to the

*Indicates portion of the procedure usually performed by a physician.

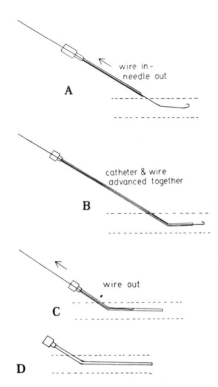

Figure 66.2 Seldinger technique of catheter insertion (wire-guided). (American Heart Association, 1983: 142. Reprinted by permission.)

hub or until resistance is met. At this point, the needle should have traversed the vein.

4. *While aspirating with the syringe, pull the needle back until blood is freely aspirated. (If only a blood sample is desired, aspirate the desired quantity and withdraw the needle. Apply pressure to the site for 5 minutes).

5. Pass a flexible J-wire through the needle into the vein. Make a small incision in the skin where the needle enters. This will facilitate catheter insertion.

6. *Withdraw the needle while holding the J-wire firmly to assure that it remains in the vein. See Figure 66.2a.

7. *Thread the catheter or dilator/catheter combination over the J-wire into the vein. See Figure 66.2b. If used, remove the dilator once the catheter has passed into the vein. When blood flows freely out of the catheter, remove the wire (Figure 66.2.c) and connect primed IV tubing to the catheter (Figure 66.2.d).

8. The IV fluid should flow freely. Catheter position in the vein can be verified by lowering bag below body level and noting blood reflux into the IV tubing. (**Note:** After any unsuccessful punctures apply pressure at the site for 5 minutes.)

9. *Suture the catheter to the skin.

10. Apply antibiotic ointment to the puncture site (optional) and a clear occlusive or gauze dressing over the puncture site and catheter.

11. Secure the tubing to the leg with tape. Do not tape directly over the catheter hub or the IV tubing connection to facilitate future tubing changes.

COMPLICATIONS

1. Hematoma at the puncture site from the vein or femoral artery
2. Infection, systemic or local
3. Thrombosis
4. Phlebitis
5. Arterial-venous fistula
6. Inadvertent cannulation of femoral artery

(American Heart Association, 1987)

PATIENT TEACHING

1. Avoid flexion of involved leg.
2. Report any wetness felt at the site or blood on the dressing.
3. Report any pain, numbness, or tingling in the leg.

REFERENCES

American Heart Association. 1987. *Textbook of Advanced Cardiac Life Support.* Dallas: American Heart Association.

Daily, R.H. 1988. Venous Access. In J.E. Tintinalli (ed). *Emergency medicine: A comprehensive study guide,* New York: McGraw Hill; 11–20.

Grossman, W. 1986. *Cardiac catherization and angiography.* Philadelphia: Lea & Febiger.

Rosen, P., & Sternbach, G.L. 1983. *Atlas of emergency medicine,* 2nd ed. Baltimore: Williams & Wilkins.

67

Venous Cutdown

Linell M. Jones, RN, BSN, CEN, CCRN

INDICATIONS

1. To provide venous access when peripheral sites are either unavailable or inadequate.
2. To administer very large volumes of fluid rapidly.

CONTRAINDICATIONS AND CAUTIONS

1. Bacteremia as a result of the catheter insertion via cutdown may have up to a ninefold increase over those inserted by direct venipuncture. The strictest aseptic technique should be used (American Heart Association, 1987).
2. Cannulation of the lower extremity (saphenous vein) has a greater incidence of phlebitis (American Heart Association, 1987).

EQUIPMENT

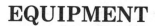

IV set up (fluid and tubing)
Large bore IV catheter or cannula.
    (Infant feeding tubes or an
    IV extension set with the
    distal end cut at a bevel are
    frequently used.)
Antiseptic solution
5-ml syringe with 18-G and 27-G
    needles
Local anesthetic
Scalpels #11 and #15 blades with
    handles
Tissue scissors (iris or metzenbaum)
Tissue forceps

Vein retractor
Hemostats
Needleholder
Silk suture 1-0 to 4-0
Gauze dressings
Transparent dressing (optional)
Antibiotic ointment
Tape
Catheter introducer (optional)
(Note: Most facilities have
    prepackaged venous
    cutdown trays with most
    needed equipment already
    assembled.)

PATIENT PREPARATION

1. Assemble IV solution and tubing
2. *Cleanse the chosen site with antiseptic solution. The sites most commonly used are the cephalic vein, just above the antecubital fossa on the dorsal-radial aspect of the upper arm (Figure 67.1); the saphenous vein, just anterior and superior to the medial malleolus of the tibia (Figure 67.2); and the femoral vein (Figure 67.3).
3. *Infiltrate the area over the vein with local anesthetic if the patient is conscious and if time permits.

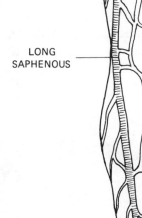

Figure 67.1 Anatomy of the veins of upper extremity.
(American Heart Association, 1987: 143. Reprinted by permission.)

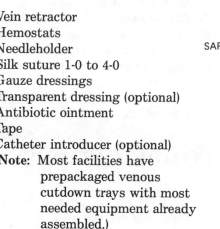

Figure 67.2 Anatomy of the long saphenous vein of the leg.
(American Heart Association, 1987: 144. Reprinted by permission.)

213

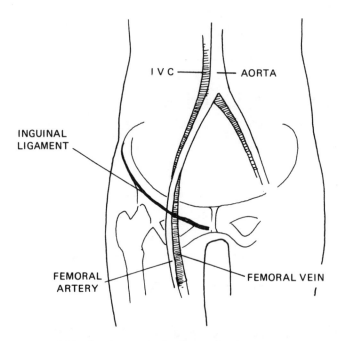

Figure 67.3   Anatomy of the femoral vein.
(American Heart Association, 1987: 146. Reprinted by permission.)

4. *Make a transverse skin incision over the vein. See Figure 67.4.a.
5. *Bluntly dissect down to the vein. See Figure 67.4.b.
6. *Isolate the vein with silk ligatures proximally and distally. See Figure 67.4.c.
7. *Tie the distal ligature.
8. *Make a small incision into the vein between the ligatures and insert the catheter toward the heart. See Figure 67.4.d. A catheter introducer may facilitate this procedure.
9. *Tie the proximal ligature to secure the catheter in place.
10. Connect the IV tubing to the catheter and begin the infusion.
11. *Suture the skin around the catheter.
12. Apply antibiotic ointment and dressing.
13. Tape the tubing securely.
14. Observe closely for signs of swelling from hematoma formation or fluid infiltration.

COMPLICATIONS

1. Inadvertent "cannulation" of a tendon or artery
2. Ligatures become loose with resultant bleeding and hematoma formation.
3. Phlebitis of the cannulated vein
4. Thrombosis and infection
5. Sepsis (late)

REFERENCES

American Heart Association. 1987. *Textbook of advanced cardiac life support.* Dallas: American Heart Association.
Wilkins, E.W. (ed). 1989. *Emergency medicine: Scientific foundations and current practice* 3rd ed., Baltimore: Williams & Wilkins.

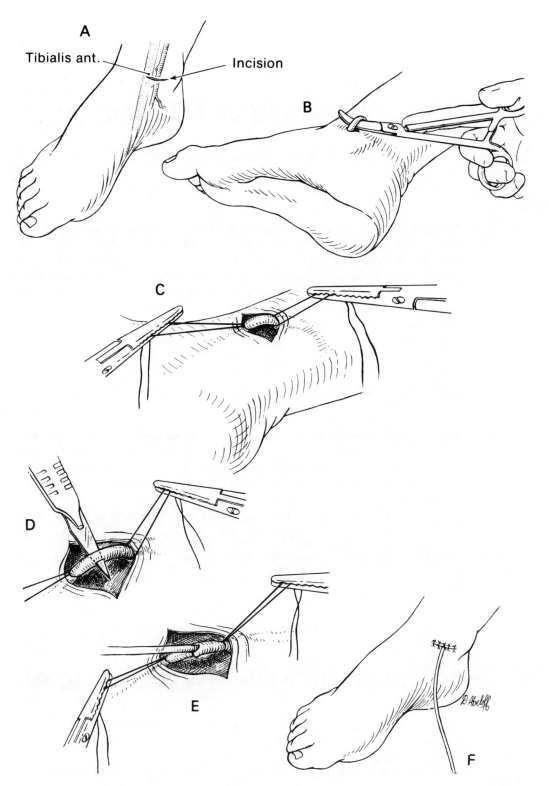

A

Tibialis ant.   Incision

B

C

D

E

F

Figure 67.4 Saphenous vein cutdown.
(Rosen, 1989: 89. Reprinted by permission.)

68

Intraosseous infusion is also known as bone marrow infusion.

Intraosseous Infusion

Marilyn K. Bourn, RN, MSN, REMTP

This technique is widely recommended for use in the pediatric population (Chameides, 1988; Smith, 1988). Recently however, some clinicians have begun to consider it's use in the adult population (Iverson, 1989). For this reason, this technique is included for your consideration as an adult procedure. The information presented is based primarily on animal and adult human research studies. Current articles, however, deal primarily with pediatric indications and techniques. As this technique is studied further in the adult population, indications and recommendations many change.

INDICATIONS

Intraosseous infusion is indicated in any emergency situation that may require rapid access to circulation for the administration of fluids or medications. Intraosseous infusion should be utilized anytime intravenous cannulation is either too difficult or too time-consuming to accomplish (Trocantins, 1940; Rogers, 1985). Some specific indications include

1. Initial bolus of colloids or crystalloids for resuscitation in shock states. Flow rates may not be sufficient, however, to fully treat severe hypovolemia or hemorrhagic shock (Hodge, 1987; Valdez, 1977).
2. Administration of medications (e.g., catecholamines, calcium, lidocaine, atropine, and sodium bicarbonate) during cardiac arrest (Berg, 1984; Chameides, 1988).
3. Administration of medications for the treatment of critical conditions such as status seizures, epiglottitis, or sepsis (Bourn, 1988).

CONTRAINDICATIONS AND CAUTIONS

Since intraosseous infusion is indicated only in serious, life-threatening situations, the contraindications are few, when the alternative may be death (Rogers, 1985).

1. Intraosseous infusion is not recommended for patients with lower extremity fractures due to risk of infiltration of fluids into the surrounding tissue (Bourn, 1985).
2. If possible, avoid placing the intraosseous line through burned tissue to decrease the risk of infection.
3. General contraindications may include patients with bone disorders such as osteopetrosis, osteogenesis imperfecta, and cellulitis (Hodge, 1985).
4. Avoid placing the needle in a site with obvious soft tissue infection present (Rogers, 1985).
5. Do not infuse marrow toxic (e.g., certain antibiotics) medications via the intraosseous route (Rogers, 1985).

EQUIPMENT

Sandbag for leg placement
Antiseptic solution
Local anesthetic (optional)
Several large bore (16-G or larger)
    needles (spinal or
    intraosseous) of various
    sizes (needle must have a
    stylet)

Syringe for aspiration
Normal saline for irrigation
Tape
Arm/leg board or hemostats for
    stabilization of needle
Gauze dressings
IV tubing and fluid bag/bottle
Pressure infusion bag (optional)

PROCEDURAL STEPS

1. Select the potential site for infusion. Consider the patient's age, size, accessibility, and other procedures needed. The sternum has been recommended for adults because it is easily accessible. It may however, be associated with serious complications (see below). Closed chest massage (CPR) is very difficult, at best, in these situations. The medial malleolus (approximately 2 cm proximal to the tip of the medial malleolus) may also be used (Rogers, 1985). The tibial plateau has become the most popular site in pediatric resuscitation (Chameides, 1988). See Figures 68.1, 68.2, and 68.3.

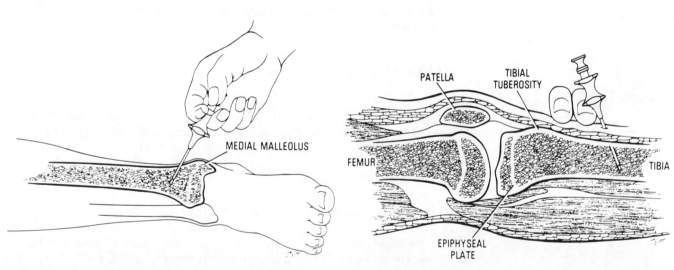

Figure 68.1   The medial malleolus may be used as an intraosseous site in the adult patient. The needle should be placed approximately 2–3cm proximal to the medial malleolus and directed slightly cephalad.
(Roberts & Hedges, 1985: 341. Reprinted by permission.)

Figure 68.2   When placing an intraosseous needle in the tibial plateau, insert the needle two fingerbreaths below the tibial tuberosity and slightly medial. The needle should be angled distally to avoid the epiphyseal growth plate.
(Roberts & Hedges, 1985: 341. Reprinted by permission.)

2. Stabilize the area with sandbags if necessary.
3. Cleanse the area with antiseptic solution.
4. *Anesthetize the area; this may not be necessary in moribund or obtunded patients.
5. *With the needle pointed slightly cephalad, puncture the skin and with a rotary motion push the needle into the bony cortex.
6. *Feel for a "pop." The needle will feel firm in the bone, but *not* stable.
7. Remove the stylet and confirm placement. This may be done by aspirating blood or marrow contents or irrigating with normal saline. In addition, the IV fluid should run steadily.

*Indicates those portions of the procedure usually performed by a physician.

Figure 68.3 A hemostat may be placed on the shaft or hub of the needle and then taped to the ankle or leg to stabilize the needle in place. Be careful not to clamp the needle too tightly. Opposing hemostats will further increase the stability of the needle.

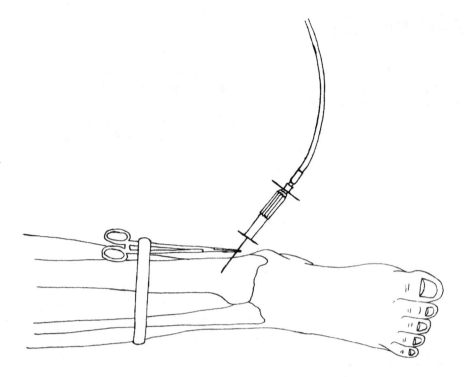

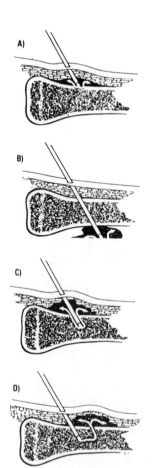

8. Connect syringe or IV tubing.
9. Apply a sterile dressing and stabilize the needle and tubing. Stabilize with tape and dressings or hemostats. See Figure 68.4.
10. Reassess patency.

COMPLICATIONS

Complications associated with intraosseous infusion are relatively rare. Most of the complications cited in the literature are related to prolonged use of the intraosseous needle or inappropriate placement of the needle.

1. Fat embolism from use of high pressure volume infusions (O'Neill, 1945).
2. Injection of fluid into the pleural space may be associated with the sternal approach (Papper, 1942). In addition, underlying tissues and organs may be damaged. Fatalities have been associated with sternal perforation.
3. Osteomyelitis, the most commonly noted complication, appears to be associated with prolonged continuous infusions (Heinild, 1947).
4. Fluid leakage from the infusion site. See Figure 68.4.

REFERENCES

Figure 68.4 Placement should be carefully assessed in order to avoid leakage or fluid around the insertion site. (a) incomplete penetration of the bony cortex; (b) penetration of the posterior cortex; (c) fluid escaping around the needle through the puncture site; (d) fluid leaking through a nearby previous puncture site.
(Roberts & Hedges, 1985: 341. Reprinted by permission.)

Berg, R.A. 1984. Emergency infusion of catecholamines into bone marrow. *American Journal of Diseases in Children*, 138:810–811.

Bourn, M.K. 1988. Intraosseous infusion: An innovation of the 1980s? *Emergency Nursing Reports*, 3, 5:1–8.

Chameides, L. (ed). 1988. *Textbook of Pediatric Advanced Life Support*, Dallas: American Heart Association; 37–46.

Heinild, S., Sondergaard, T., & Tudvad, F. (1947). Bone marrow infusion in childhood. *The Journal of Pediatrics*, 30:400–412.

Hodge, D. 1985. Intraosseous infusions: A review. *Pediatric Emergency Care*, 1:215–218.

Hodge, D., Delgado-Paredes, C., & Fleisher G. 1987. Intraosseous infusion flow rates in hypovolemic "pediatric" dogs. *Annals of Emergency Medicine*, 16:305–307.

Iverson, K.V. 1989. Intraosseous infusion in adults. *The Journal of Emergency Medicine,* 7:587–591.

O'Neill, J.F. 1945. Complications of intraosseous therapy. *Annals of Surgery,* 2:266.

Papper, E.M. 1942. The bone marrow route for injecting fluids and drugs into the general circulation. *Anesthesiology,* 3:307–313.

Roberts, J.R., & Hedges, J.R. 1985. *Clinical procedures in emergency medicine.* Philadelphia: Saunders.

Rogers, S.N., & Benumof, J.L. 1985. Intraosseous infusions. In J.R. Roberts, & J.R. Hedges (eds). *Clinical Procedures in Emergency Medicine.* Philadelphia: Saunders; 339–343.

Smith, R.J., Keseg, D.P., Manley, L.K., & Standeford, T. 1988. Intraosseous infusion by prehospital personnel in critically ill pediatric patients. *Annals of Emergency Medicine,* 17:491–495.

Tocantins, L.M., & O'Neill, J.F. 1941. Infusions of blood and other fluids into the general circulation via the bone marrow. *Surgery, Gynecology and Obstetrics,* 73:281–287.

Valdez, M.M. 1977. Intraosseous fluid administration in emergencies. *Lancet,* 2:1235–1236.

69

Accessing Preexisting Central Venous Catheters

Cass Robertson, RN, CRNI

There are many types of preexisting central venous catheters, including: Hickman/Broviac/right atrial catheter, Groshong catheter, peripherally inserted central catheter (PICC), or hemodialysis catheter (Mahurkar, Vas-Cath, Hemed, Quinton). Most are available in single or multilumen configurations. See Table 69.1 for specific descriptions. For the latest information, contact the manufacturer of the specific catheter.

INDICATIONS

To gain venous access in patients with pre-existing central venous catheters for
1. Administration of IV fluids, medications, blood, or blood products
2. Obtaining venous blood samples

CONTRAINDICATIONS AND CAUTIONS

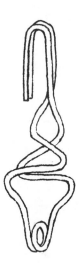

Figure 69.1 Bulldog catheter clamp.

1. Use aseptic technique and follow universal barrier precautions when handling any IV catheter. See Ch. 1: Universal Barrier Precautions.
2. Use only a clamp without teeth or a padded clamp on central venous catheters. Other clamps may sever the catheter. Bulldog clamps are safe and convenient. See Figure. 69.1.
3. If the catheter breaks or is damaged, clamp the catheter between the damaged portion and the patient. Repair kits are available from the manufacturer for most catheters.
4. To prevent air embolism, clamp the catheter or place the patient in the supine position and ask the patient to perform the Valsalva maneuver any time catheter is disconnected.
5. When inserting a needle into the male adapter plug of a central venous catheter, use needles of 1-inch length or less. Longer needles may puncture the catheter.
6. Tape all connections to prevent inadvertent disconnection and resulting air embolism.
7. For PICC lines, when administering whole blood or packed red blood cells, it may be necessary to use a pump, add 50 ml of normal saline to the blood bag, or run normal saline simultaneously with the blood to reduce viscosity and improve flow rates.
8. When performing central venous pressure (CVP) monitoring using a Groshong catheter, subtract the "valve closing pressure" from the manometer reading (5.44 cm water or 4 mm mercury) to give the true CVP reading (Groshong, 1990).

EQUIPMENT

Bulldog or other suitable clamp
Nonsterile gloves
10-ml syringe to withdraw blood for discard, or extra blood specimen tube if using vacuum tubes
Sampling syringes for blood specimens
Blood specimen tubes
Antiseptic swabs
Sterile normal saline for injection
Heparin flush, as needed (See Table 69.1 for recommended flush protocol for various catheters.)

Table 69.1 Selected central venous catheters.

Catheter Type/Name	Description of Catheter	Recommended Flush Protocol	Comments
Right Atrial Catheter (Hickman, Broviac)	Tunneled silicon catheter, (see Figure 69.2) surgically inserted. Most common location is subclavian vein, may also use femoral vein access into inferior vena cava. Available in single-, double-, or triple-lumen configurations.	Heparin 10–100units/ml, 2.5–5 ml every 12–24 hours or after each use. Flush each lumen separately.	Check for closed clamp. Do not flush vigorously or against resistance – catheter may rupture.
Groshong	Tunneled silicon catheter, surgically inserted. Available in single-, double-, and triple-lumen configurations. Has a 3-way slit valve which helps prevent air intake or bleeding if catheter comes apart (see Figure 69.3).	Heparin is not necessary. Flush after each use or once per week with 5 ml sterile normal saline for injection (use 20 ml after blood draw). Flush each lumen separately.	Need to flush with enough turbulence to clear blood from the closed tip of the catheter. No clamp is needed due to the 3-way valve.
PICC Line (Peripherally Inserted Central Catheter)	Silicon or polyurethane catheter with insertion site near antecubital fossa and catheter tip threaded into central vein. All catheters may not have tip placed in a central vein. Many brands are available in several sizes, in single- or double-lumen	Heparin 10–100units/ml, 1–2.5 ml every 12 hours or after each use. Flush each lumen separately.	Patient may have documentation regarding catheter type and placement. Care must be taken during resuscitation efforts that excessive pressures are not applied while administering IV push medications. Do not use affected arm for blood pressure

Table 69.1 continues on page 222.

Table 69.1 Selected central venous catheters. (*Continued*)

Catheter Type/Name	Description of Catheter	Recommended Flush Protocol	Comments
PICC (*cont'd.*)	configurations. Catheter flow rates may be restricted and are dependent on brand and size (see Table 69.2).		reading, venipuncture for IV, or lab draw.
Hemodialysis Catheter (Mahurkar, VasCath, Hemed, Quinton)	Usually subclavian or femoral access. Catheters are generally maintained by dialysis personnel. Not routinely used for IV therapy if other venous access is available.	Heparin flush dose and strength should be by specific physician order only. Typical dose is heparin 1000–5000units/ml, 1.5 ml instilled into each lumen after flushing with 20 ml of normal saline for injection.	To avoid heparin-induced coagulopathy, aspirate heparin from catheter before use. Most hemodialysis catheters will tolerate higher flow rates and pressures and provide good access for resuscitation efforts.

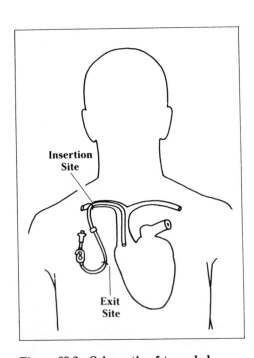

Figure 69.2 Schematic of tunneled catheter.
(*Patient Guide: How to care for your Hickman or Broviac Catheter* Publication no. 79010M. Cranston, RI: Davol, Inc; 2–3. Reprinted by permission.)

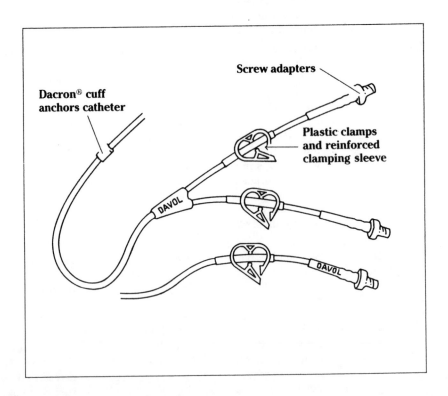

PROCEDURAL STEPS

For fluid administration

1. Prepare appropriate fluids and tubing.
2. Clamp the catheter and remove the male adapter plug from the hub of the catheter if a continuous IV is to be administered.

Table 69.2 Maximum flow rates for selected catheters as recommended by the manufacturer.

Catheter type/Name	Maximum Flow Rate
Hickman 9.6 Fr. (1.6 mm)	>500 ml/hr
Hickman 1.3 mm	>500 ml/hr
Broviac 6.6 Fr. (1.0 mm)	>500 ml/hr
Broviac 4.2 Fr. (0.7 mm)	205 ml/hr
Broviac 2.7 Fr. (0.5 mm)	49 ml/hr
Groshong 4 Fr. (18 G)	>500 ml/hr (PICC or tunneled)
Per-Q-Cath PICC 1.9 Fr. (23 G)	125 ml/hr (2 ml/min)
Per-Q-Cath PICC 2.8 Fr. (20 G)	>250 ml/hr (4 ml/min)
Per-Q-Cath PICC 3.8 Fr. (18 G)	>350 ml/hr (6 ml/min)
Per-Q-Cath PICC 4.8 Fr. (16 G)	>450 ml/h (7 ml/min)

Gesco Per-Q-Cath package insert. January 1990. San Antonio: Gesco International.

Hickman subcutaneous ports and Hickman/Broviac catheters wall poster. Cranston, RI: Davol.

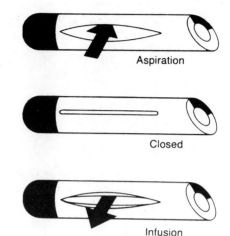

Figure 69.3 The Groshong three-position valve.
(*Hickman, M.R.I and Dome Ports: Instructions for use* 1990. Publication no. 902R, Cranston, RI: Davol, Inc; 3. Reprinted by permission.)

3. Attach the primary tubing to the hub of the catheter.
4. Unclamp the catheter and adjust IV flow to the prescribed rate.

For medication administration

1. Check for compatibility of the prescribed medication with heparin. If there is any question of the compatibility or if the medication is not compatible with heparin, flush the catheter with 5 ml of sterile normal saline for injection prior to administering the medication.
2. Flush the catheter with 5 ml of sterile normal saline for injection after the administration of the medication prior to administering the heparin flush.
3. Some catheters may have restricted flow rates, such as the Per-Q-Cath PICC line. Follow manufacturer's guidelines. See Table 69.2. Excessive pressure applied during IV push administration may cause the catheter to rupture, especially catheters constructed of silicon elastomer material.

For blood withdrawal using a syringe

1. If a continuous IV infusion is running, stop the infusion for 1 minute before drawing blood specimens.
2. Clamp the catheter and remove the tubing or male adapter plug.
3. Attach an empty syringe to the hub of the catheter, unclamp the catheter, and withdraw 10 ml of blood and discard (Plumer, 1987).
4. Aspirate gently because forceful aspiration may collapse the catheter. To facilitate blood return, have the patient raise arms, cough, perform Valsalva maneuver, or change position.
5. Withdraw the needed amount of blood and inject into the appropriate tube(s).
6. After the blood is drawn, flush the catheter with 10 ml of sterile normal saline for injection (20 ml for the Groshong catheter).
7. Reestablish IV fluids or administer appropriate heparin flush through a new male adapter plug.

For blood withdrawal using vacuum tubes

(Note: Vacuum tubes may collapse the catheter. In this instance, use the syringe method as described above.
1. Turn off infusion for 1 minute prior to withdrawing blood specimens.
2. Leave the male adapter plug on the catheter. Clean the injection port with an antiseptic swab.

3. Place the vacuum tube in the tube holder and insert the needle into the injection port of the catheter.
4. Withdraw 10 ml of blood into an extra tube and discard.
5. Draw the appropriate number and types of tubes needed.
6. After the blood is drawn, flush the catheter with 10 ml of sterile normal saline for injection (20 ml for the Groshong catheter).
7. Reestablish IV fluids or administer appropriate heparin flush through a new male adapter plug.

COMPLICATIONS

1. Infection
2. Damage to the catheter (rupture, tear, cracked hub)
3. Occlusion of the catheter with blood or precipitate if the catheter is not flushed appropriately
4. Air embolism
5. Central vein thrombosis

REFERENCES

Groshong, C.V., (1990.) *Nursing Procedure Manual,* (Publication no. CTC250013). Cranston, RI: Davol, Inc.
Plumer, A.L., & Consentino, F. 1987. *Principles and practice of intravenous therapy,* 4th ed. Boston: Little, Brown.

SUGGESTED READINGS

D'Angelo, H.H., & Welch, N.P. (eds). 1988. *Medication administration and I.V. therapy manual.* Springhouse, PA: Springhouse.
LaRocca, J.C., & Otto, S.E. 1989. *Pocket guide to intravenous therapy.* St. Louis: Mosby.

70

Accessing Implanted Venous Port Devices

Cass Robertson, RN, CRNI

An implanted port consists of a tunneled catheter attached to an injection port with a self-sealing septum. See Figure 70.1. The device is implanted under the skin and must be accessed through the skin. Although most frequently used for venous access, implanted ports may also be placed intra-arterial, epidural, or intraperitoneal. Catheter tip placement must be determined before use of the port.

There are many brands of implanted ports including: Hickman Port, Port-a-cath, Infuse-a-port, A-Port, S.E.A.-Port, Davol Port with or without Groshong Catheter attached, and others. Many ports are available in single or double port/lumen configuration. The septum(s) are located on the top of the port, except the S.E.A.-port, in which the septums are located on either side of the port. See Figure 70.2. The patient may carry written information about their port.

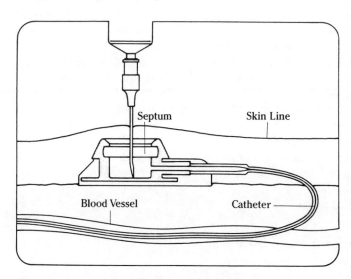

Figure 70.1 Implantable port configuration.
(*Davol Implanted Ports: Patient Information,* Publication No. 99020M. Cranston, RI: Davol, Inc.; 4. Reprinted by permission.)

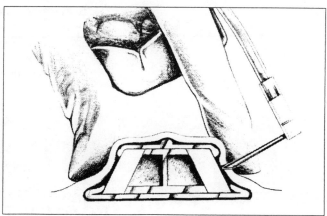

Figure 70.2 S.E.A.-Port implantable port.
(*Harbor S.E.A.-Port Instruction Manual.* Publication No. P/N 200-00241 REV. B. Boston: Harbor Medical Devices, Inc.; 5 and 22. Reprinted by permission.)

INDICATIONS

To gain venous access in patients with implanted venous ports for
1. Administration of IV fluids, medications, blood, or blood products;
2. Obtaining venous blood samples;
3. Performing routine heparin flush to maintain catheter patency.

CONTRAINDICATIONS AND CAUTIONS

1. Use strict sterile technique to avoid patient infection, because the patient would require a surgical procedure to have the device removed.
2. Use only non-coring or Huber point needles to access an implanted port, because other needles may damage the port septum, leading to extravasation of fluids or medications (Plumer, 1987). See Figure 70.3. Non-coring needles are available in 19, 20, or 22 gauge sizes and in two configurations: straight for one-time access, or 90 degree angled with or without an attached extension set for continuous infusion. If blood samples are desired, use an 19 gauge non-coring needle.
3. Although the port is sutured in place, it is possible for it to flip over. Palpate the port to ensure it is right side up before attempting needle insertion.
4. If the patient feels pain or abnormal sensation at the port site during infusion, it may indicate that the medication has extravasated. The infusion should be stopped immediately until patency has been determined. A chest x-ray will help verify catheter placement if no blood return is obtained when the port is accessed. When patency of the port is uncertain, the only conclusive method to determine patency of the port is to perform radiographic studies while injecting contrast media into the port.
5. To administer whole blood or packed red blood cells, it may be necessary to use an infusion pump or add 50 ml of normal saline to the blood bag or run normal saline concomitantly with the blood to reduce viscosity and improve flow rates.
6. For routine heparin flush of the port, use 5 ml of heparin 100 units/ml. Other concentrations of heparinized saline (10 to 1000 units/ml) may be used based on the patient's medical condition, laboratory tests, and home care or physician protocols (Plumer, 1987).
7. To avoid air embolism, the patient should be supine and perform the Valsalva maneuver, or the extension set should be clamped any time the IV line is disconnected.
8. When not accessed, the port should be flushed once per month with 5 ml of heparin 100 units/ml (Plumer, 1987). Ports placed in the hepatic artery are flushed weekly (D'Angelo, 1988).
9. Some ports with a metal portal chamber may preclude the patient from undergoing magnetic resonance imaging (MRI) procedures.

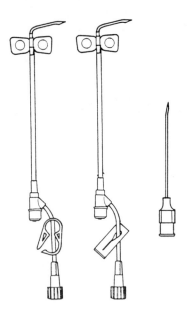

Figure 70.3   Non-coring (Huber) needle configuration. (Burron Medical Inc. Cranston, RI. Reprinted by permission.)

EQUIPMENT

2 pairs of sterile gloves
3 antiseptic swabsticks
Sterile fenestrated drape
Non-coring or Huber needle
Luer-locking T-extension set or short extension set if not already attached to the needle
Bull-dog or padded clamp if not provided on the extension set (See Figure 69.1.)

Sterile normal saline for injection
Two 10-ml syringes with needles
Dressing materials if port will remain accessed: skin tapes, transparent dressing, sterile gauze 2-✕-2 dressings, tape
IV solution as prescribed or male adapter plug
Blood specimen tubes, if needed
5 ml of heparin 100 units/ml, if heparin lock is needed

PROCEDURAL STEPS

1. Prepare all supplies on a sterile field.
2. Expose and identify the implanted port by palpating the outer perimeter of the port. Locate the septum(s) in the middle of the port by palpation (S.E.A.-port septums are located on either side of the port. See Figure 70.2.
3. Using sterile technique, clean the skin over the port with an antiseptic swabstick, working outward in a spiral motion to cover an area 5 inches in diameter (Pharmacia Deltec, 1988). Clean with the second and third swabsticks in the same manner. Allow to air dry.
4. Apply the sterile fenestrated drape, leaving only the area over the port exposed.
5. Change gloves.
6. Fill the 5-ml syringes with sterile normal saline for injection. Attach the extension set to the non-coring needle, if necessary, and prime the needle/extension set-up with the saline to purge all air. Leave the syringe attached to the needle/extension set.
7. Stabilize the port with the forefinger and thumb (one on each side of the port). Insert the non-coring needle through the skin and into the middle of the septum. Hold the needle perpendicular to the port and apply only downward pressure. **Do not twist, rock, or manipulate the needle sideways during or after needle insertion, because this may core the septum and cause leaking from the port.** Continue downward pressure on the needle until it hits the back of the septum and will go no further. See Figure 70.4.

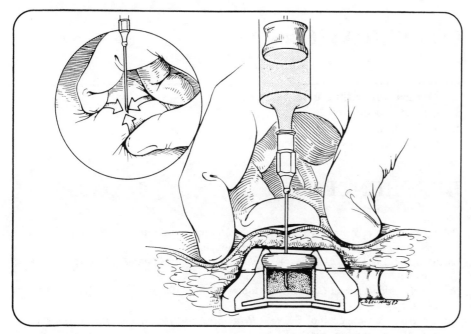

Figure 70.4   Accessing an implanted port.
(*Hickman Subcutaneous Port: Use and Maintenance*. Publication no. 11905M. Cranston, RI: Davol, Inc; 6. Reprinted by permission.)

8. Aspirate 5 ml of blood to confirm port patency. To facilitate blood return, have the patient raise arms, cough, perform Valsalva maneuver, or change position.
9. **If no blood return is obtained:** The needle may be to the side of the septum over the outer periphery of the port. If unable to achieve a blood return, remove the needle and try again with a new needle. If there is visual confirmation that the needle is in the port, attempt to irrigate the

port with 10 ml of sterile normal saline for injection (LaRocca, 1989). If there is no resistance when irrigating, proceed with the infusion (IV fluid should drip by gravity if the needle is in the port) while monitoring the patient for signs of extravasation. To assess for extravasation, place the patient on his/her back and compare both breasts, sides of the chest, and neck. Observe for asymmetry, swelling, or patient complaint of tenderness. A chest x-ray will help to confirm catheter placement and integrity.

10. **To draw blood specimens from the port:** If a continuous IV is running, stop the infusion for 1 minute. Aspirate and discard 10 ml of blood from the port (Plumer, 1987). Attach the sampling syringe and withdraw the needed amount of blood and place in appropriate specimen tubes.

11. After port patency is confirmed and/or needed blood specimens have been obtained, flush the port with 10 ml of normal saline.

12. **Dressing application:** If the port is to remain accessed
    a. Tape all connections that will be under the dressing with sterile tape.
    b. Place a sterile folded 2 × 2 gauze pad under the angled needle to provide support as needed.
    c. Place skin tapes over the needle to secure in place. To facilitate patient assessment, do not obscure the needle insertion site.
    d. Cover the entire set-up with a transparent dressing, leaving only the end of the extension set with the clamp exposed.
    e. Label the dressing with the date of insertion and needle size.

13. **To remove the needle from the port:**
    a. Flush the port with 10 ml of normal saline for injection.
    b. Flush the port with 5 ml of heparin 100 units/ml.
    c. Stabilize the port with the thumb and forefinger of one hand while removing the needle with the other hand.
    d. Clean the injection site and apply a dressing.

COMPLICATIONS

1. Infection
2. Medication or fluid extravasation
3. Catheter occlusion
4. Air embolism
5. Central vein thrombosis

REFERENCES

D'Angelo, H.H., & Welch, N.P. (eds). 1988. *Medication administration and I.V. therapy manual.* Springhouse, PA: Springhouse.

LaRocca, J.C., & Otto, S.E. 1989. *Pocket guide to intravenous therapy.* St. Louis: Mosby.

Nursing Protocol: Port-a-Cath Implantable System. 1988. St. Paul, MN: Pharmacia Deltec.

Plumer, A.L., & Consentino, F. 1987. *Principles and Practice of Intravenous Therapy,* 4th ed. Boston: Little, Brown.

71

Pneumatic Antishock Garment

Marilyn K. Bourn, RN, MSN, REMTP

The pneumatic antishock garment (PASG) is also known as military anti-shock trouser (MAST), shock pants.

The mechanism of action of the pneumatic antishock garment (PASG) is controversial (McSwain, 1989; Pepe, 1986). Current research suggests that the PASG may increase peripheral vascular resistance; increase tissue perfusion; help control intra-abdominal, pelvic, and lower-extremity hemorrhage; and stabilize fractures of the pelvis and lower extremities.

INDICATIONS

1. To augment blood pressure in the presence of shock secondary to
   a. Massive external hemorrhage (Jorden & Barkin, 1988);
   b. Hypovolemia secondary to trauma (Mannix, 1988);
   c. Hypotension secondary to anaphylaxis (Lindzon & Silvers, 1988);
   d. Post operative hemorrhage (Frumkin, 1985);
   e. Hemorrhage due to obstetrical-gynecological emergencies (Frumkin, 1985);
   f. Hypotension secondary to GI bleeding.
2. To help stabilize pelvic (Cwinn, 1988) and lower-extremity fractures (Pepe, 1986; Mannix, 1988; Frumkin, 1985)
3. To help distend upper extremity veins for the placement of intravenous catheters in the hypotensive patient (Mannix, 1988).

CONTRAINDICATIONS AND CAUTIONS

1. Pulmonary edema and congestive heart failure are absolute contraindications. The PASG increases venous return, decreases vital capacity, and elevates pulmonary wedge pressures which aggrevate pre-existing pulmonary congestion (Frumkin, 1985).
2. Caution should be exercised when using the PASG in abdominal eviscerations, abdominal impaled objects, and lumbar spine fractures. Inflation of the PASG in patients with suspected lower-extremity compartmental syndrome may exacerbate the condition.
3. The PASG may be used with caution with a pregnant female. Attempt to stabilize the pregnant patient utilizing the leg compartments only.
4. In cases of multiple trauma including head injuries, the head injury should not preclude the application of the PASG for the treatment of shock.

EQUIPMENT

Pneumatic antishock garment
Long spine board or scoop stretcher
Foot pump or inflation device (optional)
Board straps or cravats

(Note: PASG application should always be used in combination with oxygen administration and IV fluid resuscitation.)

PATIENT PREPARATION

1. If mechanism of injury warrants immobilization, place the patient on a long spine board or scoop stretcher. Refer to Ch. 109: Spinal Immobilization. Position the garment on the board or scoop stretcher before placing the patient on the board. The patient may be log rolled onto the garment (Method 1), or alternatively, the garment may be slid onto the patient like trousers (Method 2).
2. Remove all clothing below the waist. Expose the remainder of the body as necessary.

PROCEDURAL STEPS FOR INFLATION

1. Place the garment on the patient.

    Method 1

    a. Release the leg and abdominal velcro closures. Lay the garment out flat. Maintain in-line spinal immobilization if indicated. See Figure 71.1.

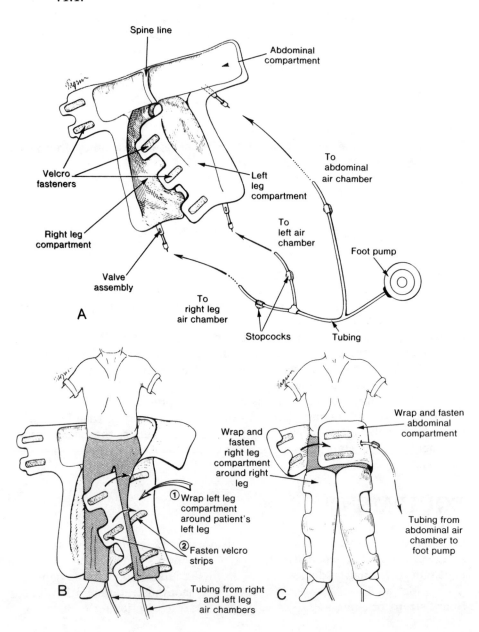

Figure 71.1   The pneumatic antishock garment (PASG).
(Wilkins, 1989: 5. Reprinted by permission.)

b. One or more persons may then slide the garment underneath the patient. Raise the feet and slide under the buttocks. Elevate the buttocks slightly to place the pants properly.

c. Match velcro straps on the leg compartments and secure. (**Note:** some models have color-coded velcro closures.) Fasten the velcro strips to close the abdominal compartment.

2. The abdominal compartment should be placed just below the rib cage so that vital capacity is not reduced and respiration impaired.

Method 2   This method is contraindicated in persons with suspected or confirmed spinal fractures.

a. Lay the garment out flat near the patient. Match velcro closures. Loosely fasten velcro on all three compartments.

b. Position (at least) one person on each side of the patient near the patient's hips. If additional help is available, they may help elevate the hips or feet. Simultaneously elevate the feet carefully while sliding the trousers over the feet and up the legs. Elevate the hips to allow proper placement of the garment.

c. Readjust velcro to ensure a snug fit.

3. **Close** the stopcock to the abdominal compartment and **open** the stopcocks to the leg compartments.

4. Attach the tubing from the foot pump to the three compartments. (**Note:** some models have color-coded tubing.)

5. Inflate the leg compartments with the pump until the pressure gauge (if present) indicates appropriate amount of pressure. The minimum amount of inflation pressure should be used to restore adequate blood pressure (25 mm Hg to 40 mm Hg). As much as 100 mm Hg may be required however, to have a positive effect on the blood pressure (Kaback, 1984). When the garment is used to control bleeding in pelvic fractures, approximately 40 mm Hg to 60 mm Hg pressure should be used (Bass, 1983). (**Note:** If the foot pump is not available, sufficient inflation may be obtained by orally inflating the compartments.)

6. Recheck the vital signs. Inflation should be stopped when the systolic pressure exceeds 100 mg Hg (Frumkin, 1985).

7. If the systolic pressure has not increased to ≥ 100 mm Hg, inflate the abdominal compartment. (**Note:** Pregnancy is a relative contraindication to inflation of the abdominal compartment.)

8. Recheck vital signs and respiratory effort. Document time and vital signs on the patient record.

9. Secure the patient to the long board or scoop stretcher as necessary.

PROCEDURAL STEPS FOR DEFLATION

1. All patients who have had the PASG applied and inflated must be stabilized prior to deflation of the garment. Stabilization may be accomplished via intravenous fluids, hemorrhagic control, vasopressors, and/or surgical intervention.

2. Document vital signs while the garment is inflated.

3. Gradually release air from the abdominal compartment and recheck the vital signs. If the blood pressure has dropped more than 5 mm Hg, deflation should be stopped and more fluids administered (if necessary) to restore pressure (Frumkin, 1985). In addition to a drop in blood pressure, some protocols suggest stopping deflation if the heart rate increases by 10 beats per minute after deflation. If pressure is not restored inflate the abdominal compartment again.

4. Continue to release air from the abdomen, assess vital signs each time. Although not fully researched or documented, some protocols suggest waiting 5 minutes between each step of deflation.

5. Release air from one leg at a time, following the same procedure as above. If one leg is injured, release pressure from the **uninjured** leg first.
6. Frequently reassess the patient after deflation.
7. Do not remove the deflated garment from the patient, in case rapid reapplication is necessary.

COMPLICATIONS

1. Sudden and severe hypotension may ensure following sudden removal of the garment (Jorden, 1988; Frumkin, 1985).
2. Metabolic acidosis may develop after prolonged use of the garment as a result of a release of lactic acid from peripheral tissues (Jorden, 1988; Frumkin, 1985).
3. Respiratory compromise may occur due to decreased vital capacity or pulmonary congestion; see Contraindications (Frumkin, 1985).
4. Decreases in renal blood flow may result in a decline in renal perfusion, glomerular filtration rate, and urine output (Frumkin, 1985).
5. Inflation of the abdominal compartment may aggravate lumbar instability due to the circumferential compartment expansion (Frumkin, 1985).
6. Bass et al. (1983) reviewed several cases and articles which found that the lower extremities were at risk of developing compartmental syndromes after application of the PASG. The precise etiology and pathophysiology are unknown.
7. Increased bleeding from upper extremity wounds may develop due to increase in the blood pressure (Frumkin, 1985).
8. Skin breakdown and decubitus ulceration may occur (Frumkin, 1985).
9. Application of the PASG prevents further examination of the abdomen, pelvis, and lower extremities.

REFERENCES

Bass, R.R., Allison, E.J., Reines, H.D., Yaeger, J.C., & Pryor, W.H. 1983. Thigh compartment syndrome without lower extremity trauma following application of pneumatic antishock trousers. *Annals of Emergency Medicine,* 12:382–384.

Cwinn, A.A. 1988. Multiple trauma. In P. Rosen, F.J. Baker, G.R. Braen, R.H. Dailey, & R.C. Levy (eds). *Emergency medicine: Concepts and clinical practice,* 2nd ed. St. Louis: Mosby; 817–838.

Frumkin, K. 1985. The pneumatic antishock garment (PASG). In J.R. Roberts & J.R. Hedges (eds). *Clinical procedures in emergency medicine* Philadelphia: Saunders; 403–414.

Jorden, R.C., & Barkin, R.M. 1988. Multiple trauma. In P. Rosen, F.J. Baker, G.R. Braen, R.H. Dailey, & R.C. Levy (eds). *Emergency Medicine: Concepts and Clinical Practice,* 2nd ed. St. Louis: Mosby; 159–177.

Kaback, K.R., Sanders, A.B., & Meislin, H.W. 1984. Mast suit update. *Journal of the American Medical Association,* 252:2598–2603.

Lindzon, R.D., & Silvers, W.S. 1988. Multiple trauma. In P. Rosen, F.J. Baker, G.R. Braen, R.H. Dailey, & R.C. Levy (eds). *Emergency medicine: Concepts and clinical practice,* 2nd ed. St. Louis: Mosby; 203–231.

Mannix, F.L. 1988. Multiple trauma. In P. Rosen, F.J. Baker, G.R. Braen, R.H. Dailey, & R.C. Levy (eds). *Emergency medicine: Concepts and clinical practice,* 2nd ed. St. Louis: Mosby; 179–202.

McSwain, N.E. 1989. Pneumatic antishock garment: Does it work? In *Prehospital and Disaster Medicine,* 4, 1:42–44.

Pepe, P.E., Bass, R.R., & Mattox, K.L. 1986. Clinical trials of the pneumatic antishock garment in the urban prehospital setting. *Annals of Emergency Medicine,* 15:1407–1409.

Wilkins, E.W., Jr. (ed). 1989. *Emergency medicine: Scientific foundations and current practice.* Baltimore: Williams & Wilkins.

72

Administration of Blood Products

Dean M. Kelly, RN, BSN, CEN

This chapter contains procedures for administering packed red blood cells (PRBCs), whole blood, platelets, plasma, and cryoprecipitate. Information regarding blood filters can be found in Ch. 73. The following list gives general principles that pertain to all of the blood components in this section.

1. The intended recipient must be positively identified before transfusion is started.
2. The plastic blood-component container should not be vented.
3. A clot filter must be used in the transfusion.
4. Components should be mixed thoroughly before administration.
5. No medications or solutions may be added to or transfused concurrently with blood components except 0.9% sodium chloride injection. Plasma or other suitable plasma expanders may be used with approval of the physician.
6. Lactated Ringers or other electrolyte solutions containing calcium should never be administered concurrently with a blood-component mixed with an anticoagulant containing citrate, because calcium binds to citrate.
7. If, upon visual inspection, the fitness of any component is questioned, it should be returned to the blood bank for further evaluation.
8. If the blood-component container is entered for any reason, the component expires after 4 hours at room temperature.
9. Blood components may be warmed to no more than 38° C (100.4° F).
10. The patient's religious beliefs may prohibit the administration of blood or blood products.

(This list was adapted from American Association of Blood Banks, 1986.)

1. PACKED RED BLOOD CELLS

Packed red blood cells (PRBCs) are prepared by removing plasma from whole blood. Therefore, there are no significant amounts of clotting factors or platelets in PRBCs. Each unit contains 250 to 300 ml.

INDICATIONS

To increase the oxygen carrying capacity of the blood in the presence of acute or chronic blood loss.

CONTRAINDICATIONS AND CAUTIONS

1. Because the plasma has been removed, there is a reduced chance of adverse reactions with PRBCs compared to whole blood. However, transfusion reactions may still occur.
2. Always check typing, crossmatching, and client identification with a

second nurse or physician, and document according to hospital policy. Most major and fatal transfusion reactions result from type mismatches caused by clerical error, administration of blood to the wrong patient, or incorrect identification of the blood component (Greenburg, 1989).

3. Carefully monitor fluid balance in patients at risk for fluid overload.
4. Do not allow PRBCs to stand at room temperature longer than 30 minutes prior to administration.
5. Infusion time should not exceed 4 hours. The longer packed RBCs are left at room temperature, the greater is the danger of bacterial proliferation and RBC hemolysis (AABB, 1990).

EQUIPMENT

Blood administration set, Y-type,
     (170 micron filter)
IV catheter, 20-gauge or larger
Normal saline IV solution
IV starting equipment

PATIENT PREPARATION

1. Complete a blood administration consent form, if required by your institution. See Figure 72.1 for an example.
2. Establish venous access using Y-blood tubing and normal saline. See Ch. 62–70.
3. Assess and document vital signs including temperature.
4. Document pre-existing hematuria; chest, back, or abdominal pain.

PROCEDURAL STEPS

1. Check expiration date on blood.
2. Identify the patient following your hospital procedure. Double check the unit of PRBCs with another nurse or physician. Then match the unit with the patient's blood identification band.
3. Gently invert PRBCs several times to suspend red blood cells.
4. Spike the PRBCs with the other tail of the Y-blood set. Ensure upper drip chamber is half full to prevent damage to red blood cells. See Figure 72.2.
5. Close the roller clamp on the normal saline tail and open the roller clamp on the PRBCs. A gentle squeeze on the filter will help start the flow of blood.
6. Infuse slowly for the first 15 minutes observing the patient for reactions. Most hemolytic reactions occur within this time. This step assumes the patient is not in need of multiple rapid, life sustaining transfusions (Millar, 1985).
7. After 15 minutes reassess vital signs and adjust the flow rate to the desired speed.
8. Continued assessment of patient and vital signs are performed throughout the transfusion as needed according to the patient's condition and number of units being administered.
9. After infusion is completed, reassess vital signs and flush tubing with normal saline. If transfusion therapy is complete either discontinue the IV or hang the prescribed solution with new IV tubing.

COMPLICATIONS

1. *Hemolytic transfusion reactions* can be either immediate or delayed. Acute hemolysis can occur when recipient plasma antibodies react with donor red blood cell antigens. Both acute and delayed hemolytic reactions are potentially life-threatening events. Hemolytic reactions occur one in every 6,000 units of blood. A fatal transfusion reaction occurs in 1 in every 100,000 units (Greenburg, 1989).

    a. Signs and symptoms of hemolytic reactions occur almost immediately and include chills; apprehensions; headache; fever; pain in the back, abdomen, chest, or at infusion site; respiratory distress; hypotension, peripheral circulatory collapse, and shock. Hemoglobin will be present in the plasma and urine.

    b. Immediately stop the transfusion. Prime new IV tubing with normal saline and replace the blood-filled tubing.

    c. Save the blood bag and tubing, notify the blood bank, and follow your hospital policy on transfusion reactions.

    d. Contact the physician for further orders.

    e. Administer IV fluids to achieve a urine output of 100ml/hr to help prevent renal failure (AABB, 1990).

2. Allergic reactions and fever occur in about 1 in every 100 units of blood. These usually occur due to allergens in donor plasma (Greenburg, 1989).

    a. Signs and symptoms commonly include skin rash, urticaria, edema, and puritis. Less frequently, dyspnea, wheezing, and occasionally, anaphylaxis can occur.

    b. Immediately stop the transfusion.

    c. Save blood bag and tubing, notify the blood bank, and follow your hospital policy for transfusion reaction.

    d. Contact physician and report findings. Usually a parenteral antihistamine will be ordered.

3. Circulatory overload

4. Hyperkalemia (See Ch. 74: Massive Transfusion.)

5. Hypocalcemia (See Ch. 74: Massive Transfusion.)

6. Microaggregates—which can lodge in the pulmonary circulation and contribute to adult respiratory distress syndrome—are usually eliminated with the use of a 170 micron filter. See Ch. 73: Blood Filters.

7. Infectious diseases such as hepatitis, cytomegulovirus, Epstein-Barr virus, and human immunodeficiency virus may be transmitted via blood products.

8. Bacterial contamination of donor blood (very rare).

PATIENT TEACHING

1. Immediately report any chills, itching, feeling of warmth, difficulty breathing, pain in back, abdomen, chest, or at IV site.

2. WHOLE BLOOD

Whole blood may either be stored or fresh. In most hospitals it is very difficult to find whole blood. Its use is rarely indicated now that all clotting factors, plasma, red blood cells, and platelets are available as individual components. Because platelets are short-lived, whole blood is platelet poor.

Figure 72.1 Blood product consent form.
(St. Elizabeth Hospital Medical Center, Lafayette, IN. Reprinted by permission.)

INFORMED CONSENT TO TRANSFUSION OF BLOOD OR BLOOD PRODUCTS

In the course of your treatment, it may become necessary to administer a transfusion of blood products. This form provides basic information concerning this procedure and, if signed by you, authorizes the administration of a transfusion of blood products by qualified medical personnel attending you.

DESCRIPTION OF PROCEDURE: Blood or a blood product is introduced into one of your veins, commonly in the arm, using a sterilized hypodermic needle. Depending on your physician's assessment of what you need, the transfusion may be of whole blood, plasma, or some other blood product. The amount of blood or blood product transfused is a judgment your physician will make based on your particular needs. The material to be transfused will be cross-matched to maximize the safety of the transfusion.

RISKS: Transfusion is a common procedure of low risk. Basically, two levels of risk are involved:

MINOR AND TEMPORARY REACTIONS ARE NOT UNCOMMON, including slight bruise, swelling, or local infection in the area where the needle pierces your skin. Nonserious reactions to the transfused material itself could include headache, fever, or a mild skin reaction, such as itching or rash.

A SERIOUS REACTION TO THE TRANSFUSED MATERIAL IS POSSIBLE, but very unlikely. The most common such reaction is SERUM HEPATITIS, an inflammatory infection of the liver. Hepatitis is a serious disease, often requiring a lengthy treatment and recuperative period. It can cause death. But the likelihood of hepatitis infection in properly administered transfusions is extremely low, approximately 1-2 percent. Transfusion of blood of the wrong type can be fatal; but this too is highly unlikely, given the care that is taken in standard blood bank practice prior to transfusion. Blood Products may also contain a virus, HTLV-III LAV, commonly known as the AIDS virus. Blood Products are screened by their manufacturer or the blood bank involved in supplying them to the hospital. The screening test presently being used detects antibodies to the virus and is very effective. It is, however, not 100% effective in eliminating Blood Products contaminated with the virus, and a small risk of infection with the virus from transfusion of blood products does exist.

ALTERNATIVE: Blood is essential to the body's functioning, to life. Care is taken to limit a patient's loss of blood and thus, to reduce the need for a transfusion. However, if one's level falls too low, he may go into shock or a coma and suffer very serious harm, or even death. If low blood level poses such a threat in the course of your treatment, there is NO EFFECTIVE ALTERNATIVE TO A TRANSFUSION.

PATIENT'S ACKNOWLEDGMENT AND CONSENT:

I, _____, have (read) (Have read to me) the above. I understand the factors bearing on the decision whether to authorize a transfusion of blood or blood products. I have no questions which have not been answered to my full satisfaction. I hereby consent to such transfusion(s) as the qualified medical personnel attending me may decide is/are necessary or advisable in the course of my treatment.

_____
Date

_____
Patient's Signature

_____
Witness

INDICATIONS

1. To increase the oxygen carrying capacity of the blood;
2. To replace volume in shock;
3. To replace a blood component that is unavailable individually.

CONTRAINDICATIONS AND CAUTIONS

1. The same contraindications and cautions are valid as for packed red blood cells.
2. Whole blood has a volume of 500 ml and places the patient at higher risk for fluid overload than PRBCs.
   The equipment, patient preparation, procedural steps, complications, and patient teaching steps are the same as those for packed red blood cells.

3. PLATELET CONCENTRATION

Platelets play an important role in blood coagulation and thrombus formation. Platelets are obtained by centrifugation of whole blood. They are available in single or multiple dose units in a 30–50-ml bag. They are usually ordered 4 to 10 units at a time. Your hospital's blood bank may pool the entire order into one bag.

INDICATIONS

To increase platelets in the presence of thrombocytopenia (low platelet count) of any etiology.

CONTRAINDICATIONS AND CAUTIONS

1. Platelets must be infused rapidly or they loose their viability.
2. Transfusion reactions are possible due to the plasma that platelets are stored in.
3. Platelets must be transfused through a filter (AABB, 1990; Persons, 1987).
4. Multiple unit packs must be infused within 4 hours of mixing. Call the blood bank only when you are ready to administer the platelets.
5. Check the unit for clumps or aggregates. If found, knead the unit gently until clumps disappear. If clumps do not disappear with gentle kneading, return the unit to the blood bank.

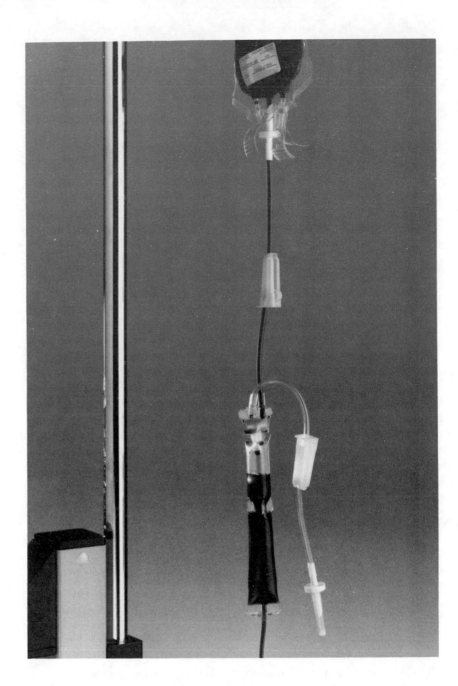

Figure 72.2
Packed red blood cells
on Y-tubing with upper
chamber half full.

EQUIPMENT

Blood administration set, Y-type
    with filter
250-ml bag, or larger, normal saline
IV catheter

IV dressing supplies
3-way stopcock
60-ml syringe

PATIENT PREPARATION

1. Assess and document vital signs.
2. Have patient review and sign blood products consent form, if required by your institution.

PROCEDURAL STEPS

1. Initiate IV line with 3-way stopcock screwed into catheter hub and IV line into other end of stopcock.
2. Check platelet blood type versus the patient's blood type. Although it is not necessary to have the same ABO type, it is preferred.
3. Hang platelet pack on the other tail of the Y-set.
4. Close normal saline line roller clamp and open platelet line.
5. Each unit of platelets must be administered within 1 to 10 minutes. Consult physician's order.
6. If platelets do not run at a sufficient speed, attach syringe onto 3-way stopcock. See Figure 72.3.
7. Turn stopcock off to patient and withdraw the platelets into syringe.
8. Close stopcock to IV line and open to the patient and inject platelets at 10 ml/min.
9. When platelet pack is empty, close its roller clamp and open normal saline, and flush line to infuse all platelets.
10. Assess and document vital signs.

See Section 1 in this chapter for Complications and Patient Teaching.

4. FRESH FROZEN PLASMA

Fresh frozen plasma (FFP) is an unconcentrated source of all clotting factors except platelets. It comes in a 100–300-ml bag.

INDICATIONS

1. To correct coagulation deficiencies for which specific factor concentrates are unavailable.
2. To correct a bleeding tendency of unknown cause or one associated with liver failure.
3. To expand intravascular volume. (This is an unusual use for FFP and carries the risk of virus transmission.)

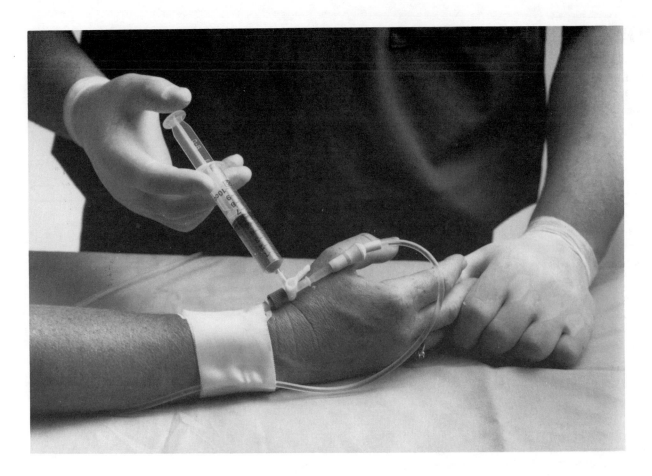

**Figure 72.3
Platelets on Y-tubing
with syringe and
3-way stopcock.**

CONTRAINDICATIONS AND CAUTIONS

1. FFP requires 30–40 minutes to thaw.
2. FFP must be transfused through a filter.
3. Transfusion reactions can occur.
4. FFP must be given within 6 hours of thawing.

EQUIPMENT

Blood administration set, Y-type
IV catheters and dressing supplies
0.9% normal saline IV fluid

PATIENT PREPARATION

1. Assess and document vital signs.
2. Have patient review and sign blood product consent form, if required by your institution.

PROCEDURAL STEPS

1. Initiate IV line with normal saline and Y-blood set.
2. Identify patient and blood type and double check the unit of plasma with another nurse or physician. It should be the same type.

3. Spike plasma with the other tail of the Y-set.
4. Close roller clamp on normal saline, open up plasma, and regulate drip rate.
5. The flow rate will be determined in part by the reason for administration. If the infusion is for clotting factor replacement, the rate will be as fast as the patient can tolerate. FFP administration should not exceed 1–2 hours.
6. Assess and document vital signs.

See Section 1 in this chapter for Complications and Patient Teaching.

5. CRYOPRECIPATATED ANTIHEMOPHILIAC FACTOR (CRYOPRECIPITATE)

Cryoprecipitate is prepared from fresh frozen plasma. On average each single donor unit or bag contains 80 or more units of factor VIII (antihemophilic factor or AHF) and at least 150 mg of fibrinogen (factor I), all in 10–15 ml of plasma. The dosage is dependent on the patient's size and degree of AHF deficiency.

INDICATIONS

To control bleeding by replacing clotting factors in the presence of
1. Hemophilia A
2. Factor VIII
3. von Willebrands' disease
4. Hypofibrinogenemia

CONTRAINDICATIONS AND CAUTIONS

1. Infuse only at room temperature.
2. Use only plastic syringe because factor VIII may bind to surface of a glass syringe.
3. Cryoprecipate must be given through a filter.
4. Transfusion reactions can occur.

EQUIPMENT

Blood administration set, Y-type
        with filter
IV catheter and supplies.
0.9% normal saline IV fluid
3-way stopcock.
30-cc *plastic* syringe.

PATIENT PREPARATION

1. Assess and document vital signs.
2. Have patient review and sign blood product consent form, if required by your institution.

PROCEDURAL STEPS

1. Initiate an IV line with normal saline and Y-blood set at a keep vein open (KVO) rate.
2. Hang cryoprecipitate on the other Y-blood set tail. (**Note:** Cryoprecipate is usually given in doses greater than one unit (often 10 units in adults). Cryoprecipate is usually diluted in the lab when the units are packed together.)
3. Adjust drip rate, diluted cryoprecipatate is administered at 10 ml per minute.
4. If necessary the 3-way stopcock and syringe may be used to infuse. Refer to platelet administration for details.
5. Flush IV line with normal saline after crycoprecipatate is finished.
6. Assess and document vital signs.

See Section 1 in this chapter for Complications and Patient Teaching.

REFERENCES

American Association of Blood Banks (AABB). 1990. *Technical manual.* Arlington, VA: Am. Assoc. of Blood Banks.

American Association of Blood Banks, American Red Cross and Council of Community Blood Centers. 1986. *Circular of information for the use of human blood and blood components.* Arlington, VA: Am. Assoc. of Blood Banks.

Berkow, R., & Fletcher, A.J., 1987. *The Merck manual of diagnosis and therapy,* 15th ed. Robway, NJ: Merck & Co.

DeLoor, R.M., & Schreibes, M.J. 1985. Blood and blood component administration. In S. Millar, L.K. Sampson, & M. Soukoup (eds). *AACN Procedure manual for critical care,* 2nd ed. Philadelphia: Saunders: 407–523.

Greenburg, A.G. 1989. Indications for transfusion. In American College of Surgeons (Ed). *Care of the surgical patient: Vol. 1. Emergency Care, Chap. 1* New York: Scientific American, Inc.

Millar, S., Sampson, L.K., & Soukoup, M. 1985. *AACN procedure manual for critical care.* Philadelphia: Saunders.

Perry, A.G., & Potter, P.A. 1990. *Clinical nursing skills and techniques,* 2nd ed. St. Louis: Mosby.

Persons, C.B. 1987. *Critical care procedures and protocols.* Philadelphia: Lippincott.

73

Blood Filters

Dean M. Kelly, RN, BSN, CEN

INDICATIONS

To remove clots and debris from blood and blood components. All blood products should be administered through a filter (170–260 microns) (AABB, 1990).

CONTRAINDICATIONS AND CAUTIONS

1. Microaggregate filters (20–40 microns) will slow down the infusion rate and are not indicated for use during rapid infusion of blood (AABB, 1990).
2. Blood-filled filters should not be reused after 4 hours.
3. Each filter may be used for 2 to 4 units of blood (AABB, 1990).
4. To prevent air entrainment into the filter, never squeeze the drip chamber with the tubing clamp open.

EQUIPMENT

(Note: Blood filters come in two sizes. The standard filter has a pore size of approximately 170–260 microns. Microaggregate filters have an effective pore size of 20–40 microns. Standard y-blood sets (Travenol, Abbott, and others have 170–260 micron filters. See Figure 73.1).

Microaggregate filters, Pall, See Figure 73.2. 20–40 micron filters are an addition to the IV line. Microaggregate filters trap microaggregates which form in blood after 5 days or more in storage (AABB, 1990). Microaggregate filters efficiently remove leukocytes and their antigens from packed red blood cells, which reduces the incidence of nonhemolytic febrile reactions (Pall, 1985).

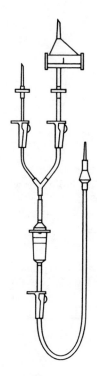

Figure 73.1 Y-bloodset tubing by Travenol.
(Reprinted by permission of Travenol.)

PROCEDURAL STEPS

Microaggretate Filter on Y-Tubing

1. Most in-line Y-blood sets prime like normal IV tubing. Fill the drip chamber half full.
2. To fill the Pall filter shown in Figure 73.2, first prime Y-blood tubing with normal saline.
3. Insert Y-tubing spike into outlet port of filter.
4. Insert filter spike into blood bag.
5. Close the patient clamp and hold the blood bag and filter upright and below level of the normal saline. Slowly open blood clamp to allow saline to fill filter. Close the solution clamp. See Figure 73.3.
6. Suspend blood bag and open blood clamp to desired rate.

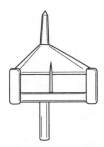

Figure 73.2 Pall filter.
(Reprinted by permission of Pall Biomedical Products.)

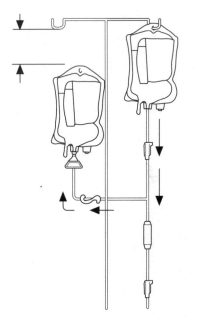

Figure 73.3 Priming Pall filter with Y-tubing.
(Reprinted by permission, of Pall Biomedical Products.)

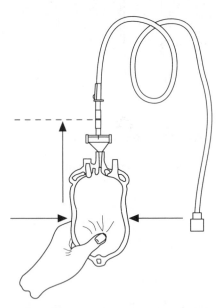

Figure 73.4 Priming Pall filter with non Y-tubing.
(Reprinted by permission of Pall Biomedical Products.)

Microaggregate Filter on Straight Tubing

1. Close the patient clamp.
2. Spike the outlet port of filter with the spike on the IV administration set. See Figure 73.4.
3. Insert the blood filter spike into the blood bag.
4. Hold the IV administration set vertically above the blood bag and open the patient clamp. Squeeze the blood bag with one firm motion until the desired blood level is obtained in the drip chamber. While maintaining pressure on the blood bag, close the patient clamp. See Figure 73.4.
5. Hang bag on IV pole and prime tubing with blood. Then attach to the IV catheter hub or 3-way stopcock.

COMPLICATIONS

1. If blood and/or its components are not administered through a filter, the subsequent micro emboli and debris may cause adult respiratory distress syndrome (ARDS) or other pulmonary dysfunction (American Association of Blood Banks, 1990). This belief is controversial.
2. During rapid resuscitation the filter may clog up, making it necessary to change the filter/tubing to achieve desired flow rates.

REFERENCES

American Association of Blood Banks (AABB). 1990 *Technical manual.* Arlington, VA: Am. Assoc. of Blood Banks.

Pall Biomedical Products Corporation, 1985. Glen Cove: N.Y.

Plummer, A.L., & Cosentino, F. 1987. *Principles and practice of intravenous therapy,* 4th ed. Boston: Little, Brown.

74

Massive Transfusion

Dean M. Kelly, RN, BSN, CEN

Note: The information in this chapter should be used in conjunction with the information in Ch. 72: Administration of Blood Products.

Massive blood transfusion is defined as the administration of a volume of blood or blood components equal to or exceeding the recipient's total blood volume within a 24-hour period (AABB, 1990; Kurskal, 1988). Massive transfusion may also be defined as a replacement of 50% or more of the patient's calculated blood volume in a 3-hour period (Sheehy, 1989).

INDICATIONS

To treat severe hypovolemic shock—Class III or Class IV hemorrhage, which is characterized by a blood loss of 2000ml, pulse rate greater than 120, respirations greater than 30, decreased blood and pulse pressure, and an altered level of consciousness.

CONTRAINDICATIONS AND CAUTIONS

1. The patient's religious beliefs may prohibit the administration of blood or blood products.
2. Warm all fluids administered during massive transfusion. See Ch. 75: Fluid Warmers.

EQUIPMENT

IV fluid (warm normal saline or blood, as ordered)
IV tubing (Y-blood or trauma tubing)

IV catheter (large bore: 14-gauge or larger; 7.5-French or larger)
Fluid warmer
Pressure infusor or pressure bags

PATIENT PREPARATION

1. Ensure patient has had blood sent for type and crossmatch (T & C) and has a blood bank identification band on.
2. Establish peripheral IV access before considering a central line (American College of Surgeons, 1988). If peripheral circulation has collapsed, then proceed to a cutdown, a percutaneous femoral approach, or central approach. See Ch. 62–68 dealing with venous access.
3. While establishing IV access, have an assistant spike the IV fluid on Y-blood or trauma tubing. Other types of IV tubing have smaller internal diameters and are unsuitable for massive transfusions. **If the IV fluid is to be infused under pressure, the air in the fluid bag should be removed with a needle and syringe to avoid air emboli.** Micropore filters are not used in emergency massive transfusions because they slow infusion rates (Moore, 1989).

PROCEDURAL STEPS

1. Give the initial crystalloid fluid bolus of 20 ml/kg or 1–2 liters as rapidly as possible. Assess the patient's response to the fluid bolus (American College of Surgeons, 1988).
2. If there is a no response or a transient response, repeat the fluid bolus and check on the availability of cross-matched blood with lab.
3. When crystalloid infusion exceeds 50 ml/kg, blood should be administered (Moore, 1989). See Ch. 72: Blood Product Administration. When possible, typed and cross-matched blood is preferred. Next in order of preference is type-specific blood. In emergent cases, O-negative packed red blood cells (PRBCs) may be used in any patient. O-positive PRBCs may be used in males and females past child-bearing age (Greenburg, 1989).
4. If available due to thoracic injury, blood from the chest may be auto-transfused. See Ch. 77–80. One to two liters of autotransfused red blood cells can be infused before significant problems are observed (Greenburg, 1989).
5. Frequent assessment of vital signs, skin perfusion, and urinary output should be used to assess the patient's response to fluid resuscitation.
6. The cause of the fluid/blood loss must be identified and corrected as soon as possible.

COMPLICATIONS

1. Platelet and coagulation factor deficiencies are seen in some patients during and after massive transfusion (Kruskall, 1988). Prothrombin time, partial prothrombin time, specific clotting factors, and platelet count should be monitored during resuscitation to help determine whether corrective therapy is indicated. Platelet transfusion is indicated when the platelet count is 100,000/mm³ or less and hemodynamic instability persists after administration of crystalloid, packed red blood cells, and two units of plasma.
2. Hypothermia if fluids are not warmed.
3. Hypocalcemia (caused by citrate binding of ionized calcium) does not occur until the blood transfusion rate exceeds 100ml/min (1 unit/5 min). Calcium gluconate (10mg/kg slow IV) should be reserved for cases in which there is ECG evidence of ST interval prolongation, or, *rarely*, for

REFERENCES

Addonizio, V.P., & Stahl, R.F. 1989. Bleeding (Ch. 7). In American College of Surgeons (ed). *Care of the surgical patient. Vol. 1. Emergency care, Section 7.* New York: Scientific American, Inc.

American Association of Blood Banks (AABB). 1990. *Technical manual.* Arlington, VA. Am. Assoc. of Blood Banks.

American College of Surgeons, Committee on Trauma. 1988. *Advanced trauma life support course: Student manual.* Chicago: Am. College of Surgeons.

Greenburg, A.G. 1989. Indications for transfusion (Ch. 6). In American College of Surgeons (ed). *Care of the surgical patient, Vol. 1. Emergency care, Section 1.* New York: Scientific American, Inc.

Kruskall, M.S., Mintz, P.D., Bergin, J.J., Johnston, M., Klein, H.G., Millar, J.D., Rutman, R., & Silberstein, L. 1988. Transfusion therapy in emergency medicine. *Annals of Emergency Medicine,* 17:327–334.

Moore, F.A., & Moore, E.E. 1989. Trauma resuscitation. In American College of Surgeons (ed). *Care of the surgical patient, Vol. 1. Emergency care Section 1.* New York: Scientific American, Inc.

Sheehy, S.B., Marvin, J.A., & Jimmerson, C.L. 1989. *Manual of clinical trauma care.* St. Louis: Mosby.

75

Fluid Warmers

Dean M. Kelly, RN, BSN, CEN

INDICATIONS

To warm IV fluids and blood products in the following situations:
1. Hypothermia
2. Rapid administration of intravenous fluids (including blood) when treating hypovolemia, (i.e., hypovolemic and distributive shocks.)
(**Note:** Warming blood transfusions helps reduce the incidence of hypothermia and transfusion reactions (Persons, 1987).)

EQUIPMENT

IV fluid or blood as ordered.
IV administration set compatible
  with warmer

Blood-fluid warmer of choice
18-G needle
20–50-ml syringe

PATIENT PREPARATION

Establish venous access. See Ch. 62–70.

PROCEDURAL STEPS

Fenwal Blood Warmer (Baxter, Deerfield, Illinois)

1. Plug in warmer with door closed. If unit does not activate, press reset switch at the rear of unit. Approximately 2 minutes are required for unit to warm to 32–37°C.
2. Obtain Fenwal Blood Warmer tubing. Close the clamp on tubing.
3. Open the warmer. Hold warmer bag so outlet chamber (which goes up) is in left hand and the right edge in right hand.
4. Mount bag on top and bottom support pins of blood warmer. See Figure 75.1.
5. Ensure that bag is flat and smooth against back panel of warmer.
6. Close the door and fasten latch. (**Note:** *Do not* open door once you have infused fluid/blood through warming bag, because you will not be able to close warming door again.)
7. Prime blood administration set with normal saline and attach to Fenwal tubing.
8. Open clamp on upper tubing with drip chamber of Fenwal tubing. Squeeze this drip chamber and hold until normal saline appears in chamber at point of white line (on blood warmer); release chamber and flush remainder of tubing.

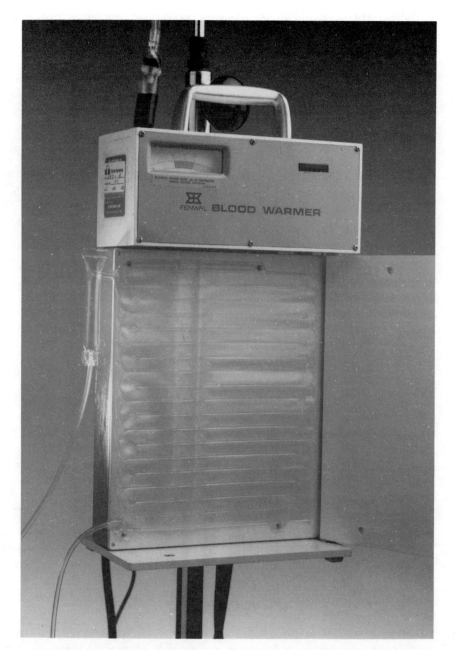

Figure 75.1   Fenwal warmer with tubing.

9. Attach tubing to IV site.
10. Hang blood and infuse as ordered.
11. After the blood is infused, flush warming tubing with normal saline to remove all blood.

Level One Fluid Warmer (Level 1 Technologies, Inc., Marshfield, MA)

1. Push bottom end of heat exchanger into socket labeled 1. See Figure 75.2.
2. Insert heat exchanger into guide. Slide top socket, labeled 2, down over the top of the tube until it clicks. See Figure 75.2.
3. Insert filter/air eliminator into its holder, labeled 3. See Figure 75.2.
4. Plug in and turn on the machine. The display panel should read "system operational."
5. Ensure that all tubing connections are tight.

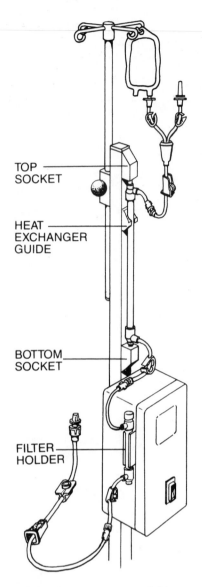

TOP
SOCKET

HEAT
EXCHANGER
GUIDE

BOTTOM
SOCKET

FILTER
HOLDER

Figure 75.2 Level one fluid warmer

6. **When infusing fluid under pressure, remove all air from fluid bag by withdrawing air with needle and syringe to avoid an embolism.**
7. Close all IV line clamps, spike the IV bag, and hang it on IV pole.
8. Open the clamp above the drip chamber and squeeze the drip chamber until it is half full.
9. Open the last two clamps, remove the end cap, and prime remaining tubing.
10. Close the distal clamp, and the filter/air eliminator will self prime. Tap filter/air eliminator against cabinet to remove all trapped air.
11. Connect directly to IV catheter to achieve optimal flow rate. The Level One System 250 can warm blood to 35°C at a rate of 250 ml/min. The Level One System 500 can warm blood to 35°C at a rate of 735 ml/min. (Smith, 1989).

COMPLICATIONS

1. Hemolysis
2. Sepsis
3. Equipment failure leading to overheating of blood or IV fluid (Millar, 1985)

PATIENT TEACHING

1. Report any discomfort associated with infusion.

REFERENCES

Persons, C.B. 1987. *Critical care procedures and protocols.* Philadelphia: Lippincott.
Smith, J.S., & Snider, M.T. 1989. Improved technique for rapid infusion of warmed fluid using a Level 1 fluid warmer. *Surgery, Gynecology & Obstetrics,* 168:273–274.

SUGGESTED READINGS

Millar, S., Sampson, L.K., & Soukoup, M. (eds). 1985. *AACN procedure manual for critical care,* 2nd ed. Philadelphia: Saunders.
Plummer, A.L., & Consentino, F. 1987. *Principles and practice of intravenous therapy,* 4th ed. Boston: Little, Brown.

76

Blood and Fluid Pumps

Dean M. Kelly, RN, BSN, CEN

INDICATIONS

To rapidly infused packed red blood cells and/or IV fluids to treat hypotension due to intravascular volume deficit or electromechanical dissociation (EMD).

CONTRAINDICATIONS AND CAUTIONS

1. Elderly patients or those with chronic disease (renal, liver, heart failure) must be fluid resuscitated with caution due to their impaired ability to deal with fluid overload.
2. Frequent assessment of blood pressure, pulse, skin temperature, capillary refill, urinary output, central venous pressure, or pulmonary artery wedge pressure (if available) is required to determine response to fluid resuscitation.
3. Glass IV containers cannot be used.

EQUIPMENT

Manual pressure cuff *or*
Automatic pressure infusor (Alton Dean) (See Figure 76.1.)
Blood administration set or trauma tubing
20-cc syringe with 21-G needle attached

(**Note:** There is a significant flow difference in flow rates among regular, pump, and trauma or blood tubings. For rapid administration, use blood or trauma tubing.

PATIENT PREPARATION

Establish IV access, preferably with a 14-G or larger catheter. See Ch. 62–70.

PROCEDURAL STEPS

Manual cuff

1. Invert and insert IV bag (already spiked) through lower opening of pressure cuff.
2. Insert loop at the top end of pressure cuff through the eye of the IV bag. **Withdraw air from bag of solution with 20cc syringe and needle to prevent air embolism.**

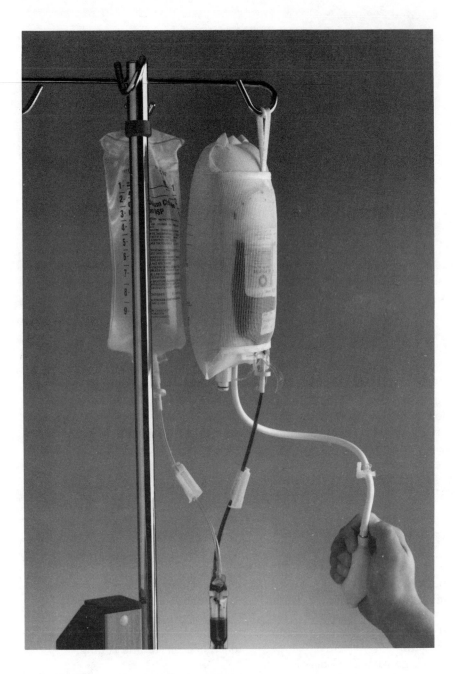

Figure 76.1 Manual pressure cuff.

3. Suspend cuff and solution bag by strap on IV pole.
4. Check security of IV tubing connections at bag and at IV site.
5. Inflate to desired pressure, usually 300 mm Hg. There is no clinically significant hemolysis at this pressure (Floccare, 1990).
6. Maintain desired pressure by squeezing bulb pump as blood is infused (Millar, 1985).
7. Remove empty solution bag by releasing pressure in bag.
8. After removing bag, finish deflating the pressure bag manually. This facilitates insertion of the next bag of solution.
9. Continually assess the patient's hemodynamic status to prevent fluid overload.

Automatic Pressure Infusor (Alton Dean Medical, Inc. North Salt Lake, Utah)

1. Turn on/off switch to off position.
2. Plug air hose into air or oxygen outlet.

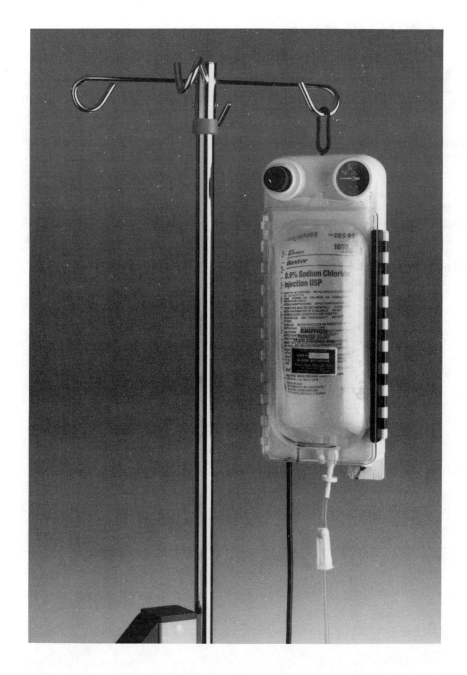

Figure 76.2 Alton Dean pressure infusor.

3. Remove air from IV bag with needle and syringe.

4. Open door and hang IV solution bag on hang tab.

5. Close the door and lock with latch.

6. Hang pressure infusor on IV pole.

7. Turn on/off switch to on position. A hissing sound will be heard as air bladder behind solution bag fills.

8. Monitor the pressure gauge. If pressure exceeds 300 mm Hg, turn off the infusor. Then pull out the pressure regulator and turn it counterclockwise one complete turn. Turn the infusor on and monitor pressure. Repeat adjustment if necessary.

9. To increase the pressure (do not turn infusor off), pull out regulator knob and turn clockwise 1/4 turn at a time setting the pressure where desired. Do not exceed 300 mm Hg (Alton Dean, 1989).

10. To remove IV bag, turn the infusor off. Open the door and remove the bag. Replace with a new bag and repeat Steps 3 to 8.

COMPLICATIONS

1. Air embolization
2. Volume overload
3. Infiltration of intravenous fluid

REFERENCES

Alton Dean Infusor: Instructions for Use, 1989. North Salt Lake, UT: Alton Dean Medical, Inc.

Flocare, D.J., Kelen, G.D., Altman, R.S., Hassett, J.M., Bahjat, Q., Ness, P.M., & Silverstone, K.T. 1990. Rapid infusion of additive red blood cells: Alternative technique for massive hemorrhage. *Anals of emergency medicine,* 19:129–133.

Millar, S., Sampson, L.K., & Soukoup, M. 1985. *AACN procedure manual for critical care.* 2nd ed. Philadelphia: Saunders.

77

General Principles of Autotransfusion

Stephanie Kitt, RN, MSN
Jean A. Proehl, RN, MN, CEN, CCRN

Autotransfusion is also known as autologous blood transfusion.

In a broad sense, autotransfusion also includes preplanned donation of blood prior to elective surgery. This procedure describes emergency autotransfusion only.

INDICATIONS

To return shed autologous blood to the patient with a massive hemothorax.

CONTRAINDICATIONS AND CAUTIONS

1. If contamination of blood with abdominal contents is suspected, the patient may not be a candidate for autotransfusion. The risk of sepsis is significant when blood contaminated with intestinal contents is autotransfused. When the possibility of communication exists between the abdomen and chest (i.e., diaphragmatic disruption from a gunshot or stab wound), autotransfusion may not be considered. However, the physician must weigh the risks of autotransfusion in the exsanguinating patient.
2. Blood from injuries more than 4 hours old should not be autotransfused because of the risk of bacterial colonization.
3. Pre-existing disorders such as coagulopathies, malignant neoplasms, and infections are considered contraindications to autotransfusion. However, these disorders may not be known in the emergency situation.
4. Only blood collected in the autotransfusion unit should be reinfused. Blood collected in the chest drainage device should not be reinfused. The Atrium system is an exception because the blood is collected in a sterile chamber and later transferred to a bag for reinfusion.
5. Blood must be reinfused within 4 hours after collection has started.
6. If blood is being collected from the sternal area during a thoracotomy, the usual amount of suction via the chest drainage device will be insufficient to siphon blood. You may be able to circumvent this by connecting the collection chamber directly to the suction outlet.

PROCEDURAL STEPS

1. *Insert the chest tube(s). See Ch. 42.
2. Prepare the autotransfuser for blood collection. See Ch. 78, 79, and 80.
3. Inject citrate phosphate dextrose (CPD), an anticoagulant, into the collection unit. A ratio of 1 ml of CPD for every 7 ml of blood is recom-

*Indicates portions of the procedure usually performed by a physician.

255

mended. Because it is difficult to estimate the amount of blood in a patient's chest, one approach is to instill enough CPD to anticoagulate one unit of blood initially (60–70 ml). When 1 unit (about 500 ml) of blood has been collected, it may be reinfused or additional CPD may be added to continue collection. CPD injection is facilitated by the use of a volume control IV chamber; run the desired amount of CPD into the chamber and then infuse the CPD via IV tubing to the injection port. CPD may be infused before or during blood collection.

4. Collect blood.
5. When 500–1000 ml of blood has been collected, prepare for reinfusion. See Ch. 78, 79, and 80.
6. Ongoing evaluation of the patient who is being autotransfused includes evaluation of laboratory data to include hematocrit, PT, PTT, platelets, and arterial blood gases.

COMPLICATIONS

1. Massive autotransfusion (greater than 25% estimated blood volume) has been associated with the development of coagulopathies. A reduction in platelets, fibrinogen, and clotting factors may significantly alter normal clotting (Napoli, et al., 1987). For this reason, the amount of blood autotransfused should generally not exceed 2000 ml.
2. Electrolyte abnormalities may occur with massive autotransfusion. Hyperkalemia occurs secondary to red blood cell hemolysis. Hemolysis results from mechanical irritation of the blood during collection, preparation, and reinfusion. Hypocalcemia may occur when more than 3 units of blood are reinfused. Citrate, contained in the anticoagulant, binds calcium in the blood making the ionized or unbound portion of calcium insufficient for normal metabolic processes. Patients exhibiting signs of hypocalcemia (prolonged QT intervals, T-wave inversion, circumoral numbness and tingling, muscle cramping, hyperreflexia, carpopedal spasms, tetany, seizures) may require calcium replacement.

REFERENCE

Napoli, V.M., Symbas, P.J., Vroon, D.H., et al. (1987). Autotransfusion from experimental hemothorax: Levels of coagulation factors. *Journal of Trauma*, 27:296–300.

SUGGESTED READINGS

Barriot, P., Rious, B., & Viars, P. (1988). Prehospital autotransfusion in life-threatening hemothorax. *Chest*, 93:522–526.
Birdsall, C., Carpenter, K., & Considine, R. (1988). How is autotransfusion done? *American Journal of Nursing*, 88:108–110.
Butler, S. (1989). Current trends in autologous transfusion. *RN*, 52, 11:44–54.
Hallett, J.W. (1989). Minimizing the use of homologous blood products during the repair of abdominal aortic aneurysms. *Surgical Clinics of North America*, 69:817–826.
Timerlake, G.A., & McSwain, N.E., Jr., (1988). Autotransfusion of blood contaminated by enteric contents: A potentially life-saving measure in the massively hemorrhaging trauma patient? *Journal of Trauma*, 28:855–857.

78

Autotransfusion Using the Pleur-evac System

Stephanie Kitt, RN, MSN

INDICATIONS

Refer to Ch. 77: General Principles of Autotransfusion.

CONTRAINDICATIONS AND CAUTIONS

Refer to Ch. 77.

EQUIPMENT

Pleur-evac chest tube drainage system and autotransfusion unit

Citrate phosphate dextrose solution (CDP), 500 ml

Volumetric chamber IV solution set or 60-cc syringe

18-G needle

Blood filter

Blood pump (optional)

Suction device

Connector tubing for suction to drainage system

Clamp for chest tube

Normal saline 1000 IV solution

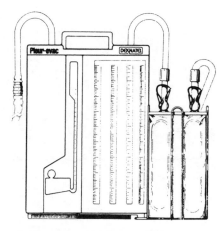

Figure 78.1   Pleur-evac (Deknatel) autotransfuser, set up to collect blood.
(*Pleur-evac—Instructions for Use (A-6000)*. **Deknatel, 1988, Fall River, MA: Pfizer Hospital Products Group. Copyright 1988 by Pfizer Hospital Products Group. Reprinted by permission.)**

PROCEDURAL STEPS

1. *Insert a large chest tube. See Ch. 42: Chest Tube Insertion.
2. Prepare the chest drainage unit. See Ch. 50: Pleur-evac Chest Drainage Device.
3. Attach the autotransfusion bag. The autotransfusion bag (A-1500) is attached to the side of the Pleur-evac chest tube drainage system using the foot hook and ATS hanger on the side of the unit. See Figure 78.1.
   a. Close the two white clamps on the top of the A-1500 replacement bag.
   b. Close the white clamp on the Pleur-evac patient tubing and milk blood distally from the tubing into the Pleur-evac.
   c. Disconnect the red and blue connectors.
   d. Remove the red protective cap from the collection tubing on the A-1500 replacement bag and connect it to the patient chest drainage tubing using red connectors.
   e. Remove the blue protective cap from the tubing on the A-1500 replacement bag and connect to the Pleur-evac tubing using blue connectors.
   f. Open all clamps and make sure all connections are air tight.
   g. Inject CPD into the collection bag so that the ratio of CPD to blood is 1 to 7.

4. To discontinue collection:
   a. Use the high negativity relief valve to reduce excessive negativity.
   b. Close the white clamps on the patient tubing and on top of the auto-transfusion bag.
   c. Disconnect all red and blue connectors.
   d. Attach red and blue connectors on top of the autotransfusion bag.
   e. Securely attach red and blue connectors joining the patient tube (red) to the Pleur-evac tube (blue).
   f. Open the white clamps on the patient tube and patient drainage will be collected in the Pleur-evac.
   g. Remove the autotransfusion bag from the Pleur-evac by removing the collection bag frame from the hanger on the side of the unit. Disconnect the foot hook from the Pleur-evac unit and prepare to autotransfuse.
5. To change the autotransfusion bag, refer to preceding Steps 3a through 3g.
6. To prepare for reinfusion:
   a. Invert the bag so the spike port points upward, remove the protective cap, and insert a blood filter into the spike port using a constant twisting motion. See Ch. 73: Blood Filters.
   b. Remove air from the bag. Keeping the unit inverted, gently squeeze the autotransfusion bag, allowing blood to slowly prime the reinfusion filter. Continue squeezing until the filter is saturated with blood and the drip chamber is half-full.
      (Note: Priming the filter with normal saline prior to this step facilitates this process.) Carefully squeeze all air from the bag through the filter and drip chamber assembly. Close the infusion set clamp, invert the autotransfusion bag, suspend from an IV pole using the plastic strap, open infusion set, and carefully flush the administration line to remove all air.
   c. Reinfusion: Attach the distal end of the infusion set assembly to the appropriate patient line and infuse blood according to the approved hospital procedure, using gravity or pressure reinfusion. (Note: a blood pump that wraps around the bag is best suited for the A-1500 replacement bag when pressure reinfusion is requested.

COMPLICATIONS

Refer to Ch. 77: General Principles of Autotransfusion.

Air embolism is a potential complication during autotransfusion with this system. To reduce the risk of air embolism, the collected blood must be properly prepared for reinfusion by removing all air from the blood bag prior to hanging for reinfusion.

SUGGESTED READINGS

Butler, S., & Moriarty, M.B. 1989. Current trends in autologous transfusion. *RN*, November. Medical Economics Company.

Product Insert: Delknatel, Inc., A Pfizer Company. *Pleur-evac adult-pediatric single use chest drainage unit.*

Thompson, J.M., McFarland, G.K., Hirsch, J.E., Tucker, S.M., & Bowers, A.C. 1986. Chest tubes and chest drainage systems. In *Clinical Nursing*, St. Louis: Mosby; 242–245.

79

Autotransfusion Using the Thora-Klex System

Stephanie Kitt, RN, MSN

INDICATIONS

Refer to Ch. 77: General Principles of Autotransfusion.

CONTRAINDICATIONS AND CAUTIONS

Refer to Ch. 77.

EQUIPMENT

Thora-Klex Autotransfusion Kit 7756

Thora-Klex 2500-ml collection unit (2150-ml collection unit and 4000-ml collection units can be used in conjunction with the autotransfusion kit)

Blood filter and tubing

Citrate Phosphate Dextrose (CPD)

Volumetric chamber IV tubing or 60-cc syringe

18-G needle

PROCEDURAL STEPS

1. *Insert a large chest tube. See Ch. 42.
2. Prepare the chest drainage unit. See Ch. 51.
3. Disconnect the Thora-Klex Chest Drainage Unit from suction.
4. Attach the autotransfusion unit.
   a. Remove the protective seal from the quick disconnect locking connector located midway on the Thora-Klex unit patient tube. See Figure 79.1.
   b. Clamp or crimp the chest tube to stop the flow of blood.
   c. Separate connector by twisting the quick disconnect locking connector counterclockwise and pulling apart.
   d. Using aseptic technique, remove the red cover from the filter of the autotransfusion unit and insert the corresponding red color-coded connector of the patient tube to the filter, making sure that the connector is locked into place by twisting clockwise. Repeat by inserting and locking the blue connector into the bottle cap. See Figure 79.2.
   e. Release the clamp from the patient's chest tube.
   f. Reconnect to suction.
   g. Inject CPD through the anticoagulant port on the filter so that the

*Indicates portions of the procedure usually performed by a physician.

**Location of Quick Disconnect on
Patient Tube of the Thora-Klex®
Chest Drainage Unit.**

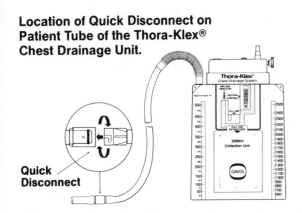

Figure 79.1   Thora-Klex chest drainage system.
(Product insert, *Thora-Klex autotransfusion kit
quick reference guide.* C.R. Bard, Inc. Cranston,
RI. Reprinted by permission.)

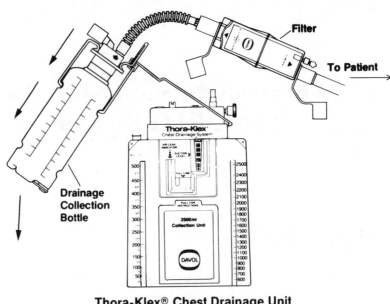

**Thora-Klex® Chest Drainage Unit
and Autotransfusion Kit.**

Figure 79.2   Thora-Klex chest drainage unit and autotransfusion kit.
(Product Insert, *Thora-Klex autotransfusion kit quick
reference guide.* C.R. Bard, Inc. Cranston, RI. Reprinted by
permission.)

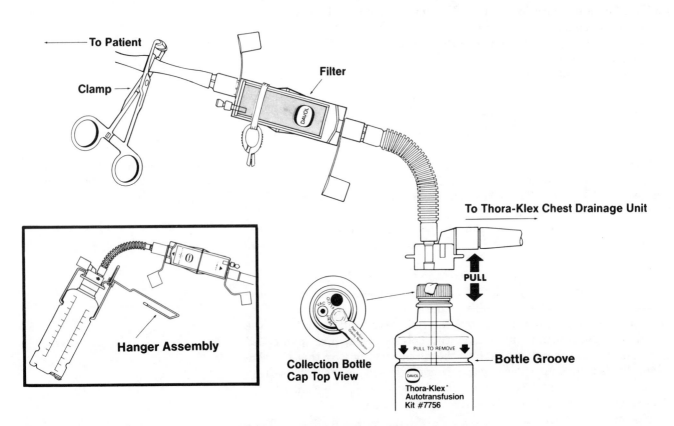

Figure 79.3   Replacing the bottle.
(Product insert, *Thora-Klex autotransfusion kit quick reference guide.* C.R. Bard,
Inc. Cranston, RI. Reprinted by permission.)

ratio of CPD to blood is 1 to 7. Add the anticoagulant by inserting a needle through the latex injection port of the filter housing. Alternatively, twist and remove injection port fitting and insert luer lock to add anticoagulant.

5. To prepare for reinfusion. See Figure 79.3.
    a. Disconnect the Thora-Klex chest drainage unit from suction.
    b. Clamp the patient tube above the filter.
    c. Separate the patient tube from the filter connector by rotating quick disconnect locking connector counterclockwise and pulling apart.
    d. Similarly, separate Thora-Klex chest drainage patient tube at the bottle cap by rotating the quick disconnect locking connector counterclockwise.
    e. Join the patient tubes together at the quick disconnect locking connector or attach another collection bottle as discussed in steps 4b through 4g.
    f. Release the clamp from the patient tube.
    g. Reconnect to suction.
    h. Remove the spike adapter package from the side of the bottle.
    i. Remove the hanger from the bottle.
    j. Grasp the bottle cap and pull away from the bottle exposing the rubber stopper.
    k. Discard the bottle cap and filter.
    l. Using aseptic technique, remove the IV spike adapter from the package and insert it into the spike of the blood filter. See Ch. 73: Blood Filters.
    m. Remove the protective cap from the adapter and insert the adapter firmly into the port marked "fluid" until the adapter is firmly seated against the rubber stopper.
    n. Remove the protective seal from the air vent on the bottle stopper.
    o. Invert the bottle and hang from an IV pole using the hanger loop. See Figure 79.4.
    p. Prime the blood administration set to remove air.
    q. Infuse the collected blood using gravity. For faster infusion, encase the blood bottle in a pressure bag.

6. To replace the collection bottle: See steps 4b through 4g.

7. To replace the macro filter, see Figure 79.5.
    a. Clamp the patient tube above the filter.
    b. Remove the used filter by twisting both quick disconnect locking connectors counterclockwise.

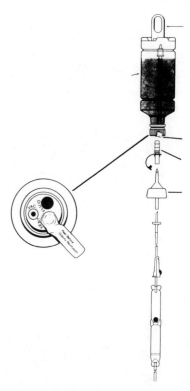

Figure 79.4   Preparation for gravity infusion.
(Product Insert, *Thora-Klex auto-transfusion kit quick reference guide.* C.R. Bard, Inc. Cranston, RI. Reprinted by permission.)

Figure 79.5   Filter replacement.
(Product Insert, *Thora-Klex auto-transfusion kit quick reference guide.* C.R. Bard, Inc. Cranston, RI. Reprinted by permission.)

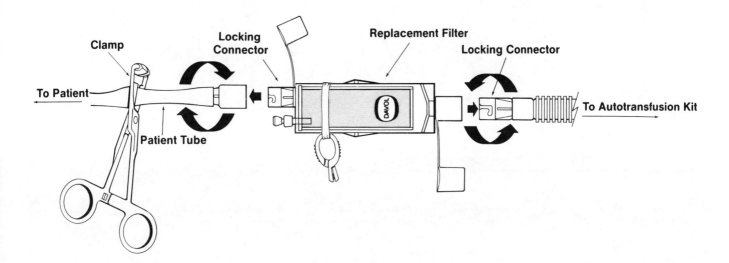

c. Remove the protective caps from the quick disconnect locking connectors on the replacement filter.

d. Attach the new filter by twisting the quick disconnect locking connectors clockwise.

e. Release the clamp from the patient tube.

COMPLICATIONS

Refer to Ch. 77.

REFERENCE

Information adapted from Product Insert: *Thora-Klex Autotransfusion kit quick reference guide.* C.R. Bard, Inc. Cranston, RI 02920.

80

Autotransfusion Using the Atrium System

Valerie Novotny-Dinsdale, RN, MSN, CEN

The Atrium system is also known as blood recovery system 2050.

INDICATIONS

Refer to Ch. 77: General Principles of Autotransfusion.

CONTRAINDICATIONS AND CAUTIONS

Refer to Ch. 77.

EQUIPMENT

Atrium 2050 blood recovery system
Atrium ATS blood recovery bag
Blood filter and tubing
Citrate Phosphate Dextrose (CPD)
    anticoagulant solution
Sterile water

18-G needle
60-mL syringe or IV tubing with
    volumetric chamber
Antiseptic solution
Suction setup (optional)

PROCEDURAL STEPS

1. *Insert a chest tube. See Ch. 42.
2. Prepare 2050 blood recovery chest drainage unit as described in Ch. 53: Atrium Chest Drainage Device.
   (**Note:** Sterile water must be used for blood recovery procedures. This unit has an additional access line for autotransfusion (ATS Access Line), which allows access to the drainage without disconnecting the chest drain or interrupting patient drainage. See Figure 80.1.)
3. Add the CPD to the drainage collection chamber through the grommet located on the face or top of the collection chamber. The manufacturer recommended controlled dose is 14 ml CPD solution to 100 ml of collected autologous blood (Atrium Medical Corporation, 1989).
4. Remove the ATS blood recovery bag from sterile wrap and affix a label containing the patient's name, number, and date and time of collection.
5. Prior to connecting the ATS blood recovery bag, clamp off the access line and remove the spike port cap. See Figure 80.2 on page 265.
6. Clamp off the ATS access line on the drainage system.
7. Insert the ATS blood recovery bag spike into the chest drainage access line using a firm twisting motion.
8. Position the ATS blood recovery bag below the chest drain and open both clamps.

*Indicates portions of the procedure usually performed by a physician.

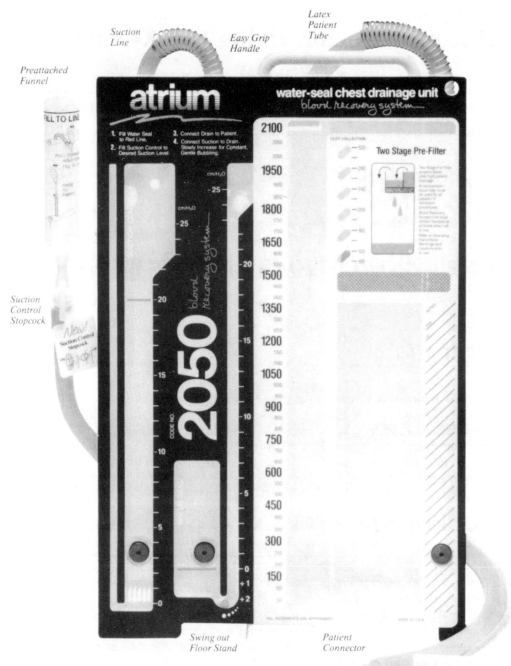

Labels on figure:

Preattached Funnel

Suction Line

Easy Grip Handle

Latex Patient Tube

atrium

water-seal chest drainage unit
blood recovery system

Suction Control Stopcock

1. Fill Water Seal to Red Line.
2. Fill Suction Control to Desired Suction Level.
3. Connect Drain to Patient.
4. Connect Suction to Drain. Slowly Increase for Constant, Gentle Bubbling.

2050

blood recovery system

CODE NO. 2050

Two Stage Pre-Filter

Swing out Floor Stand

Patient Connector

Figure 80.1   Atrium 2050 blood recovery system.
(*Atrium 2050 blood recovery system instruction sheet.* Copyright 1989 by Atrium Medical Corporation. Reprinted by permission.)

9. Hold the ATS blood recovery bag 2–4 inches below the base of the chest drain and gently bend the bag upward as indicated on the bag. This activates the blood transfer. See Figure 80.3.

   (**Note:** Blood transfer without suction to the chest drain provides a more rapid transfer than with suction. It takes approximately 40 seconds to collect 450 ml of blood (Atrium Medical Corporation, 1989). Once full, displace any residual air into the chest drain by gently squeezing the ATS blood bag.)

10. Once the blood transfer to the ATS blood bag is complete, reconnect the suction to the chest drain (if previously disconnected).

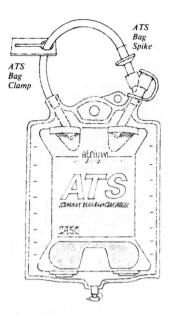

Figure 80.2   Autotransfusion blood recovery bag.
(*Atrium 2050 blood recovery system instruction sheet.* Copyright 1989 by Atrium Medical Corporation. Reprinted by permission.)

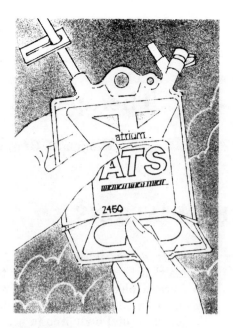

Figure 80.3   Autotransfusion blood recovery bag.
(*Atrium 2050 blood recovery system instruction sheet.* Copyright 1989 by Atrium Medical Corporation, Hollis, NH. Reprinted by permission.)

11. Clamp both the ATS bag and the drainage unit and remove the ATS bag spike. Replace the access line spike port cap.
12. Connect a blood filter and tubing to the base of the ATS blood recovery bag prior to connecting the IV set.
13. Prime filter by gently squeezing the ATS blood recovery bag. This allows blood to move from the bag to the filter and into the IV line.

     (**Note:** Air must be purged from the filter and IV set prior to patient connection. The ATS blood bag has a filtered air vent with a tethered plug for reclosure after use. The air vent must be open for nonpressure infusion and closed for manual or automatic pressure infusion. Maximum ATS blood bag infusion pressure is 150 mm Hg) (Atrium Medical Corporation, 1989).
14. When the infusion is complete, close the ATS air vent by replacing the tether plug (if open). Disconnect the ATS blood bag from the blood filter and replace the tethered cap from the blood filter port.

COMPLICATIONS

Refer to Ch. 77: General Principles of Autotransfusion.

REFERENCE

Atrium 2050 blood recovery system instruction sheet. 1989. Hollis, NH: Atrium Medical Corporation.

81

Therapeutic Phlebotomy

Manjula D. Gray, RN, BSN, MA, CCRN

INDICATIONS

1. To decrease circulating volume in the presence of severe pulmonary edema that is refractory to other therapies.
2. To decrease blood volume in the presence of an increased hematocrit secondary to a disease process (i.e., polycythemia vera).
3. To decrease total body iron in hemochromotosis (Plumer, 1987).
4. To provide relief from porphyria cutanea (a dermatological condition). The mechanism of relief is unknown (Plumer, 1987).

CONTRAINDICATIONS AND CAUTIONS

1. Phlebotomy is not the first line treatment for pulmonary edema and is used only after other therapies have failed.
2. Monitor patients with bleeding disorders or on anticoagulant medications closely.
3. Do not remove more than 500 ml of blood at one time (Guyton, 1986).

EQUIPMENT

500–1000-ml vacuum bottle (a 1000-ml bottle may create too much negative pressure and collapse the vein)
Phlebotomy tubing with needles on both ends
or
Safti donor set (36-inch tubing with a 17-G needle on one end and a 15-G stopper piercing needle on the other end)
Blood pressure cuff or tourniquet
Antiseptic solution
Local anesthesia (optional)
Occlusive dressing (e.g., Op-site)
Gauze dressing
Hemostat

PROCEDURAL STEPS

1. Apply the tourniquet or blood pressure cuff and locate the most suitable antecubital vein.
2. Remove the tourniquet or deflate the blood pressure cuff.
3. Cleanse the site with antiseptic solution.
4. Clamp the tubing with the hemostat at the patient's end and insert the other end into the vacuum bottle. If using Safti donor set, connect the 15-G stopper piercing needle to the bottle. Clamping the tubing maintains the vacuum in the bottle.
5. Reapply the tourniquet or inflate the blood pressure cuff to a pressure between the patient's systolic and diastolic readings.

6. Inject 1–2 ml of local anesthetic intradermally at the venipuncture site or spray the site with ethyl chloride (optional).
7. Perform the venipuncture with the needle on the proximal end of the tubing.
8. Tape the needle in place and cover with occlusive dressing.
9. Unclamp the hemostat and collect the desired amount of blood in the collection bottle.
   a. If the blood return is slow, have the patient pump his or her hand. Reapply the tourniquet or blood pressure cuff. Increase the distance between the patient and the collection bottle. Check the position of the needle.
   b. If the blood collection takes longer than 10–15 minutes, a blood pressure cuff will be more comfortable than a tourniquet. Release the cuff every 10–15 minutes.
10. Reclamp the tubing with the hemostat.
11. Release tourniquet or deflate the cuff.
12. Withdraw the needle and apply pressure with a gauze dressing until the bleeding stops.
13. Assess and document vital signs.

COMPLICATIONS

1. Adverse effects include: fainting, nausea, vomiting, muscular twitching. In the event of adverse effects, clamp the tubing and notify the physician.

PATIENT TEACHING

1. Rest for 15 minutes before moving to a sitting or standing position.
2. Drink tepid fluids, unless contraindicated.

REFERENCES

Guyton, A.C. 1986. *Textbook of medical physiology,* 7th ed. Philadelphia: Saunders.
Plumer, A.L., & Consentino, F. 1987. Therapeutic phlebotomy. In A.L. Plumer (ed)., *Principles and practice of intravenous therapy,* 4th ed. Boston: Little, Brown, 214–223.

82

Rotating Tourniquets

Manjula D. Gray, RN, BSN, MA, CCRN

INDICATIONS

To redistribute circulating volume in the presence of severe pulmonary edema that is refractory to other therapies.

CONTRAINDICATIONS AND CAUTIONS

1. Contraindicated in peripheral vascular disease, bleeding disorders, embolus, infection, or ischemia to extremities and shock (Frantz & Gladys, 1978).
2. Rotating tourniquets are not the treatment of choice unless the benefits outweigh the complications and other therapies are unavailable or ineffective.

EQUIPMENT

Automatic rotating tourniquets
    machine
or
Blood pressure cuffs (2 for the
    upper extremities and 2 for
    the lower extremities)
or

Tourniquets (4)
Stethoscope
Dry wash cloths (4)
or
Cast padding
Felt tip marker

PATIENT PREPARATION

1. Remove clothing at tourniquet sites.
2. Place dry wash cloths or cast padding on all extremities, approximately 2 inches below the axilla and 4 inches below the groin. Do not prepare an extremity proximal to an IV line.
3. Place the patient in Fowler's or semi-Fowler's position.
4. Assess and document blood pressure.
5. Mark the peripheral pulse sites with a felt tip marker.

PROCEDURAL STEPS

Automatic tourniquet application

1. Apply the pressure cuffs to all four extremities.
2. Attach the proper hose from the machine to each of the cuffs.
3. Turn the machine on, and set the pressure dial between 20–50 mm Hg.

4. Adjust the pressure on the machine to allow for arterial flow to the extremities. You should be able to palpate peripheral pulses at all times.
5. Monitor vital signs at least every 15 minutes (Frantz & Gladys, 1978).

Manual application

1. Apply tourniquets to three of the extremities or apply blood pressure cuffs to all 4 extremities. If using cuffs, inflate only 3 of them to just below the patient's diastolic reading. You should be able to palpate peripheral pulses at all times.
2. Release 1 tourniquet or deflate 1 cuff every 15 minutes and apply a tourniquet or inflate the cuff to the previously free extremity. Document rotation intervals and clinical findings.
3. Continue to rotate the tourniquet or the cuff in a clockwise pattern every 15 minutes. See Figure 82.1. Rotate the tourniquet or cuff in the elderly every 5 minutes to prevent gangrene (Brunner & Suddarth, 1988).
4. Monitor vital signs at least every 15 minutes.
5. To discontinue rotating tourniquets, remove one tourniquet or cuff every 15 minutes (every 5 minutes for the elderly) in a clockwise rotation, until all are removed. Removal of all tourniquets or cuffs at the same time may result in recurrence of pulmonary edema (Brunner & Suddarth, 1988).

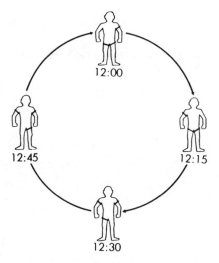

Figure 82.1 Clockwise rotation of tourniquets.
(Brunner & Suddarth, 1988: 580. Reprinted by permission.)

COMPLICATIONS

1. Lower the cuff pressure or loosen the tourniquet if peripheral pulses are not palpable.
2. Bleeding in the extremities, thrombophlebitis, tissue ischemia, and myocardial infarction.
3. Respiratory distress due to metabolic acidosis or pulmonary embolus.
4. Permanent damage can occur to the blood vessels and the tissues of the extremities involved, if the Automatic Rotating Tourniquet machine is used for more than 3–4 hours (Frantz & Gladys, 1978).
5. Circulatory overload if all the tourniquets and cuffs are removed at once (Brunner & Suddarth, 1978).

PATIENT TEACHING

Immediately report any chest pain or increased shortness of breath.

REFERENCES

Frantz, A., & Gladys, M. 1978. Keeping up with automatic rotating tourniquets. *Nursing,* 78:31–35.

Brunner, L.S., & Suddarth, D.S. (1978). *Lippincott manual of nursing practices,* 2nd ed. Philadelphia: Lippincott.

Brunner, L.S., & Suddarth, D.S. 1988. *Textbook of medical-surgical nursing,* 6th ed. Philadelphia: Lippincott.

83

Pericardiocentesis

Valerie Novotny-Dinsdale, RN, MSN, CEN

Pericardiocentesis is also known as pericardial tap.

INDICATIONS

1. To assist in the diagnosis of pericardial tamponade in patients with decreased cardiac output, elevated central venous pressure with jugular vein distention, muffled heart tones, and hypotension (also known as Beck's triad) because they have sustained blunt or penetrating trauma to the chest.
2. To relieve pericardial tamponade secondary to infection, tumor, bleeding diathesis, or recent intracardiac instrumentation such as pacemaker insertion.
3. To assist in the diagnosis and treatment of patients in electromechanical dissociation.

CONTRAINDICATIONS AND CAUTIONS

1. Extreme caution is necessary for patients on anticoagulant medication.
2. All equipment must be secured and properly grounded to prevent delivering current to the myocardium, which could cause ventricular fibrillation (Thompson, 1986).

EQUIPMENT

16- or 18-G spinal needle or 6-inch
    over-the-needle catheter
50-ml syringe
Alligator clamps
Kelly clamp
Tape
12-lead ECG machine
3-way stopcock
Antiseptic solution

Gauze dressings
Local anesthetic (optional)
10-ml syringe, 18-G and 27-G
    needles (optional)
Sterile gloves
Gown and mask
Cardiac resuscitation equipment at
    the bedside

PATIENT PREPARATION

1. If possible, complete chest x-rays and 12-lead ECG prior to procedure.
2. Place patient in a semi-Fowler's position to facilitate pooling of blood in the apex of the heart and lower the diaphragm and abdominal organs.
3. Insert a nasogastric tube to decompress the stomach. See Ch. 98: Insertion of Orogastric and Nasogastric Tubes.
4. Connect the patient to the 12-lead ECG limb leads.

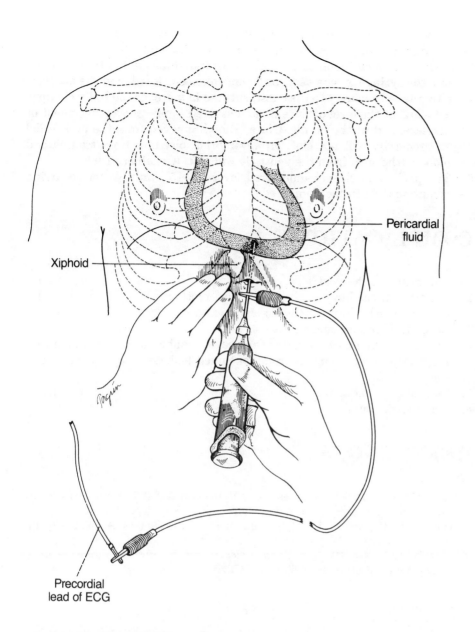

Xiphoid

Pericardial
fluid

Precordial
lead of ECG

**Figure 83.1 Pericardiocentesis.
(Wilkins, 1989: 1017. Reprinted by
permission.)**

PROCEDURAL STEPS

1. Cleanse the patient's chest with antiseptic solution from the left costal
    margin to the xiphoid.
2. *Infiltrate the area with local anesthetic (if indicated).
3. Attach the spinal needle to a 50-ml syringe with a 3-way stopcock.
4. Attach the alligator clamp to the metal hub of the needle and to the an-
    terior chest ECG lead. The V lead is then recorded to monitor for punc-
    ture of the ventricle.
5. *Insert the needle below the xiphoid at a 30–45° angle and direct it to-
    ward the tip of the left shoulder. See Figure 83.1.
6. *Gently aspirate the plunger on the syringe as the needle is advanced.
7. *Once a blood flash is seen, the following may occur
    a. If blood is obtained, and the monitor does not show S-T segment or T-
        wave changes, large widened QRS complexes, or PVC's, then as much
        blood/fluid as possible is withdrawn.
    b. Should any of the above ECG changes occur, (indicating that the nee-
        dle is in the epicardium or myocardium), the needle is slowly with-
        drawn until the patient's baseline rhythm returns. It is important to

*Indicates portions of the procedure
usually performed by a physician.

note that myocardial scarring due to an infarction or disease may prevent an injury pattern from occurring (Callaham, 1895).

8. *After as much blood as possible is aspirated (anywhere from 10–150-ml), the syringe is removed, the 3-way stopcock closed, and the needle is either taped securely to the chest, sutured in place, or the Kelly clamp is attached at the level of the skin and secured to prevent advancement or displacement of the needle. (**Note:** Blood removed from the pericardial sac generally will not clot. However brisk bleeding from trauma and blood withdrawn from the ventricle will clot) (Callaham, 1985).

9. The patient is closely monitored (every 5–15 minutes) for recurring symptoms of cardiac tamponade.

COMPLICATIONS

1. Laceration of the ventricle
2. Puncture of the lung resulting in a pneumothorax.
3. Cardiac dysrhythmia, including cardiac arrest
4. Laceration of a coronary artery or vein
5. Puncture of the aorta, inferior vena cava, esophagus, or peritoneum
6. Decreased cardiac output from continued leakage into the pericardial sac
7. Venous air embolism
8. Pericarditis (late)

REFERENCES

Callaham, M. 1985. Pericardiocentesis. In J.R. Roberts, & J.R. Hedges (eds). *Clinical procedures in emergency medicine.* Philadelphia: Saunders.

Thompson, J., McFarland, G., Hirsch, J., Tucker, S., & Bowers, A. 1986. *Clinical nursing.* St. Louis: Mosby.

Wilkins, E.W., Jr. (ed). 1989. *Emergency medicine: Scientific foundations and current practice.* Baltimore: Williams & Wilkins.

SUGGESTED READING

Budassi, S., & Barber, J. (1984). *Mosby's manual of emergency care practices and procedures,* 2nd ed. St. Louis: Mosby.

Cosgriff, J., & Anderson, D. 1984. *The practice of emergency care,* 2nd ed. Philadelphia: Lippincott.

Kite, J. 1987. Cardiac and great vessel trauma: Assessment, pathophysiology and intervention. *Journal of Emergency Nursing,* 13, 6:346–351.

Kitt, S., & Kaiser, J. (1990). *Emergency nursing: A physiologic and clinical perspective.* Philadelphia: Saunders.

Rea, R.E., (ed). (1991). *Trauma nursing core course (provider) manual,* 3rd ed. Chicago: Award Printing Corporation.

84

Defibrillation

Barbara E. Gamrath, RN, MN, CEN

Defibrillation is also known as direct current (DC) countershock, external shock, cardiac defibrillation, transthoracic defibrillation, ventricular defibrillation, semi-automatic defibrillation, unsynchronized cardioversion.

INDICATIONS

1. To terminate ventricular fibrillation. Defibrillation is accomplished by passage of an appropriate electrical current through the heart to sufficiently depolarize a critical mass of the myocardium (Garrey, 1914).
2. To terminate pulseless ventricular tachycardia. If a patient is *severely* unstable (which may be defined as pulselessness, pulmonary edema, unconsciousness, or severe hypotension) and presents with ventricular tachycardia, unsynchronized countershock is recommended. Delivery of an unsynchronized countershock avoids delays inherent in synchronized countershock and may be safer for the patient (American Heart Association, 1987; Ewy, 1986).
3. To terminate an unclear rhythm which may or may not be asystole but may possibly be ventricular fibrillation. If only 1 lead in a 3-lead system is monitored, ventricular fibrillation may masquerade as asystole or low amplitude fibrillation may be misdiagnosed as asystole (Ewy, 1982).

CONTRAINDICATIONS AND CAUTIONS

Factors which have a major influence on successful defibrillation include: defibrillation electrode size, electrode placement, electrode-skin interface, electrode pressure, interelectrode distance, amount of delivered energy, previous defibrillations, duration of ventricular fibrillation, and condition of the myocardium.

1. The optimal defibrillation electrode size for adults is 13cm (Kerber, 1980). The optimal defibrillation electrode size for pediatrics is 4.5cm in diameter for infants and 8.0cm in diameter for children (American Heart Association, 1987). For defibrillation both hard defibrillation paddles and disposable defibrillation electrodes may be used. Some defibrillators use pregelled disposable defibrillation electrodes. Disposable defibrillation electrodes have the ability to monitor, defibrillate, and synchronize cardiovert allowing the clinician to deliver hands-off defibrillation.
2. Another important factor in determining the success of defibrillation is electrode placement (Ewy, 1978). Either the anterior/lateral electrode placement or the anterior/posterior placement can be used. There is inadequate evidence to indicate that one electrode placement is superior to another (Kerber, 1981). Specific electrode placement is described in Procedural Steps.
3. Electrode-skin interface influences the success of the defibrillation. Conductive medium between the skin and the electrode surface lowers the transthoracic resistance (also known as transthoracic impedance) allowing better delivery of energy to the cardiac muscle. Too little conductive medium may cause burns while excessive conductive medium may lead to current arcing across the paddles (Cronin, 1982). If arcing occurs,

there is potential for a decrease in therapeutic energy delivered to the patient (Cronin, 1982). Disposable defibrillation electrodes are pregelled with conductive medium.

4. Electrode pressure against the chest wall also influences the transthoracic resistance when hard defibrillation paddles are used (Kerber, 1981). Recommended paddle pressure is 25 pounds per paddle (American Heart Association, 1987). The pressure should be sufficient to assure that the entire surface of the paddle is in contact with the chest.

   The adhesive qualities of disposable defibrillation electrodes allow consistent electrode pressure when using this method of defibrillation and additional pressure to disposable defibrillation electrodes should not be applied.

5. Interelectrode distance influences defibrillation success. Adequate paddle pressure on the hard paddles and proper placement of the disposable defibrillation electrodes maintains appropriate interelectrode distance, which decreases the transchest resistance to energy (Kerber, 1981).

6. The amount of energy needed to successfully defibrillate the heart is dependent on several factors:

   a. Body size influences the amount of energy required to successfully defibrillate the heart. However, it should be noted that over the weight range of most adults, body size does not seem to influence energy requirements for successful defibrillation. A weight-related dose of 1 joule per pound (2 joules per kilogram) is recommended for pediatric patients (Gutgesell, 1976).

   b. Transthoracic resistance decreases with successive countershocks (Geddes, 1975), thus increasing the success rate with successive countershocks. Recommendations for the initial countershock is 200 joules. If a second shock is necessary, it should be delivered at 200 to 300 joules. The third shock should be delivered at up to 360 joules (Weaver, 1982). In the event of refibrillation, the same energy level that last converted the patient should be used.

7. The sooner defibrillation can be delivered to a patient with ventricular fibrillation or pulseless ventricular tachycardia the better the chance of success. Success of defibrillation is related to the rapidity of electrical therapy (Eisenberg, 1979; Weaver, 1984; Cobb, 1982). The success of electrical therapy for defibrillation decreases over time.

8. The condition of the myocardium also determines the success of defibrillation. Factors that may hinder successful defibrillation include severe hypothermia, hypoxia, acidosis, or electrolyte imbalance.

EQUIPMENT

Cardiac monitor
Direct Current (DC) defibrillator
ECG electrodes
ECG cable
Strip chart recorder
Strip chart recording paper
Hard defibrillation paddles or disposable defibrillation electrodes
Defibrillation conductive medium (gel or pads)

Adapter/cable for disposable defibrillation electrode connection to the monitor/defibrillator (Needed to operate defibrillators that offer "hands-off" defibrillation capabilities.)

PATIENT PREPARATION

1. Patients with ventricular fibrillation or pulseless ventricular tachycardia are not generally alert enough for extensive preparation. A hard copy ECG strip should be obtained if possible.

PROCEDURAL STEPS

1. Identify ventricular fibrillation through a 3-lead ECG system (Lead I, II and/or III), through hard paddles, or through disposable defibrillation electrodes.

    If a pulseless ventricular tachycardia is identified, it should be treated the same as ventricular fibrillation.
2. Apply conductive medium to defibrillation electrode surfaces or conductive pads to the patient's chest. Disposable defibrillation electrodes are pregelled, thus eliminating the need to apply additional conductive medium.
3. Assure proper hard paddle placement and pressure. Twenty-five pounds of pressure on each hard paddle is recommended (American Heart Association, 1987). Assure proper placement and adequate adherence on the chest of disposable defibrillation electrodes. Both hard paddles and disposable defibrillation electrodes may be placed in either of the following positions:

    Anterior/lateral placement:
    The anterior defibrillation electrode is placed to the right of the upper sternum in the second or third intercostal space. The lateral defibrillation electrode is placed in the anterior axillary line at the level of the apex of the heart (to the left of the nipple).

    Anterior/posterior placement:
    The anterior defibrillation electrode is placed over the precordium (left sternal at the fourth intercostal space) and the posterior electrode is placed behind the heart at the left scapular line at the inferior angle of the scapula. See Figure 84.1.
4. Turn on the defibrillator.
5. Select the appropriate energy level. The American Heart Association's recommendation for the first shock in adults is 200 joules. If unsuccessful, the first shock should be followed by a 200–300 joule shock. If unsuccessful, the second shock should be followed by a third shock delivering up to 360 joules. The highest energy level used should be repeated as necessary.
6. Charge the defibrillator by depressing charge button.
7. After verbally requesting that personnel "clear" from the patient, visually check that all personnel have no direct or indirect contact with the patient.
8. Deliver a countershock by depressing both discharge buttons simultaneously.
9. Obtain a hard copy of the post-shock rhythm and palpate for a pulse.

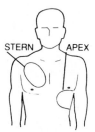

APEX-STERNUM
PLACEMENT

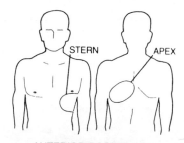

ANTERIOR-POSTERIOR
PLACEMENT

**Figure 84.1 Placement of defibrillation electrodes.
(Physio-Control Corporation, Redmond, WA. Reprinted with permission.)**

SPECIAL SITUATIONS

1. **AICD** An AICD is an implantable electronic device used in patients that have survived an episode of sudden cardiac death resulting from ventricular fibrillation or ventricular tachycardia. An AICD may also be

used in patients with recurrent, refractory life-threatening ventricular arrythmias (ventricular tachycardia or ventricular fibrillation) (Cooper, 1987). The AICD includes a pulse generator and leads. An AICD is designed to monitor cardiac rhythms and deliver a countershock if ventricular fibrillation or ventricular tachycardia is identified. An AICD is capable of giving up to 3–4 shocks in increasing energy increments (Cardiac Pacemakers, Inc., 1987). If the last internal countershock is unsuccessful, external countershock and advanced life support measures should be implemented. Once the rhythm is converted to a nonshockable rhythm, the AICD will reset itself automatically. During internal shocks, electrical voltage may be felt if the patient is touched. It is unlikely that the clinician would be harmed by touching the patient with an active AICD (Cooper, 1987).

If the two electrodes (patches) on the heart are large, difficulty in cardioverting and defibrillating the patient externally may occur (Walls, 1986). The outside surface of the patches act as an insulator around the heart (Moser, 1987). If external defibrillation is necessary and found to be unsuccessful in one paddle position, move the paddles to an alternative position. Increased energy requirements may be necessary because of the position of the internal defibrillating patch leads (Cooper, 1987). External defibrillation should not harm the AICD (Cooper, 1987).

2. **Permanent pacemaker** If a patient with a permanent pacemaker needs to be externally defibrillated, it is recommended that the hard paddles or the disposable defibrillation electrodes be placed at least 5 inches from the pulse generator of the permanent pacemaker (Levin, 1983). Although unlikely, there remains a risk that the current shunting occurring during external defibrillation may cause damage to the electrode-myocardial interface and increase pacemaker stimulation thresholds (Levin, 1983).

3. **Noninvasive pacemaker** Defibrillation may become necessary during noninvasive pacing. This may require turning off the pacemaker before external defibrillation may be done. Some manufacturers provide pacemakers that automatically turn off with the initiation of defibrillation. Defibrillating a noninvasively paced patient may actually require disconnecting the pacemaker from the patient before externally defibrillating. This is device dependent and manufacturer recommendations should be followed.

If hard paddle defibrillation becomes necessary and disposable defibrillation electrodes have already been applied, do not place the hard paddles on top or touching the disposable electrodes. This may result in diversion of energy away from the patient and provide a fire hazard.

COMPLICATIONS

1. Skin irritation, redness, or burns may result if inadequate conductive medium is used or with multiple countershocks.
2. Arcing of current may occur if defibrillation gel or conductive medium is spread across the chest wall. Nitroglycerin ointment may also allow an inappropriate path for current and should be removed prior to defibrillation.
3. Direct or indirect contact with the patient during defibrillation may result in ventricular fibrillation or skin burns in bystanders.

Cardiac Pacemakers, Inc. 1987. *Patient manual-for the automatic implantable cardioverter defibrillator system.*

Cobb, L.A., & Hallstrom, A., 1982. Community based cardiopulmonary resuscitation: What have we learned? *Annals New York Academy of Science,* 382:330–341.

Cooper, D.K. 1987. Care of the patient with the automatic implantable cardioverter defibrillator: A guide for nurses. *Heart and Lung,* 16:640–648.

Cronin, K., Haagsma, J., & Lane, G., 1982. Defibrillation. *Critical Care Nurse,* Nov/ Dec, 32–35.

Eisenberg, M.A., Bergner, L., & Hallstrom, A., 1979. Paramedic programs and out-of-hospital cardiac arrest: Factors associated with successful resuscitation. *American Journal of Public Health,* 69:30–38.

Ewy, G.A. 1978. Cardiac arrest and resuscitation: Defibrillators and defibrillation. *Current Problems in Cardiology,* 2:1.

Ewy, G.A. 1982. Defibrillating cardiac arrest victims. *The Journal of Cardiovascular Medicine,* 7:28–49.

Ewy, G.A. 1986. Electrical therapy of cardiovascular emergencies. *Circulation,* 74 (supplement IV), IV–111.

Garrey, W.E. 1914. The nature of fibrillatory contraction of the heart: Its relation to tissue mass and form. *American Journal of Physiology,* 33:397.

Geddes, L.A., Tacker, W., Cabler, D., Chapman, R., Riviera, B., & Kidder, H. 1975. Decrease in transthoracic resistance during successive ventricular defibrillation trials. *Medical Instrumentation,* 9:179.

Gutgesell, H.P., Tacker, W., Geddes, L., et al. 1976. Energy dose for defibrillation in children. *Pediatrics,* 58:898.

Kerber, R.E., Grayzel, J., Hoyt, R., Marcus, M., & Kennedy, J. 1984. Transthoracic resistance in human defibrillation: Effects of body weight, chest size, serial same energy shocks, paddle size, and paddle pressure, abstracted. *Circulation,* 63:676.

Kerber, R.E., Jensen, S., Grayzel, J., et al. 1981. Elective cardioversion: Influence of paddle-electrode location and size on success rates and energy requirements. *The New England Journal of Medicine,* 305:658–662.

Levin, P.A., Barvold, S., Fletcher, R., & Talbot, P. 1983. Adverse acute and chronic effect of electrical defibrillating and cardioversion on implanted unipolar cardiac pacing system. *Journal of American Cardiac Care,* 6:1413.

Moser, S.A. 1987. AICD technology and therapy advances. *Cardiac Pacemakers Incorporated, Second Quarter Report,* 4.

American Heart Association. 1987. *Textbook of Advanced Cardiac Life Support.* Dallas: American Heart Association.

Walls, J.T. 1986. Adverse effect of permanent cardiac internal defibrillator on external defibrillation. Presented at 1986 World Congress of Cardiology, Washington D.C.

Weaver, W.D., Cobb, L., Copass, M., & Hallstrom, A. 1982. Ventricular defibrillation—A comparative trial using 175 J and 320 J shocks. *New England Journal of Medicine,* 307:1101.

Weaver, W.D., Copass, M., Buffi, D., et al. 1984. Improved neurologic recovery and survival after defibrillation. *Circulation,* 69:943.

85

Synchronized Cardioversion

Barbara E. Gamrath, RN, MN, CEN

Synchronized cardioversion is also known as "sync," electrical cardioversion, synchronized cardioversion, synchronized countershock, synchronous defibrillation.

INDICATIONS

1. To terminate unstable ventricular tachyarrythmias in patients with a pulse.

    If the patient with ventricular tachycardia has a pulse but is **moderately unstable** (which may be defined as having any of the following: chest pain, dyspnea, systolic blood pressure <90mm Hg, congestive heart failure, ischemia, or infarction) or is refractory to intravenous antiarrhythmic medications, synchronized cardioversion is the therapy of choice.

    If the patient with ventricular tachycardia is **severely unstable**, asynchronous cardioversion is recommended.

    If the patient with ventricular tachycardia is **stable**, oxygen and antiarrhythmic medication is the first line of treatment. Synchronized cardioversion follows unsuccessful conversion of pharmacological measures (American Heart Association, 1987).

2. To terminate unstable supraventricular tachyarrythmias.

    If a patient with a supraventricular tachycardia is hemodynamically unstable or is refractory to antiarrhythmic medications, synchronized cardioversion is warranted (American Heart Association, 1987).

    Devices that deliver synchronized countershocks have the ability to deliver energy on the QRS complex. Delivery of the energy at this point in the cardiac cycle decreases the energy requirements and the complications associated with electrical therapy (Lown, 1962). One major complication associated with countershock is delivery of energy on the T wave which is the vulnerable phase of the cardiac cycle. If this occurs, inducement of ventricular fibrillation is possible. Delivery of energy on the QRS complex prior to the vulnerable period reduces the chance of inducing this deteriorating rhythm. During synchronized cardioversion electrical current passes through and depolarizes the myocardium. This current flow allows the sinus node to resume its pacemaker function.

CONTRAINDICATIONS AND CAUTIONS

1. When the patient's condition permits, a standard 12-lead electrocardiogram (ECG) should be obtained prior to synchronized cardioversion. A 12-lead ECG may be helpful for future electrophysiology testing (American Heart Association, 1987).
2. Protection of the airway to avoid aspiration may be necessary especially if the patient has been sedated prior to synchronized cardioversion.
3. Deterioration of hemodynamic stability may occur while preparing for synchronized cardioversion preparation. An unsynchronized countershock should be delivered immediately if the patient's status deteriorates.

Cardiac monitor
Direct current (DC) defibrillator
    (with synchronized
    cardioversion feature)
ECG electrodes
ECG cable
Strip chart recorder
Strip chart recording paper
Hard defibrillation paddles or
    disposable defibrillation
    electrodes

Defibrillation conductive medium
    (gel, pads)
Adapter/cable for disposable
    defibrillation electrode
    connection to
    monitor/defibrillator
    (Needed to operate manual
    defibrillator that offers
    hands-off defibrillation.)

PATIENT PREPARATION

1. Administer sedation and/or analgesia as indicated for the conscious, stable patient (Kowey, 1988).
2. Document the preshock rhythm. If preparing to synchronize cardiovert with hard paddles, a 3-lead ECG (electrocardiograph) should be used to confirm a shockable rhythm.

Fig.

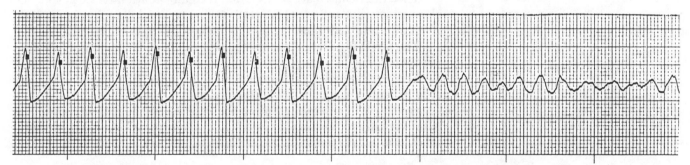

Figure 85.1 Appropriate "SYNC" marker placement.
(Physio-Control Corporation, Redmond, WA. Reprinted by permission.)

PROCEDURAL STEPS

1. Depress the "sync" button to activate the synchronized cardioversion mode. Some defibrillators default to the asynchronous mode after energy discharge and the "sync" button must be depressed before each individual synchronized cardioversion. Some devices retain their "sync" mode after discharge and the "sync" button needs to be disengaged before an asynchronous countershock can be delivered.
2. Adjust the ECG gain setting (size) to assure "sync" markers on each QRS complex. The QRS complex is often simply referred to as the R wave. See Figure 85.1. Both upgoing and downgoing R waves will be detected as the monitor searches for certain criteria such as the slope and amplitude that distinguishes a QRS complex from other components of the ECG such as P or T waves.
3. Apply conductive medium to hard paddles or conductive pads to the patient's chest. Disposable defibrillation electrodes are pregelled and this step may be omitted.
4. Assure proper placement and pressure of the hard paddles. If disposable defibrillation electrodes are used, assure proper placement and adherence on the chest. Both hard paddles and disposable defibrillation electrodes may be placed in either of the following positions:

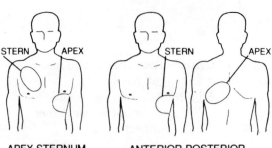

STERN · APEX · STERN · APEX · STERN · APEX ·

Figure 85.2 Placement of defibrillation electrodes.
(Physio-Control Corporation, 1989, Redmond, WA. Reprinted by permission.)

APEX-STERNUM
PLACEMENT

ANTERIOR-POSTERIOR
PLACEMENT

Anterior/lateral placement:
The anterior defibrillation electrode is placed right of the upper sternum in the second or third intercostal space. The lateral defibrillation electrode is placed in the anterior axillary line at the level of the apex, to the left of the nipple. See Figure 85.2.

Anterior/posterior placement:
The anterior defibrillation electrode is placed over the precordium (left sternal at the fourth intercostal space) and the posterior electrode is placed behind the heart at the left scapula line at the inferior angle of the scapula.

5. Turn on the defibrillator.
6. Select the appropriate energy level.

The American Heart Association recommendation for both ventricular tachycardia and atrial flutter is 50 joules in adults followed by 100, 200, and up to 360 joules as repeated countershocks if necessary.

The atrial fibrillation energy recommendation is 200 joules followed by 360 joules.

For paroxysmal supraventricular tachycardia (PSVT), the initial energy recommendation is 75–100 joules.

7. Charge the defibrillator and place the paddles on the patient's chest.
8. After verbally requesting that personnel clear from the patient, visually check that all personnel have no direct or indirect contact with the patient.
9. Depress discharge buttons simultaneously and hold until synchronized countershock has been delivered (on the next sensed QRS complex).
10. Obtain a hard copy of the postshock rhythm and palpate for a pulse.

COMPLICATIONS

1. Inappropriate sensing of the R wave (by improper ECG size adjustment) may cause improper timing of the discharge on the vulnerable period of the cardiac cycle and induce ventricular fibrillation. Unsynchronized countershock should be given immediately if ventricular fibrillation occurs.
2. Arcing of the current may occur if defibrillation gel or conductive medium is spread across the chest wall. Nitroglycerin ointment may also allow an inappropriate path for current and should be removed prior to synchronized cardioversion.
3. Direct or indirect contact with the patient during cardioversion may result in ventricular fibrillation or skin burns in bystanders.
4. Cardioversion will not be effective in arrhythmias induced by digitalis toxicity. In the presence of overdigitalization, cardioversion may provoke serious rhythm disturbances (Lown, 1965).
5. Skin redness, irritation, and burns may occur if inadequate conductive medium is used or if multiple countershocks are necessary.

If episodes of ventricular or supraventricular tachycardias occur, they may be experienced as an irregular heart rate, dizziness or syncope. Seek medical assistance immediately.

REFERENCES

American Heart Association. 1987. *Textbook of Advanced Cardiac Life Support.* Dallas: American Heart Association.

Kowey, P.R. 1988. The calamity of cardioversion of conscious patients. *The American Journal of Cardiology,* 61:1106–1107.

Lown, B. 1962. New methods for terminating cardiac arrhythmias: Use of synchronized capacitor discharge. *Journal of the American Medical Association,* 182:621–627.

86

Noninvasive Cardiac Pacing

Barbara E. Gamrath, RN, MN, CEN

Noninvasive cardiac pacing is also known as external cardiac pacing, transcutaneous pacing, precordial cardiac pacing, temporary pacing, external transthoracic pacing.

INDICATIONS

1. To provide temporary cardiac stimulation in the presence of the following:
   a. **Symptomatic bradycardia**
      i. Symptomatic, in this context, is defined as decreased cardiac output, altered level of consciousness, hypotension, congestive heart failure, chest pain, or shortness of breath (Eisenberg, 1987).
      ii. Bradycardiac rhythms may include sinus node dysfunction, second degree heart block (Mobitz Type II), third degree heart block, or an idioventricular rhythm.
   b. **Asystole** (including postdefibrillation asystole)
2. To provide temporary *noninvasive* cardiac stimulation therapy for patients in which temporary *invasive* pacing is undesirable or potentially dangerous (Noe, 1986; Crockett, 1989).

   Patients included in this category are those patients at increased risk for developing infections, for example, immune system depression (Crockett, 1989); patients with bleeding disorders, or patients on medications that predispose them to bleeding problems, for example, thrombolytics.
3. To provide standby temporary pacing for patients that have the potential for developing life-threatening dysrhythmias. Standby noninvasive pacing may benefit patients with an acute myocardial infarction demonstrating signs of increased degree of heart block, those undergoing cardiac catheterization, those undergoing anesthesia (Eisenberg, 1987), those with postdefibrillation bradycardia, those with asymptomatic bradycardia, or those with asymptomatic digitalis toxicity (Eisenberg, 1987). Standby use of a noninvasive pacemaker eliminates the need for unnecessary prophylactic transvenous pacemaker insertion.
4. To provide overdrive pacing to patients with recurrent ventricular fibrillation, recurrent ventricular tachycardia, atrial tachycardia, or torsades des pointes (Eisenberg, 1987).

CONTRAINDICATIONS AND CAUTIONS

1. Pacing will be less effective if the patient presents with a prolonged cardiac arrest time (Paris, 1985), extensive myocardial damage, electromechanical dissociation (EMD), chronic metabolic disturbances, or extensive cardiac trauma. Early implementation is recommended when initiating noninvasive pacing (Syverud, 1986; Hedges, 1984).
2. Noninvasive pacing is contraindicated with open chest wounds (Eisenberg, 1987).

EQUIPMENT

Noninvasive pacemaker (demand
   and/or nondemand)
Cardiac monitor/defibrillator
Pacing electrodes
Pacing cable

ECG electrodes
ECG cable
ECG strip chart recorder and paper
Advanced Cardiac Life Support
   (ACLS) equipment

PATIENT PREPARATION

1. A simple explanation of the purpose and procedure for noninvasive pacing is important. Relaxation and deep breathing techniques should be emphasized in the conscious patient. Sedation and analgesia options should be discussed. A description of the possible discomfort associated with noninvasive pacing may help the patient. Sensations of noninvasive pacing have been described at lower currents as a superficial tingling sensation and at higher current levels as a deeper thumping sensation. Continuous reassurance during this unfamiliar procedure is important.
2. Administer sedatives/analgesics as indicated/ordered.
3. If time allows, prepare the patient's skin by cleaning with soap and water. Alcohol or benzoin on the skin may induce chemical reactions that interfere with pacing and use of these agents should be avoided. Clipping the chest hair at electrode site may also be necessary to improve adherence of the electrodes. Shaving the skin may cause small superficial lacerations and is not recommended. Lacerations caused by shaving may change the impedance of the chest and cause increased discomfort for the patient.
4. Attach ECG cable (which must be connected to a cardiac monitor for interpretation of electrical capture) to ECG electrodes and apply to patient's clean, dry skin.
5. Obtain a hard copy strip of patient's baseline rhythm along with the patient's vital signs.

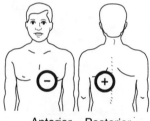

Anterior – Posterior

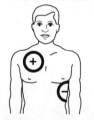

Anterior – Anterior

Figure 86.1 Noninvasive pacing electrode placement. (Crockett & McHugh, 1989: 19. Reprinted by permission.)

PROCEDURAL STEPS

1. Attach pacing cable (which must be connected to a noninvasive pacemaker) to pacing electrodes and apply to patient's clean, dry skin in the anterior/posterior or anterior/anterior position. See Figure 86.1.
2. Select the pacing mode (demand or nondemand)

   Demand

   If demand (synchronous, variable) mode is selected and the patient has an intrinsic QRS complex, assure proper sensing of intrinsic cardiac activity. This is most often done by adjusting the ECG gain setting (size) until a sense (or sync) marker is noted on each intrinsic R wave. Some noninvasive pacemakers have an "auto gain" built in to the device and this step may be deleted. Once sensing has been properly adjusted, the pacemaker will sense any intrinsic cardiac activity and deliver a pacing stimulus only when needed. As the pacemaker senses an intrinsic beat, it inhibits delivery of a pacing stimulus. If no intrinsic beat is sensed, the pacing stimulus will be delivered at the preselected rate. See Figure 86.2.

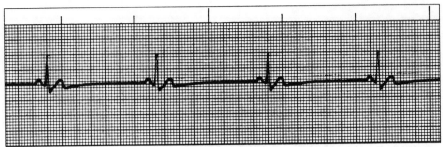

Patient is bradycardic with a heart rate of 40 BPM.

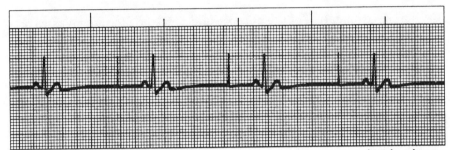

Demand pacing at 60 BPM. Pacemaker senses intrinsic beats. Fires only when heart rate drops below 60 BPM.

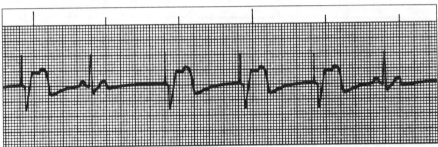

Figure 86.2 Demand pacing. (Crockett & McHugh, 1989: 11. Reprinted by permission.)

Current turned up until capture occurs. Paced beats and intrinsic beats give patient a pulse of 60 BPM.

Nondemand

If nondemand (asynchronous, fixed) mode is selected, the pacemaker disregards the patient's intrinsic cardiac activity and delivers a pacing stimulus at the preselected rate. Theoretically, if an intrinsic QRS complex existed and no adjustment of ECG gain setting was done, the pacing pulse may be delivered on the vulnerable period of the cardiac cycle (T wave) and induce ventricular fibrillation. Nondemand pacing has utility in a clinical setting where excessive motion artifact exists and accurate sensing is unrealistic. It may also be used for overdrive pacing to terminate tachyarrythmias and with electromechanical dissociation (EMD) See Figure 86.3.

3. Select the pacing rate. The rate range in which pacing is typically set for a bradycardic or asystolic patient is 60–100 beats per minute.

4. Activate the pacemaker with the current at the lowest setting. Increase the current until electrical and mechanical (ventricular) capture have been verified. Capture thresholds typically range from 60–120 milliamperes (mA).

Electrical capture represents the depolarization and repolarization of the ventricle. Electrical capture is evidenced by a wide QRS at least 0.14 milliseconds in length followed by a tall T wave (Eisenberg, 1987). See Figure 86.4.

The wide QRS complex of electrical capture should not be confused with the narrow preceding pacing spike (sometimes referred to as the

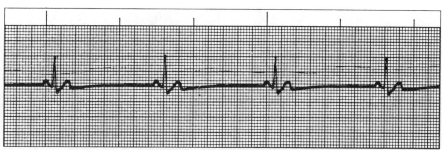

Patient is bradycardic with a heart rate of 40 BPM.

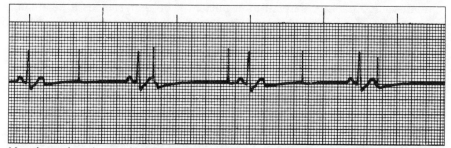

Non-demand pacing at 60 BPM. Intrinsic beats are ignored.

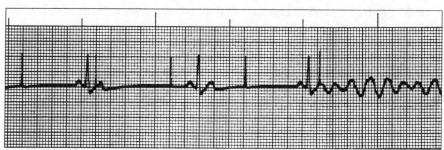

Pacemaker fires on T-wave, triggering ventricular fibrillation.

Figure 86.3 Nondemand pacing. (Crockett & McHugh, 1989: 10. Reprinted by permission.)

ELECTRICAL CAPTURE

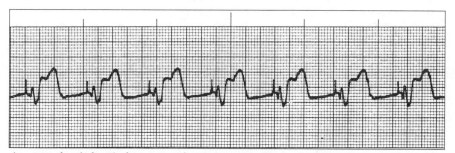

An example of electrical capture, showing a wide QRS and tall T-wave.

Figure 86.4 Electrical capture. (Crockett & McHugh, 1989: 21. Reprinted by permission.)

pacing artifact). The clinician must also distinguish the wide QRS complex of electrical capture from the wave form distortion that may appear following a pacing spike. This distortion may be generated from the pacing pulse and does not represent electrical capture (Dunn, 1989). See Figure 86.5.

Mechanical capture, which represents the contraction of the myocardium, is realized by palpating a pulse. The ability to palpate a pulse with concurrent skeletal muscle contraction may be difficult. Increased blood pressure, improved arterial pressure measurements, increased skin temperature and color, or increased levels of consciousness may assist in identifying mechanical capture.

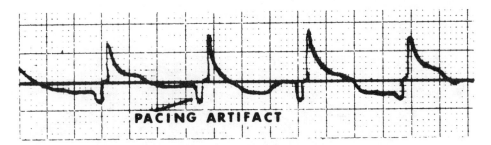

Figure 86.5 Wave form distortion during pacing. Note the 40-mSec pacing spike (also referred to as pacing artifact) followed by wide ECG distortion. This type of ECG distortion needs to be differentiated from the wide QRS that occurs with electrical capture.
(Dunn, 1989: 26. Reprinted by permission.)

5. Acquire a hard copy strip to document findings.
6. Prepare for follow-up treatment with transvenous pacemaker. Successful noninvasive pacing, defined as a patient who experiences a perfusing, pacemaker-dependent rhythm, should be followed up by insertion of a tranvenous pacemaker (Eisenberg, 1987).

COMPLICATIONS

1. Induction of ventricular fibrillation is unlikely. The amount of energy needed to induce ventricular fibrillation has been studied in the animal model and it is approximately 12 times that amount needed to pace the heart (Voorhees, 1984). However, a defibrillator should be available when implementing noninvasive pacing.
2. Discomfort may be experienced as cutaneous nerve stimulation and skeletal muscle stimulation. Analgesia or sedation may be necessary.
3. Minor skin erythema may occur at the electrode site.
4. Short-term use of noninvasive pacing appears to be safe to the myocardium (Kicklighter, 1985). Cardiac enzymes and ECGs acquired in animal testing indicate that no cardiac ischemia or infarction occurs with noninvasive pacing (Kicklighter, 1985).
5. There is little risk to the operator performing CPR and other hands-on procedures during noninvasive pacing. CPR should continue to be performed in the event that mechanical capture is not identified. The clinician may feel a slight tingling sensation during pacing procedures.
6. Defibrillation may be necessary during pacing. To defibrillate a patient who is being noninvasively paced, either the pacemaker may need to be turned off and/or disconnected from the patient or the pacing functions will automatically turn off when the defibrillator is charged. This will vary with difficult pacemakers and manufacturers' recommendations need to be consulted. Defibrillation should then proceed per protocol.

PATIENT TEACHING

1. Discuss realistic expectations of the discomfort associated with pacing and available measures to alleviate it.
2. Reinforce to the patient and the family that during routine noninvasive pacing there is no risk of electrocution (Crockett, 1989).

REFERENCES

Crockett, P., & McHugh, L.G. 1989. *Noninvasive pacing: What you should know.* Physio-Control Corporation, Redmond, WA.
Dunn, D.L. 1989. Noninvasive temporary pacing: Experience in a community hospital. *Heart and Lung,* 18:23–28.

Eisenberg, M., & Cummins, R. (1987). Emergency cardiac pacing: transcutaneous pacing, transvenous pacing, and transthoracic pacing. In Eisenberg, M. Cummins, R., & Ho, M. (eds). *Code blue: Cardiac arrest and resuscitation.* Saunders: Philadelphia; 99–102.

Hedges, J.R. 1984. Developments in transcutaneous and transthoracic pacing during bradycardiac arrest. *Annals of Emergency Medicine,* 13:822–827.

Kicklighter, E.J. 1985. Pathological aspects of transcutaneous cardiac pacing. *American Journal of Emergency Medicine,* 3:108–112.

Noe, R., Crockwell, W., Moses, H., Dove, J., & Batchelder, J. 1986. Transcutaneous pacemaker use in a large hospital. *Pace,* 9:101–104.

Paris, P.M. 1985. Transcutaneous pacing for bradycardic cardiac arrest in prehospital cardiac arrest. *Annals of Emergency Medicine,* 14:320–323.

Syverud, S.A. 1986. Transcutaneous and transvenous cardiac pacing for early bradyasystolic cardiac arrest. *Annals of Emergency Medicine,* 15:121–124.

Voorhees, W.D. 1984. Safety factor for precordial pacing: Minimum current thresholds for pacing and for ventricular fibrillation by vulnerable-period stimulation. *Pace,* 7:356–360.

Zoll, P.M. 1981. External noninvasive electrical stimulation of the heart. *Critical Care Medicine,* 9:393–394.

87

Temporary Transthoracic Pacemaker Insertion

Ruth Altherr Giebel, MS, RN

INDICATIONS

To pace the heart when external or transvenous pacing is not immediately available in the following situations (Roberts & Greenberg, 1981)
1. Asystole
2. Severe bradycardia
   a. Pulseless idioventricular rhythm
   b. Atrioventricular dissociation with inadequate ventricular response or recurrent ventricular fibrillation or ventricular tachycardia
3. Unstable sinus bradycardia, junctional bradycardia, and atrial fibrillation with a high degree of atrio-ventricular block.

CONTRAINDICATIONS AND CAUTIONS

1. Transthoracic pacing is contrainindicated in stable or awake patients or in conditions that may be quickly or easily corrected by medication, or transvenous or external pacing due to the seriousness of the potential complications (Roberts & Greenberg, 1981).
2. Advanced cardiac life support (ACLS) equipment, including medications and a defibrillator, should be present during insertion.
3. Equipment should be kept grounded to prevent electrical shock. Routine equipment checks can help to ensure that all equipment has been properly grounded.
4. Place any noninsulated exposed metal parts of the generator or pacing wire in a rubber glove.
5. Wear rubber gloves when handling the connective ends of the pacing wire.

PATIENT PREPARATION

1. Connect patient to ECG monitor for continuous ECG monitoring. See Ch. 57: ECG Monitoring.
2. Cleanse the left chest wall just below the left nipple area with antiseptic solution and shave if necessary. See Figure 87.1.

EQUIPMENT

Antiseptic solution
Gauze dressings
Sterile towels and drapes
Sterile gloves
Gowns

Masks
Caps
Transthoracic pacing kit, which contains the pacing wire and connectors.

Extension cable
Temporary pacemaker generator
New 9-volt battery
3-0 suture with needle

Needle holder
Scissors (suture)
Tape
ACLS equipment

289
Ch. 87 Temporary Transthoracic
Pacemaker Insertion

PROCEDURAL STEPS

1. Obtain a 12-lead ECG. See Ch. 58: 12-Lead ECG.
2. *Drape the area with sterile towels.
3. *Insert the needle/stylet transthoracically into the ventricle through the fourth intercostal space. See Figure 87.1.

*Indicates portions of the procedure usually performed by a physician.

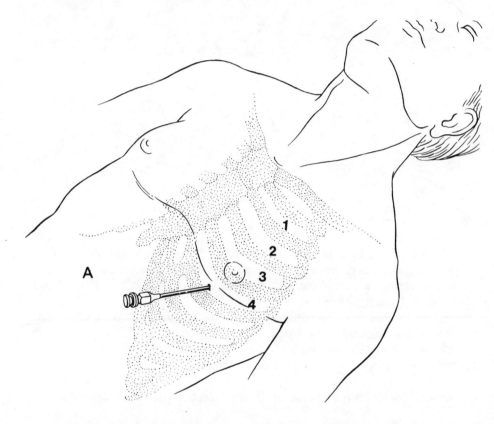

Figure 87.1 Emergency transthoracic cardiac pacemaker insertion: transthoracic needle insertion. (Rosen & Sternbach, 1983: 103. Reprinted by permission.)

4. *Insert the pacing wire through the needle after removing the stylet. Withdraw the needle over the pacing wire.
5. *Secure the pacing wire in place with suture or tape.
6. Attach the wire to the extension cable and temporary pacemaker generator using the connecting adaptor. The proximal end of the pacing wire is inserted into the adaptor and both locks are tightened. The distal lead is then connected to the negative pole on the pacing generator and the proximal lead is connected to the positive pole. See Figure 87.2.
7. Turn on the external generator.
8. Adjust the settings on the pacing generator as indicated by the physician.

Rate:

The pacemaker rate will be set above the patient's intrinsic rate, usually between 80–100 depending on the patient's clinical condition.

Output:

The output will be increased until continuous capture is seen. This point is called the pacing threshold. The output is then set at 2 to 3 times the threshold.

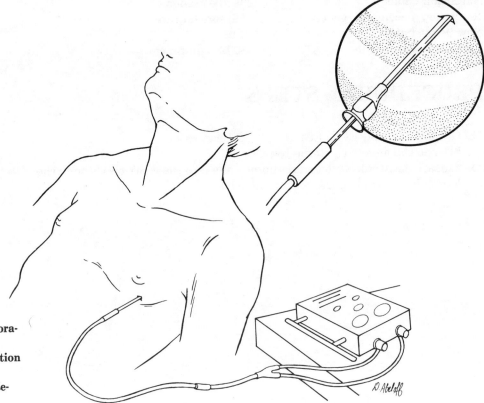

Figure 87.2 Emergency transthoracic cardiac pacemaker insertion:
pacing lead insertion and connection
to external generator.
(Rosen & Sternbach, 1983: 103. Reprinted by permission.)

Sensitivity:
The sensitivity is usually set somewhere between the maximum setting,
which allows the pacemaker to function in a demand mode, and the minimum setting, which allows the pacemaker to function in a fixed mode.
(Love & Paraskos, 1987)

9. Assess the patient's response to the pacing mode using vital signs, neurologic checks, and urine output.
10. Monitor the ECG continuously for pacemaker function.
11. *The pacing wire may be sutured to the skin.
12. Place a sterile dressing over the insertion site. The pacing leads are then
secured by looping and taping them to the outside of the dressing.

COMPLICATIONS

1. Cardiac tamponade
2. Myocardial hematoma
3. Myocardial laceration
4. Coronary artery laceration
5. Pneumothorax
6. Cardiac arrhythmias
7. Liver or stomach puncture
(Roberts & Greenberg, 1981)

PATIENT TEACHING

1. Bed rest is required while the temporary pacemaker is in place. Request
assistance before changing positions.

2. Report any symptoms of dizziness, lightheadedness, or weakness immediately.
3. The transthoracic pacemaker is temporary and may be replaced with a transvenous or permanent pacemaker.

REFERENCES

Love, J.A., & Paraskos, J.A. 1987. Emergency cardiac pacing. *Hospital Medicine,* 19, 10:149–167.

Roberts, J.R., & Greenberg, M.I. 1981. Emergency transthoracic pacemaker. *Annals of Emergency Medicine,* 10:600–612.

Rosen, P., & Sternbach, G.L. 1983. *Atlas of Emergency Medicine,* Baltimore: Williams & Wilkins.

SUGGESTED READING

Braun, A.E. 1986. Transthoracic pacing in the emergency department. *Journal of Emergency Nursing,* 12:354–359.

88

Temporary Transvenous Pacemaker Insertion

Ruth Altherr Giebel, MS, RN

INDICATIONS

1. To maintain an adequate heart rate in the presence of symptomatic bradydysrhythmias unresponsive to drug therapy. Bradydysrhythmias may result from myocardial infarction with atrioventricular block or right bundle branch block with left anterior hemiblock, drug toxicity, or electrolyte disturbance (Benjamin, 1985).
2. To terminate paroxysmal supraventricular tachycardia, atrial flutter, or ventricular tachycardia (Benjamin, 1985).

CONTRAINDICATIONS AND CAUTIONS

1. Advanced cardiac life support (ACLS) equipment to include emergency medications and defibrillator should be present during insertion.
2. Equipment in patient area should be grounded to prevent electrical shock. Routine equipment checks can help to ensure that all equipment is properly grounded.
3. Place any noninsulated metal parts of the generator or pacing wire in a rubber glove.
4. Wear rubber gloves when handling the connective ends of pacing wires.

PATIENT PREPARATION

1. Position patient on the fluoroscopy table if applicable.
2. Place patient on continuous ECG monitoring. See Ch. 57: ECG Monitoring.
3. Shave the insertion site.
4. Cleanse the site with antiseptic solution.

EQUIPMENT

10-ml syringe
2–22-G needles
Local anesthetic
Alcohol wipes
Antiseptic solution
Gauze dressings
Scalpel blade #11
Cutdown tray (for antecubital insertion)

Percutaneous insertion kit (for jugular or subclavian insertion)
Sterile towels and drapes
Sterile gloves
Gowns
Masks
Caps
Needle holder

Scissors (suture)
2-0-3-0 silk suture on needles
Tape
Temporary pacemaker generator
New 9-volt battery
Extension cable
Pacing lead (A bipolar lead is
normally used, however
unipolar leads are also
available.)

Cardiac monitor/defibrillator
12-lead ECG machine (well
grounded)
Male-to-male connector or alligator
clamp (optional)
Fluoroscopy equipment (optional)
ACLS equipment

PROCEDURAL STEPS

1. Obtain a baseline 12 lead ECG. See Ch. 58: 12-Lead ECG.
2. *Drape the area with sterile towels.
3. *Insert the pacing wire via the percutaneous or cut-down technique. See Ch. 64: Subclavian Venous Access, Ch. 65: Internal Jugular Venous Access, Ch. 67: Venous Cutdown.
4. *Once the pacing lead is in the vessel, advance it approximately 10–12 centimeters (Benjamin, 1985).
5. To monitor the pacemaker lead placement by ECG, connect the distal terminal of the pacing lead to the V-lead of the ECG machine by a male-to-male connector or by an insulated wire with alligator clips on each end. The pacing catheter is then advanced quickly and smoothly while monitoring the V-lead to determine location of the pacing lead as described in Figure 88.1. Consistent ST segment elevation indicates that the pacemaker lead is seated against the endocardial surface.
6. To monitor the pacemaker lead placement by fluoroscopy, advance the pacing lead through the vessel to the right ventricle of the heart. The tip is advanced until contact is made with the endocardial surface.
7. Monitor the patient's tolerance of the procedure and vital signs every 5 minutes.
8. *During the pacemaker insertion, if catheter induced ectopy occurs, withdraw the catheter slightly until the ectopy subsides and then readvance the pacing lead.
9. Intravenous lidocaine may be given to prevent ventricular ectopy during placement.
10. Once endocardial placement is achieved with ECG guidance or under fluoroscopy, connect the pacing lead to the pacing generator or extension cable. See Figure 88.2.
11. Adjust the settings on the pacing generator as indicated by the physician. See Figure 88.3.

    Rate:
    The pacemaker rate will be set above the patient's intrinsic rate, usually between 80–100 depending on the patient's clinical condition.

    Output:
    The output will be increased until continuous capture is seen. See Figure 88.4. This point is called the pacing threshold. The output is then set at 2 to 3 times the threshold.

    Sensitivity:
    The sensitivity is usually set somewhere between the maximum setting, which allows the pacemaker to function in a demand mode, and the minimum setting, which allows the pacemaker to function in a fixed mode (Love & Paraskos, 1987).
12. Assess the patient's response to the pacing mode using vital signs, neurological checks, and urine output.
13. Monitor the ECG continuously.

*Indicates portions of the procedure usually performed by a physician.

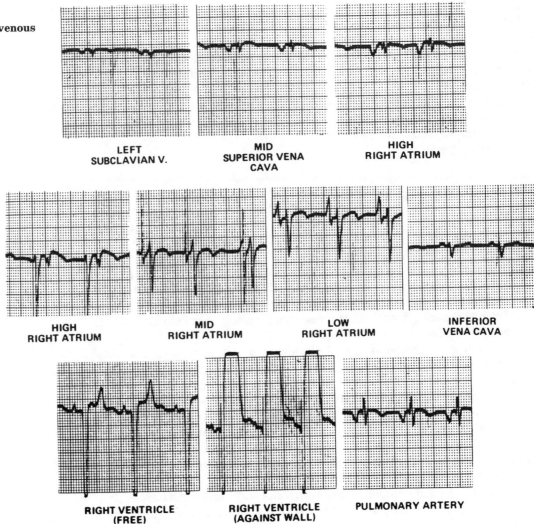

LEFT
SUBCLAVIAN V.

MID
SUPERIOR VENA
CAVA

HIGH
RIGHT ATRIUM

HIGH
RIGHT ATRIUM

MID
RIGHT ATRIUM

LOW
RIGHT ATRIUM

INFERIOR
VENA CAVA

RIGHT VENTRICLE
(FREE)

RIGHT VENTRICLE
(AGAINST WALL)

PULMONARY ARTERY

Figure 88.1 Pacemaker placement by electrocardiographic monitoring. "As the pacing catheter approaches the right atrium, the amplitude of the P waves increases progressively. Since atrial depolarization is inferiorly directed in this patient, P waves recorded above the atria have a negative deflection whereas those low in the atria and in the inferior vena cava are positive. As the catheter enters the ventricle, the QRS amplitude increases markedly, and a QS complex is inscribed. When the catheter tip touches the endocardial surface, marked ST-segment elevation is seen. As the electrode passes into the pulmonary artery, the QRS amplitude diminishes, and a negative P wave is inscribed since the catheter tip is again above the level of the atria."
(Bing, et al., 1972: 651. Reprinted by permission.)

14. *Secure the pacing catheter to the skin with suture.
15. Place a sterile dressing over the insertion site. The pacing leads are then secured by looping and taping them to the outside of the dressing.
16. Obtain a chest x-ray to verify lead placement and evaluate the patient for complications.
17. Keep the patient in bed while the temporary pacing lead is in place.

COMPLICATIONS

Related to insertion

1. Hemothorax
2. Pneumothorax
3. Myocardial perforation, which may lead to cardiac tamponade
4. Myocardial irritability, which may cause ventricular dysrhythmias (Love & Paraskos, 1987).

Related to hemodynamic response

1. Loss of the contribution of atrial contraction, which occurs with ventricular pacing, may lead to decrease in blood pressure, urine output, and level of consciousness (Zipes & Duffin, 1984).

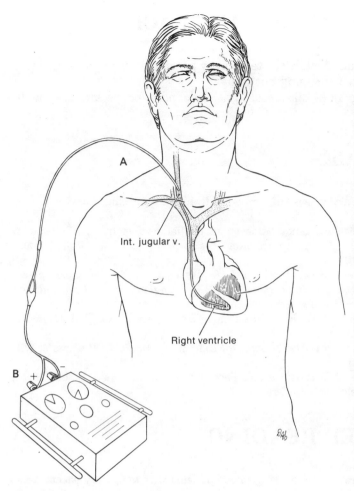

Figure 88.2 Internal jugular placement and setup for temporary transvenous cardiac pacing.
(Rosen & Sternbach, 1983: 101. Reprinted by permission.)

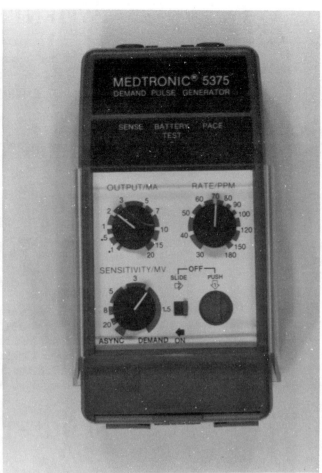

Figure 88.3 An example of a temporary external pacemaker generator.
(Courtesy of Community Hospitals Indianapolis, Indianapolis, Indiana.)

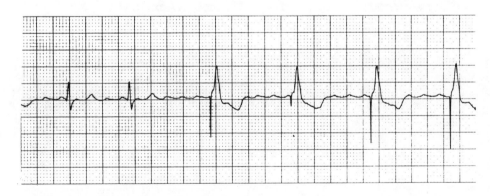

Figure 88.4 An example of an ECG strip documenting appropriate capture of a ventricular pacemaker.

Related to catheter maintenance

1. Sepsis
2. Thrombophlebitis

Related to equipment

1. Generator battery failure may result in a failure to fire, capture, or sense.
2. Lead displacement may result in a failure to sense or capture.
3. Poor connections may result in a failure to fire, sense, or capture (Belshaw, 1989).

PATIENT AND FAMILY TEACHING

1. Bed rest is required while the temporary pacemaker is in place. Request assistance before changing positions.
2. Report symptoms of dizziness, lightheadedness, or weakness immediately.

REFERENCES

Belshaw, M. 1989. Making sense of temporary transvenous pacing. *Nursing Times,* 85, 1:39–41.

Benjanim, G.C. 1985. Emergency transvenous cardiac pacing. In J.R. Roberts, & J.R. Hedges (eds). *Clinical procedures in emergency medicine.* Philadelphia: Saunders; 170–191.

Bing, O.H.L., McDowell, J.W., Hantman, J., & Messer, J.V. 1972. Pacemaker placement by electrocardiographic monitoring. *New England Journal of Medicine* 287:651.

Love, J.A., & Paraskos, J.A. 1987. Emergency cardiac pacing. *Hospital Medicine,* 19, 10:149–167.

Rosen, P., & Sternbach, G.L. (1983). *Atlas of Emergency Medicine.* Baltimore: Williams and Wilkins.

Zipes, D.P., & Duffin, E.G. 1984. Cardiac Pacemakers. In Braunwald, E. (ed). *Heart Disease.* Philadelphia: Saunders.

SUGGESTED READING

Eldredge, T. 1983. Protocol for nursing care of patients with temporary pacemakers. *Critical Care Nurse,* 3, 3:47–50.

89

Emergency Thoracotomy and Internal Defibrillation

Stephanie Kitt, RN, MSN

Emergency thoracotomy and internal defibrillation is also known as chest cracking.

INDICATIONS

1. To tamponade internal bleeding in trauma patients with actual or impending hypovolemic cardiac arrest.
2. To resuscitate patients with significant thoracic or abdominal injury who, in spite of massive fluid resuscitation, remain unconscious and severely hypotensive (systolic blood pressure below 60 mm Hg) for 5–10 minutes. This can be accomplished through thoracic aortic occlusion and open cardiac massage (Wahlstrom, 1986).
3. To employ maximal resuscitative efforts for the patient who suffers major trauma, arrives in cardiac arrest, and remains unresponsive after medical resuscitative efforts.
4. To relieve a pericardial tamponade in patients where pericardiocentesis has been ineffective and cardiac arrest has occurred or is imminent.

CONTRAINDICATIONS AND CAUTIONS

1. Emergency thoracotomy is not indicated for patients with massive central nervous system injuries or cardiogenic shock (Wahlstrom et al., 1986).
2. While emergency thoractomies at times need to be performed in the emergency department, ideally they are performed in the operating room. Only when the patient is too unstable to be transported to the OR, should a thoracotomy be performed in the ED.
3. A major risk associated with thoracotomy in the patient who has intra-abdominal bleeding is release of abdominal tamponade before aortic control can be achieved. This results in rapid exsanguination and death.
4. If the patient is presumed or known to have been in cardiac arrest for a prolonged period of time, the chance for survival after emergency thoracotomy is small. Indicators of poor prognosis include multiple major injuries, blunt trauma to the thorax and/or abdomen, absent pupillary reflexes, no respiratory effort, and no palpable pulse (Wahlstrom et al., 1986). The best prognosis following emergency thoracotomy is after thoracic stab wound where the survival is estimated at 30–40% (Wahlstrom, 1986).
5. Rarely, patients regain consciousness during thoracotomy. In this event, chemical and physical restraint will be required immediately to prevent the patient from causing further injury by pulling on clamps, tubes, etc.

EQUIPMENT

Antiseptic solution
Sterile gown, gloves, mask, and
 protective eyewear
Suction, long (30-foot) extension
 tubing, and a Yankauer tip
Sterile thoracotomy tray consisting
 of minimally:
 Knife handles (2 long and 2
  short)
 #11 blade
 Rib cutter
 Rib retractor (Finochietto,
  Scapular, Tuffier,
  Harrington, or Richardson,
  selected based on physician
  preference)
 Long scissors (Mayos), curved
  and straight
 Vascular clamps (Mixters),
  extra long, medium long
  and regular Satinsky clamp
 Needle holders, regular, 9″
  vascular

Tissue forceps (Russians,
 Debakeys, thoracic
 Debakeys)
Toothed forceps (Brown, 8″
 Peons)
Noncrushing clamps (bronchial
 clamps)
Lepske knife and mallet
 (optional)
Lap pads (sterile gauze sponges
 used to absorb blood,
 packed in fives, and each
 marked with a blue tab for
 ease in counting
Cardiac monitor
Internal defibrillator paddles and
 cable
Pledgets
Sterile saline
Gauze dressings
Nonabsorbable suture (e.g., 3-0 silk)

PATIENT PREPARATION

1. If time allows, prep the chest by scrubbing with an antiseptic solution, wipe with a sterile towel, and apply antiseptic as a paint solution. In most situations time does not allow for thorough skin cleansing and in these situations, pouring full strength antiseptic solution on the chest prior to the incision is acceptable.
2. Ventilation via an endotracheal tube with a bag-valve-mask device must be in progress.
3. For patients in cardiac arrest, external cardiac massage must continue until the thoracic incision is made.
4. Attach ECG leads to the patient's limbs. See Ch. 57: ECG Monitoring.

PROCEDURAL STEPS

*Indicates portions of the procedure usually performed by a physician.

1. Turn on full strength suction and attach via extension tubing to a sterile Yankauer.
2. *Make an anterolateral incision in the fourth or fifth intercostal space. See Figure 89.1.
3. *Incise the skin and subcutaneous tissue to the intercostal muscles. See Figure 89.2.
4. *Enter the pleural space by pushing the index finger through the intercostal space near the sternal border and then posteriorly, running along the superior border of the rib. See Figure 89.3. Ventilations should be interrupted until the incision is complete.
5. *Insert a rib retractor and expose the pleural cavity. Pick up the pericardium with toothed forceps and open it with scissors, taking care not to sever the phrenic nerve. See Figure 89.4.

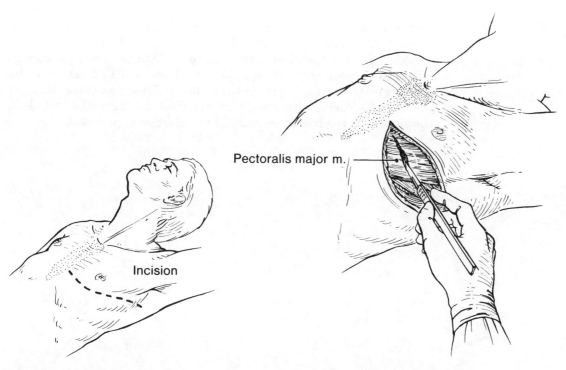

Pectoralis major m.

Figure 89.1 Anterolateral incision for thoracotomy.
Rosen, & Sternbach, 1983: 51. Reprinted by permission.)

Figure 89.2 Intercostal muscle dissection.
Rosen & Sternbach, 1983: 51. Reprinted by permission.)

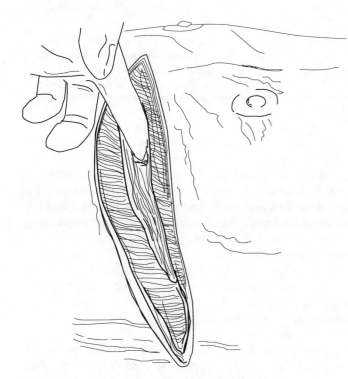

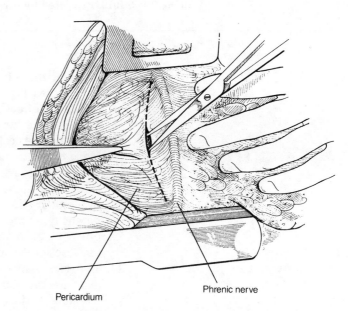

Pericardium

Phrenic nerve

Figure 89.3 The fastest way to enter the pleural space without risking injury to the underlying lung is to push the index finger through the intercostal space near the sternal border and then forcefully push it posteriorly, running it along the superior border of the rib.
(Wahlstrom et al., 1980: 25. Reprinted by permission.)

Figure 89.4 Release of pericardial tamponade.
(Wilkins, 1989: 1019. Reprinted by permission.)

6. *Inspect the heart. If there is a penetrating injury, it can be temporarily occluded with direct pressure by placing a finger into the hole. See Figure 89.5. Alternatively, a large Foley catheter (e.g., 28-French) can be inserted and the inflated balloon used to occlude the hole. Be sure to inflate the balloon with sterile fluid. Also, blood and IV fluid can be infused directly into the heart via the catheter. The defect is then sutured with nonabsorbable suture and pledgets. Pledgets are used to help hold the sutures in the friable myocardial muscle. See Figure 89.6.

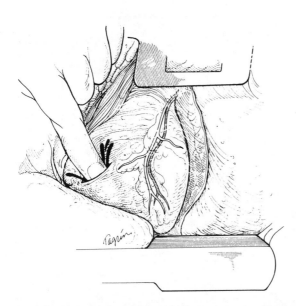

Figure 89.5   Occlusion of bleeding after a penetrating injury to the myocardium.
(Wilkins, 1989: 1019. Reprinted by permission.)

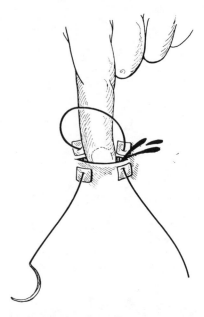

Figure 89.6   Use of Teflon felt pledgets to close a myocardial defect.
(Wilkins, 1989: 1020. Reprinted by permission.)

7. *Cardiac massage may be performed either with two hands or with one by compressing the heart against the sternum. Compress in a superior to inferior direction to mimic normal blood flow from atria to ventricles.
8. *Retract the lung and visualize the descending aorta. The descending aorta may be occluded until the intravascular volume is restored and the blood pressure returned to normal. This is accomplished by compressing the aorta against the spine or cross clamping. See Figure 89.7.
9. **Document the time the aorta is clamped.**
10. *Pulmonary injuries may be controlled by use of a clamp across the parenchyma proximal to the injury, across the hilus of the lung (see Figure 89.8), or by wrapping the hilus with a Penrose drain and then providing traction to occlude the vessels and control hemorrhage.
11. To perform internal defibrillation:
    a. Place the sterile paddles on the sterile field and have the physician hand off the connector end of the cable to plug into the monitor/defibrillator.
    b. Turn the defibrillator on and charge the paddles (usually 30 watt/sec for adults). Internal paddles are programmed to deliver no more than 50 watt/sec.
    c. *Place the paddles on opposite sides of the myocardium. See Figure 89.9. Make sure all personnel clear the cart, state "all-clear," and discharge the current into the paddles.

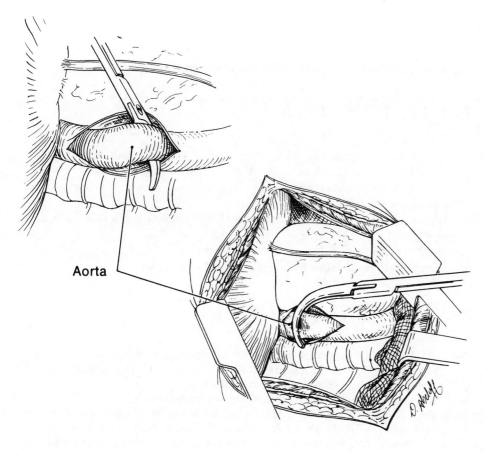

Aorta

Figure 89.7 Cross clamping of the aorta.
(Rosen & Sternbach, 1983: 56. Reprinted by permission.)

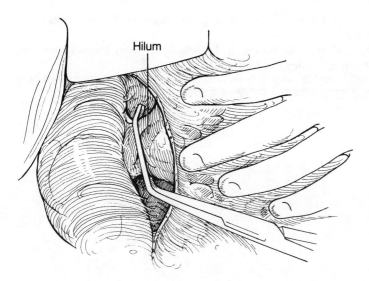

Hilum

Figure 89.8 Clamping of the hilus of the lung with an appropriate vascular clamp. A Satinsky clamp is shown.
(Wilkins, 1989: 1020. Reprinted by permission.)

(Note: Some monitor/defibrillators require a second person to discharge the paddles from the defibrillator. In this instance, the physician holding the paddles should say "all clear" before the paddles are discharged.

Saline soaked gauze dressing between the paddles and myocardium may be used to improve conduction and decrease myocardial injury.

d. Monitor the ECG for improvement in rhythm and repeat above steps as necessary.

12. If the patient appears to be salvageable, prepare for stat transport to the operating room. In anticipation of the transfer notify the OR, place IV

poles on the bed, secure portable oxygen and a cardiac monitor, and transfer all IV lines and monitor cables, from permanent fixtures to the transport stretcher. Instruct security to clear the corridors and secure an elevator in order to expedite the transfer.

COMPLICATIONS

1. Inadvertant lung injury while incising down to the pleural space.
2. Phrenic nerve transection causing diaphragmatic paralysis.
3. Injury to coronary arteries while suturing lacerations or attempting to relieve a pericardial tamponade.
4. Injury to the heart while performing CPR against a fractured sternum or rib.
5. Hemorrhage from internal mammary arteries.
6. Organ and tissue ischemia from aortic clamping.

SUGGESTED READINGS

Bayer, M.J. 1980. Emergency thoracotomy and internal cardiac massage. In S.A. Budassi, J.J. Bander, L. Kimmerle, & K.F. Eie (eds). *Cardiac arrest and CPR assessment, planning, and intervention*, 91–98.

Lockhart, C.G. 1986. Thoracic trauma. *Critical Care Quarterly*, 9, 3:32–40.

McQuillan, K.A., & Wiles, C.E. 1988. Initial management of traumatic shock. In V.D. Cardona, P.D. Hurn, P.J.B. Bastnagel Mason, A.M. Scanlon-Schilpp, & S.W. Veise-Berry, *Trauma nursing from resuscitation through rehabilitation*, (eds). 166.

Rosen, P., & Sternbach, G.L. 1983. *Atlas of emergency medicine*, 2nd ed. Baltimore: Williams & Wilkins.

Wahlstrom, H.E., Carroll, B.J., & Phillips, E.H. 1986. Emergency thoracotomy: Indications and technique. *Surgical Rounds*, 9:23–34.

Wilkins, E.W., Jr. (ed). 1989. *Emergency medicine: Scientific foundations and current practice*, 3rd ed. Baltimore: Williams & Wilkins.

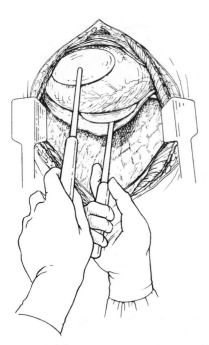

Figure 89.9 Internal defibrillation. (Rosen & Sternbach, 1983: 55. Reprinted by permission.)

90

Central Venous Pressure Measurement Via Manometer

Manjula D. Gray, RN, BSN, MA, CCRN
Anjula D. Littleton, RN, BSN, CCRN

Central venous pressure measurement via manometer is also known as CVP, right atrium pressure (RAP).

INDICATIONS

1. To monitor hemodynamic status in patients with cardiogenic shock, septic shock, hypovolemic shock, and congestive heart failure.
2. To guide the administration of fluids, diuretics, and vasoactive drugs.

CONTRAINDICATIONS AND CAUTIONS

1. Pneumothoraces, positive pressure ventilation, and increased airway resistance (as a result of asthma or COPD) cause increases in intrathoracic pressure and give false high CVP readings.
2. Dislocation of the tip of the central venous line from the superior vena cava causes inaccurate readings.

EQUIPMENT

Central venous pressure water manometer

Intravenous fluid and tubing
Felt tip marker

PATIENT PREPARATION

1. See Ch. 64: Subclavian Venous Access or Ch. 65: Internal Jugular Venous Access for information on inserting central venous lines.
2. Place patient in the supine position with the head of the bed flat or elevated no greater the 30 degrees.
3. Locate the phlebostatic angle (also known as the phlebostatic axis). This angle is located at the junction of the midaxillary line and the fourth intercostal space.
4. Mark this point with a felt tip marker, to be used as the zero reference point, to be used for all readings.

PROCEDURAL STEPS

1. Turn the stopcock off to the manometer and flush the tubing with IV fluid. See the left part of Figure 90.1.
2. Attach the manometer tubing to the central venous line and flush the central venous line to assure patency.

3. Position the zero mark on the water manometer at the phlebostatic angle. The manometer can be either secured to an IV pole or hand held at the point of reference.
4. Turn the stopcock off to the patient. Allow the manometer to fill up to the 25-cm level with IV fluid. Note that the faster the IV fluid is running, the faster the manometer will fill. Avoid letting the fluid run out the top of the manometer as contamination of the manometer may result. See the center part of Figure 90.1.

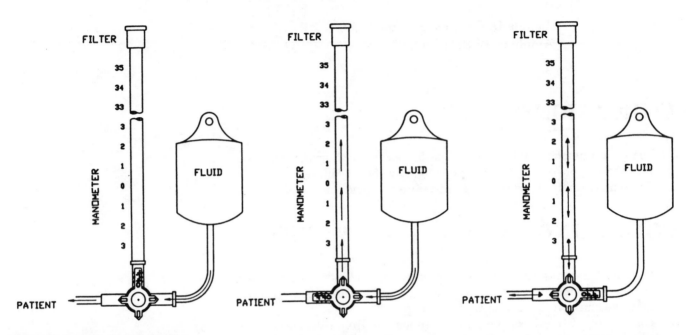

Figure 90.1 *Left:* Stopcock off to monometer to flush tubing. *Center:* Stopcock off to patient to fill manometer. *Right:* Stopcock off to IV fluid to read CVP.
(Courtesy of Medex, Inc., Hilliard, OH. Reprinted by permission.)

5. Turn the stopcock off to the IV fluid. The fluid level will fall and fluctuate with respirations. See the right part of Figure 90.1.
6. Take the CVP reading when the fluid level stabilizes. The reading should be taken at the base of the meniscus at the end of expiration.
7. Turn the stopcock off to the manometer and run the IV fluids through the central venous line as prescribed. See Figure 90.1.
8. Document the reading and the patient's position.
9. Normal CVP ranges from 5–10cm of water pressure. When monitoring CVP, it is the trend of the reading that is most significant. The trend of the CVP combined with the clinical assessment will determine the appropriate interventions.

COMPLICATIONS

1. Occlusion of the catheter due to improper positioning of the stopcock will result in too slow or no administration of IV fluids through the central venous line.
2. Hemorrhage due to disconnection of tubing from the central venous catheter.

PATIENT TEACHING

Immediately report any tubing disconnections or blood in the tubing.

SUGGESTED READINGS

American Heart Association. 1987. Invasive monitoring techniques: Bedside pulmonary artery catherization. *Textbook of advanced cardiac life support.* Dallas: American Heart Association; 167–181.

Bush, C.A. 1987. Nursing interventions for insertion, maintenance, and removal of invasive catheter. K.J. Loach, & N.B. Thomson, Jr. (eds). *Hemodynamic monitoring.* Philadelphia: Lippincott, 21–83.

Roberts, R.R., & Hedges, J.R. 1985. *Clinical procedures in emergency medicine.* Philadelphia: Saunders.

91

Arterial Line Insertion and Monitoring

Stephanie Kitt, RN, MSN

Arterial line is also known as a-line, art line.

INDICATIONS

1. To accurately and continuously monitor arterial pressure of patients who are or have the potential to become hemodynamically unstable. Because Korotkoff sounds may be inaudible in hypotensive patients, determination of blood pressure by conventional means is not always possible. In addition, ongoing arterial pressure evaluation is useful in noting abrupt changes.
2. To continuously monitor response to vasoactive drugs.
3. To facilitate frequent arterial blood gas sampling.
4. To determine derived hemodynamic parameters, such as mean arterial pressure (MAP), in patients, such as those with head injury who benefit from maintaining MAP at 50 mm Hg or higher, to maintain cerebral perfusion pressure.

CONTRAINDICATIONS AND CAUTIONS

1. A major catastrophe may occur should separation of the system take place. Extreme caution is necessary in order to prevent disconnections and subsequent blood loss.
2. Close patient monitoring is necessary for any patient with an a-line in place and monitor alarms should always be on to alert the nurse of hemodynamic change or system malfunction.
3. Avoid use of extremities with injuries that may compromise distal circulation.

EQUIPMENT

20-G 1½- or 2-inch angiocath
Antiseptic solution
Tincture of Benzoin
Adhesive tape
4-0 nylon sutures
Transducer
500 cc flush solution (NS or lactated ringer's solution may be used with 500 to 5000 units of heparin based on your institution's policy)
Pressure tubing with continuous
flush device and an extension set
Pressure administration bag or cuff
3-way stopcock
Dead end caps for stopcock ports
Cardiac monitor with hemodynamic monitoring capability
Transducer cable
(**Note:** Prepackaged pressure tubing with flush device and disposable transducer is available.

PATIENT PREPARATION

1. Establish cardiac monitoring.
2. Check with the physician regarding the site to be cannulated. Either the radial, brachial, or femoral artery may be selected. The radial artery is most commonly used for arterial pressure monitoring because it usually has good collateral circulation, is easily accessible, and does not require extremity immobilization that restricts patient movement as much as other suitable sites. The patient's collateral circulation to the hand should be assessed prior to insertion of the radial line. This can be done by performing the Allen test (see Ch. 17: Drawing Arterial Blood Gases) or using a Doppler ultrasound device.
3. Position the extremity properly and cleanse the area to be cannulated with antiseptic solution. Prior to insertion of a radial line, the patient's hand is supinated and the wrist restrained in a position of mild hyperextension. See Figure 91.1.

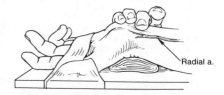

Figure 91.1   Slight hyperextension of wrist for radial artery catheter insertion.
(Rosen & Sternbach, 1983: 97. Reprinted by permission.)

PROCEDURAL STEPS

1. Turn on the hemodynamic monitor according to the manufacturer's directions and allow the system to warm up.
2. Prepare the pressure monitoring system as follows: (Refer to Figure 91.2.)
   a. Prepare the flush solution according to your institution's policy.
   b. Attach the flush solution to the administration part of the IV pressure tubing.
   c. Attach a stopcock to the end of the pressure tubing and add the extension set.
   d. Connect the transducer to the pressure tubing proximal to the continuous flush device.
   e. Prime the line and transducer by opening the roller clamps and activating the flush device according to the manufacturer's directions. Be sure to clear all air from the line, flush device, and transducer.
   f. Place the flush solution in the pressure bag or cuff and hang the bag on an IV pole. Pump pressurize the bag to 300 mm Hg.
   g. Secure the transducer either on the IV pole or cart at the level of the right atrium (midaxillary line) and fourth intercostal space.
   h. Open the transducer to air and zero the system according to the manufacturer's directions. Once zeroed, the system can be closed to air.
3. *Infiltrate the insertion site with local anesthetic (optional).
4. *Cannulate the artery with the teflon catheter and remove the inner wire. Allow the catheter to back fill with blood. See Figure 91.3.
5. Connect the pressure tubing to the catheter and secure tightly via a leur-lock connection.
6. Activate the flush device to clear the line of any blood resulting from backflow.
7. *Suture the catheter in place.
8. Clean the site with an antiseptic solution, apply Benzoin around the insertion site, and tape securely.
9. Observe the pressure waveform (Figure 91.4) on the monitor and note the digital blood pressure reading. Check cuff pressure to assure accuracy of hemodynamic measurement.
10. Turn on monitor alarms to limits based on the patient's clinical condition.
11. Attach the dead end caps to open pressure line ports.

*Indicates portions of the procedure usually performed by a physician.

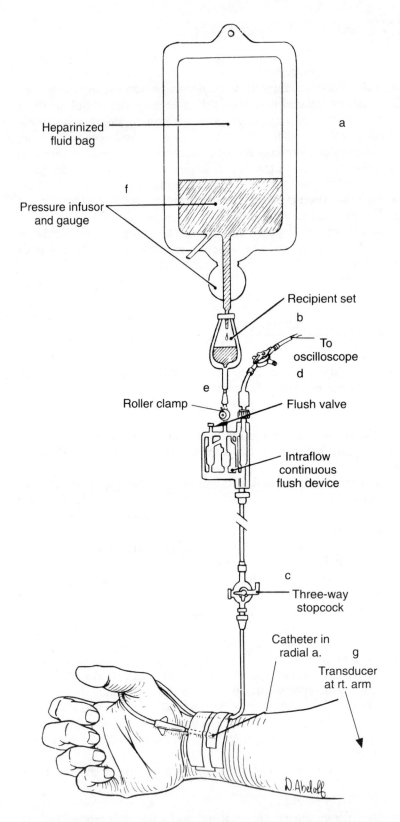

Heparinized fluid bag

a

f

Pressure infusor and gauge

Recipient set

b

To oscilloscope

d

Roller clamp

e

Flush valve

Intraflow continuous flush device

Three-way stopcock

c

Catheter in radial a.

g

Transducer at rt. arm

D.Abeloff

Figure 91.2 Arterial pressure line assembly. See text for explanations (Rosen & Sternbach, 1983: 97. Reprinted by permission.)

12. Withdraw blood for blood gas analysis by performing the following steps:
    a. Attach a 5-ml syringe to the stopcock port most proximal to the catheter site.
    b. Turn the stopcock off to the monitoring system and on to the patient and withdraw approximately 5 ml of blood to clear the line of any heparinized blood.
    c. Turn the stopcock halfway toward the original position and discard the waste syringe.

d. Attach the 3- or 5-ml heparinized syringe to the port, turn the stopcock off to the monitoring system, and withdraw the ABG specimen.

e. Turn the stopcock to the original position, remove the blood gas syringe from the port, and remove any air bubbles from the syringe before capping and sending it to the laboratory for analysis.

f. Using the flush device, flush the system to the patient followed by a flush to clear the access port by turning the stopcock off to the patient.

g. Turn the stopcock to the original position and recap with a dead end cap.

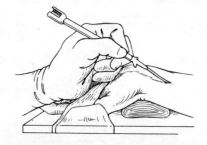

Figure 91.3   Radial artery cannula insertion.
(Rosen & Sternbach, 1983: 97. Reprinted by permission.)

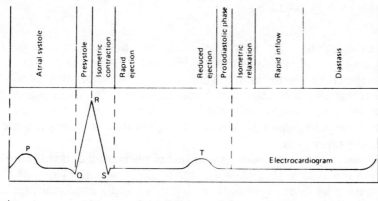

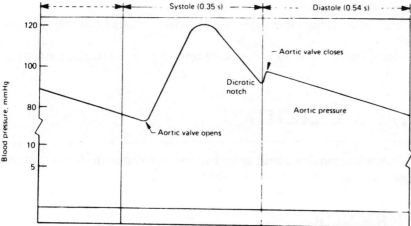

Figure 91.4   Arterial pressure waveform.
(Smith, 1988: Reprinted by permission.)

COMPLICATIONS

1. An air embolism can be introduced into the circulation if the tubing and transducer are not flushed properly prior to connection to the cannula. If air bubbles persist despite tight connections, check the flush device and stopcocks for cracks.

2. Severe blood loss or exsanguination may occur if the connections are not tightly secured or the catheter is dislodged.

3. Inaccurate pressure readings may occur if the transducer is incorrectly placed. If the transducer is above the level of the right atrium, the pressure reflected on the monitor will be lower than the patient's true blood pressure. Conversely, if the transducer is below the level of the right atrium, the pressure reflected on the monitor will be higher than the patient's true blood pressure. The transducer should be recalibrated if it is moved.

4. Damping of the waveform (Figure 91.5) may occur as a result of the cannula lodging against the vessel wall, clot formation, kinking of the cathe-

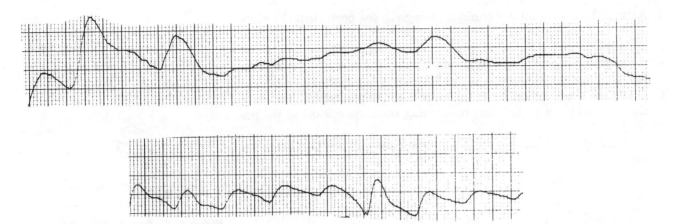

Figure 91.5 Arterial pressure wave-form damping.

ter, or air trapped between the transducer diaphragm and the dome diaphragm. Slight readjustment of the cannula may free it from its position against the vessel wall. If a clot is suspected, aspirate with a syringe in attempt to remove the clot. Never inject into the line because a clot may become dislodged into the circulation. If air is entrapped in the transducer and cannot be cleared, refer to manufacturer's instructions on dome placement.

5. Infection may occur if poor aseptic technique is used or if there are openings in the system that allow culture of bacteria (e.g., blood not cleared from the port after blood draw or failure to apply dead end caps to unused ports).

6. Median nerve damage may occur if the wrist remains dorsiflexed (Lake, 1990).

7. Hematoma with possible nerve compression at the insertion site may occur.

PATIENT TEACHING

1. Use care when moving about in bed so as not to disconnect the system.
2. Report any disconnections immediately.

REFERENCES

Beck-Sague, C.M., & Jarvis, W.R. 1989. Epidemic bloodstream infections associated with pressure transducers: A persistent problem. *Infection Control Hospital Epidemiology*, 10, 2:54–59.

Curry, K., Scott, L., Kearney, R., & Rosemurgy, A.S. 1989. Appropriate use of hospital monitoring capabilities. *Nursing Management*, 20, 5:112I–112P.

Henneman, E.A., & Henneman, P.L. 1989. Intricacies of blood pressure measurement: Reexamining the rituals. *Heart & Lung*, 18, 3:263–273.

Lake, C.L. 1990. *Clinical Monitoring*. Philadelphia: Saunders.

Mermel, L.A., & Maki, D.G. 1989. Epidemic bloodstream infections from hemodynamic pressure monitoring: Signs of the times. *Infection Control Hospital Epidemiology*, 10, 2:47–53.

Smith, R.N., & de Asla, R.A. 1988. Instrumentation. In M.R. Kinney, D.R. Packa, & S.B. Dunbar, (eds). *AACN's Clinical Reference for Critical Care Nursing*, 2nd ed. St. Louis: Mosby; 38–50.

92

Pulmonary Artery Catheter Insertion

Anjula D. Littleton, RN, BSN, CCRN

Pulmonary artery catheter is also known as Swan-Ganz catheter and balloon-tipped, flow-directed pulmonary artery catheter.

INDICATIONS

1. To provide a continuous and reliable method of monitoring right atrial, pulmonary artery, and pulmonary artery wedge pressure in hemodynamically unstable patients.
2. To determine cardiac output using the thermodilution method.
3. To guide and calculate the administration of fluid replacements, diuretics, and vasoactive medications.
4. To obtain mixed venous blood samples for analysis of intrapulmonary shunt, oxygen consumption, and extracardiac shunts.

CONTRAINDICATIONS AND CAUTIONS

Patients with bleeding disorders must be monitored carefully for hemorrhage.

EQUIPMENT

Pressure bag
IV pole
*Disposable transducer with double
    pressure tubing allowing
    two ports to be monitored
    with a single transducer.
*Pressure monitor with compatible
    transducer cable
Flush solution—500-cc of normal
    saline with 500 units of
    heparin.
Felt tip marker
ECG monitoring equipment
Sterile gloves, gowns, and masks
Sterile sheet and towels

Pulmonary artery catheter
Plastic catheter sleeve
Introducer
Suture
Sterile basin, gauze dressings, and
    antiseptic solution
Sterile saline
Local anesthetic (e.g., lidocaine)
3-ml syringes
25-G ¹/₂-inch needle
Scalpel
Occlusive dressing
Antibiotic ointment
Tape

*Familiarization with the manufacturer's recommendations for proper use of this equipment is necessary.

PATIENT PREPARATION

1. Attach patient to the ECG monitor and obtain a good waveform. See Ch. 57: ECG Monitoring.
2. Insert an intravenous line because insertion of a pulmonary artery cath-

eter may cause dysrhythmias requiring treatment. See Ch. 62: Peripheral Intravenous Cannulation.

3. Check with the physician for insertion site and place patient in the proper position. For the internal jugular or femoral vein, the patient is positioned in the supine position. For the subclavian approach, the patient is placed in a slight Trendelenburg position with a rolled towel along the spine on the side of cannulation.

4. Locate the level of right atrium or phlebostatic axis. The phlebostatic axis is located at the junction of the fourth intercostal space and midway between the outermost point of sternum to outermost point of posterior chest. With the patient supine, this is the midaxillary line (American Heart Association, 1987). It is important to mark this point using a felt tip marker to ensure zero reference point consistency for all measurements. See Figure 92.1.

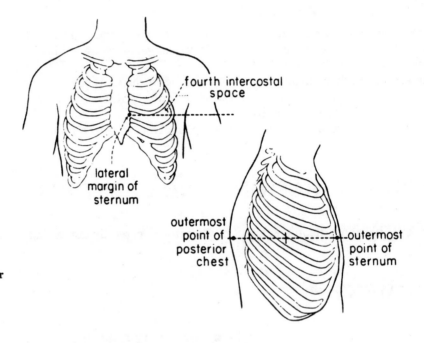

Figure 92.1   Level of right atrium or phlebostatic axis.
(Wood, 1976: 84. Reprinted by permission.)

PROCEDURAL STEPS

1. Turn on the hemodynamic monitor according to the manufacturer's guidelines and allow the system to warm up for a minimum of 15 minutes. Place the monitor on the 40–60 mm Hg scale. Attach cable to hemodynamic monitor.

2. Prepare the pressure monitoring system as follows: See Figure 92.2.
   a. Attach the flush solution (500 cc normal saline with 500 units of Heparin) to the macrodrip chamber of the pressure tubing set.
   b. Flush the pressure tubing and transducer according to the manufacturer's guidelines to remove all air from the system.
   c. Place the flush solution in the pressure bag and hang the bag on an IV pole. Pressurize the bag to 300 mm Hg.
   d. Attach cable to disposable transducer.
   g. Zero reference and calibrate the transducer/monitor.
      – Secure the transducer to the IV pole so that the air-fluid interface (stopcock used to open the system to atmospheric pressure) is at the level of the patient's phlebostic axis.
      – Open the stopcock to air to zero balance and calibrate the monitor/transducer system using monitor instructions.
      – Close the stopcock to air. Cover with a nonvented cap.

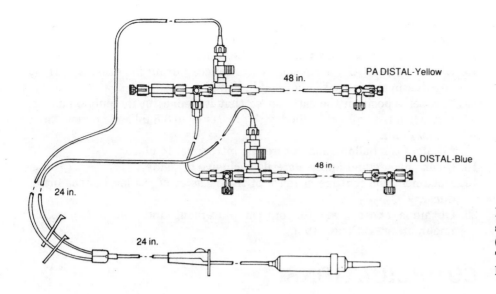

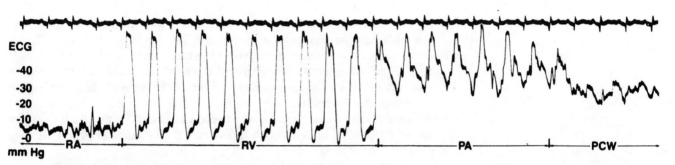

Figure 92.2 Pulmonary artery pressure monitoring system.
(Abbott Critical Care Systems the Transpac disposable transducer. Reprinted by permission.)

Figure 92.3 Pressure waveforms recorded as pulmonary artery catheter is advanced through right atrium (RA) and right ventricle (RV) into pulmonary artery (PA) and to pulmonary artery wedge (PCW) position.
(American Heart Association, 1987: 173. Reprinted by permission.)

Other pressure monitoring systems may be used. If only a single pressure tubing system is available, then it is necessary to set up two systems, one for the distal port and another for the proximal port. Another option is to use a single pressure tubing system to monitor the distal port and attach a 10-cc syringe of heparinized (10 units per cc) flush solution to the proximal port during insertion. Later, intravenous solution or a monitoring system can be attached to the proximal port.

3. *Check the catheter balloon for leaks by inflating it to the recommended inflation volume, which is indicated on the catheter shaft, and plunging the balloon in a sterile basin of normal saline.
4. Connect the distal and proximal lumens of the catheter to the proper pressure tubing and flush the catheter by activating the fast flush device.
5. *Place the sterile sleeve over the catheter.
6. During insertion the transducer must be set up to monitor the distal lumen pressure.
7. Cleanse the skin at the insertion site using antiseptic solution.
8. *Infiltrate the insertion site with local anesthetic.
9. *Cannulate the vein as per central line insertion technique. See Ch. 64: Subclavian, Ch. 65: Internal Jugular Vein, Ch. 66: Femoral.
10. *Insert the introducer.
11. *Advance the catheter through the introducer until it is at the 15–20-cm mark for the internal jugular or subclavian approach. The catheter should be in the right atrium (RA) and the RA waveform should be visible (American Heart Association, 1987). See Figure 92.3.
12. *Inflate the balloon with the recommended volume of air when the catheter is in the right atrium.
13. *While monitoring the pressure waveform advance the catheter from the RA into the right ventricle (RV), and into the pulmonary artery (PA).

*Indicates portions of the procedure usually performed by a physician.

The change in waveform will guide in the advancement of the catheter through each chamber of the heart and into the PA. See Figure 92.3.

14. Document the pressures in the RA, RV, and PA.
15. Observe the ECG for rhythm disturbances during insertion and treat any dysrhythmia that is not self-limiting.
16. *Properly position the catheter so that it wedges in the pulmonary artery when the balloon is filled with greater than 0.8 ml and no more than 1.5 ml of air.
17. *Deflate the balloon and suture the introducer in place.
18. Clean the site and apply a sterile occlusive dressing.
19. Document the centimeter mark of the catheter at the level of the introducer.
20. Obtain a chest x-ray to confirm placement and rule out possible pneumothorax (Straw, 1986).

COMPLICATIONS

1. A pneumothorax may result if the introducer pierces the apex of the thorax when the internal jugular or subclavian vein is used.
2. Hematoma or hemothorax may develop due to transection of an artery. If a hematoma occurs on one side of the neck, it would be hazardous to attempt puncture on the other side of the neck, because this may lead to an airway obstruction.
3. An air embolism can be introduced into the circulation if the introducer is not allowed to backfill with blood and if the catheter is not flushed properly prior to insertion.
4. Dysrhythmias (PACs, PVCs, atrial fibrillation, ventricular tachycardia, and fibrillation) may occur due to the irritation of the endocardium by the catheter.
5. The pulmonary artery may be perforated due to the advancement of the catheter with an uninflated balloon or due to an overinflated balloon during wedge pressure measurement.
6. Damage to intracardiac structures may occur if the catheter is withdrawn with the balloon inflated.
7. Knotting and coiling of the catheter can occur when smaller 5-French catheters are used (American Heart Association, 1987).
8. Cardiac tamponade can occur from the perforation of the right atrium or right ventricle in patients with a noncompliant ventricle.
9. A balloon rupture can occur if the catheter is inserted for a prolonged period of time (greater than 72 hours) or if there have been multiple balloon inflations.
10. Pulmonary infarction can occur when balloon inflation is prolonged or due to distal migration of the catheter. When obtaining the wedge pressure measurement, slowly inflate the balloon and leave inflated for no more than 15 seconds or 3 respiratory cycles (Darovic, 1987).
11. Hemorrhage may occur if stopcocks are left open to the atmosphere (Sanderson & Kurth, 1983).
12. An infection can result from poor aseptic technique or fluid contamination (i.e., through stopcock ports, nondisposable transducers, or nonocclusive dressing) (Masters, 1989).

PATIENT TEACHING

1. Request assistance when changing positions so that the catheter is not displaced.
2. A supine position with the head of the bed raised no more than 20 de-

grees (in acutely ill patients) is necessary when obtaining measurements in order to ensure reproducibility.

3. Report any tubing disconnections immediately.

REFERENCES

American Heart Association. 1987. *Textbook of Advanced Cardiac Life Support.* Dallas: American Heart Association.

Darovic, G.O. 1987. *Hemodynamic monitoring.* Philadelphia: Saunders.

Masters, S. 1989. Complications of pulmonary artery catheters. *Critical Care Nursing,* 9:82–90.

Sanderson, R.G., & Kurth, C.L. 1983. *The cardiac patient: a comprehensive approach,* 2nd ed. Philadelphia: Saunders.

Straw, M.M. 1986. *Critical care nurse's knowledge of pulmonary artery pressure measurement.* Unpublished master thesis. University of Washington, Seattle, Washington.

Wood, S.L., & Mansfield, L.W. 1976. Body position upon pulmonary artery and pulmonary capillary wedge pressures in noncritically ill patients. *Heart & Lung,* 5:83–90.

SUGGESTED READINGS

Bush, C.A. 1987. Nursing interventions for insertion, maintenance, and removal of invasive catheters. In J. Loach & N.B. Thomson, Jr. (eds). *Hemodynamic Monitoring* Philadelphia: Lippincott; 21–83.

Etling, T., Hudson, J., & Lantiegne, K. 1976. Invasive monitoring of heart, circulation. *AORN Journal.* 23:199–205.

Halpenny, C.J. 1985. *Cardiac nursing.* Philadelphia: Lippincott.

Niemczura, J. 1985. Rules to remember when caring for the patient with a Swan-Ganz catheter. *Nursing,* 15, 3:38–41.

Runkel, R., & Burke, L. 1983. Troubleshooting Swan-Ganz catheters, *Heart & Lung,* 12:591–594.

Visalli, F. & Evans, P. 1981. Swan-Ganz catheter: A program for teaching safe, effective use. *Nursing,* 11, 1:42–47.

Positioning the Patient with Increased Intracranial Pressure

Ruth L. Schaffler, RN, MA, CEN

INDICATIONS

1. To minimize increased intracranial pressure (ICP) in the presence of head trauma, brain lesion, or other neurological disorders.
2. To facilitate venous drainage from the brain (Hickey, 1986).

CONTRAINDICATIONS AND CAUTIONS

1. Avoid supine, prone, or Trendelenburg positions.
2. Do not rotate the head or flex the neck.
3. Minimize sensory stimuli. Warn the patient before touching, explain procedures, and use gentle movements. Do not jar the bed, make loud noises, or use bright lights.
4. Plan turning or positioning activities separately from other nursing interventions. Allow at least 15 minutes between each activity to avoid a cumulative effect of ICP increases (Miller, 1989).
5. Elevating the head of the bed greater than 40 degrees may contribute to postural hypotension and decreased cerebral perfusion (Stewart-Amidei, 1988).
6. Head elevation is contraindicated in hypotensive patients because it may compromise cerebral perfusion (cerebral perfusion pressure = mean arterial pressure − intracranial pressure).
7. Remove from spinal immobilization only after the cervical spine has been cleared by a physician.

EQUIPMENT

Stretcher or hospital bed
Towel roll

Cervical collar (optional)
Soft restraints (per physician order)

PROCEDURAL STEPS

1. Place the patient in a supine position.
2. Maintain the head in a neutral position without flexion or rotation by placing a towel roll under the shoulders (Stewart-Amidei, 1988). If a cervical collar is prescribed, be sure it does not obstruct venous return via the jugular veins.
3. Elevate the head of the bed to 15–30 degrees. See Figure 93.1.

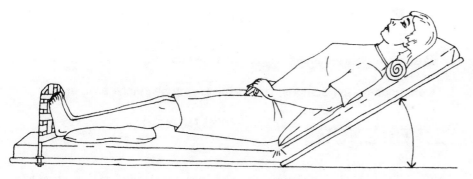

**Figure 93.1 Head of bed elevated to
30 degrees.**

4. Align torso and lower extremities, with hip flexion less than 90 degrees (Mitchell & Mauss, 1978).
5. Place a padded foot board at the end of the stretcher or bed to prevent the patient from sliding or shifting position.
6. Pad side rails and maintain seizure precautions.
7. If full spinal immobilization must be maintained, position the patient on the backboard in a reverse Trendelenburg position (Stewart-Amidei, 1988). See Figure 93.2.

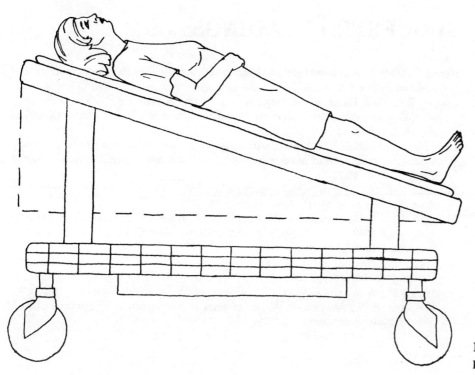

**Figure 93.2 Reverse Trendelenberg
position.**

COMPLICATIONS

1. Flexion, extension, or rotation of the head will increase ICP by obstructing venous outflow.
2. Abnormal posturing may be stimulated by the position of the head in relation to gravity or by excessive noxious stimuli (Palmer & Wyness, 1988).
3. Agitation and the use of restraints may result in increased ICP.
4. Pooling of secretions or skin breakdown may occur if the patient is not turned every two hours (Hickey, 1986).

PATIENT TEACHING

1. Positioning is used along with other interventions to control intracranial pressure.
2. Conscious patients should report increasing headache or nausea.

REFERENCES

Hickey, J.V. (ed). 1986. *The clinical practice of neurological and neurosurgical nursing*, 2nd ed. Philadelphia: Lippincott.

Miller, E.R. 1989. Nursing care of the head-injured patient. In D.P. Becker & S.K. Gudeman, (eds). *Textbook of head injury*. Philadelphia: Saunders; 386–419.

Mitchell, P.H., & Mauss, N.K. 1978. Relationship of patient-nurse activity in intracranial pressure variations: A pilot study. *Nursing Research, 27*, 1:4–10.

Palmer, M., & Wyness, M.A. 1988. Positioning and handling: Important considerations in the care of the severely head-injured patient. *Journal of Neuroscience Nursing, 20*, 1:42–49.

Stewart-Amidei, C. 1988. What to do until the neurosurgeon arrives. . . . *Journal of Emergency Nursing, 14*:296–301.

SUGGESTED READINGS

Berrol, S. 1988. Risks of restraints in head injury. *Archives of Physical Medicine and Rehabilitation, 69*:537–538.

Cooper, P.R. 1982. *Head injury*. Baltimore: Williams & Wilkins.

Gardner, D. 1986. Acute management of the head-injured adult. *Nursing Clinics of North America, 21*:555–562.

Lipe, H.P., & Mitchell, P.H. 1980. Positioning the patient with intracranial hypertension: How turning and head rotation affect the internal jugular vein. *Heart & Lung, 9*:1031–1037.

Mitchell, P.H. 1986. Intracranial hypertension: Influence of nursing care activities. *Nursing Clinics of North America, 21*:563–575.

Mitchell, P.H. 1988. Neurologic disorders. In M. Kinney, D. Packa, & S. Dunbar, (eds). *AACN's Clinical Reference for Critical-Care Nursing*, 2nd ed. New York: McGraw-Hill; 971–1028.

Rea, R.E. (ed). 1991. *Trauma nursing core course provider manual*, 3rd ed. Chicago: Award Printing Corporation.

Shogan, S.H., & Kindt, G.W. 1985. Injuries of the head and spinal cord. In G. Zuidema, R. Rutherford, & W. Ballinger. *The Management of Trauma*, 4th ed. Philadelphia: Saunders; 207–228.

94

Lumbar Puncture

Janet A. Neff, RN, MN, CEN, CCRN

Lumbar puncture is also known as LP, spinal tap.

INDICATIONS

1. To assist in the diagnosis of meningitis or encephalitis in febrile patients exhibiting an acute alteration in mental status.
2. To assist in the diagnosis of subarachnoid hemorrhage (SAH). If SAH is highly suspected and the CT scan is negative, LP may be required for diagnosis, because approximately 4% of fresh SAHs are not detected on CT (Marshall, 1990).
3. To instill medication, air, blood, or radiopaque contrast material into the subarachnoid space.

CONTRAINDICATIONS AND CAUTIONS

1. If a lumbar puncture is performed in the presence of elevated intracranial pressure, supratentorial or foramen magnum herniation may occur and result in serious injury or death, because fluid drainage increases the pressure gradient between the supratentorial and lumbar spaces. In the patient with a history of a progressive deterioration of mental status, a worsening headache, localizing neurologic signs, or papilledema, a computed tomography scan should precede the LP.
2. Positioning patients, especially children, with excessive neck flexion may lead to respiratory compromise. Monitoring oxygen saturation via pulse oximetry can alert the nurse to problems during the procedure.
3. Performing an LP in anticoagulated patients may result in a spinal epidural hematoma.

EQUIPMENT

Lumbar puncture kit including:
  Sterile drape and towels
  Gauze dressings
  21–25-G 2½–3-inch spinal
    needle with stylet
  1% Lidocaine with epinephrine
  25-G ⅝-inch and 21–22-G
    1½-inch needles for
    anesthetic infiltration

3–5-ml syringe
Manometer with 3-way stopcock
  (extension tubing optional)
4 Collection tubes
Adhesive gauze patch
Antiseptic solution

PATIENT PREPARATION

1. Assist the patient into a lateral decubitus position, with the shoulders and pelvis perpendicular to the stretcher. The patient should then flex or

curl the back maintaining this position in order to separate the lumbar spinous processes. It may help to provide a small pillow for the head. The nurse should remain to assist with proper positioning, especially in children or uncooperative adults.

2. If the patient has bony deformities or is obese, a sitting position with head and arms resting over a padded bedside table may help to identify landmarks. Some physicians will proceed with the tap in this position.

PROCEDURAL STEPS

*Indicates portions of the procedure usually performed by a physician.

1. *Palpate the back to identify the spinous process levels. The level of L3–4, L4–5, or L5–S1 can safely be used as they avoid the spinal cord which ends at the level of L2–L3. The posterior iliac crest is even with L3–4. See Figure 94.1. The site may be marked with an indentation from a fingernail or a ball point pen with the ink cartridge retracted.

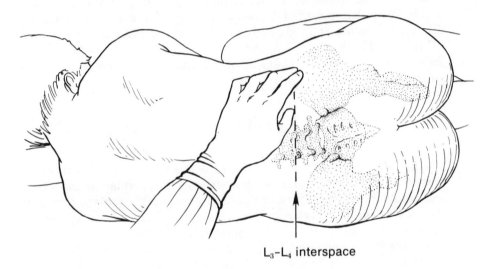

L₃–L₄ interspace

Figure 94.1 Patient position for lumbar puncture and relationship of posterior iliac crest with spinous processes.
(Rosen & Sternbach, 1983: 149. Reprinted by permission.)

2. *Cleanse the back with antiseptic solution in a circular fashion.
3. *Apply the sterile drape to the patient's back with the adhesive strips.
4. *Prepare patient for a sharp sensation. Infiltrate the anesthetic into the skin and subcutaneous tissue using the 25-gauge needle and into the interspinous spaces with the 22-gauge needle at the intended puncture site.
5. *Identify the intended puncture site and insert the spinal needle in the midline with the bevel parallel to the axis of the spine. The needle is often angled slightly cephalad. The patient will feel pressure, but should not feel pain.
6. *A pop may be felt once the needle passes the ligamentum flavum and it is advised that the stylet be removed to check for cerebrospinal fluid (CSF) every 2 mm or so to avoid passing through the subarachnoid space into the ventral epidural space.

    If the epidural space is entered, the patient may feel pain from puncture of a nerve root and a traumatic tap is likely due to the venous plexus within the epidural space (Sternbach, 1988).

7. *Once CSF is noted at the hub of the needle, attach the manometer and 3-way stopcock to measure the CSF opening pressure. Normal CSF pressure is 70–180 mm H_2O (Simon & Brenner, 1987). Extension tubing may be used between the needle and manometer to allow greater flexibility. Relaxation of legs and neck by the patient will help avoid falsely elevated pressures. To decrease the risk of herniation, do not withdraw CSF

samples if the opening pressure is greater than 350 mm H$_2$O (Rosen & Sternbach, 1983).

8. *Collect CSF specimens in the 4 collection tubes. See Figure 94.2. Fluid from the manometer may be drained into the first tube. Usually 1–2 ml are placed in each tube. The first tube is sent for culture, sensitivity, and gram stain and red blood cell count (if a traumatic tap is suspected, comparison with tube 4 is needed); the second for glucose and protein determination; the third tube may be used for cytology or other specialized exams, (i.e., tuberculosis or fungal cultures); and the last tube is examined for cell count (white and red cell). A blood serum specimen for glucose should be drawn just prior to the L.P.

Normal CSF findings include (Kooiker, 1985; Sternbach, 1988):

a. Clear fluid (turbidity usually appears when ≥400 cells/mL are present).

b. Cell count: 0–5 lymphocytes/mL.

c. Total protein count = 20–45mg/dl (adults), up to 150 in infants. Numerous processes elevate protein including blood in the CSF, but levels above 500 mg/dL may indicate meningitis or other disease.

d. Glucose is normally 60–80% of the blood level; a decreased level may implicate CNS disease and is helpful in differentiating viral from bacterial meningitis.

Table 94.1 will assist with the differentiation of viral from bacterial meningitis.

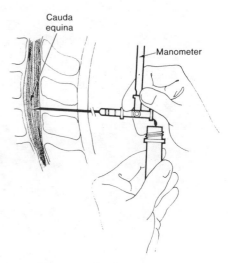

Figure 94.2 Technique for collection of CSF samples from spinal needle with manometer attached (the manometer may also be removed and fluid collected directly from the spinal needle hub.)
(Simon & Brenner, 1987; 168. Reprinted by permission.)

Table 94.1   Basic differentiation of CSF findings in viral and bacterial meningitis.

	Viral	Bacterial
WBC	Elevated, lymphocytes predominant	Very high, neutrophils predominant
Protein	Normal to mild increase	High
Glucose	Usually normal	Low (<60% of blood value)

9. *Reinsert the stylet and slowly remove the spinal needle. Apply pressure to the site with a gauze pad, and then apply the adhesive gauze pad.

10. The patient should remain flat for 3–4 hours. Prone positioning may help reduce CSF leakage and thereby decrease the likelihood of postlumbar puncture headache (Simon & Brenner, 1987).

11. Observe the patient for any changes in level of consciousness (in case of worsening meningitis or possible herniation), altered motor or sensory status in the lower extremities or bladder dysfunction (spinal subdural hematoma), or complaints of headache.

COMPLICATIONS

1. Traumatic tap (compare the cell count from first tube to last tube—if a decrease is noted, it was likely a traumatic tap instead of a subarachnoid bleed.) CSF would usually be xanthochromic from hemolyzed blood if the bleed occurred at least 4 hours earlier.

2. A spinal subdural hematoma may occur in thrombocytopenic patients or in the elderly in whom the CSF was taken off too rapidly or in too large a volume.

3. Headache, often associated with use of a large spinal needle, which creates a greater chance of CSF leakage. Sometimes a blood patch (injection of autologous blood into the epidural space) may be required.

4. A spinal epidural hematoma is rare but may occur in anticoagulated patients.
5. A dry tap (no CSF obtained).
6. Infection is usually related to inadequate aseptic technique or puncture through irritated or infected tissue. A local infection, meningitis, or epidural or subdural empyema may result.

PATIENT TEACHING

1. Monitor temperature and report if > 100°F.
2. Take mild analgesic or prescribed medication for headache.
3. Remain flat for 4 hours after the procedure. A prone position may help prevent a spinal headache.

REFERENCES

Kooiker, J.C. 1985. Spinal puncture and cerebral spinal fluid examination. In J.R. Roberts, & J.R. Hedges (eds). *Clinical procedures in emergency medicine*. Philadelphia: Saunders; 860–876.

Marshall, S.B., Marshall, L.F., Vos, H.R., & Chestnut, R.M. 1990. *Neuroscience Critical Care*. Philadelphia: Saunders.

Rosen, P., & Sternbach, G.L. 1983. *Atlas of emergency medicine*, 2nd ed. Baltimore: Williams & Wilkins.

Simon, R.R., & Brenner, B.E. 1987. *Emergency procedures and techniques*, 2nd ed. Baltimore: Williams & Wilkins.

Sternbach, G.L. 1988. Lumbar puncture. *Topics in Emergency Medicine*, 10, 1:1–7.

95

Burr Holes

Marijane Smallwood, RN, BSN,

Burr holes are also known as skull trepanation, twist drill holes.

(Note: Burr holes are rarely placed in the emergency department setting. With the advent of computerized tomography (CT), the diagnosis of subdural or epidural hematoma can be readily confirmed. In most settings, the CT scan is obtained, the neurosurgeon consulted, and a decision is made to provide immediate surgical intervention in the operating room. However, not all hospitals have CT scanners immediately available and, therefore, must transfer the patient to a trauma center. A delay in the treatment of an epidural or subdural hematoma may significantly increase morbidity/mortality. For this reason, temporal burr hole placement will be discussed in this chapter.)

INDICATIONS

1. To relieve increased intracranial pressure (ICP) in the patient with a suspected epidural or subdural hematoma when
   a. The patient is nonresponsive to conventional first-line interventions to decompress the brain tissue and prevent brain herniation such as hyperventilation, hyperosmolar, or diuretic therapy. Hyperventilation reduces carbon dioxide levels and promotes vasoconstriction of intracranial vessels. Hyperosmolar agents and diuretics act to decrease fluid volume, which decreases intracranial pressure.
   b. The patient exhibits rapidly deteriorating neurological status.
   c. CT is unavailable and transport time is lengthy.
2. To place an intracranial pressure monitoring device.

CONTRAINDICATIONS AND CAUTIONS

1. Burr holes are usually placed in the emergency department as a final effort to maintain a patient's life. The optimal environment for the procedure is in the controlled atmosphere of an operating room.
2. Ensure a patent airway prior to insertion of burr holes. Intubation is preferred to provide hyperventilation and maximize oxygenation.
3. Burr holes should not be attempted in patients with intracranial hematomas not demonstrating signs of tentorial herniation (Lang, 1985).
4. Patients with a past history of hemophilia or use of anticoagulants require special treatment. Obtain baseline coagulation studies and prepare to administer 20 mg of vitamin K and fresh frozen plasma to decrease intracranial bleeding (Lang, 1985).

EQUIPMENT

Burr hole/craniotomy tray
Instruments per physician
    specifications:
    Hand drill with bits (or twist
      drill)
    #4 Knife handle
    #11 Blade
    2 Curved hemostats
    Dural suction tip
    Scalp/dural hook
    Self-retaining retractors
    Sterile towels/drapes

Local anesthetic with epinephrine
    (optional)
10-cc syringe
18-G needle
25-G needle
Electric hair clippers or razor
Antiseptic solution
Gauze dressings
Sterile saline for irrigation
Hemostatic agents (i.e., Gelfoam,
    bone wax)

PATIENT PREPARATION

1. Assess and document baseline neurological status.
2. Maintain cervical spine precautions if injury has not been radiologically ruled out. If no cervical spine precautions are needed, place the patient in the supine position with the head of the bed elevated 20–30 degrees. Turn the side of the head with the dilated pupil upward. Pupillary changes occur on the same side as the hematoma in 80% of patients (Lang, 1985). If possible, place a sandbag or rolled towel under the patient's shoulder to help prevent kinking of the neck and venous outflow obstruction, which may increase ICP.
3. Insert a nasogastric tube to decompress the stomach and help prevent aspiration.

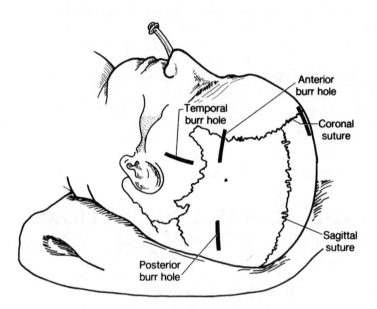

Figure 95.1 Placement of burr holes and incision sites. (Simon & Brenner, 1987: 160. Reprinted by permission.)

4. Shave the insertion site. If an epidural hematoma is suspected following trauma, a temporal burr hole is usually attempted first on the side of the dilated pupil. If no hematoma is located, an anterior or posterior burr hole may be placed (Simon, 1987). See Figure 95.1.
5. Cleanse the scalp with antiseptic solution.
6. Administer sedatives/paralytics as indicated/ordered.

PROCEDURAL STEPS

1. *Anesthetize the site with local anesthetic with epinephrine. (This is optional depending on the level of consciousness of the patient.)
2. *Drape the area to provide a sterile field.
3. *The temporal burr hole site is located just above the midpoint of the zygomatic arch and one finger breadth anterior to the external ear (Simon, 1987). See Figure 95.2.

    Using the scalpel, make a 3–4 mm vertical skin incision at the temporal site. See Figure 95.1. Minimal bleeding is usually encountered and may be controlled by applying direct pressure with gauze dressings.
4. *Expose the burr hole site and place a self-retaining retractor. See Figure 95.3.
5. *Using either the standard hand-held drill or twist drill, (see Figure 95.4), introduce the drill bit perpendicular to the site and rotate drill in a

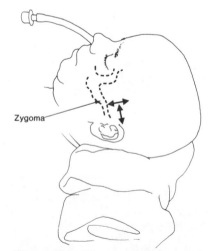

Figure 95.2 The temporal burr hole is placed just above the midpoint of the zygomatic arch and one finger breadth anterior to the external ear. (Simon & Brenner, 1987; 161. Reprinted by permission.)

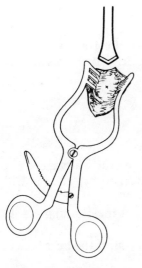

Figure 95.3 Use of self-retaining retractor to expose burr hole site. (Simon & Brenner, 1987; 161. Reprinted by permission.)

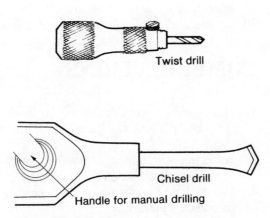

Twist drill

Chisel drill

Handle for manual drilling

Figure 95.4 Top: hand-held twist drill; bottom: chisel drill bit. (Simon & Brenner, 1987: 160. Reprinted by permission.)

clockwise motion to penetrate the inner table of the skull. Use bone wax to control any bleeding from the bone.

6. *Gently irrigate bone dust from the site using a saline-filled syringe.

7. *Visualize the extradural site for a hematoma. Dark red, clotted, blood usually indicates an epidural hematoma. Use the dural suction tip to assist in evacuation of the clotted material. See Figure 95.5. Bright red blood indicates an active bleed which should be located and clamped until further surgical intervention can be provided. Strips of Gelfoam may also be placed as a temporary measure to stop the bleeding (Lang, 1985).

*Indicates portions of the procedure usually performed by a physician.

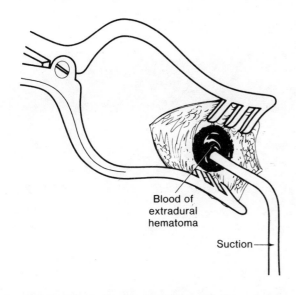

Blood of extradural hematoma

Suction

Figure 95.5 Once the extradural space is entered, a hematoma may be visualized. Use suction to remove any clots or hemorrhaging present. (Simon & Brenner, 1987: 162. Reprinted by permission.)

8. *A bluish tinge usually indicates a subdural hematoma. Insert the dural hook through the outer layer of the dura, pull upward, and incise with a #11 blade to release the accumulated blood. Suction may be needed to evacuate the clot. Use a low vacuum setting to prevent damage to brain

tissue. If bleeding continues, small pieces of thrombin-soaked Gelfoam may be applied to the area (Lang, 1985).

9. Apply a loose gauze dressing over site and prepare for transport to the operating room or a tertiary care facility for definitive treatment.
10. Assess and document neurological status.

COMPLICATIONS

1. Damage may occur to underlying brain tissue if the drill is advanced too far while placing the burr hole. This can be prevented by using a drill stop.
2. Infection or subdural empyema may result from not maintaining sterile technique throughout the procedure.
3. Laceration of an artery or sinus perforation may occur if the burr hole is incorrectly placed.

REFERENCES

Lang, R. 1985. Emergency neurosurgical procedures. In J. Roberts, & J. Hedges (eds). *Clinical procedures in emergency medicine*, Philadelphia: Saunders; 843–855.

Simon, R., & Brenner, B. 1987. *Emergency procedures and techniques*, 2nd ed. Baltimore: Williams & Wilkins.

96

Tong Insertion for Cervical Spine Traction

Marijane Smallwood, RN, BSN

Tongs for cervical spine traction are also known as Gardner-Wells tongs, skull tongs, caliper traction, Heifetz tongs.

INDICATIONS

1. To reduce and realign fractured and/or dislocated cervical vertebrae.
2. To provide continuous traction and stabilization for a cervical spine fracture and/or dislocation, to prevent any further damage to the underlying spinal cord and nerves (Millar, 1985).

CONTRAINDICATIONS AND CAUTIONS

1. Addition or deletion of traction weights should be supervised by a physician.
2. Avoid sudden movements of the traction apparatus, patient, or bed.
3. Cervical tongs usually take 24 hours to become seated. Assess and document the stability of the tongs hourly for the first 24 hours.
4. Tongs are not recommended for stable compression fractures of the vertebral bodies or cervical spinous processes unless associated with severe ligamentous disruption (Lang, 1985).
5. Tongs should not be inserted directly over a skull fracture (Lang, 1985).
6. Keep the cervical collar in place until traction placement is complete.
7. Obtain x-ray confirmation of alignment whenever weight is added or deleted.

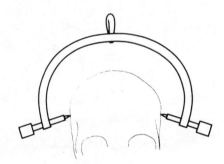

Figure 96.1 Gardner-Wells tongs. (Simon & Brenner, 1987: 172. Reprinted by permission.)

EQUIPMENT

Sterile tong set
Local anesthetic with epinephrine
Antiseptic solution
Gauze dressings
10-cc syringe
18-G needle

25-G 1½-inch needle
Razor
Bed with pulley/traction system attached
Weights: assorted sizes 1#, 2#, 5#
Weight holder

(Note: Various tongs are available for insertion. This procedure will discuss Gardner-Wells and Heifetz tongs. Gardner-Wells tongs feature spring-loaded points for assisting in cervical traction (Gardner, 1973) and are easily placed on the patient in the emergency department. See Figure 96.1.

Similarly, the Heifetz tong is readily inserted in the emergency department with minimal preparation by alternating the advancement of 3 drill bolts into the skull. See Figure 96.2. Heifetz tongs maintain a constant position and do not allow flexion or extension as the Gardner-Wells tong do (Simon & Brenner, 1987). Tong selection is usually by physician preference or availability.

If magnetic resonance imaging (MRI) is ordered or anticipated, special nonmagnetic tongs are necessary.

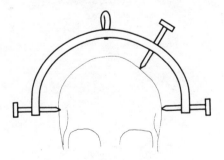

Figure 96.2 Heifetz tongs. (Simon & Brenner, 1987: 173. Reprinted by permission.)

PATIENT PREPARATION

1. Assess and document neurological status.
2. Shave a small area of hair from the scalp approximately 2 cm above the top of each ear.
3. Cleanse the area with antiseptic solution.
4. *Infiltrate the pin insertion sites with local anesthetic.
5. Instruct the patient to immediately report any increased pain, parathesia, or difficulty in breathing during or following the insertion.

PROCEDURAL STEPS

Gardner-Wells tongs

*Indicates portions of the procedure usually performed by a physician.

1. *Apply points of tongs below the temporal ridges and in line with the external auditory meatus (Rosen & Sternbach, 1983). Tighten each side alternately until the spring loaded mechanism extends approximately 1 mm on each side. See Figure 96.3. This indicates a squeezing pressure of 30 pounds (Simon & Brenner, 1987).

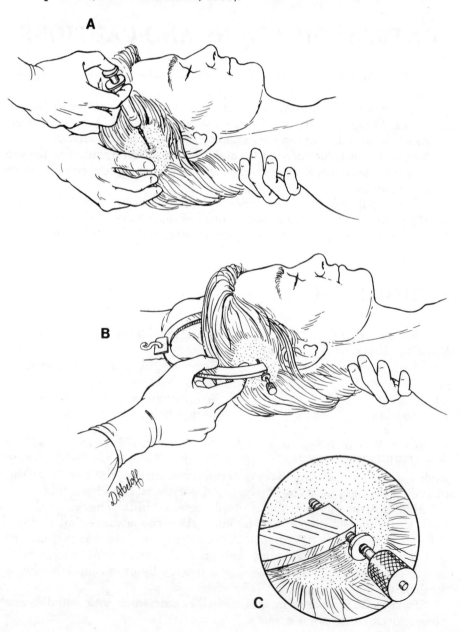

Figure 96.3 a. Anesthetizing the insertion site; b. placement of Gardner-Wells tongs; c. indicator of spring-loaded pins extends 1 mm on each side when a squeeze pressure of 30 pounds has been obtained. (Rosen & Sternbach, 1983: 153. Reprinted by permission.)

2. *Gently rock the tong back and forth to ensure that it is securely seated in the scalp.
3. *Connect the S-hook on the tongs to the pulley rope. Cervical flexion and extension may be obtained by adjusting the height of the pulley (Gardner, 1973).
4. *Place the desired amount of weights onto the weight holder. Approximately 5 pounds per disc space is required for reduction (i.e., 15 pounds for a C-3 fracture) (Cerullo & Quigley, 1985).
5. Obtain an x-ray to check alignment.
6. Sandbags or rolled towels may be placed on each side of the patient's head to provide additional stability.
7. A small towel may be folded and placed under the neck for patient comfort. Do not hyperextend the neck.
8. Place antiseptic-soaked dressings around each pin site.

Heifetz tongs

1. *Place the Heifetz tongs in position along the calvarium.
2. *Advance the 2 temporal bolts until they meet the skull. Note that the bolt drill is marked in 2-mm increments.
3. *Advance the temporal bolts 2–3 mm into the outer table of the skull by alternately screwing one bolt drill 3 complete turns clockwise and then unscrewing it 2 complete turns counterclockwise (Simon & Brenner, 1987).
4. *When insertion is complete, rotate the bolt so that the flat side is facing the patient's feet.
5. *Tighten the parietal bolt to maintain the position of the temporal bolts.
6. Apply traction as described for the Gardner-Wells tongs.
7. Place antiseptic soaked dressings around each pin site.

COMPLICATIONS

1. Excessive traction may result in additional neurological impairment.
2. Perforation of the inner table of the skull has been reported with Gardner-Wells tongs (Lang, 1985).
3. The tongs may loosen and pull out if not checked regularly for integrity. The points may require additional tightening.
4. Infection or localized erythema may develop at the pin insertion site. Observe for redness, swelling, or purulent drainage, and keep the site clean.
5. If traction is released, additional cord damage may result. This may accidentally occur if the weights gradually pull the patient to the head of the bed and rest on the floor. The weights should always hang freely.

PATIENT TEACHING

1. Report increased pain at the insertion site, neck, or across the shoulders.
2. Avoid sudden movements to voice or visual stimulation as mobility of the neck and head is severely restricted.

REFERENCES

Cerullo, L.J., & Quigley, M.R. 1985. Management of cervical spinal cord injury. *Journal of Emergency Nursing,* 11:182–187.
Gardner, W. 1973. The principle of spring-loaded points for cervical traction. *Journal of Neurosurgery,* 39:543.

Lang, R. 1985. Insertion of cervical traction devices. In J. Roberts, & J. Hedges (eds). *Clinical Procedures in Emergency Medicine.* Philadelphia: Saunders; 838–842.

Millar, S., Sampson, L., & Soukoup, M. 1985. *AACN Procedure Manual for Critical Care,* 2nd ed. Philadelphia: Saunders.

Rosen, P., & Sternbach, G.L. 1983. *Atlas of Emergency Medicine,* 2nd ed. Baltimore: Williams & Wilkins.

Simon, R., & Brenner, B., 1987. *Emergency Procedures and Techniques.* 2nd ed. Baltimore: Williams & Wilkins.

97

Peritoneal Lavage

Jean A. Proehl, RN, MN, CEN, CCRN

Peritoneal lavage is also known as belly tap, peri dial, peri lavage, or diagnostic peritoneal lavage (DPL).

INDICATIONS

1. To help diagnose intra-abdominal bleeding or viscous perforation after abdominal trauma, especially in patients unable to contribute to the physical exam because of paralysis, unconsciousness, intoxication, etc.
2. To evaluate patients at risk for intra-abdominal trauma who are about to undergo lengthy anesthesia for nonabdominal surgical procedures.
3. To help diagnose patients with unexplained hypotension following trauma.
4. To provide core rewarming for severely hypothermic patients (core temperature <32°C or 90°F).

CONTRAINDICATIONS AND CAUTIONS

1. If abdominal surgery is already indicated by physical exam or clinical presentation, there is no need to perform peritoneal lavage.
2. Multiple prior abdominal surgeries increase the risk of adhesions, which may cause the intestines to adhere to the abdominal wall and result in viscous perforation when the catheter is introduced.
3. Pregnancy greater than 12 weeks gestation is a relative contraindication.
4. Because pelvic fractures may result in false positive results, a supraumbilical insertion site should be chosen.
5. Because insertion of the catheter through a hematoma may cause false positive results, an alternative site should be chosen.
6. Peritoneal lavage is not helpful in diagnosing retroperitoneal injuries unless the peritoneum is disrupted.

EQUIPMENT

Sterile gloves
Masks
Razor
Antiseptic solution
#11 scalpel
Mosquito forceps
Gauze sponges
Local anesthesia (with epinephrine)
Alcohol wipes
5-ml syringe, 18-G needle, 25–27-G needle for anesthesia
1000 ml warmed (36.6°C to 37.7°C) normal saline or lactated

Ringer's solution (20 ml/kg for children)
Peritoneal dialysis catheter (with or without trocar) or catheter/dilator/spring wire guide assembly (commercially available in preassembled kits)
Nonvented IV tubing without a backcheck valve or single chamber cystoscopy tubing
Sterile drapes or towels
20-ml syringe

331

Blood collection tubes
Needle holder
4-0 nylon sutures
Scissors
Antibiotic ointment

Adhesive tape
(Note: Preassembled kits
containing much of this
equipment are also
available.)

PATIENT PREPARATION

1. Insert an indwelling urinary catheter to decompress the bladder and prevent bladder perforation when the catheter is introduced.
    (Note: The peritoneal lavage catheter should never be inserted until the preceding step is completed.)
2. Insert a gastric tube to decompress the stomach and prevent stomach perforation during catheter introduction.
3. If possible, complete any abdominal x-rays before the procedure, because air may enter the abdomen and confuse any future abdominal films.
4. Place the patient in the supine position.
5. *Shave the abdomen and prep with antiseptic solution. The usual site for catheter insertion is midline, one-third of the distance between the umbilicus and the symphysis pubis.

PROCEDURAL STEPS

*Indicates portions of the procedure usually performed by a physician.

1. *Drape the abdomen with sterile towels.
2. *Infiltrate the area with local anesthetic (optional). In general, an anesthetic containing epinephrine is used to help control bleeding at the site. Absolute hemostasis at the site is essential to help prevent false positive results.
3. *Incise through the abdominal skin and subcutaneous tissue and insert the catheter through the abdominal wall. If conscious, the patient may assist by tensing the abdominal muscles as the catheter is inserted. This will facilitate catheter passage through the muscles and help prevent viscous perforation. If desired, towel clips may be used to provide traction on the abdomen of unconscious or uncooperative patients. The catheter may be inserted over a trocar or a spring wire guide. The spring wire guide is less likely to result in damage to intra-abdominal contents and is recommended for use in children to help prevent evisceration of abdominal contents through the larger opening necessitated by the trocar technique (Matlak, 1985).
4. *To provide core rewarming, two catheters may be inserted. One will be used to constantly infuse warmed solution, and the other to drain the solution from the abdomen. This is more time efficient than infusing and draining via the same catheter.
5. If the lavage is being performed for diagnostic purposes, the catheter is now aspirated with a 20-ml syringe. If more than 5–10 ml of blood or any gastric/bowel contents are aspirated, the lavage is considered positive and stopped at this point (American College of Surgeons, 1988).
6. Attach the primed IV tubing to the catheter. See Figure 97.1. The IV tubing should not contain a backcheck valve, because this will prevent the fluid from being siphoned out of the abdomen. If the tubing is vented, the fluid may leak from the vent or a water seal may form and prevent fluid return.
    Cystoscopy tubing will allow much faster installation and drainage. To connect the tubing, push the end of the connecting tubing into the

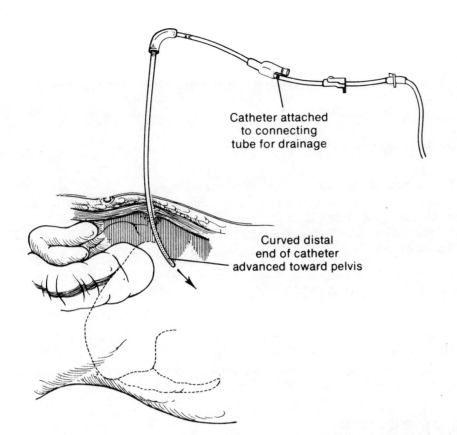

Catheter attached
to connecting
tube for drainage

Curved distal
end of catheter
advanced toward pelvis

Figure 97.1 Lavage catheter in peritoneal space.
(Wilkins, 1989: 1031. Reprinted by permission.)

latex sleeve of the cystoscopy tubing. Tying a suture around the distal end of the latex tubing will tighten the connection.

7. Infuse sterile warmed normal saline or lactated Ringer's solution. Room temperature solutions may cause or worsen pre-existing hypothermia. 1000 ml of fluid is usually infused for adults and 10–20 ml/kg in children (American College of Surgeons, 1988; Matlak, 1985; Rea, 1986).

8. Allow the fluid to remain in the peritoneal space for 5–10 minutes. Palpate the abdomen or gently rock the patient from side to side to help distribute the fluid throughout the peritoneal cavity.

9. Lower the IV bag to the floor and allow the fluid to siphon out of the abdomen. If fluid does not return, make sure the appropriate IV tubing has been used. If necessary, cut off a backcheck valve or vent and drain the fluid into a basin. Then try repositioning the patient or the catheter. Additional fluid may also be instilled to encourage fluid return. Any fluid left in the abdomen will be absorbed by the peritoneum and should be added to the patient's parenteral fluid intake.

10. Laboratory specimens are obtained from the returned fluid. Commonly ordered tests include red blood cell count (RBC), white blood cell count (WBC), hematocrit (Hct), bilirubin, SGOT, amylase, alkaline phosphatase, culture and sensitivity, and gram stain. The fluid is placed in the same specimen tubes that would be used if the tests were being performed on blood. The fluid may also be submitted in the IV bag or syringes.

11. Positive findings include (based on 1000 ml infused):

     RBC > 100,000 per cubic millimeter in blunt trauma
     RBC > 10,000 per cubic millimeter in penetrating trauma
     WBC > 500 per cubic millimeter
     Hct > 2% within the first hour after trauma
     Amylase > 100–200 somogyi units
     Any bile, bacteria, or fecal material
     (American College of Surgeons, 1988; Rea, 1991).
     A less sensitive method is to attempt to read newsprint through the

fluid in the IV bag. If the fluid is so bloody that newsprint cannot be read, the lavage is considered positive.

12. *The catheter is then removed and the wound sutured.
13. Place a thin layer of antibiotic ointment and a sterile dressing over the wound.

COMPLICATIONS

1. Perforation of abdominal organs or blood vessels
2. False positive results, which may occur secondary to bleeding at the insertion site, bleeding within the muscle sheath, or pelvic fractures.
3. Wound infection or dehiscence (late)
4. Incisional hernia (late)

PATIENT TEACHING

1. Keep the wound clean and dry and observe for signs of infection.
2. Have the sutures removed in 8–10 days.
3. Notify the nursing or medical staff immediately if abdominal pain, tenderness, rigidity, or fever increase.

REFERENCES

American College of Surgeons, Committee on Trauma, 1988. *Advanced trauma life support course.* Chicago: American College of Surgeons.

Matlak, M.E. 1985. Abdominal injuries. In T.A. Mayer (ed). *Emergency management of pediatric trauma.* Philadelphia: Saunders; 328–340.

Rea. R.E. (ed). (1991). *Trauma nursing core course (provider) manual,* 3rd ed. Chicago: Award Printing Corporation.

Wilkins, E.W., Jr. 1989. *Emergency Medicine: Scientific Foundations and Current Practice,* 3rd ed. Baltimore: Williams and Wilkins.

SUGGESTED READINGS

Budassi, S. 1981. Peritoneal lavage. *Journal of Emergency Nursing,* 7, 1:27–29.

Burney, R.E. 1986. Peritoneal lavage and other diagnostic procedures in blunt abdominal trauma. *Emergency Medical Clinics of North America,* 4:513–526.

Simon, R.R., & Brenner, R.E. 1987. *Emergency procedures and techniques,* 2nd ed. Baltimore: Williams & Wilkins.

98

Insertion of Orogastric and Nasogastric Tubes

Dawn M. Swimm, RN, CEN

Orogastric and nasogastric tubes are also known as Levin, Salem-sump, Ewald, Levacuator, and feeding tubes.

INDICATIONS

1. To remove air and/or gastric contents from the stomach.
2. To instill fluid (lavage fluid, tube feedings, etc.) into the stomach.

CONTRAINDICATIONS AND CAUTIONS

1. Maxillofacial injury or anterior fossa skull fracture offer the potential for inadvertent penetration of the brain via the cribiform plate or ethmoid bone if the tube is inserted nasally. The orogastric route is recommended for such patients.
2. Esophageal varices place the patient at risk for esophageal rupture and/ or hemorrhage as a result of tube placement.

EQUIPMENT

Piston or catheter tip syringe (60-cc)
Lubricating jelly
Stethoscope
Emesis basin
Tape
Orogastric or nasogastric tube (See Figure 98.1).

(Note: The type and size of the tube relate to the reason for placement. The Salem sump has a two-lumen system. The smaller blue pigtail is an extension of the vent lumen. The major advantage of the double-lumen tube is that the constant airflow allows for a controlled suction force at the drainage eyes.)

PROCEDURAL STEPS

1. If alert, have the patient sit upright or in the high Fowler's position. Obtunded or unconscious patients should be head down, semi-prone, preferably lying on the left side.
2. Measure the tube either from the tip of the nose to the tip of the earlobe and down to the xiphoid process, or from the tip of the nose to the umbilicus and mark the length. See Figure 98.2.

Nasogastric placement
a. Lubricate the tube, choose the largest nare and thread the tube through the nose, aiming down and back. See Figure 98.3.
b. When the tube reaches the pharynx, have the patient flex the head forward to facilitate swallowing.

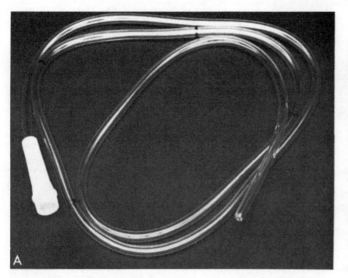

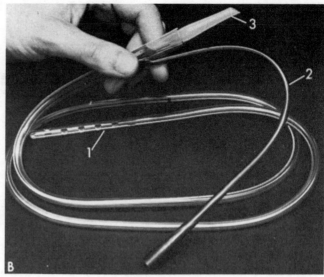

Figure 98.1 Two types of gastric tubes.
(Roberts & Hedges, 1985: 754. Reprinted by permission.)

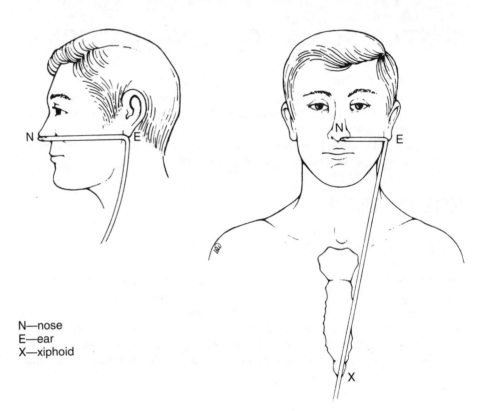

N—nose
E—ear
X—xiphoid

Figure 98.2 Measuring the nasogastric tube.
(Brunner & Suddarth, 1986: 413. Reprinted by permission.)

(Note: Flexing the head forward is desirable for tube passage in the alert, unconscious, or obtunded patient.)

c. Advance the tube while the patient swallows (either a small amount of water or mimicking) until reaching the previously noted mark.

Orogastric placement

a. If the patient is uncooperative, place an airway or biteblock in the mouth to prevent the patient from biting the tube (preventing passage or occluding flow). See Ch. 6: Oral airway insertion.

b. Lubricate the tip of the tube and pass it through the lips, over the tongue, aiming down and back towards the pharynx with the patient's head flexed forward. See Figure 98.4.

336

c. Advance the tube with the patient's swallowing motion until reaching the previously noted mark.
3. Verify position either by aspirating gastric contents and/or auscultating the stomach with a stethoscope while injecting 15–20 cc of air into the tube.
4. Center and tape the tube in place with hypoallergenic tape or secure with a gastric tube holder. Do not tape to the forehead because this places undue pressure on the nares.

COMPLICATIONS

1. Epistaxis may occur from trauma to the nasopharynx.
2. Vagal response secondary to gagging may cause respiratory or cardiac compromise.
3. Inadvertent intubation of the trachea can cause hypoxia, cyanosis, or respiratory arrest.
4. Prolonged nasogastric tube placement can cause skin erosion, sinusitis, esophagitis, esophagotracheal fistula, gastric ulceration, pulmonary or oral infections. (Roberts et al., 1985)
5. Vomiting and aspiration.

PATIENT TEACHING

Assure the patient that the discomfort will subside.

REFERENCES

Brunner, L.S., & Suddarth, D.S. 1986. *The Lippincott manual of nursing practice,* 4th ed. Philadelphia: Lippincott.
Roberts, J.R., & Hedges, J.R. 1985. *Clinical procedures in emergency medicine.* Philadelphia: Saunders.
Smith, S., & Duell, D. 1989. *Clinical nursing skills,* 2nd ed. Norwalk, CT: Appleton & Lange.

SUGGESTED READINGS

Budassi, S.A., & Barber, J.M. 1985. *Emergency nursing: Principles and practice.* 2nd ed. St. Louis: Mosby.

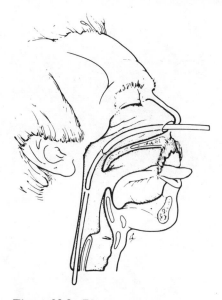

Figure 98.3   Placement of a nasogastric tube.
(Smith & Duell, 1989: 361. Reprinted by permission.)

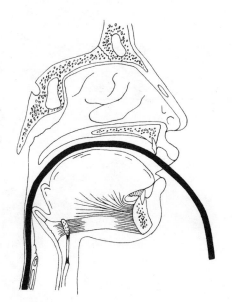

Figure 98.4   Orogastric tube in place.

99

Gastric Lavage for Gastrointestinal Bleeding

Valerie Novotny-Dinsdale, RN, MSN, CEN

INDICATIONS

1. To control an acute upper gastrointestinal hemorrhage when other interventions are not immediately available.

    Other interventions may include: electrocoagulation; injection sclerotherapy (sodium morrhuate, ethanolamine oleate); photocoagulation (laser technology); vasoactive infusion (usually Vasopressin); and transcatheter embolization (Cosgriff & Anderson, 1984).

    (Note: Although gastric lavage is still being performed to control acute gastrointestinal hemorrhage, its therapeutic value has not been proven. In many facilities, emergency departments have access to endoscopy units capable of performing esophagogastroduodenoscopy, which has become the primary method of identifying the site of upper gastrointestinal hemorrhage.)

2. To remove irritating gastric secretions and prevent nausea and vomiting through gastric decompression.
3. To obtain information on the site and rate of bleeding.
4. To help evacuate clots.

CONTRAINDICATION AND CAUTIONS

1. In the presence of GI hemorrhage, irrigation can knock the clot off a bleeding vessel and cause further bleeding, resulting in shock. Consider prophylactic pneumatic anti-shock garment (PASG) application without inflation unless indicated. See Ch. 71.
2. If the patient has a gag reflex but is obtunded, or does not have a gag reflex, there is risk of aspiration if vomiting occurs during lavage. Consider endotracheal intubation to protect the airway.
3. Controversy continues to exist regarding the use of iced or cold saline. Some authors believe that iced saline causes a local vasoconstriction resulting in decreased bleeding and clot formation (Civetta, 1988). Others maintain that cold temperatures stimulate hydrochloric acid production, thereby adding to gastric irritation (Strange, 1987).

EQUIPMENT

Gastric tube of physician's choice (usually a large 32–26-French gastric lavage tube)

Gloves, protective apron or gown, goggles, mask

Lubricating jelly

60-ml catheter tip syringe

Irrigation tray

Stethoscope

Tape

Tincture of Benzoin

Irrigating solution of physician's choice (usually saline)

Bite block

Suction equipment

PATIENT PREPARATION

1. Protect patient's airway from accidental aspiration by endotracheal intubation if indicated.
2. Have suction equipment readily available.
3. Place patient on cardiac monitor and assess vital signs every 5–10 minutes.
4. Insert at least one large bore IV line.
5. Insert stomach tube in mouth or nose using lubricating jelly. If inserting via the mouth, a bite block with a hole for the tube to pass through is preferable. See Ch. 98: Inserting Orogastric and Nasogastric Tubes.

PROCEDURAL STEPS

1. Pour cool, normal saline solution and ice (optional) into irrigation container (Cosgriff & Anderson, 1984; Civetta et al., 1988).
2. Draw up solution using a 60-ml syringe and inject it into the tube as rapidly as possible. Infuse approximately 200–300 ml.
3. Aspirate the solution from the stomach and discard into a measured basin.
4. Repeat until active bleeding stops or until the patient is transferred to endoscopy.
5. Measure the differences in volumes of irrigant and aspirant and document as intake/output.

COMPLICATIONS

1. Perforation of esophageal varices.
2. Mallory-Weiss tear resulting from repeated vomiting, a sharp increase in intra-abdominal pressure from over-distention of the stomach, or aggressive insertion of the lavage tube.
3. Aspiration of gastric contents into an unprotected airway.
4. Systemic hypothermia if the lavage is prolonged or large quantities of cold irrigant are used.

REFERENCES

Civetta, J., Taylor, R., & Kirby, R., 1988. *Critical care.* Philadelphia: Lippincott.

Cosgriff, J., & Anderson, D. 1984. *The practice of emergency care,* 2nd ed. Philadelphia: Lippincott.

Strange, J., 1987. Acute upper gastrointestinal bleeding. In J.M. Strange (ed). *Shock trauma care plans.* Springhouse, PA: Springhouse Corporation; 107–111.

SUGGESTED READINGS

Budassi, S., & Barber, J. 1984. *Mosby's manual of emergency care: Practices and procedures,* 2nd ed. St. Louis: Mosby.

O'Boyle, C., Davis, K., Russo, B., & Kraf, T. 1985. *Emergency care: The first 24 hours.* Norwalk, CT: Appleton-Century-Crofts.

Persons, C. 1987. *Critical care procedures and protocols: A nursing process approach.* Philadelphia: Lippincott.

100

Gastric lavage for removal of toxic substances is also known as gastric emptying, stomach pumping.

Gastric Lavage for Removal of Toxic Substances

Dorothy M. Schulte, RN, MS

INDICATIONS

To remove potentially toxic ingested substances from patients who
1. have a decreased level of consciousness or do not have a gag reflex;
2. have been given ipecac but have failed to produce emesis;
3. are uncooperative and refuse ipecac therapy;
4. are awake but who, by history, have ingested a lethal amount of a highly toxic substance making instillation of charcoal an important therapy (Haddad & Winchester, 1983);
5. have ingested substances known to cause a rapid deterioration in level of consciousness where ipecac is contraindicated (i.e., tricyclics, antidepressants, propoxyphene, camphor, narcotics).

CONTRAINDICATIONS AND CAUTIONS

1. Do not lavage patients who have ingested a caustic (alkali or acid) substance or petroleum distillate.
2. Do not lavage patients who are actively convulsing, because the passage of the tube may increase severity and frequency of seizures (Poisindex, 1989).
3. Excess fluid administration through the lavage tube may push stomach contents into the duodenum and increase the absorption of the ingested substance. No more than 100–300 ml of fluid should be instilled at one time and it should be removed by gravity or syringe as quickly as possible (Dreisbach & Robertson, 1987).
4. Assure proper tube placement prior to instillation of fluid to prevent aspiration.
5. The use of gastric lavage as the standard of care for removing toxic substances is controversial and is of questionable value for patients who present to the emergency department greater than one hour after exposure to the poison. Research has indicated that patients have a satisfactory clinical outcome without gastric emptying, because administration of activated charcoal and aggressive supportive care are sufficient treatment (Kulig, 1985).

EQUIPMENT

Gastric tubes 22–36 French (average size for adult is 32–36) with at least two through-and-through holes at distal end

60-ml irrigating syringe with catheter tip
Endotracheal tube (optional)
Enema or douche bag with straight

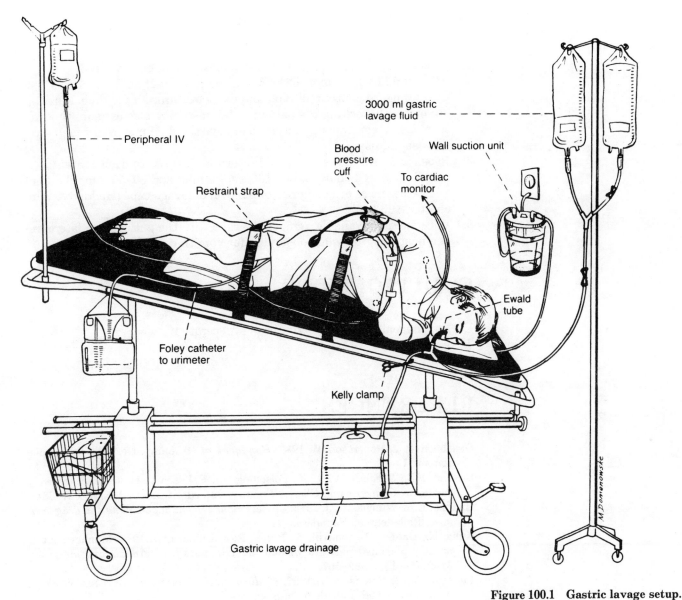

Peripheral IV

3000 ml gastric
lavage fluid

Blood
pressure
cuff

Wall suction unit

To cardiac
monitor

Restraint strap

Ewald
tube

Foley catheter
to urimeter

Kelly clamp

Gastric lavage drainage

**Figure 100.1 Gastric lavage setup.
For illustration purposes the patient
is shown uncovered with the siderails down. The patient should be
covered to preserve body temperature and the siderails should be up
for safety.**
(Luckman & Sorenson, 1987: 1934.
Reprinted by permission.)

connector or
premanufactured lavage kit
Room temperature normal saline or
tap water (Epstein & Eilers,
1988)

Restraints (optional)
Bucket or basin
Pharyngeal suctioning equipment

PATIENT PREPARATION

1. Set up and turn on continuous pharyngeal suctioning equipment. See Ch. 31.
2. Restrain the patient as indicated/ordered. See Ch. 178: Application of Restraints.
3. Endotracheal intubation is required for the unresponsive, comatose patient to avoid aspiration. Controversy exists regarding endotracheal intubation of the comatose, responsive patient. It is recommended that the physician use clinical judgment in the decision (Haddad & Winchester, 1983). See Ch. 10: Oral Endotracheal Intubation and Ch. 11: Nasal Endotracheal Intubation.
4. Place the patient on the left side in the Trendelenberg position to promote return of lavage fluid and help prevent aspiration. See Figure 100.1.
5. Insert a large bore gastric tube. See Ch. 98.

PROCEDURAL STEPS

1. Instill 100–300 ml warmed fluid (Dreisbach & Robertson, 1987).
2. Allow fluid to drain into the bucket using gravity. If no fluid returns, use the syringe to gently pull fluid and particles through the tube. Massaging or gently rocking the patient's abdomen may also enhance fluid return. Using continuous suction to remove the fluid may result in gastric mucosal damage.
3. Repeat Steps 1 and 2 until fluid return is clear of stomach contents.
4. Instill activated charcoal (50–100 g for adults and 30–50 g for children) and cathartic as ordered prior to removal of lavage tube (Haddad & Winchester, 1983).
5. With suction available, remove the tube with the patient in a lateral recumbent position while observing for vomiting.

COMPLICATIONS

1. Esophageal or gastric perforation or laceration
2. Aspiration
3. Gagging

REFERENCES

Dreisbach, P., & Robertson, W. 1987. *Handbook of Poisoning.* Norwalk, CT: Appleton and Lange.

Epstein, F.B., & Eilers, M. 1988. Poisoning. In, P. Rosen et al., (eds). *Emergency Medicine: Concepts and Clinical Practice,* 2nd ed. St. Louis: Mosby; 321–361.

Haddad, L., & Winchester, J. 1983. *Clinical management of poisoning and drug overdose.* Philadelphia: Saunders.

Kulig, K., Bar-Or, D., Cantrill, S., Rosen, P., & Rumack, B. 1985. Management of acutely poisoned patients without gastric emptying. *Annals of Emergency Medicine,* 14, 6:562–567.

Luckman, J., & Sorensen, K. 1987. *Medical-surgical nursing: a psychophysiologic approach,* 3rd ed. Philadelphia: Saunders.

Poisindex: a computer generated microfiche poison information service, (revised quarterly). Rumack, B.N., (ed). Denver, CO: Micromedix, Inc.

101

Ipecac Administration

Dorothy M. Schulte, RN, MS

INDICATIONS

To decrease absorption of ingested substances by emesis induction.

CONTRAINDICATIONS AND CAUTIONS

1. Do not administer if the gag reflex is absent or the patient has a decreased level of consciousness.
2. Do not give ipecac to patients who are comatose or seizing.
3. Do not administer ipecac to patients with a history of ingestion of medications that result in CNS depression within 30 minutes (i.e., propoxyphene, camphor, tricyclics, narcotics) (Poisindex, 1989).
4. Ipecac is not recommended for patients younger than 9 months.
5. Do not use ipecac for ingestions of corrosives or caustic substances.
6. Although not contraindicated in hydrocarbon ingestion, ipecac must be used with caution, weighing the risks of potential aspiration from vomiting against the seriousness of systemic toxicity from the ingested substance (Haddad & Winchester, 1983).
7. Use only **syrup of ipecac**, because fluid extract of ipecac is extremely toxic with central nervous system and cardiac effects.
8. Calculate the amount of water given to the patient, because large amounts of water may result in reflex emptying of the stomach into the small intestine, which could result in an increase in absorption of the ingested substance. Thirty-two (32) ounces (960 ml) is recommended for an adult and proportionately less for a child (Epstein & Eilers, 1988).
9. Do not administer concomitantly with charcoal, because the ipecac will be absorbed by the charcoal. Charcoal can be administered following ipecac when the patient is no longer vomiting or having dry heaves.
10. Induction of emesis by ipecac may not be beneficial if ingestion occurred longer than one hour prior to its administration, because the efficacy of removing the ingested substance decreases as the time from ingestion increases (Haddad & Winchester, 1983).

EQUIPMENT

Tongue blade
10–30-ml of syrup of ipecac
8–32-ounces (240–960 ml) of water
     or noncarbonated beverage

Glass with graduated markings
Large basin
Tissues
Waterproof pads

PATIENT PREPARATION

1. Place the patient in a sitting position with a basin on his or her lap.
2. Assess the patient's level of consciousness and determine the presence of a gag reflex with a tongue depressor.

PROCEDURAL STEPS

1. Administer ipecac dosage based on age (Epstein & Eilers, 1988).

10 ml	9–12 months
15 ml	1–12 years
30 ml	greater than 12 years

2. Follow ipecac administration immediately with water or another noncarbonated beverage (Epstein & Eilers 1988).

1–16 ounces (30–480 ml)	child
16–32 ounces (480–960 ml)	adult

3. Ambulate the patient, if possible.
4. After the first episode of vomiting, give additional fluids to prevent dry retching.
5. Stimulate the gag reflex with a tongue depressor if emesis does not occur within 20–30 minutes (Epstein & Eilers, 1988).
6. Repeat ipecac and fluids as above if no emesis results after attempting to stimulate the gag reflex.
7. Lavage may be indicated if there is no response from the second dose of ipecac.
8. Discontinue fluid administration after the first episode of clear emesis.

COMPLICATIONS

1. Aspiration
2. Prolonged contact of ipecac with the gastric mucosa may result in protracted vomiting with gastric irritation, central nervous system depression, and cardiac toxicity (evidenced by T wave flattening or inversion, QT prolongation).
3. Mallory-Weiss tear
4. Pneumomediastinum

PATIENT TEACHING

1. Vomiting may continue for 2–4 hours after ipecac administration. Nothing should be taken by mouth for two hours after the last emesis. Begin with clear fluids and progress to diet as tolerated. If vomiting returns after the first attempt to retain fluids, do not give food or fluids for another two hours.
2. Ipecac stimulates peristalsis, so you may experience some diarrhea for 3–4 hours.

REFERENCES

Epstein, F.B., & Eilers, M. 1988. Poisoning. In P. Rosen, et al. (eds). *Emergency Medicine: Concepts and Clinical Practice*, 2nd ed. St. Louis: Mosby; 321–361.

Haddad, L., & Winchester, J. 1983. *Clinical Management of Poisoning and Drug Overdose.* Philadelphia: Saunders.

Poisindex: A computer generated microfiche poison information service (revised quarterly). Rumack, B.N., (ed). Denver, CO: Micromedix, Inc.

102

Balloon Tamponade of Gastroesophageal Varices

Jean A. Proehl, RN, MN, CEN, CCRN

Balloons for the tamponade of gastroesophageal varices are also known as Sengstaken-Blakemore tube, Minnesota tube.

INDICATIONS

To control severe bleeding from gastroesophageal varices that is unresponsive to other interventions or when other interventions are unavailable or contraindicated.

Note: In the United States balloon tamponade had largely been replaced by other measures due to the potential for serious complications. However, recent European research has demonstrated that balloon tamponade is effective in more than 90% of patients as initial therapy with 10% or less experiencing complications (Feneyrou, 1988; Haddock, 1989; Panes, 1988).

CONTRAINDICATIONS AND CAUTIONS

1. Because the potential for serious complications exists, more conservative measures (i.e., intravenous Pitressin, sclerotherapy) are usually attempted first (Simon & Brenner, 1987).
2. Caution should be exercised in the patient with pre-existing esophageal disease (i.e., strictures, cancer, etc.).

EQUIPMENT

Sengstaken-Blakemore (SB) or Minnesota tube (**Note:** The SB tube is a triple-lumen, double-balloon tube. One lumen functions as a gastric tube, one is used to inflate/deflate the gastric balloon, and the third is used to inflate/deflate the esophageal balloon. The Minnesota tube is a quadruple-lumen tube. It is the same as a SB tube plus it has a lumen that terminates just proximal to the esophageal balloon. This lumen is attached to suction to remove oropharyngeal secretions that accumulate in the esophagus.)

Nasogastric (NG) tube (**Note:** The NG tube is not needed if a Minnesota tube is used.)
Lubricating jelly
50–60-ml catheter tip syringe
3 rubber shod clamps
Manometer
Intermittent suction source
Adhesive tape
Foam rubber to pad nares
Basin of ice to chill tube (optional)
Topical anesthetic (viscous lidocaine, cetacaine, cocaine, etc., optional)
Catcher's mask, football helmet, or commercial mask (optional)
Bite block (if tube is inserted orally)
Normal saline solution
Scissors

PATIENT PREPARATION

1. *Endotracheal intubation may be necessary to help prevent aspiration in the patient with a decreased level of consciousness.
2. Empty the stomach via lavage. See Ch. 99: Gastric lavage for GI bleeding. Failure to do so may result in vomiting and aspiration during tube insertion (Simon & Brenner, 1987).
3. *Anesthetize the conscious patient's nasopharynx (optional).

PROCEDURAL STEPS

1. Inflate both balloons under water to check for leaks.
2. Stiffen the tube by chilling it in a basin of ice (optional).
3. *Pass the lubricated tube through the patient's nostril or mouth to about the 500-mm marking (Buschiazzo & Possanzo, 1986; Feneyrou, 1988). The balloons are folded around the tube to facilitate its passage. If the oral route is chosen, a bite block must be placed to prevent the patient from biting through the tube.
4. Check tube placement by instilling air through the gastric lumen while auscultating over the epigastric area. At this point it is recommended that tube position be further verified by instilling 50 ml of air into the gastric balloon and obtaining a chest x-ray (McGrath, 1986; Barsan & Baker, 1988; Salam, 1986). Other options to help assure proper tube placement include insertion during direct laryngoscopy or fluoroscopy (McGrath, 1986).
5. *Instill 250–275 ml of air into the gastric balloon and double clamp the port. A manometer and Y-connector may be used to check the pressure in the balloon (see Figure 102.1), 25–30 mm Hg is optimal (Simon & Brenner, 1987). Using water in the balloons has also been recommended but makes the tube heavier and increases the risk of pressure necrosis (Simon & Brenner, 1987).

*Indicates portions of the procedure usually performed by a physician.

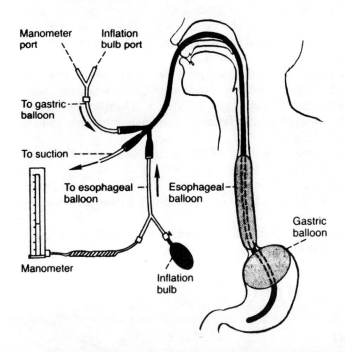

Figure 102.1 Measuring balloon pressure in a Sengstaken-Blakemore tube using a manometer. (Luckman, J., & Sorenson, K.C., 1987: 1365. *Medical-surgical nursing: A psychophysiologic approach,* 3rd ed. Philadelphia: Saunders; 1365. Reprinted by permission.)

6. *Gentle traction may be exerted on the tube to pull the gastric balloon up and compress varices in the upper stomach. The traction is maintained by fastening the tube to a football helmet or catcher's mask placed on the patient or by taping the tube to the patient's cheek or nose.

7. Attach the gastric lumen to intermittent suction to evacuate and/or lavage the stomach and assess for continued bleeding (Simon & Brenner, 1987).

8. *If bleeding continues, inflate the esophageal balloon to 25–45 mm Hg of pressure and clamp the port (Buschiazzo & Possanzo, 1986).

9. Insert a small nasogastric tube through the opposite nare to the top of the esophageal balloon and attach to low suction to remove oropharyngeal secretions and assess for proximal bleeding sites. (**Note:** This is not necessary with the Minnesota tube; simply attach the proximal port to low suction.)

10. Pad the nares with foam rubber to help prevent pressure necrosis as a result of the tube (Luckmann & Sorenson, 1987).

11. Clearly label the ports of the tube so that the gastric balloon is not inadvertently deflated (see Complications) (Brunner & Suddarth, 1986; Luckmann & Sorenson, 1987).

12. Intermittent deflation of the esophageal balloon may be ordered to help prevent esophageal pressure necrosis.

13. Lavage for GI bleeding may continue through the gastric port as ordered.

14. Restrain the patient as necessary to prevent the tube from becoming dislodged.

COMPLICATIONS

1. Airway obstruction as a result of the tube being dislodged. Never deflate the gastric balloon with the esophageal balloon inflated or while there is traction on the tube. **If the tube becomes dislodged and obstructs the airway, cut the ports for both balloons and quickly remove the tube. Always keep a pair of scissors at the bedside for this purpose** (Buschiazzo & Possanzo, 1986; Brunner & Suddarth, 1986; Luckmann & Sorenson, 1987).

2. Vomiting and aspiration of gastric contents or oropharyngeal secretions. This can usually be prevented by emptying the stomach prior to tube insertion, maintaining suction on the gastric port, and placing a proximal NG tube to remove secretions when a SB tube is used (Buschiazzo & Possanzo, 1986; Simon & Brenner, 1987).

3. Esophageal rupture as a result of excess pressure in the esophageal balloon or inflation of the gastric balloon in the esophagus (McGrath, 1986). Monitor the pressure in the esophageal balloon and verify tube placement with a chest x-ray prior to inflation of the gastric balloon to help prevent this complication.

4. Persistent hiccups. Elevate the head of the bed to help control hiccups and prevent aspiration (Simon & Brenner, 1987).

5. Esophageal erosion from prolonged pressure. Intermittent deflation may be ordered to help prevent this complication (Brunner & Suddarth, 1986).

6. Irritation or ulceration of the nares. This can be decreased by carefully padding the nares with foam rubber.

PATIENT TEACHING

1. Immediately report any chest pain, difficulty breathing, or nausea.
2. Do not pull on the tube or attempt to readjust tube position.

REFERENCES

Brunner, L.S., & Suddarth, D.S. (eds). 1986. *The Lippincott manual of nursing practice*, 4th ed. Philadelphia: Lippincott.

Buschiazzo, L., & Possanzo, C. 1986. A 57-year-old man with bleeding esophageal varices. *Journal of Emergency Nursing*, 12, 3:131–133.

Feneyrou, B., Hanana, J., Daures, J.P., & Prioton, J.B. 1988. Initial control of bleeding from esophageal varices with the Sengstaken-Blakemore tube. *American Journal of Surgery*, 155:509–511.

Haddock, G., Garden, O.J., McKee, R.F., Anderson, J.R., & Carter, D.C. 1989. Esophageal tamponade in the management of acute variceal hemorrhage. *Digestive Diseases and Sciences*, 34:913–918.

Luckmann, J., & Sorenson, K.C. 1987. *Medical-surgical nursing: A psychophysiologic approach*, 3rd ed. Philadelphia: Saunders.

McGrath, R.B. 1986. Inadvertent gastric balloon inflation within the chest in the management of esophageal varices. *Critical Care Medicine*, 14:580–582.

Panes, J., Teres, J., Bosch, J., & Rodes, J. 1988. Efficacy of balloon tamponade in treatment of bleeding gastric and esophageal varices: Results in 151 consecutive episodes. *Digestive Diseases and Sciences*, 33:454–459.

Barsan, W.G., & Baker, P.B. 1988. Upper gastrointestinal tract disorders. In P. Rosen, F.J. Baker, II, R.M. Barkin, G.R. Braen, R.H. Dailey, & R.C. Levy (eds). *Emergency medicine: Concepts and clinical practice*, 2nd ed. St. Louis: Mosby; 1403–1432.

Salam, A.A. 1986. Upper gastrointestinal bleeding: Differential diagnosis & management. In G.R. Schwartz, P. Safar, J.H. Stone, P.B. Storey, & D.K. Wagner (eds). *Principles and practice of emergency medicine*, 2nd ed. Philadelphia: Saunders; 1026–1038.

Simon, R.R. & Brenner, R.E. 1987. *Emergency procedures and techniques*, 2nd ed. Baltimore: Williams & Wilkins.

103

Urinary Bladder Catheterization

Nancy Carrington, RN, BSN, MA, CEN

INDICATIONS

1. To obtain a sterile urine specimen for diagnostic purposes when it is not practical to obtain a clean specimen, such as during a patient's menses.
2. To ascertain the amount of residual urine in the patient's bladder after voiding.
3. To continuously monitor urinary output in the critically ill patient.
4. To obtain a urine specimen for a toxicology screen in the patient who is unable or unwilling to urinate, and when it is imperative that the substance ingested or injected be known as soon as possible.
5. To empty the bladder when the patient is unable to urinate.
6. To facilitate filling of the bladder for radiologic diagnostic procedures (i.e., pelvic ultrasound, cystogram).
7. To provide a means to deal with urinary incontinence, after other methods have not been successful.
8. To decompress the bladder prior to surgical procedures such as peritoneal lavage.

CONTRAINDICATIONS AND CAUTIONS

1. Urinary catheterization should not be performed in the trauma patient with blood at the urinary meatus until a retrograde urethrogram is done.
2. Strict aseptic technique should be used at all times when inserting any device into the urinary bladder.
3. A sterile closed drainage system must be connected to all indwelling catheters.
4. Before inserting an indwelling catheter, check the balloon for leaks by inflating it with sterile water or saline.
5. Never inflate the balloon on an indwelling catheter in a male patient until urine has returned from the bladder, to prevent rupturing the urethra. Pressing gently on the suprapubic area may cause urine to flow.

EQUIPMENT

Antiseptic solution
Sterile gloves
Sterile fenestrated drape
Sterile towel
Sterile cotton balls
Sterile water-soluble lubricant
Sterile catheter either straight or
    Foley (10–22 French)
Sterile graduated receptacle
Sterile drainage bag

Sterile 10-cc syringe and sterile
    water
Sterile specimen container
Tape
(Note: Preassembled kits are
    available, which contain all
    the equipment needed for
    either urethral
    catheterization or
    indwelling catheterization.)

Female

1. Place the patient in the supine position to best visualize the urinary meatus.
2. If the patient is unresponsive, unstable, or combative, assistance may be necessary to keep the knees flexed and prevent contamination of the equipment.
3. If the patient is cooperative, but has decreased strength in her legs, have the patient flex her knees and place the bottoms of her feet together as close to her perineum as possible. This allows her knees to relax against the side rails.

Male

The patient may be in a supine position with the head elevated or flat, depending on patient comfort and ability to cooperate.

PROCEDURAL STEPS

Female

1. Put on sterile gloves and place a drape under the patient's buttocks assuring that the drape is cuffed over the gloves so they are not contaminated. Place the fenestrated drape over the perineum.
2. Pour the antiseptic solution over the cotton balls.
3. If using an indwelling catheter kit, remove the tip from the syringe filled with sterile water and attach the syringe to the balloon port. Inflate the balloon and check for leaks. Deflate the balloon and leave the syringe attached.
4. Dispense the lubricant onto a sterile surface in the kit and lubricate two to three inches of the catheter. Attach the drainage bag to the catheter if an indwelling catheter is being placed.
5. Using the nondominant hand, separate the labia majora and expose the urinary meatus. This hand is now considered contaminated and should not release the labia until catheterization is complete. See Figure 103.1.
6. Grasp an antiseptic-soaked cotton ball with the forceps and, using a downward motion with one cotton ball for each side, cleanse the labia

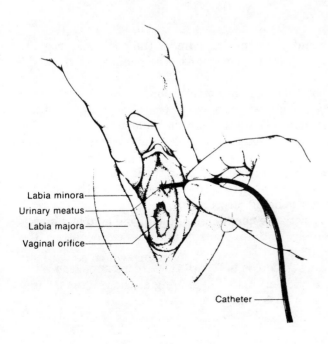

Labia minora
Urinary meatus
Labia majora
Vaginal orifice

Catheter

Figure 103.1 Exposing the urinary meatus.
(Brunner & Suddarth, 1986: 507.
Reprinted by permission.)

minora. Continue to cleanse from the top of the labia to the anus with a clean cotton ball for each pass, until all the cotton balls are used.

7. Grasp the lubricated catheter with the noncontaminated hand approximately two to three inches from the tip. Allow the distal end of the catheter to rest in the urine collection container if not attached to a drainage bag.

8. Insert the catheter gently into the urinary meatus for approximately two inches (one inch in a child) or until urine returns. Then pass the catheter another one or two inches. If the catheter does not pass easily, do not force it. Have the patient relax by taking deep breaths. If the catheter still does not pass easily, seek assistance.

9. Grasp the catheter with the hand that has been separating the labia to hold it in place.

10. If this is a straight catherization only, collect the amount of urine required in the specimen container and then transfer the drainage end back into the receptacle to empty the bladder. Gently remove the catheter.

11. For an indwelling catheter, follow the preceding steps except, instead of removing the catheter, inject the water or saline into the balloon port (usually 5 cc or 30 cc). Do not inject more than the amount specified on the catheter (many kits provide more than is needed.)

12. Hang the drainage bag below the level of the patient's bladder.

13. Anchor the catheter to the upper leg.

To use the Quik-cath or Fem-cath to obtain a urine specimen in female patients:

1. Open the kit onto a flat surface.

2. Put on the sterile gloves provided, open the antiseptic solution, and dispense the sterile lubricant onto a sterile surface.

3. Pull the tip of the catheter beyond the plastic container it is in until four to six inches of the catheter is free.

4. Using the nondominant hand, separate the labia majora and expose the urinary meatus.

5. Using the dominant hand, cleanse the labia minora and urinary meatus with the antiseptic-soaked prep sticks using one for each pass.

6. Lubricate the tip of the catheter with the lubricant and gently insert it into the urethra until urine returns into the container holding the catheter.

7. Gently remove the catheter from the urethra and then from the container. Close the top of the container.

Male

1. Put on sterile gloves and place the drape under the penis and over the thighs. The fenestrated drape should go over the penis and expose the penis and pubis.

2. Pour the antiseptic solution over the cotton balls.

3. If using an indwelling catheter kit, remove the tip from the syringe filled with sterile water and attach the syringe to the balloon port. Inflate the balloon and check for leaks. Deflate the balloon and leave the syringe attached.

4. Dispense the lubricant onto a sterile surface in the kit and lubricate the catheter six inches from the tip. Attach the drainage bag to the catheter if an indwelling catheter is being placed.

5. Grasp the penis firmly with the nondominant hand, and hold at a ninety degree angle to the body. If the patient is uncircumcised, retract the foreskin. See Figure 103.2.

6. Grasp an antiseptic-soaked cotton ball with the forceps and cleanse the meatus and glans in a circular motion beginning at the meatus using a clean cotton ball for each pass until all are used.

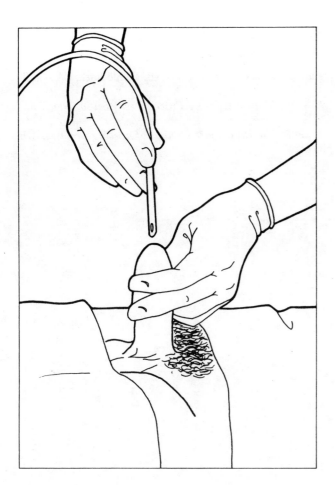

Figure 103.2   Holding the penis at a
90° angle.
(Belland & Wells, 1986: 253. Reprinted by permission.)

7. Exert a slight upward pull with the hand holding the penis and grasp
   the lubricated catheter in the other hand approximately eight inches
   from the tip of the catheter, while gathering the remainder of the tubing
   in the same hand. Insert the catheter into the meatus. Advance the catheter until urine flows (about eight inches in the adult and about one inch
   in the small child.) The catheter may need to be inserted to the junction
   of the balloon port.
8. Grasp the catheter with the hand that has been holding the penis and
   hold it in place.
9. If this is a straight catheterization only, collect the amount of urine required in the specimen container and then transfer the drainage end
   back into the receptacle to empty the bladder. Gently remove the catheter.
10. For an indwelling catheter, follow the preceding steps except, instead of
    removing the catheter, inject the water or saline into the balloon port
    (usually 5 cc or 30 cc). Do not inject more than the amount specified on
    the catheter (many kits provide more than is needed).
11. Hang the drainage bag below the level of the patient's bladder.
12. Anchor the catheter to the upper leg.

COMPLICATIONS

1. Urethral damage including rupture
2. Urinary tract infection
3. Sepsis

SUGGESTED READINGS

Kozier, B., & Erb, G. 1987. *Fundamentals of nursing,* 3rd ed. Menlo Park, CA: Addison-Wesley.

Belland, K.H., & Wells, M.A. 1986. *Clinical Nursing Procedures.* Boston: Jones and Bartlett.

Brunner, L., & Suddarth, D. 1986. *The Lippincott manual of nursing practice,* 4th ed. Philadelphia: Lippincott.

104

Pelvic Examination

Nancy Carrington, RN, BSN, MA, CEN

INDICATIONS

1. To assist in the diagnosis of intra-abdominal pathology in the female patient with abdominal pain.
2. To obtain specimens to diagnose vaginal and uterine infections.

CONTRAINDICATIONS AND CAUTIONS

1. If cultures or other specimens are to be obtained for study, use warm water on the speculum instead of lubricant.
2. Be careful not to pinch the labia or vagina in the speculum.
3. To prevent the spread of gonococcal infection or blood from the vagina to the rectum, change gloves before doing a rectal exam.
4. When using a tube of lubricant, squirt some lubricant onto a convenient surface prior to doing the examination (such as the wrapper in which the speculum was wrapped) to prevent cross-contamination.
5. When examining a virgin or a child, a nasal speculum can be used if the smallest vaginal speculum available is too large.
6. The ovaries are not usually palpable three to five years after menopause.

EQUIPMENT

Good light source
Vaginal speculum (appropriate size
    for the patient)
Lubricating jelly (water based)
Gloves

Ring forceps
Gauze dressings
Specimen collection supplies
Damp, warm wash cloth and towel

PATIENT PREPARATION

1. Have the patient empty her bladder.
2. Assist the patient into a lithotomy position.

PROCEDURAL STEPS

1. *Inspect the external genitalia, observing for swelling, inflammation, discharge, skin changes.
2. *Insert a speculum moistened with warm water carefully into the introitus by gently pressing down on the perineal body. Initially, insert the speculum perpendicular to the vaginal opening and gently rotate it as it

*Indicates portions of the procedure usually performed by a physician.

is inserted, to avoid excessive trauma and discomfort to the patient. See Figure 104.1.

3. *Remove your fingers from the perineal body and assure that the speculum is fully inserted into the vagina. Open the blades of the speculum and tighten the thumb screw to hold the blades open. See Figure 104.2.

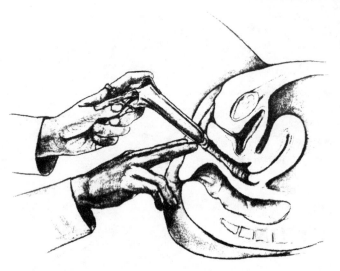

Figure 104.1 Inserting the speculum perpendicular to the vaginal opening.
(Bates, 1990: 233. Reprinted by permission.)

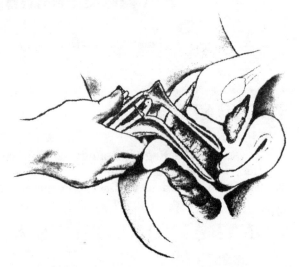

Figure 104.2 Opening the blades of the speculum and tighten the thumb screw to hold the blades open.
(Bates, 1990: 234. Reprinted by permission.)

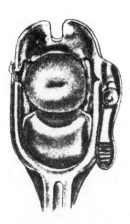

Figure 104.3 Inspect the cervix noting color, bleeding, discharge, ulcerations, and position.
(Bates, 1990: 234. Reprinted by permission.)

4. *If necessary for visualization of the cervix, gently wipe the cervix with a dry gauze dressing held by a ring forcep.

5. *Inspect the cervix noting color, bleeding, discharge, ulcerations, and its position. See Figure 104.3. The cervix is more anterior when the uterus is retroverted. Bluish discolorations of the cervix (Chadwick's sign) may be seen as early as the sixth week of pregnancy.

6. *Obtain specimens as indicated. Commonly performed laboratory tests include culture for gonorrhea, culture for chlamydia, Gram's stain, wet mount, and KOH prep.

7. *Release the thumb screw and gradually withdraw the speculum, inspecting the vaginal walls and mucosa for color, lacerations or ulcers, inflammation or discharge.

8. *Perform a bimanual examination by first inserting the lubricated index finger of the dominant hand gently into the vagina. If space in the vagina allows, as it should in most women except virgins and children, also insert the middle finger into the vagina. The fourth and fifth fingers are flexed on the palm and the thumb is extended away from the perineum.

9. *Distinguish the position (anterior or posterior), consistency (soft or firm), mobility, and any tenderness of the cervix.

10. *Place your nondominant hand on the abdomen between the symphysis pubis and umbilicus. Press gently toward the fingers in the vagina to palpate the uterus between the two hands to identify size, position, tenderness, and masses. See Figure 104.4.

11. *Continue to palpate with the hand on the abdomen in the right lower quadrant with the fingers in the vagina to the right of the cervix, and likewise on the left. Palpate the ovary on each side and any masses that might be present.

12. Offer the patient a warm, damp washcloth and towel with which to clean her perineum following the examination.

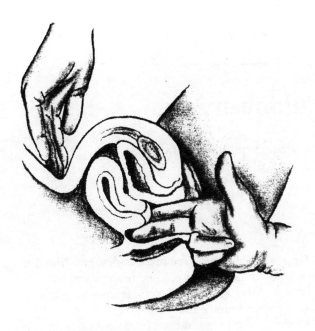

Figure 104.4 **Place the nondominant hand on the abdomen between the symphysis pubis and umbilicus. (Bates, 1990: 236. Reprinted by permission.)**

COMPLICATIONS

1. Vaginal or labial laceration
2. Incorrect specimen collection, thereby inaccurate results
3. Ruptured ovarian cyst with vigorous palpation

PATIENT TEACHING

1. Instruct the patient how to obtain the results of laboratory tests.
2. Further teaching is centered on the diagnosis derived from the pelvic examination and should be individualized accordingly.

REFERENCES

Bates, B. (1990). *Physical examination,* 5th ed. Philadelphia: Lippincott.
Bobak, I., Jensen, M., & Zalar, M. (1989). *Maternity and gynecologic care,* 4th ed. St. Louis: Mosby.

105

Culdocentesis

Nancy Carrington, RN, BSN, MA, CEN

INDICATIONS

1. To help determine if a female patient has free intra-abdominal blood in the cul-de-sac, which might be indicative of ectopic pregnancy.
2. To establish the diagnosis of intra-abdominal hemorrhage in blunt or penetrating trauma to the gravid female abdomen.
3. To help diagnose intra-abdominal disease in female patients (i.e., ovulatory bleeding, ruptured ovarian cyst, acute salpingitis, pelvic abscess, perforation of gastric or duodenal ulcer, ruptured gallbladder, acute pancreatitis, or ruptured urinary bladder).

CONTRAINDICATIONS AND CAUTIONS

1. Should not be performed in late pregnancy to avoid perforating the uterus.
2. Usually not considered as accurate as ultrasound.
3. May reveal a false negative.
4. May be useful when ultrasound is not immediately available for an unstable patient.

EQUIPMENT

Antiseptic solution
Sterile vaginal speculum (largest size possible)
Tenaculum
Ring forceps
Gauze dressings
20-ml syringe (preferably glass ring syringe)

Spinal needle (the size will vary from a 10-gauge for aspirating contents such as pus for diagnosis of disease to 18-gauge for aspiration of blood only.)

PATIENT PREPARATION

1. Have the patient empty her bladder.
2. If not contraindicated by the patient's condition, assist her in sitting up for five to ten minutes to allow blood or fluid to pool in the cul de sac.
3. Assist the patient into a lithotomy position.
4. Administer analgesia or sedation as ordered.
5. Local anesthetic is optional. If used, usually a paracervical block is chosen.

PROCEDURAL STEPS

1. *Gently insert the speculum into the vagina.
2. *Cleanse the vagina with gauze dressings soaked in antiseptic solution and held with the ring forceps.
3. *Place a tenaculum on the posterior lip of the cervix and elevate the cervix.
4. *Expose the posterior fornix and cleanse with antiseptic solution.
5. *Insert the spinal needle with attached syringe one centimeter below the junction of the cervix and vaginal mucosa. See Figure 105.1. The needle should be inserted to a depth of approximately 2 cm (Cavanaugh, 1982).

*Indicates portions of the procedure usually performed by a physician.

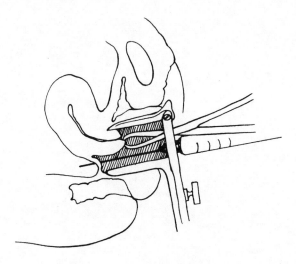

Figure 105.1 **Performing a culdocentesis.**
(Klippel & Anderson, 1979: 337. Reprinted by permission.)

6. *Attempt to aspirate fluid.
   a. Intra-abdominal bleeding is diagnosed if nonclotting blood is obtained.
   b. If no blood or fluid is obtained, the procedure is repeated.
   c. Blood that clots within 5 minutes is indicative of a traumatic tap. The needle probably was inserted into the posterior wall of the uterus. (Cavanaugh et al., 1982.) A dry tap should not be considered normal, only nondiagnostic. A positive tap should be considered in conjunction with other pertinent findings to make the final diagnosis.

COMPLICATIONS

1. Uterine perforation
2. Bowel perforation
3. Perforation of an artery or vein
4. Local infection at the puncture site (rare and late)
5. Damage to the fetus

PATIENT TEACHING

Report increasing abdominal pain, chills, or fever. (Most teaching centers on the diagnosis; there are rarely sequelae from the procedure itself.)

REFERENCES

Cavanaugh, D., Woods, R.E., O'Connor, T.C.F., & Knuppel, R.A. 1982. *Obstetric Emergencies*, 3rd ed. Philadelphia: Harper & Row.

Honigman, B. 1988. Ectopic pregnancy. In P. Rosen, F.J. Baker, R.M. Barkin, G.R. Braen, R.H. Dailey, & R.C. Levy (eds). *Emergency medicine: Concepts and clinical practice*, 2nd ed. St. Louis: Mosby; 1591–1603.

Klippel, A.P., & Anderson, C. 1979. *Manual of Emergency and Outpatient Techniques*. Boston: Little and Brown.

Sheehy, S.B. & Barber, J. 1985. *Emergency nursing: Principles and practice*, 2nd ed. St. Louis: Mosby.

106

Assessing Fetal Heart Tones

Nancy Carrington, BSN, MA, RN, CEN

Fetal heart tones are also known as FHTs, heart tones, fetal heart rate (FHR).

INDICATIONS

1. To assess fetal status when the pregnant patient is ill or injured.
2. To assess fetal status when the pregnant patient presents with a complication of pregnancy such as placenta abruptio, placenta previa, or prolapsed cord.

CONTRAINDICATIONS AND CAUTIONS

1. It is important to differentiate between *fetal* heart rate and *maternal* heart rate by simultaneously feeling the mother's pulse while auscultating fetal heart rate.
2. If unable to auscultate fetal heart tones, reassure the patient that it is not unusual to have difficulty locating the heart tones.
3. To prevent supine hypotension (venacaval syndrome) and potential fetal distress, do not permit a third trimester pregnant woman to remain in a supine position. A folded sheet under her right hip will also prevent this problem from occurring if it is necessary that she remain supine for an extended period of time.
4. The position of the baby will impact where fetal heart tones are found (e.g., breech position baby will have fetal heart tones above the umbilicus).
5. Prior to the third trimester, fetal position will be difficult to ascertain.
6. Any compromise to the mother compromises the fetus (i.e., hypoxia).
7. Abnormal heart rate (< 120 or > 160) may indicate fetal distress and should be reported immediately to the physician.
8. A "whooshing" sound is the placental circulation being auscultated. It is usually the same rate as the maternal pulse.
9. If an obstetrical nurse is available, it is preferable to use her or his expertise in assessing fetal heart tones.

EQUIPMENT

Doppler device
Conductive gel

Watch or clock with second hand

PATIENT PREPARATION

Ask the patient where fetal heart tones were heard last time she saw her doctor.

PROCEDURAL STEPS

1. With the patient in the supine position, confirm fetal position via palpation.
2. Place the conductive gel on abdomen or on Doppler device.
3. Place Doppler device on abdomen where flat surface has been palpated. This is the baby's back and is usually located in the mother's right or left lower abdominal quadrant.
4. Move the Doppler device until fetal heart tones can be heard. Changing the direction by angling the probe may help elicit fetal heart tones.
5. Count rate for a full minute noting any accelerations or decelerations. Compare the fetal heart rate to the maternal heart rate. Normal fetal heart rate is 120–160 per minute.
6. Record rate and rhythm (regular or irregular).
7. Recheck fetal heart tones each time mother's vital signs are checked.

COMPLICATIONS

Supine hypotension

SUGGESTED READING

Brunner, L., & Suddarth, D. (1986). *The Lippincott manual of nursing practice,* 4th ed. Philadelphia: Lippincott.

107

Emergency Childbirth

Nancy Carrington, RN, BSN, MA, CEN

Emergency childbirth is also known as birth-on-arrival (BOA), precipitous (precip) delivery.

INDICATIONS

To deliver an infant when birth is imminent, i.e.:
1. The woman is pushing, or grunting and bearing down with contractions.
2. The perineum is bulging and the infant's head is visible at the vaginal opening even between contractions.

   In a woman who has had previous vaginal deliveries, visibility of the baby's head at any time signals imminent delivery.

CONTRAINDICATIONS AND CAUTIONS

1. Remain calm and controlled to help reassure the delivering mother. Remember, this birth will occur with or without your presence.
2. Attempt to control the expulsion of the infant to minimize perineal tearing and to prevent rapid pressure changes in the baby's skull. The infant may suffer dural or subdural tears as a result of an explosive delivery.
3. Because newborns are wet, they chill very quickly. Carefully dry the baby and keep it warm after delivery to avoid neonatal complications such as hypothermia and acidosis.
4. Keep your fingers out of the vagina to help prevent maternal infections.
5. Do not violently stimulate the baby to cry by holding it upside down or slapping its buttocks.
6. If sterile equipment is not available, defer cutting the umbilical cord.
7. Sterility (except of instruments as listed below) is difficult to attain during a delivery such as this and one should strive for cleanliness.
8. A side-lying or knee-chest position will assist in slowing down fetal descent.
9. Keep the mother on a cart for the delivery. If she is walking or in a wheelchair without time to move to a stretcher, ease her to the floor for the delivery.

EQUIPMENT

Gloves, preferably sterile
Bulb syringe
Cloth towels
Dry baby blanket
Sterile bandage scissors
Two sterile cord clamps or Kelly forceps

(Note: Most departments have a sterile OB or "precip pack" with the listed equipment included, except the gloves.)

PATIENT PREPARATION

The mother will be having extremely intense contractions every 1.5–2 minutes lasting 60–90 seconds at this stage of labor. She will not be receptive to most teaching. Give instructions firmly and with confidence at important times in the delivery, such as when trying to control an explosive delivery of the head, or when attempting to suction the baby's mouth and nose after delivery of the head.

Assist the mother in using active breathing techniques so she can better control the delivery. If she has had prenatal classes, attempt to ascertain the type of breathing she was taught so you can help her use that technique. If she has had no classes, instruct her in deep, abdominal breathing. She should breathe in through her mouth, and exhale slowly through pursed lips. You may need to breathe with her in order to gain her cooperation.

PROCEDURAL STEPS

1. Position the mother on her side (preferably left) or in a dorsal recumbent position (Figure 107.1.)
2. Cleanse the patient's perineum with soap and water or pour antiseptic solution over the area.
3. Place a clean towel or drape under buttocks.
4. *Use a towel or sterile gauze dressings to support the perineum just above the anus. As the head delivers, this area will be slipped over the baby's head (Figure 107.2).

*Indicates portions of the procedure usually performed by a physician.

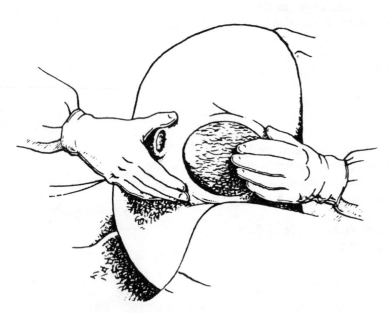

Figure 107.1   Placement of hands on perineum with the mother in the side-lying position.
(Roberts & McGowan, 1985: 127. Reprinted by permission.)

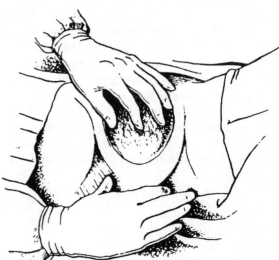

Figure 107.2   Placement of hands to control the emerging fetal head.
(Roberts and McGowan, 1985: 128. Reprinted by permission.)

5. *As the head emerges, use the hand not on the perineum to firmly support the caput with the palm of the hand (Figure 107.2).
    (**Note:** The head should never be held back from delivering. Gentle pressure is applied with the palm only to prevent an explosive delivery.)
6. As the head is being delivered, instruct the mother to pant to control expulsion.

7. As soon as the head is delivered, instruct the mother to continue to pant or to blow to allow time to suction the infant's nose and mouth. The bulb syringe should be compressed and placed in the infant's mouth and nose. As the bulb is released, the fluid in the mouth and nose is drawn into the bulb. This fluid should be squeezed out of the bulb before suctioning the mouth or nose again. Gently repeat the procedure until the majority of fluid is removed, but be very gentle and avoid over-suctioning or traumatizing the infant's mouth and nose. A gauze dressing wrapped around the index finger can also be used to clear secretions from the mouth.

8. *Check with your fingers to ascertain if the umbilical cord is around the neck. If it is, slip it over the head. If this is not possible, slip it over the shoulders as the delivery proceeds. If it is tightly circling the neck, it will be necessary to clamp the cord in two places and cut it between the clamps with sterile scissors before proceeding with the delivery.

9. It is not necessary to turn the infant's head to the side to complete the delivery. This will occur naturally with the contractions. Support the head as it turns.

10. *The infant will turn and face one of the mother's thighs with one of the next contractions. Place the palms of the hands over the side of the child's head and apply gentle downward traction (Figure 107.3) to deliver the anterior shoulder.

11. *Apply gentle upward traction (Figure 107.4) to allow delivery of the posterior shoulder.

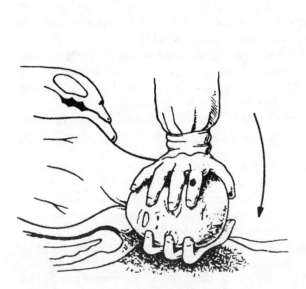

Figure 107.3 Delivery of the anterior shoulder. (Roberts & McGowan, 1985: 128. Reprinted by permission.)

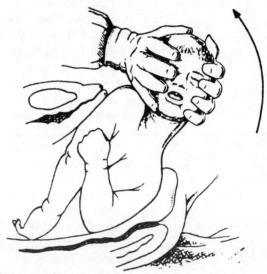

Figure 107.4 Delivery of the posterior shoulder. (Roberts & McGowan, 1985: 129. Reprinted by permission.)

12. *At this point the baby will slip out very rapidly and it will be very slippery. Be careful not to drop the baby!

13. Note the time of delivery.

14. Suction the infant's nose and mouth again. Dry the baby as quickly as possible and place on the mother's abdomen, skin-to-skin, and cover them both with a dry blanket. Make sure the infant's head is covered.

15. Assess the infant and proceed with any necessary resuscitation.

16. Determine Apgar score at one minute and five minutes after birth (Figure 107.5).

17. *When the cord has stopped pulsating, place a sterile clamp on the umbilical cord about six inches from the infant's abdomen. Place the other

Figure 107.5 Apgar chart.

Apgar Score	0	1	2
Heart rate	Absent	Less than 100	Over 100
Resp. effort	Absent	Slow, irregular	Good cry
Muscle tone	Limp	Some flexion	Active motion
Reflex irritability	No response	Grimace	Cry
Color	Pale	Body pink, extremities blue	All pink

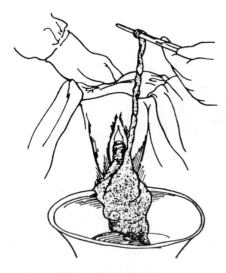

Figure 107.6 Allow the placenta to be delivered into a basin. (Klippel & Anderson, 1979: 330. Reprinted by permission.)

clamp about two or three inches distal to the first. Using sterile scissors, cut the cord between the clamps.

    (**Note:** If sterile equipment is not available, it is not necessary to perform this step.

18. If possible, place the infant to the mother's breast to nurse to assist in the third stage of labor (expulsion of the placenta).
19. *Watch for the signs of separation of the placenta (i.e., a spurt of blood from the vagina or lengthening of the cord coming from the vagina). Using very gentle pressure on the cord and asking the mother to bear down, allow the placenta to be delivered into a basin (Figure 107.6). Save the placenta (do not use Formalin). The placenta is saved in case there are problems with the infant that could be better diagnosed with pathology studies of the placenta.
20. Do not exert more than gentle pressure on the cord or perform any other maneuvers if the placenta does not deliver easily. Transport the mother to the labor and delivery suite for placental delivery if necessary.
21. Obtain the mother's vital signs and continue to assess the newborn.
22. Check the condition of the fundus of the uterus. This is vital to prevent postpartum hemorrhage. Place the open palm of one hand just above the symphysis pubis and the open palm of the other hand at the umbilicus. Exert gentle downward pressure with the hand at the umbilicus so that the fundus is between both hands. The fundus should feel about the size and firmness of a grapefruit. If it feels like that, do not massage it. If it does not feel like a grapefruit, massage your hands together until the uterus firms up and is felt between your palms. When it becomes firm, do not over-massage. Check the firmness of the fundus every five minutes to assure that it is remaining firm.
23. Place a sterile sanitary napkin to the mother's perineum after washing off the blood and antiseptic.
24. Transport the mother and infant to the labor and delivery suite.

COMPLICATIONS

1. Maternal hemorrhage
2. Fetal distress (i.e., hypothermia, aspiration, etc.)
3. Perineal tearing

4. Retained placenta
5. Shoulder dystocia
6. Vaginal lacerations
7. Meconium aspiration: The infant should be suctioned using a DeLee suction apparatus to clear the airway of meconium.
8. Fetal death

(Note: For any complications in the emergency department, an obstetrician should be contacted immediately. The mother should have high-flow oxygen via mask. She should be placed on her left side or with a folded sheet under her right buttocks to increase blood return to the right side of the heart, thereby maximizing circulation to the fetus. If it is safe to do so, transfer the mother to the labor and delivery suite as quickly as possible.

PATIENT TEACHING

To achieve maternal-infant bonding, it is vital to provide physical and emotional contact between the mother and newborn as soon as possible after birth. The nurse can serve as the liaison to assure that this occurs in the emergency department setting, if both mother and infant are stable.

REFERENCES

Roberts, J., & McGowan, N. (1985). Emergency birth. *Journal of Emergency Nursing,* 11:125–131.

Bobak, I.M. Jensen, M.D. & Zalar, M.K. (1989). Maternity and gynecologic care, 4th ed. St. Louis: Mosby.

Klippel, A.P., & Anderson, C. (1979). *Manual of emergency and outpatient techniques.* Boston: Little, Brown.

108

Dilatation and Curettage

Nancy Carrington, RN, BSN, MA, CEN

Dilatation and curettage is also known as D&C, suction curettage.

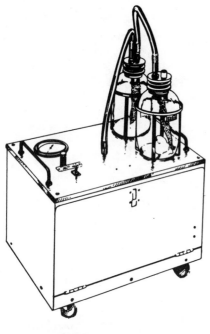

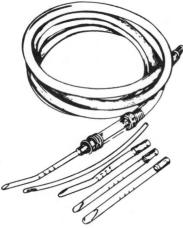

Figure 108.1   An example of the suction machine, tubing, swivel handle, and curettes used in suction curettage.
(Klippel & Anderson, 1979: 335. Reprinted by permission.)

INDICATIONS

To empty the contents of the uterus following an incomplete or inevitable abortion.

CONTRAINDICATIONS AND CAUTIONS

1. This procedure should be carried out soon after diagnosis of incomplete abortion to avoid possibility of hemorrhage or sepsis (Bland, 1986).
2. This procedure should always be preceded by a thorough pelvic examination to ascertain uterine position and size.
3. The patient should have stable vital signs and be afebrile. (The patient is usually taken to the operating room if these criteria are not met.)
4. The procedure should be discontinued if patient is unable to cooperate due to anxiety or pain. The decision must be made at this time whether patient should have the procedure done in the operating room.
5. When grasping the cervix with the tenaculum, avoid the highly vascular area at 3 and 9 o'clock on the cervix.
6. Perforation of the uterus is most likely to occur when the uterine sound or dilators are inserted.
7. Suction curettage is used for pregnancies of 12 weeks duration or less (Tatum, 1987).

EQUIPMENT

10-ml syringe
Spinal needle (usually 20- or 22-G)
Sterile vaginal speculum
Tenaculum
Ring forceps
Gauze sponges
Uterine sound
Curettes
Pathology specimen container with
          preservative

Hegar or Hank dilators
Sterile drapes
Antiseptic solution
For suction curettage:
          Suction machine (Figure 108.1.)
          Sterile tubing
          Sterile plastic suction cannulas
               (8–12 mm in diameter)
               (Figure 108.1)
          Sterile swivel handle

PATIENT PREPARATION

1. Teach the patient active relaxation techniques.
2. Have the patient empty her bladder prior to the procedure. Insert an indwelling urinary catheter if she is unable to void.

3. Place patient in dorsal lithotomy position.
4. Start an IV line, preferably 18-G or larger.
5. Draw blood for ABO and Rh type.
6. Administer analgesia/sedation as ordered.

PROCEDURAL STEPS

1. *Perform a paracervical block (optional).
2. *Drape the pubic area and inner thighs. Place a sterile towel under the buttocks.
3. *Using a speculum, visualize the cervix.
4. *Grasp the anterior lip of the cervix with the tenaculum.
5. *Using gentle traction, bring the cervix down toward the vaginal opening.
6. *Visualize the cervix and examine thoroughly.
7. *Gently insert uterine sound into the cervix and advance into uterine cavity. (**Note:** This is accomplished using information about size and position of uterus found on pelvic examination.)
8. *Note depth of uterine cavity.
9. *Beginning with largest dilator cervix will accommodate, insert progressively larger dilators until adequate dilatation is achieved.
10. *If performing sharp curettage, use the largest sharp curette that will fit through the dilated cervix and scrape the anterior, lateral, and posterior walls. Use a firm pressure proceeding in a systematic fashion from the top of the fundus down to the internal os.

    If performing suction curettage, the diameter of the cannula in millimeters should be about 1 mm less than the weeks of gestation from the last menses. The cannula should be inserted only to the level of the lower uterine segment. The suction machine is turned on, and the uterine contents are then evacuated by rotation of the cannula.
11. Save all tissue obtained to be sent to pathology. Tissue should be placed in preservative as soon as possible.
12. Wash antiseptic and blood from the perineal area.
13. Place a sterile perineal pad and lower the patient's legs gently to the table.
14. Send tissue to the laboratory.

*Indicates portions of the procedure usually performed by a physician.

COMPLICATIONS

1. Uterine perforation
2. Uterine hemorrhage
3. Sepsis
4. Incomplete curettage with retained products of conception

PATIENT TEACHING

1. The patient can expect to go through a grieving process for the loss of the pregnancy.
2. Do not use tampons until reexamined by your physician.
3. Avoid intercourse and do not douche until cleared by your physician.
4. Notify your physician for fever, chills, abdominal pain, or vaginal bleeding that is heavier than a normal menstrual period.
5. Instructions regarding Rhogam if ordered and administered.

REFERENCES

Bland, E.H. 1986. Uterine curettage in the emergency department. *Journal of Emergency Nursing,* 12:41–43.

Klippel, A.P. & Anderson, C.B. 1979. *Manual of emergency and outpatient techniques.* Boston: Little, Brown.

Malinak, L.R. & Wheeler, J.M. 1987. Therapeutic gynecologic procedures. In M.L. Pernoll, R.C. Benson (eds). *Current obstetric and gynecologic diagnosis and treatment.* Norwalk, CT: Appleton & Lange; 822–823.

Mattingly, R.F. & Thompson, J.D. 1985. *Operative gynecology,* 6th ed. Philadelphia: Lippincott, 526–531.

Jones, H.W., Wentz, A.C. & Burnett, L.S. 1988. *Novak's textbook of gynecology,* 11th ed. Baltimore: Williams & Wilkins.

Tatum, H.J. 1987. Contraception and family planning. In M.L. Pernoll, & R.C. Benson, (eds). *Current obstetric and gynecologic diagnosis and treatment.* Norwalk, CT: Appleton & Lange; 586–611.

109

Spinal Immobilization

Jean A. Proehl, RN, MN, CEN, CCRN

INDICATIONS

To immobilize the spine of a patient with actual or potential spinal injury. The decision to immobilize the spine is most often based on mechanism of injury and not physical findings. A high index of suspicion should accompany the following mechanisms and patient presentations:

Motor vehicle accidents

Falls

Head/neck/facial trauma

Multiple trauma

Trauma in the presence of unconsciousness or intoxication

If in doubt, immobilize!

CONTRAINDICATIONS AND CAUTIONS

1. Pre-existing spinal deformities secondary to arthritis, ankylosing spondylitis, etc., may require modification of the following procedures (Butman & Paturas, 1986; Proehl, 1992).
2. If realignment maneuvers cause additional pain or muscle spasm, stop immediately and immobilize the patient in the position found (Butman & Paturas, 1986).
3. If the patient holds the head rigidly angulated or is unable to move the head, realignment is contraindicated and the patient should be immobilized in the position found (Butman & Paturas, 1986).
4. Evacuation should precede immobilization in the presence of an environmental hazard such as fire, noxious fumes, etc. (Worsing, 1984).
5. Placing the patient on a backboard should be deferred until life-threatening problems (i.e., airway, breathing, circulation) are addressed and a secondary survey completed. See Ch. 2: Primary Survey and Ch. 3: Secondary Survey. Stabilization of the head with tape and towel rolls or foam blocks should be employed during initial resuscitative efforts.
6. Suction should be immediately available in the event the immobilized or partially immobilized patient begins to vomit.

EQUIPMENT

Stiff cervical collar of appropriate size for the patient

3-inch adhesive tape

Towel rolls, foam blocks, or blankets to provide lateral head support

Long backboard

Straps or cravats

Large bore continuous oral suction (preferable)

4–5 Team members

PATIENT PREPARATION

1. Manually stabilize the head in the position found and instruct the patient not to move. Large bore oral suction should be immediately available in case the patient vomits.
2. Instruct the patient to remain as still as possible and let the health care providers do all of the work.
3. Instruct the patient to alert you immediately if any of the maneuvers causes increased neck pain or numbness/tingling of the extremities.
4. Assess and document neurological status including movement and sensation of all extremities.

PROCEDURAL STEPS

1. Return the patient's head to a neutral position with gentle inline traction. The traction pull should be just enough to support the head (Butman & Paturas, 1986). Place your thumbs under the mandible and your index and middle fingers on the occipital ridges to avoid soft tissue compression and secure a firm hold on the patient. See Figure 109.1. This manual stabilization should be maintained until the patient is securely immobilized to a spine board with cervical collar in place.

   (**Note:** Some sources recommend immobilizing the head in the position found. The recommendation of nationally recognized medical, nursing, and prehospital trauma curricula is to return the head to a neutral position (American College of Surgeons, 1988; Butman & Paturas, 1986; Rea, 1991). One source reports complete neurologic recovery following rapid realignment of a spinal cord injury (Brunette & Rockwold, 1987).

2. Apply a stiff cervical collar. Soft foam collars have proven inadequate for cervical spine immobilization (Aprahamian, 1984; Huerta, 1987; Podolsky, 1983). If possible, remove jewelry from the ears and neck prior to collar placement.

3. Log roll the patient to a supine position on a long backboard. The team leader should maintain alignment of the head and coordinate the team's movements. A useful landmark for maintaining head position is to keep the nose aligned with the umbilicus. At least three additional people are preferred for this movement; one to roll the shoulders and hips, one to roll the hips and legs, and one to place the backboard under the patient.

4. Remove protective headgear if indicated. See Ch. 110: Helmet Removal.

5. Pad underneath the head if necessary to prevent hyperextension when the head is lowered to the board (Butman & Paturas, 1986).

6. Stabilize the patient's head bilaterally with pillows, towel rolls, etc., and place 3-inch adhesive tape directly on the skin across the patient's forehead and onto the board. See Figure 109.2.

   The use of sandbags for lateral head stabilization is discouraged because the weight of the sandbags could increase head movement if the board is tipped to the side (Butman & Paturas, 1986). Try to avoid taping across hair or eyebrows to prevent patient discomfort and optimize immobilization. Do not place tape or straps across the patient's chin as this could lead to aspiration if vomiting occurs (Butman & Paturas, 1986; Rea, 1991).

7. Secure the torso and legs to the board with straps, sheets, or tape. Minimally, strap across the shoulders, hips, and distal thighs. See Figure 109.3.

   (**Note:** This immobilization technique is not intended for patients in the pre-hospital setting or for intrafacility transport. Further immobilization may be indicated for these patients. Refer to *Pre-hospital Trauma*

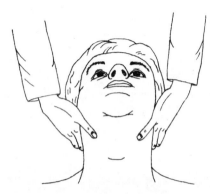

Figure 109.1 Manual stabilization of the head during cervical spine immobilization. The fingers are placed on the mandible and occipital ridges to avoid soft tissue compression and secure a firm hold on the patient.

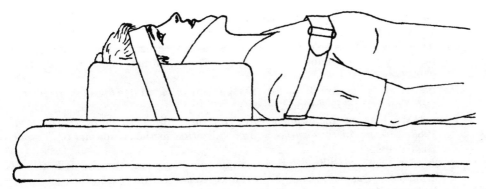

Figure 109.2 Head immobilization with adhesive tape and lateral head support.

Life Support by A. M. Butman and J. L. Paturas (eds) for more information.)

8. Assess and document the patient's neurological status including movement and sensation of all extremities.
9. Maintain immobilization until the spine is cleared by a physician.
10. Have suction available at all times and be prepared to turn the patient on the board should vomiting occur.

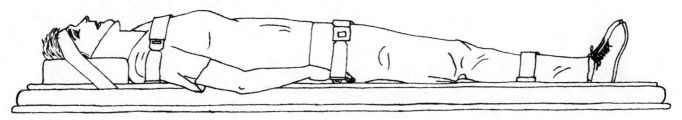

Figure 109.3 Torso and legs immobilized to backboard with straps.

COMPLICATIONS

1. Further damage to spine or spinal cord as a result of movement.
2. Respiratory compromise secondary to tight straps across the chest or aspiration of vomitus (Bauer & Kowalski, 1988; Butman & Paturas, 1986).
3. Tissue breakdown secondary to prolonged contact of bony prominences with the backboard (late).
4. Supine hypotension in pregnant patients (secondary to the pressure of the gravid uterus on the inferior vena cava). This can be minimized by tilting the backboard to the patient's left 15–20°. Care must be taken to immobilize the patient in such a way that she does not slide to the side when the board is tilted.

PATIENT TEACHING

1. Do not move until spinal injury has been ruled out.
2. Immediately report any nausea, difficulty breathing, increased pain, numbness, or tingling.

REFERENCES

American College of Surgeons, Committee on Trauma. 1988. *Advanced trauma life support course.* Chicago: American College of Surgeons.
Bauer, D., & Kowalski, R. 1988. Effect of spinal immobilization devices on pulmo-

nary function in the healthy, non-smoking man. *Annals of Emergency Medicine,* 17:915–918.

Brunette, D.D., & Rockwold, G.L. (1987). Neurologic recovery following rapid spinal realignment for complete cervical spinal cord injury. *Journal of Trauma,* 27:445–447.

Butman, A.M., & Paturas, J.L. (eds). (1986). *Pre-hospital trauma life support.* Akron, OH: Educational Direction, Inc.

Podolosky, S., Barraf, L.J., Simon, R.R., Hoffman, J.R., Larmon, R., & Ablon, W. 1983. Efficacy of cervical spine immobilization methods. *Journal of Trauma,* 23:461–465.

Proehl, J.A. 1992. Mobility: Spinal and musculoskeletal injuries. In. J. Neff & P. Kidd (eds). *Trauma nursing: The art and science.* St. Louis: Mosby.

Rea, R.E. (ed). 1991. *Trauma nursing core course (provider) manual,* 3rd ed. Chicago: Award Printing.

Worsing, R.A., Jr. 1984. Principles of prehospital care of musculoskeletal injuries. *Emergency Medicine Clinics of North America,* 2:205–217.

Helmet Removal

Jean A. Proehl, RN, MN, CEN, CCRN

INDICATIONS

To remove protective headgear (i.e., motorcycle, football helmets, etc.) from patients with potential cervical spine injuries.

CONTRAINDICATIONS AND CAUTIONS

Helmet removal may be deferred in a stable patient without airway compromise when cervical spine injury is strongly suspected. If the helmet must be rapidly removed from an unstable patient, physician assistance is preferable. An electric saw may be used to cut the helmet off if necessary (Meyer & Daniel, 1985; Rea, 1991).

EQUIPMENT

2 People skilled in this technique
(**Note:** A one-person technique has also been described (Meyer & Daniel, 1985); however, the two-person technique is the most widely endorsed (Butman, 1986; McSwain, 1981; Rea, 1991).)

PATIENT PREPARATION

1. Instruct the patient to remain as still as possible and let the health care providers do the work of removing the helmet.
2. Instruct the patient to alert you immediately if any of the maneuvers cause increased neck pain or numbness/tingling of the extremities.
3. Assess and document a neurological status including movement and sensation of all extremities.

PROCEDURAL STEPS

1. *Leader:* Stand at the patient's head and apply gentle inline traction/stabilization by placing your thumbs on the patient's mandibles and your index fingers on the occipital ridges.
   Assistant: Cut or remove any chin strap or face guard. If the helmet has snap-out ear protectors, remove them by prying them loose with a tongue blade.
2. *Assistant:* Assume inline traction/stabilization from the leader by cupping the mandible with the thumb and index finger of one hand and placing the other hand on the occipital ridge. See Figure 110.1.

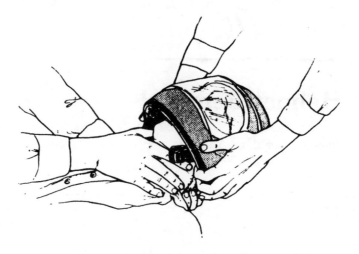

Figure 110.1 The assistant assumes traction by cupping the mandible with the thumb and index finger of one hand and placing the other hand on the occipital ridge.
(Meyer & Daniel, 1985: 332. Reprinted by permission.)

3. *Leader:* Spread the helmet laterally and gently remove it. See Figure 110.2. As it comes over the occiput it may be necessary to rotate the helmet anteriorly over the face, taking care to avoid the patient's nose.
   Assistant: **Warning** – the head will drop as the helmet is removed unless adequate support is provided to the occipital ridges.
4. *Leader:* Resume traction laterally with your fingers on the mandible and occipital ridges as described in Step 1. See Figure 110.3.

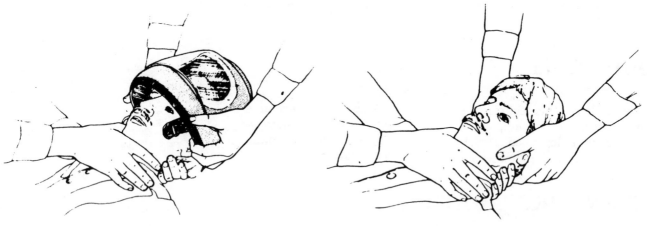

Figure 110.2 The leader spreads the helmet laterally and gently removes it.
(Meyer & Daniel, 1985: 332. Reprinted by permission.)

Figure 110.3 The leader resumes traction laterally with fingers on the patient's mandibles and occipital ridges.
(Meyer & Daniel, 1985: 332. Reprinted by permission.)

   Assistant: Assemble equipment and personnel to definitively immobilize the patient's spine. See Ch. 109: Spinal Immobilization.
5. Assess and document neurological status including movement and sensation of all extremities.

COMPLICATIONS

Further damage to spine or spinal cord as a result of movement.

PATIENT TEACHING

Do not move until instructed to do so by the nurse or physician.

Butman, A.M., & Paturas, J.L (eds). 1986. *Pre-hospital trauma life support.* Akron, OH: Educational Direction, Inc.

McSwain, N.E., Jr. 1981. Techniques of helmet removal from injured patients. *Bulletin of the American College of Surgeons,* 66:19–21.

Meyer, R.D., & Daniel, W.W. 1985. The biomechanics of helmets and helmet removal. *Journal of Trauma,* 25:329–332.

Rea, R.E. (ed.) 1991. *Trauma nursing core course (provider) manual,* 3rd ed. Chicago: Award Printing.

111

Ring Removal

Jean A. Proehl, RN, MN, CEN, CCRN

INDICATIONS

To remove a ring when upper extremity injury is present and other methods such as use of lubricant and soap have failed.

CONTRAINDICATIONS AND CAUTIONS

1. In the presence of any upper extremity injury, all jewelry should be removed from the extremity as soon as possible.
2. If vascular compromise is present or imminent, the ring should be removed with a ring cutter (see Technique A) as quickly as possible. If time permits, the ring may be removed without damage using the string technique (see Technique B).
3. Digital block anesthesia may increase the swelling at the base of the finger and cause further compromise of circulation (Rosen & Sternbach, 1983).

EQUIPMENT FOR TECHNIQUE A

Ring Cutter   Hemostat

PROCEDURAL STEPS FOR TECHNIQUE A

1. Insert the curved blade of the ring cutter under the narrowest part of the ring. See Figure 111.1. If the finger is so swollen that the ring cutter cannot be inserted under the ring, a dental drill may be used to cut the ring (Rosen & Sternbach, 1983).
2. Clamp the saw down on the ring firmly and turn the blade manually until the ring is severed.
3. Pry the ends of the ring apart and away from the finger with a hemostat.
4. Remove the ring carefully to prevent injury from the severed ring ends.

EQUIPMENT FOR TECHNIQUE B

2–3 feet of string or umbilical tape   Small, curved hemostat
Bar soap (optional)

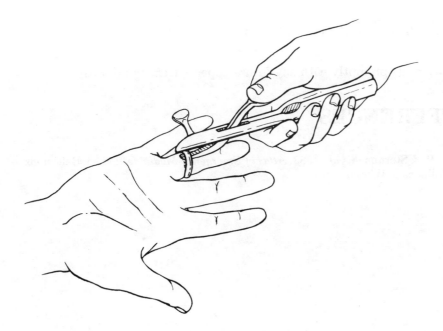

**Figure 111.1   Ring cutter.
(Rosen & Sternbach, 1983: 219. Reprinted by permission.)**

PROCEDURAL STEPS FOR TECHNIQUE B

1. Rub the bar soap along the length of the string. This step is optional but will make ring removal easier.
2. Have the patient anchor the string against his palm with his thumb. Wrap the string around the finger tightly in close, concentric circles starting next to the ring and moving toward the finger tip.
3. Pass the proximal end of the string under the ring, using the hemostat if necessary. See Figure 111.2.

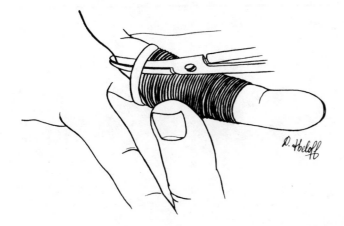

**Figure 111.2   Finger wrapped with string for ring removal.
(Rosen & Sternbach, 1983: 219. Reprinted by permission.)**

4. While pulling the distal end of the string toward the finger tip and against the ring, unwrap the string from the finger. This will move the ring over the string-wrapped finger.
5. Repeat the procedure until the ring is removed.

COMPLICATIONS

Laceration of the finger from the severed ring ends (Technique A).

PATIENT TEACHING

Remove rings promptly with any future upper extremity injuries.

REFERENCES

Rosen, P., & Sternbach, G.L. 1983. *Atlas of Emergency Medicine,* 2nd ed. Baltimore: Williams & Wilkins.

112

General Principles of Splinting

Ruth L. Schaffler, RN, MA, CEN

INDICATIONS

1. To immobilize and stabilize fractures and/or dislocations as soon as possible after an injury to prevent further soft tissue or bony damage.
2. To decrease pain from impaired neurologic function or muscle spasm.
3. To decrease swelling associated with injury by reducing blood and fluid loss into the soft tissues.
4. To immobilize injured areas after burns, bites, stings, etc.
5. To immobilize an area during healing of infectious or inflammatory processes and after surgical repair of muscles or tendons.

CONTRAINDICATIONS AND CAUTIONS

1. Handle bone fragments gently and minimize movement of the affected area in order to decrease risk of complications, i.e., compartmental syndrome, fat embolism, vascular or nerve damage.
2. Pad bony prominences adequately to avoid undue pressure and skin breakdown.
3. Immobilize the joints above and below the injury site.
4. Gentle longitudinal traction may be exerted while the splint is being applied except when the injury site involves a joint, a dislocation, or an open fracture. In these cases, splint in the position found unless circulatory compromise exists, then straighten only enough to restore distal pulses.

   (Note: It is generally agreed that traction splints should be applied in cases of open femoral fractures, this will likely cause the bone ends to slip beneath the skin. Open fractures are generally considered contaminated and wound care management becomes an urgent priority (Crenshaw, 1987; Hughes & Fitzgerald, 1986; Zuidema, 1985).)
5. Do not force the extremity to fit the splint. You may have to improvise or alter the splint to fit the deformity.
6. No zippers, knots, or attachments of the splinting device are to be placed directly over the injury site.
7. Assess and document neurovascular status before and after splinting. If deterioration occurs, the splint must be reassessed and readjusted or removed and reapplied.
8. When in doubt, splint!

EQUIPMENT

Splints are divided into four general categories: See Table 112.1 for specific indications.

Plaster splinting will not be addressed in this chapter, see Ch. 120: General

Principles of Plaster
Splinting.

1. Soft – nonrigid splints

Pillow

Foam rubber

Blanket

Cravats

Cloth

Bandaging material

Soft commercial supports

    Cervical collar

    Clavicle strap

    Sling and swathe

    Binder

**3. Hard – rigid and semirigid
splints (see Figure 112.1).**

Aluminum or other metal

Ladder splints

Cardboard

Wood, boards, backboards

Molded plastic

Leather

Plaster

Fiberglass

Vacuum

Semirigid commercial supports

    Cervical collar

    Wrist splint

    Finger splint

    Knee immobilizer

    Ankle support

    Orthopedic shoe

3. Pneumatic – inflatable splints

Air splints

Pneumatic anti-shock garment
    (PASG)

**4. Traction – capable of maintaining
longitudinal traction for
lower extremity fractures**

Hare (Dynamed, Carlsbad, CA)

Kendrick Traction Device (Medix
    Choice, El Cajon, CA)

Sager (Minto Research &
    Development, Redding, CA)

Thomas

Additional equipment may include

    Padding material

    Elastic bandage

    Roller gauze bandage

    Tape

    Safety pins

Table 112.1   Initial immobilization of orthopedic injuries.

Site	Type of Splint
Clavicle	Sling and swathe or Figure-of-8 splint
Shoulder dislocation	
anterior	Splint to the body with elastic bandage in the position found
posterior	Sling and swathe
Scapula	Sling and swathe
Humerus	Rigid splint with sling and swathe
Elbow	Rigid splint with sling and swathe in position found
Forearm	Rigid splint with sling, air splint
Wrist	Rigid splint with sling
Hand, fingers	Rigid splint in position of function
Spine	Backboard, stiff cervical collar, lateral head support
Pelvis	Backboard, PASG
Hip	Backboard, traction splint or secure the injured leg to the uninjured leg with cravats, bandages, etc.
Femur	Traction splint, rigid splint or PASG
Patella	Soft or padded rigid splint placed posteriorly in position found
Tibia/fibula	Traction splint, air splint, rigid splint
Ankle	Air splint or pillow
Foot	Air splint or pillow
Toe	Tape to adjacent digit on medial side
Great toe	Rigid, nonweight-bearing splint

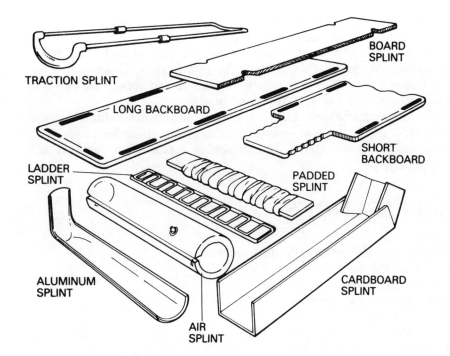

TRACTION SPLINT

BOARD
SPLINT

LONG BACKBOARD

SHORT
BACKBOARD

LADDER
SPLINT

PADDED
SPLINT

ALUMINUM
SPLINT

CARDBOARD
SPLINT

AIR
SPLINT

Figure 112.1 Types of splints.
(Campbell, 1988: 162. Reprinted by
permission.)

PATIENT PREPARATION

1. Cut away clothing over the suspected injury site, remove sharp objects from pockets or bulky material that may lie under the splint after application.
2. Assess and document neurovascular status.
3. Measure the area to be splinted on the noninjured side in order to determine the correct splint size.
4. Pad bony prominences.
5. Remove jewelry from injured extremities.
6. Remove boots or shoes from lower extremity injuries in order to assess pulses and sensation. (Footwear that is difficult to remove and is supportive to the ankle may be left on if using a traction splint, however, neurovascular status cannot be monitored.)
7. Place a sterile dressing on all open wounds.
8. Pad areas of skin-to-skin contact under the splint to absorb perspiration and prevent tissue maceration.

PROCEDURAL STEPS

1. Grasp the extremity with both hands, one hand below and one hand above the injury site, and exert gentle longitudinal traction to straighten any angulation. Maintain manual traction until the splint is secure. (**Note:** Fractures or dislocations of the joints should be splinted in the position found unless distal circulation is diminished or absent. In this situation straighten the limb only enough to restore pulses. Do not attempt to realign fractures of the shoulder, elbow, wrist, knee, or spine (Trunkey & Lewis, 1986).) Do not attempt to push protruding bone ends beneath the skin, but if bone ends slip back into the wound, document the existence of an open fracture and notify the physician.
2. Immobilize the joints above and below the injury site.
3. The splint should fit snugly but not be constrictive. Leave fingers and toes exposed.

4. Assess and document distal neurovascular status and readjust the splint as necessary if function is impaired.
5. Traction splints may be used for fractures of the proximal tibia or femur (American Academy of Orthopedic Surgeons, 1987; Hafen & Kerran, 1989; Rea, 1986). They may not be suitable if fractures of the pelvis or ankle coexist. See Ch. 115: Traction Splints.
6. Leave the splint intact until a physician establishes definitive treatment. If it is necessary to remove or readjust the splint for x-rays, reassess and document distal neurovascular status after removal and reapplication.

COMPLICATIONS

1. Decreased or absent distal pulses and sensation
2. Increased edema
3. Vascular or nerve damage
4. Compartmental syndrome
5. Fat embolism
6. Disruption of skin integrity
7. Malalignment of bone ends

PATIENT TEACHING

1. Keep the splint clean and dry to avoid irritating the skin and weakening the splint.
2. Watch for changes in fingertips and toes—cool to touch, dusky color, swelling, altered or decreased sensation.
3. Report pain that continues to increase in severity and does not respond to pain medications.
4. Elevate limb above the level of the heart to decrease edema and pain.
5. Use cold packs over the injured area to minimize bleeding and edema.
6. Limit mobility/activity in order to allow healing of the injury site.
7. Do not use coat hangers or other sharp objects to scratch inside the splint.
8. Review with the patient the length of time to wear the splinting or immobilization device and when to follow up with the physician and/or physical therapist.
9. Instruct the patient in crutch walking if indicated.
10. Assess the patient's ability to continue activities of daily living and possible need for family or professional assistance at home.

REFERENCES

American Academy of Orthopaedic Surgeons. 1987. *Emergency care and transportation of the sick and injured,* 4th ed. Chicago: American Academy of Orthopedic Surgeons.

Campbell, J.E. (ed). 1988. *Basic trauma life support: Advanced prehospital care,* 2nd ed. Englewood Cliffs, NJ: Prentice-Hall.

Crenshaw, A.H. (ed). 1987. *Campbell's operative orthopaedics,* 7th ed. St. Louis: Mosby.

Hafen, B.Q., & Kerran, K.J. 1989. *Prehospital Emergency Care and Crisis Intervention,* 3rd ed. Englewood, CO: Morton.

Hughes, S.P., & Fitzgerald, R.H., Jr. 1986. *Musculoskeletal infections.* Chicago: Year Book Medical Publishers.

Rea, R.E. (ed). 1991. *Trauma nursing core course (provider) manual*, 3rd ed. Chicago: Award Printing Corporation.

Trunkey, D.D., & Lewis, F.R. 1986. *Current therapy of trauma—2*. Philadelphia: Decker.

Zuidema, G.D., Rutherford, R.B., & Ballinger, W.F. 1985. *The management of trauma*, 4th ed. Philadelphia: Saunders.

SUGGESTED READINGS

Geiderman, J. 1983. Orthopedic injuries. In P. Rosen (ed). *Emergency medicine: Concepts and clinical practice* (Vol. 1). St. Louis: Mosby; 523–537.

Hansell, M.J. 1988. Fractures and the healing process. *Orthopaedic Nursing*, 7, 1: 43–50.

Maher, A.B. 1986. Early assessment and management of musculoskeletal injuries. *Nursing Clinics of North America*, 21:717–727.

Moore, E.E., Eiseman, B., & Van Way, C.W., III. 1984. *Critical decisions in trauma*. St. Louis: Mosby.

Redheffer, G.M. & Bailey, M. 1989. Assessing and splinting fractures. *Nursing*, 19, 6:51–59.

Tintinalli, J.E., Rothstein, R.J., & Krome, R.L. 1985. *Emergency medicine: A comprehensive study guide*. New York: McGraw-Hill.

113

Vacuum Splints

Ruth L. Schaffler, RN, MA, CEN

The information in this chapter
should be used in conjunction with
the information in Ch. 112: General
Principles of Splinting.

The information in this chapter is specific to vacuum splints and should be used in conjunction with Ch. 112: General Principles of Splinting.

INDICATIONS

1. To temporarily immobilize injured extremities. Vacuum splints are particularly useful for immobilizing an extremity in the position found. They are also lightweight and radiotranslucent.

CONTRAINDICATIONS AND CAUTIONS

1. Vacuum splints are bulky and nontransparent and may not allow access to the distal limb for reassessment after splint application.
2. Close the splint valve tightly to prevent loss of rigidity once the splint has been applied.

EQUIPMENT

Vacuum splint
Vacuum pump
Accessory straps or tape

Talcum powder or cornstarch
(optional)

PROCEDURAL STEPS

1. Lay the vacuum splint flat with all straps open and inner surface facing up. Smooth the foam beads evenly throughout the splint to assure uniform distribution.
2. Dust the splint with talcum powder or cornstarch (optional, contraindicated in the presence of open wounds).
3. Support the bone ends above and below the injury site as the splint is placed around the limb.
4. Form or shape the splint over the sides and top of the limb. See Figure 113.1.
5. Secure the splint with the attached straps or tape. (**Note:** Fold the distal portion of the splint outward as necessary to allow inspection of fingers or toes.)
6. Attach the vacuum pump to the splint and evacuate the air until the splint converts from a soft, pliable device to castlike rigidity. See Figure 113.2.
7. Twist the valve clockwise until tight before disconnecting the pump.

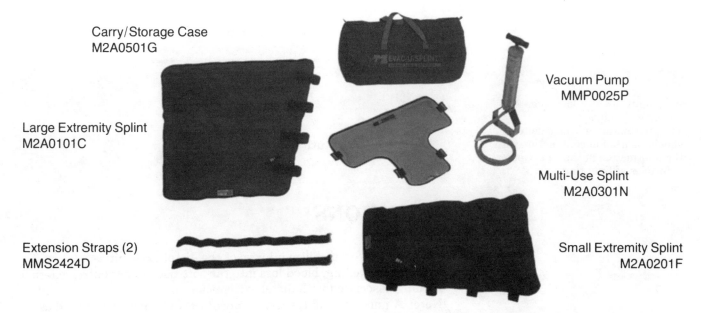

Carry/Storage Case
M2A0501G

Large Extremity Splint
M2A0101C

Extension Straps (2)
MMS2424D

Vacuum Pump
MMP0025P

Multi-Use Splint
M2A0301N

Small Extremity Splint
M2A0201F

Figure 113.1 Examples of vacuum splints. The splint forms to the extremity and becomes rigid when the air is evacuated.
(Hartwell Medical Corporation, 1989. Reprinted by permission.)

(Some models have a spring-loaded valve that is self-sealing when the pump is removed).

8. To remove the splint, open the splint valve by turning it in a counter-clockwise motion. When the splint is pliable, open the straps and carefully support the limb while the splint is detached.

COMPLICATIONS

1. Accumulation of perspiration or moisture inside the splint may cause it to adhere to the skin and create increased pain or skin maceration when removing. Dusting the interior of the splint with talcum powder or cornstarch prior to application may help decrease this.
2. The splint will loose its rigidity if punctured or torn.
3. The splint may soften during significant changes in altitude and may need to be adjusted accordingly.

SUGGESTED READINGS

American Academy of Orthopedic Surgeons. 1981. *Emergency care and transportation of the sick and injured*, 3rd ed. Chicago: American Academy of Orthopedic Surgeons.

Hafen, B.Q., & Kerran, K.J. 1989. *Prehospital emergency care and crisis intervention*, 3rd ed. Englewood, CO: Morton.

Hartwell Medical Corporation. 1989. *Product information bulletin*. San Marcos, CA: Hartwell Medical Corporation.

Jobst Institute. 1989. *Product identification information bulletin*. Toledo, OH: Jobst Institute, Inc.

Rea, R.E. (ed). 1991. *Trauma nursing core course (provider) manual*, 3rd ed. Chicago: Award Printing Corporation.

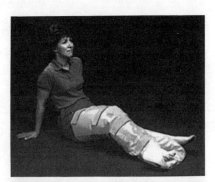

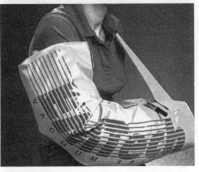

Figure 113.2 The vacuum splint forms to the extremity and becomes rigid after the air is evacuated.
(Jobst Institute, 1989. Reprinted by permission.)

114

Air Splints

Ruth L. Schaffler, RN, MA, CEN

Air splints are also known as pneumatic splints.
The information in this chapter should be used in conjunction with the information in Ch. 112: General Principles of Splinting.

INDICATIONS

1. To temporarily immobilize injuries of the distal extremities.
2. To decrease swelling, blood loss into the soft tissues, or control external bleeding associated with distal extremity injuries.

(**Note:** A pneumatic anti-shock garment (PASG) may also be used as an air splint for fractures of the pelvis or lower extremities. See Ch. 71: Pneumatic Anti-shock Garment.)

CONTRAINDICATIONS AND CAUTIONS

1. Air splints are not suitable for angulated injuries. The design of the splint only allows immobilization in anatomical position. See Figure 114.1.
2. Do not apply air splints over clothing because the pressure created by buckles, buttons, wrinkles, etc., may injure the soft tissues.
3. Do not inflate air splints with positive pressure devices such as Elder valves.
4. Overinflation of an air splint may cause circulatory compromise; underinflation may not provide enough support.
5. Air splints are not effective for fractures of the humerus or femur.
6. Air pressure within a pneumatic splint is subject to fluctuation with temperature and altitude variations. The pressure increases with warmth and ascent and decreases with cold and descent. Careful monitoring is required when using this type of splint in a changing environment (American Academy of Orthopedic Surgeons, 1987; Hafen, 1989).

EQUIPMENT

Air splint with or without zipper
Talcum powder or cornstarch
    (optional)

PATIENT PREPARATION

Remove any clothing and jewelry that would lie under the splint.

PROCEDURAL STEPS

1. Dust the interior of the splint with talcum powder or cornstarch (optional, contraindicated in the presence of open wounds).

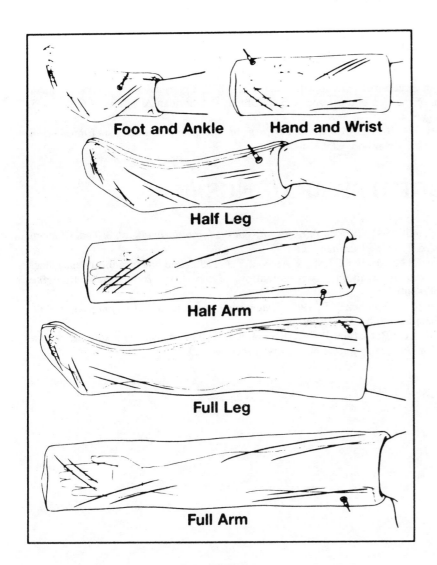

Foot and Ankle   **Hand and Wrist**

Half Leg

Half Arm

Full Leg

Full Arm

Figure 114.1   Examples of air splints.
(Hafen & Kerran, 1989: 208. Reprinted by permission.)

2. Open the zipper of the air splint. If the splint has no zipper, gather the distal portion of the splint over your arm.
3. Grasp the patient's hand or foot and apply gentle longitudinal traction (American Academy of Orthopedic Surgeons, 1987; Hafen, 1989).
4. Place the splint free of wrinkles on the patient's extremity.
5. Twist the valve on the splint in a counterclockwise motion to open it.
6. Inflate the splint by mouth to a point where your finger will make a slight dent in the outer wall.
7. Twist the valve clockwise to close it and prevent air loss.
8. Monitor the air pressure within the splint frequently. You should be able to indent the splint with your finger.

COMPLICATIONS

1. Pressure variation within the splint due to environmental factors.
2. Accumulation of perspiration or moisture inside the splint may cause it to cling to the skin and make removal difficult or cause skin maceration. Dusting the interior of the splint with talcum powder or cornstarch prior to application may help decrease this.
3. Some pneumatic splints are not transparent and wounds under the splint cannot be visualized.

REFERENCES

American Academy of Orthopedic Surgeons. 1987. *Emergency care and transportation of the sick and injured,* 4th ed. Chicago: American Academy of Orthopedic Surgeons.

Hafen, B.Q. & Kerran, K.J. 1989. *Prehospital emergency care & crisis intervention,* 3rd ed. Englewood, CO: Morton.

SUGGESTED READINGS

Rea, R.E. (ed). 1991. *Trauma nursing core course (provider) manual,* 3rd ed. Chicago: Award Printing Company.

Schneider, P.A., Mitchell, J.M., & Allison, E.J. 1989. The use of military antishock trousers in trauma—A reevaluation. *Journal of Emergency Medicine,* 7:497–500.

Simon, R.R., & Brenner, B.E. 1987. *Emergency procedures and techniques,* 2nd ed. Baltimore: Williams & Wilkins.

Tintinalli, J.E., Rothstein, R.J., & Krome, R.L. 1985. *Emergency medicine: A comprehensive study guide.* New York: McGraw-Hill.

115

Traction Splints

Ruth L. Schaffler, RN, MA, CEN

Traction splints are also known as Hare, Kendrick, Sager, and Thomas splints.
The information in this chapter is specific to traction splints and should be used in conjunction with Ch. 112: General principles of splinting.

INDICATIONS

1. To align and stabilize a fracture of the femur or proximal tibia (American Academy of Orthopedic Surgeons, 1987; Hafen & Kerran, 1989; Rea, 1991).

CONTRAINDICATIONS AND CAUTIONS

1. Traction splints are not suitable for fractures of the distal fibula, distal tibia, ankle, foot, or upper extremity.
2. Use traction splints cautiously with patients who have concomitant pelvic fractures. If pelvic pain increases after splint application, the splint should be removed.
3. Traction splints may be used with open fractures of the femur. In this case, the bone ends will usually slip back beneath the skin. Open fractures are considered surgical emergencies and are potentially contaminated (Crenshaw, 1987; Hughes & Fitzgerald, 1986).
4. Two persons are needed to apply most traction splints.
5. In general, remove clothing and footwear before applying a traction splint. If a shoe or boot is difficult to remove or if it serves as a splint for the ankle, leave it on (Rea, 1991).

EQUIPMENT

Any of the following four splints may be used.
1. **Hare Traction Splint** (Dynamed, Carlsbad, CA)
   metal frame with padded ischial bar and heel stand
   ratchet device
   ankle hitch
   elastic straps
2. **Kendrick Traction Device** (Medix Choice, El Cajon, CA)
   snap out traction pole
   thigh strap with pole receptacle
   ankle hitch
   elastic straps
3. **Sager Traction Splint** (Minto Research & Development, Redding, CA)
   ankle strap
   elastic straps
   metal bar with padded arch support for groin
   attached pulley-and-cable apparatus
4. **Thomas Splint**
   metal frame with padded ischial half-ring
   cravats (6 minimum)
Padding material
Long wooden backboard

PATIENT PREPARATION

1. Pad the anterior groin area.
2. Measure against the unaffected extremity to determine the needed length of the splint.
3. Place the patient on a backboard.

PROCEDURAL STEPS

Hare traction splint

See Figure 115.1.
1. Place the ankle hitch under the heel of the foot and cross the straps over the top of the foot.
2. Have an assistant exert longitudinal traction by placing one hand behind the heel of the patient and the other hand over the dorsum of the foot and pull firmly. (**Note**: the amount of traction required will vary, but will generally be approximately 15 pounds of pulling force) (American Academy of Orthopedic Surgeons, 1987).
3. Support the injury site while lifting the leg just high enough to slide the splint under the extremity and position the padded bar against the ischial tuberosity.
4. Fasten the groin strap around the leg and over the padding.
5. Attach the S-ring of the ratchet to the D-rings of the ankle hitch and twist the ratchet knob to tighten traction. (**Note**: Be careful not to overstretch the limb. Mechanical traction should equate the manual traction.)
6. Secure the Velcro straps, two above and two below the knee, if possible. Do not place straps directly over the injury site.
7. Lower the heel stand into place to elevate the limb.

Kendrick traction device

See Figure 115.2.
1. Adjust the plastic buckle on the thigh strap so it will be located on the anterior thigh when fastened.
2. Apply the ankle hitch slightly above the ankle and tighten the stirrup by pulling the green tab until the stirrup is snug under the heel.
3. Slide the thigh strap under the leg and position it in the crotch by using a seesaw motion. Fasten the buckle. Cinch the strap until the traction pole receptacle rests against the belt line or pelvic crest.
4. Extend the folded traction pole making sure that all joints are properly locked in position.
5. Place the traction pole beside the leg. Extend one end of the pole 8 inches beyond the bottom of the foot. Adjust the opposite end to the patient's extremity length and insert it into the traction pole receptacle on the groin strap.
6. Secure the elastic knee strap.
7. Place the yellow tab on the ankle strap over the dart end of the traction pole beyond the patient's heel.
8. Apply traction by simultaneously pulling and feeding the strap with both hands until 10% of the patients body weight in kilograms is equated in pounds of tension or to a maximum of 22–25 pounds (Simon & Brenner, 1987).
9. Apply the appropriate elastic thigh and ankle straps.
10. The legs may be tied together as needed to provide further stability.

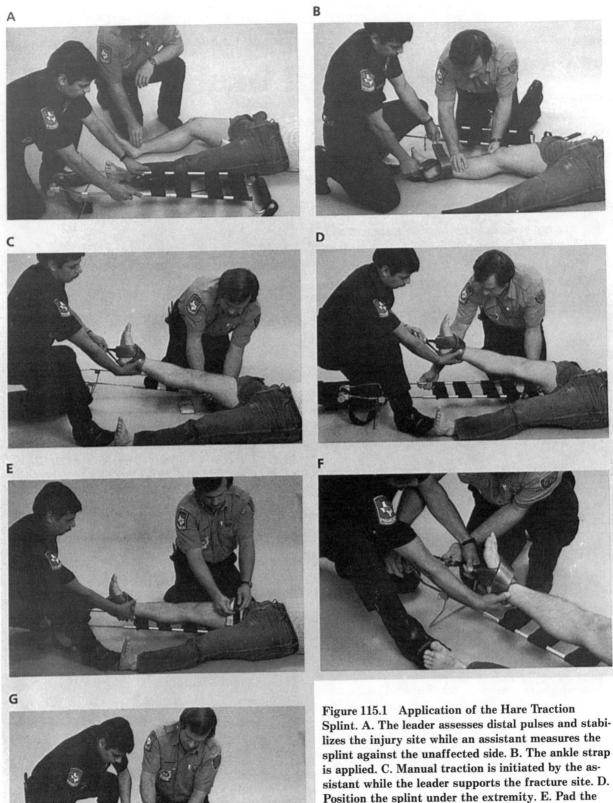

Figure 115.1 Application of the Hare Traction Splint. A. The leader assesses distal pulses and stabilizes the injury site while an assistant measures the splint against the unaffected side. B. The ankle strap is applied. C. Manual traction is initiated by the assistant while the leader supports the fracture site. D. Position the splint under the extremity. E. Pad the groin area and secure the ischial strap. F. Attach the ankle strap to the ratchet and tighten it just enough to maintain limb alignment and relieve pain. G. Fasten the support straps after proper mechanical traction has been applied.
(American Academy of Orthopedic Surgeons, 1987: 192. Reprinted by permission.)

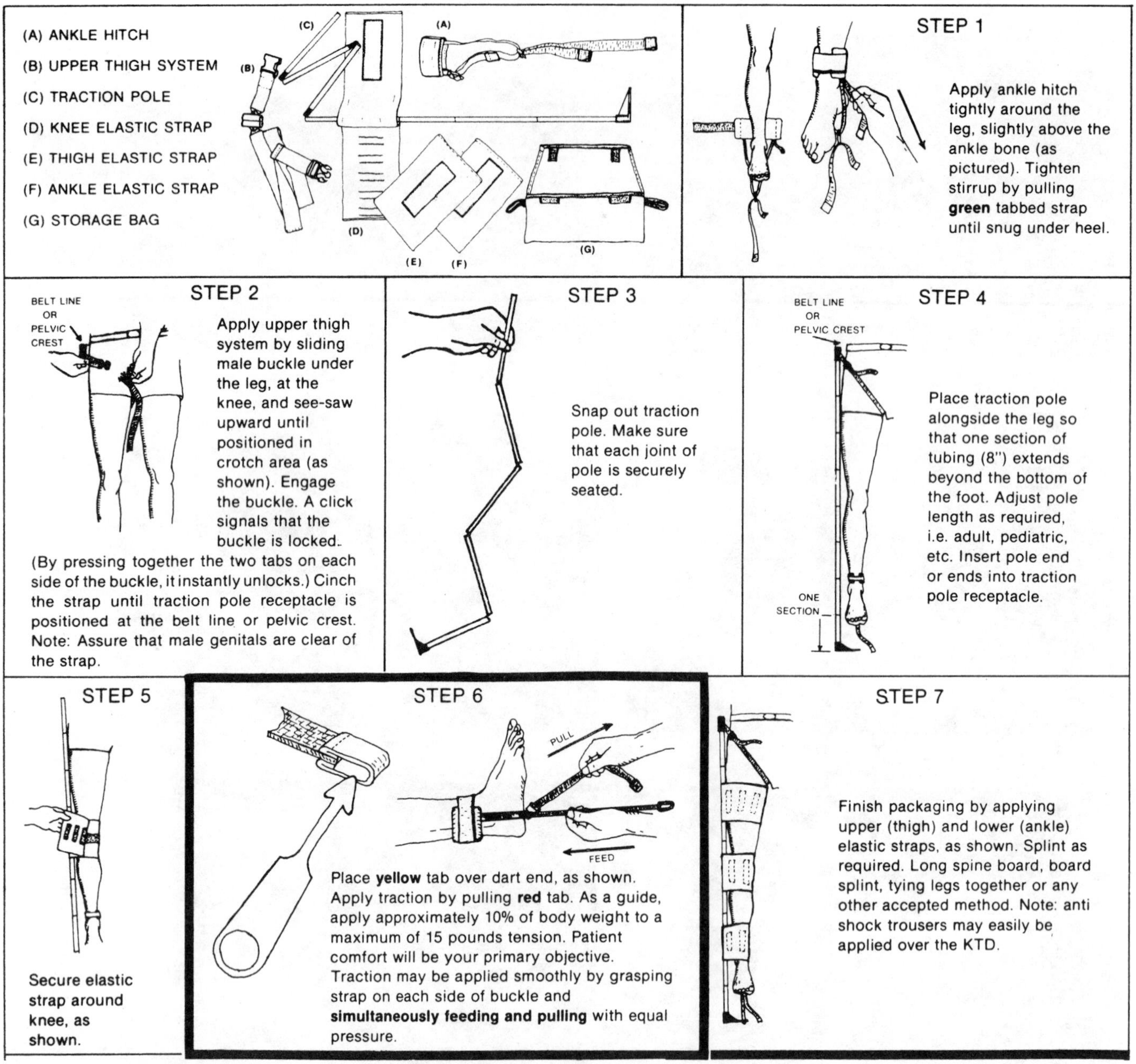
(A) ANKLE HITCH
(B) UPPER THIGH SYSTEM
(C) TRACTION POLE
(D) KNEE ELASTIC STRAP
(E) THIGH ELASTIC STRAP
(F) ANKLE ELASTIC STRAP
(G) STORAGE BAG
(A)
(B)
(C)
(D)
(E)
(F)
(G)
STEP 1
Apply ankle hitch tightly around the leg, slightly above the ankle bone (as pictured). Tighten stirrup by pulling **green** tabbed strap until snug under heel.
STEP 2
BELT LINE OR PELVIC CREST
Apply upper thigh system by sliding male buckle under the leg, at the knee, and see-saw upward until positioned in crotch area (as shown). Engage the buckle. A click signals that the buckle is locked. (By pressing together the two tabs on each side of the buckle, it instantly unlocks.) Cinch the strap until traction pole receptacle is positioned at the belt line or pelvic crest. Note: Assure that male genitals are clear of the strap.
STEP 3
Snap out traction pole. Make sure that each joint of pole is securely seated.
STEP 4
BELT LINE OR PELVIC CREST
ONE SECTION
Place traction pole alongside the leg so that one section of tubing (8") extends beyond the bottom of the foot. Adjust pole length as required, i.e. adult, pediatric, etc. Insert pole end or ends into traction pole receptacle.
STEP 5
Secure elastic strap around knee, as shown.
STEP 6
PULL
FEED
Place **yellow** tab over dart end, as shown. Apply traction by pulling **red** tab. As a guide, apply approximately 10% of body weight to a maximum of 15 pounds tension. Patient comfort will be your primary objective. Traction may be applied smoothly by grasping strap on each side of buckle and **simultaneously feeding and pulling** with equal pressure.
STEP 7
Finish packaging by applying upper (thigh) and lower (ankle) elastic straps, as shown. Splint as required. Long spine board, board splint, tying legs together or any other accepted method. Note: anti shock trousers may easily be applied over the KTD.

Figure 115.2 Application of the Kendrick Traction Device. (Medix Choice. Reprinted by permission.)

Sager traction splint

See Figure 115.3.

1. Slide the plastic buckle along the strap so that it will be positioned over the lateral thigh when fastened.
2. Place the splint next to the lateral aspect of the leg and adjust the length by measuring from the groin to the bottom of the foot. The wheel of the pulley should be at the heel of the patient. (**Note:** Tight-fitting clothing should be cut open or removed before the splint is applied.)
3. Prepare the padded ankle strap to fit around the lower leg just above the ankle. (**Note:** Additional padding may be required so that it fits snugly.)
4. Slide the thigh strap into the patient's groin so that the padded cushion on the shaft of the splint is snugly against the perineum and ischial tuberosity.
5. Tighten the thigh strap, drawing the splint to the medial side of the leg.
6. If necessary, connect the foot harness to the pulley apparatus by inserting the metal pin on the foot strap into the receptacle on the pulley cable. Apply the ankle harness snugly above the medial and lateral malleoli.

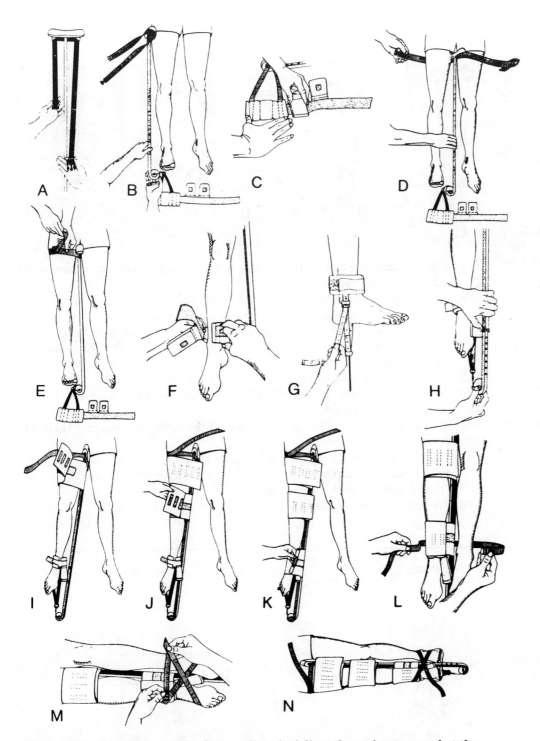

Figure 115.3 Application of the Sager splint. A. Adjust the groin strap so that the buckle will be over the lateral thigh when fastened. B. Adjust the splint shaft to the desired length. C. Prepare the ankle strap. D. Position the splint in the patient's groin with the padded bar resting against the perineum. E. Secure the thigh strap. F. Connect the ankle harness to the splint and apply the ankle strap over the malleoli. G. Pull the ankle strap through the buckle to tighten the harness. H. Extend the inner shaft of the splint until the desired amount of traction is noted on the pulley wheel markings (see text for explanation). I. Apply the longest strap around the thigh and pole. J. Apply the next longest strap around the knee. K. Apply the shortest strap around the ankle. L. Slide the long narrow strap under the ankles of both legs. M. Cross the strap over the feet in a figure-eight manner. N. The final position of the splint and straps as shown will control shifting and rotation of the bone fragments. (Simon & Brenner, 1987: 208. Reprinted by permission.)

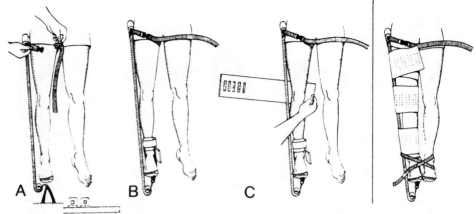

Figure 115.4 Application of the Sager splint on the outside of the leg. This method may be preferable in the case of perineal injury or pelvic fracture. A. Extend the length of the pole and place the padded bar next to the lateral thigh as shown. B. The groin strap should make a sling around the upper thigh and form an angle of about 55°. C. Apply the wide straps to the extremity as in the procedural steps for standard application. D. Secure the feet with a figure-eight strap as the final step.
(Simon & Brenner, 1987: 209. Reprinted by permission.)

7. Shorten the loop of the ankle harness by pulling on the strap threaded through the D buckle.
8. Extend the inner shaft of the splint by opening the lock and pulling the shaft out until the desired amount of traction tension is noted on the markings of the pulley wheel. (**Note:** Apply approximately 10% of the patient's body weight equated to pounds of tension to a maximum of 22–25 pounds).
9. Apply the longest 6″-wide elastic strap to the thigh.
10. Apply the second longest 6″-wide strap over the knee. Use additional padding as necessary.
11. Apply the shortest 6″-wide strap around the ankle harness and traction pole.
12. Use the remaining long narrow strap to secure the splint. Slide it under both ankles and cross it over the feet in a figure-eight manner. This will control shifting and rotation of the distal bone fragment.
13. For alternative methods of application see Figs. 115.4 and 115.5.

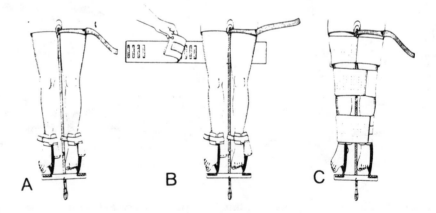

Figure 115.5 Application of the bilateral Sager splint. A. Modify the length of the splint to allow placement of a horizontal harness bar adjacent to the patient's heels. Ankle straps are applied bilaterally and secured to the harness bar as shown. B. Additional 6″-wide straps may be hooked together to achieve the desired length for encircling the legs. C. The straps are wrapped around both legs to secure them together. A figure-eight strap may be added to the ankles and feet, if needed.
(Simon & Brenner, 1987: 210. Reprinted by permission.)

Thomas splint

1. Adjust the splint to the length of the patient's leg and allow an extension of 6–8 inches beyond the foot.
2. Apply the traction strap over the patient's foot after padding the surfaces that will lie under the strap.
3. Have an assistant exert longitudinal traction on the leg by placing one hand under the patient's heel and the other over the dorsum of the foot and gently pulling. Manual traction is to be maintained until the splinting process is complete.
4. Place the splint under the patient's leg by gently lifting the leg and eas-

ing the padded half-ring against the ischium. Be sure that the buckle on the splint is to the outside and that the half-ring is turned downward.

5. Fasten the ischial strap over the thigh and padding.
6. Bring the long free end of the foot strap over and then under the top of the notched end of the splint.
7. Pass the strap through the link at the swivel in the stirrup under the patient's foot. Traction can be applied by pulling the strap toward the end of the splint. If no foot strap is available, create an improvised ankle hitch and a Spanish windlass (see Figure 115.6) to maintain traction as illustrated (see Figure 115.7).

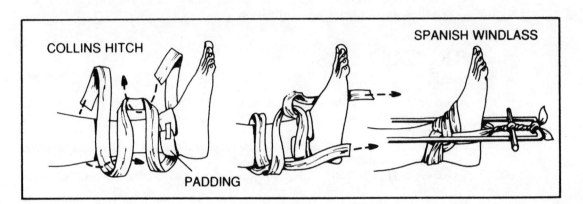

8. Slide the footrest on the splint until it rests against the bottom of the patient's foot.
9. Apply 3 or 4 cravats around the splint to support the leg. Make sure that no fastening device is directly over the injury site. Apply 2 additional cravats to support the foot and secure it to the footrest.

Figure 115.6 An improvised ankle hitch. A. Place the tail of a cravat just behind the patient's heel. **B.** Loop the remainder of the cravat as shown. **C.** Pass the tails through the loops in the directions indicated. **D.** Pull the tails to tighten around the ankle. **E.** Form a Spanish windlass by knotting the tails on the end of the splint. Insert a stick between the tails and twist to tighten until the desired amount of traction is attained. **F.** Secure the stick to the sides of the splint so that it will not unwind.
(Campbell, 1988: 166. Reprinted by permission.)

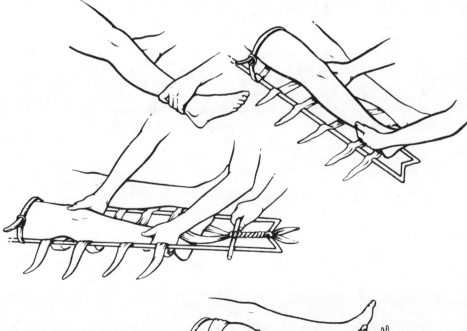

Figure 115.7 Application of the Thomas splint using a Spanish windlass (refer to text for procedural steps). Cravats lie over the splint to form a sling that supports the leg, the Spanish windlass maintains traction.
(Parcel, 1986: 165. Reprinted by permission.)

COMPLICATIONS

1. Compression of the sciatic nerve or perineal tissues.
2. Flexion and outward rotation of the proximal femur.
3. Excessive traction and overstretching of the limb.

PATIENT TEACHING

1. Report when muscle spasm subsides and pain in the injured leg decreases during traction application.

REFERENCES

American Academy of Orthopedic Surgeons. 1987. *Emergency care and transportation of the sick and injured,* 4th ed. Chicago: American Academy of Orthopedic Surgeons.

Campbell, J.E. (ed). 1988. *Basic trauma life support: Advanced prehospital care,* 2nd ed. Englewood Cliffs, NJ: Prentice-Hall.

Crenshaw, A.H. (ed). 1987. *Campbell's operative orthopaedics,* 7th ed. St. Louis: Mosby.

Hafen, B.Q., & Kerran, K.J. 1989. *Prehospital emergency care & crisis intervention,* 3rd ed. Englewood, CO: Morton.

Hughes, S.P., & Fitzgerald, R.H., Jr. 1986. *Musculoskeletal infections.* Chicago: Year Book Medical Publishers.

Parcel, G. 1986. Basic emergency care of the sick and injured, 3rd ed. St. Louis: Times Mirror/Mosby.

Rea, R.E. (ed). 1991. *Trauma nursing core course (provider) manual,* 3rd ed. Chicago: Award Printing Corporation.

Simon, R.R., & Brenner, B.E. 1987. *Emergency procedures and techniques,* 2nd ed. Baltimore: Williams & Wilkins.

SUGGESTED READINGS

Barber, J.M., & Dillman, P.A. 1981. *Emergency patient care for the EMT-A.* Reston, VA: Reston Publishing Co.

Connolly, J.F. (ed). 1981. *DePalma's the management of fractures and dislocations: An atlas,* 3rd ed. Philadelphia: Saunders.

Hansell, M.J. 1988. Fractures and the healing process. *Orthopedic Nursing,* 7:43–48.

Redheffer, G.M., & Bailey, M. 1989. Assessing and splinting fractures. *Nursing,* 19, 6:51–59.

116

Sling Application

Ruth L. Schaffler, RN, MA, CEN

The information in this chapter should be used in conjunction with the information in Ch. 112: General Principles of Splinting.

INDICATIONS

To support an injured shoulder, clavicle, or upper extremity.

EQUIPMENT

Triangular bandage measuring 40 x 40 x 55 inches

or

Commercially prepared sling or collar and cuff

Safety pin(s) or tape

PATIENT PREPARATION

Pad the axilla to absorb perspiration and prevent skin maceration if the sling is placed under the patient's clothing.

PROCEDURAL STEPS

Sling

1. Place the longest edge of a triangular bandage vertically across the anterior chest with one tip over the uninjured shoulder. The apex of the bandage should lie under the elbow of the injured arm.
2. Place the humerus on the injured side next to the lateral chest wall and bend the elbow so the hand is positioned at the opposite 4th or 5th anterior rib. See Figure 116.1.
   (Note: The weight of the arm should create an angle of slightly less than 90° at the elbow while in the sling.)
3. Bring the lower edge of the triangle over the injured arm and tie a square knot to the other end of the bandage at the side of the posterior neck (not over the cervical spine) and place a pad under the knot.
4. Fold the apex of the triangle forward and pin or tape it securely to the sling. The apex could also be twisted and knotted when snugly fitted against the elbow.
5. Position the edge of the sling to expose the ends of the fingers.

Collar and cuff

1. Secure the cuff to the patient's wrist.
2. Place the collar around the patient's neck making sure it is secure but not restrictive.
3. Loop a strap through the cuff and collar to suspend the wrist. The final position of the elbow should be 90° flexion. See Figure 116.2.

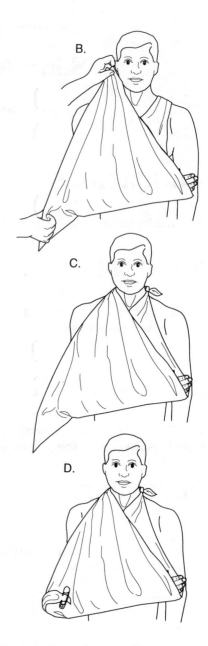

A.

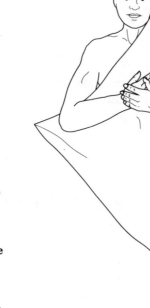

Figure 116.1   Applying a triangular bandage as a sling. A. The arm is placed across the chest and bandage as shown. B. Bring the lower end of the bandage over the arm and behind the neck. C. Tie a square knot to the opposite end at the side of the neck. D. Secure the apex of the bandage with a knot or pin. The final position of the arm should create an angle of slightly less than 90° at the elbow; fingers should be exposed.

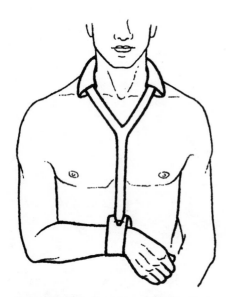

Figure 116.2   A collar and cuff. (Connolly, 1981: 695. Reprinted by permission.)

Commercial sling

1. Place the injured arm in the fabric holder with the elbow in the seamed corner.
2. Loop the attached strap across the chest toward the uninjured side, loop it behind the neck and then down the chest to the D-rings at the wrist end of the holder.
3. Pass the strap upward through the rings and secure the Velcro edges together with the elbow flexed at 90°. See Figure 116.3.

PATIENT TEACHING

1. Keep the knot positioned at the side of the neck and not directly over the spine to avoid excessive pressure on blood vessels, nerves, and spinous processes.
2. Keep the hand above elbow level to prevent or decrease swelling.

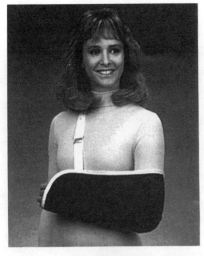 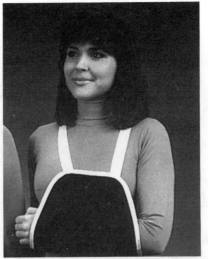

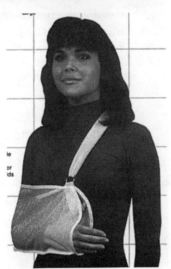 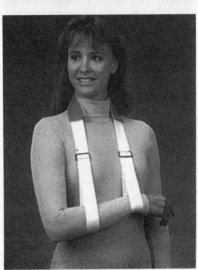

Figure 116.3 Examples of commercial slings.
(From Technol, Inc. Copyright 1989 by Technol, Inc. Reprinted by permission.)

SUGGESTED READINGS

Alvero, E.M. 1988. Life on a limb: Management of upper extremity injuries. *Journal of Emergency Medical Services*, 13, 9:42–51.

American Academy of Orthopedic Surgeons. 1987. *Emergency care and transportation of the sick and injured*, 4th ed. Chicago: American Academy of Orthopedic Surgeons.

Connolly, J.F. (ed). 1981. *DePalma's the management of fractures and dislocations: An atlas*, 3rd ed. Philadelphia: Saunders.

Hafen, B.Q., & Kerran, K.J. 1989. *Prehospital emergency care and crisis intervention*, 3rd ed. Englewood, CO: Morton.

Rosen, P., Baker, F.J., Braen, G.R., Dailey, R.H., & Levy, R.C. 1983. *Emergency medicine: Concepts and clinical practice*, Vol. 1. St. Louis: Mosby.

Simon, R.R., & Brenner, B.E. 1987. *Emergency procedures and techniques*, 2nd ed. Baltimore: Williams & Wilkins.

Tintinalli, J.E., Rothstein, R.J., & Krome, R.L. 1985. *Emergency medicine: A comprehensive study guide.* New York: McGraw-Hill.

117

Shoulder Immobilization

Ruth L. Schaffler, RN, MA, CEN

Shoulder immobilization is also known as sling and swathe, Velpeau bandage.
The information in this chapter should be used in conjunction with the information in Ch. 112: General Principles of Splinting.

INDICATIONS

1. To immobilize the clavicle, acromioclavicular joint, shoulder, or proximal humerus.
2. To immobilize unstable fractures of the proximal humerus in order to prevent recurrent dislocation as a result of contraction of the pectoralis major muscle (Velpeau bandage) (Connolly, 1981; Tintinalli et al., 1985).

EQUIPMENT

Commercial sling and swathe
2–3 triangular bandages to create a sling and swathe
3–4 rolls of 6″-wide elastic bandage or a 3–4 meter length of

stockinette to create a Velpeau bandage
Safety pins
Axillary padding (e.g., surgical dressing or "abd" pad)

PATIENT PREPARATION

Pad the axilla on the affected side, across the chest where the arm will lie and over the opposite shoulder where the dressing material will lie.

PROCEDURAL STEPS

Sling and swathe:

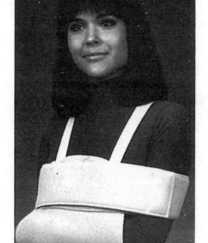

Figure 117.1   Example of a sling and swathe.
(Tecnol, Inc. Copyright 1989 by Tecnol, Inc. Reprinted by permission.)

See Figure 117.1.
1. Place the humerus next to the chest wall.
2. Place the forearm across the anterior chest wall with the elbow flexed at a right angle.
3. Apply the cloth sling to the forearm with the elbow positioned in the seamed corner, the hand extending into the open end.
4. Pass the self-fastening strap behind the neck and secure to the sling at the wrist.
5. Place the fabric swathe around the arm and chest to keep the extremity and shoulder immobilized.

Shoulder immobilizer:

See Figure 117.2.
1. Place the humerus next to the chest wall.
2. Place the forearm across the anterior chest wall with the elbow flexed at a right angle.

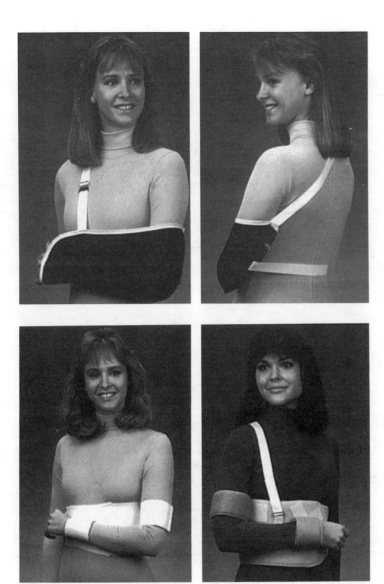

Figure 117.2   Examples of commercial shoulder immobilizers. (Tecnol, Inc. Copyright 1989 by Tecnol, Inc. Reprinted by permission.)

3. Apply the elastic band around the chest and secure with the Velcro fastener. Fasten the arm strap around the humerus and then fasten the wrist strap at the lower forearm.

Velpeau bandage

See Figure 117.3.
1. Position the affected arm across the chest so that the hand rests on the opposite shoulder.
2. Roll the bandage away from the injury beginning underneath the crossed arm in the center of the chest and pass the roll under the uninjured axilla.
3. Continue the roll diagonally behind the patient's back and over the top of the affected shoulder.
4. Roll downward diagonally over the folded arm and then loop the bandage behind the elbow and middle of the humerus.
5. Repeat the direction of the initial roll across the chest and encircle the entire thorax and arm.
6. Overlap the upper half of the first encirclement. Continue this same pattern, alternating the roll of the bandage over the shoulder and around the torso with each pass.

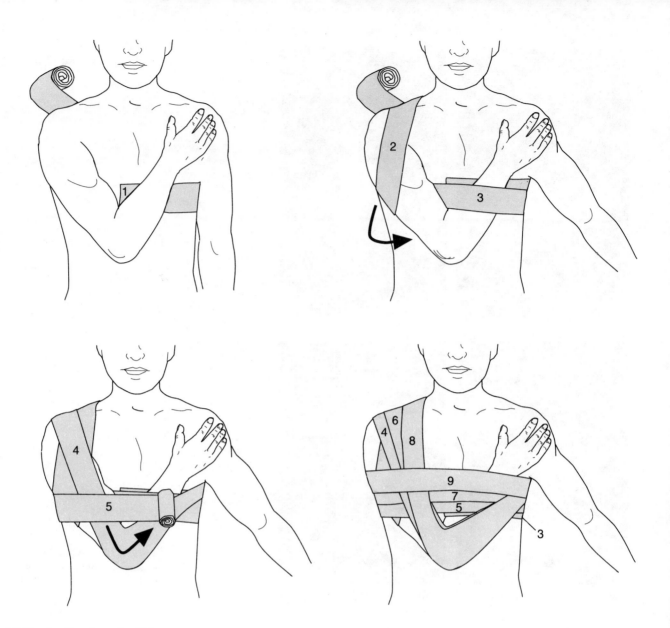

Figure 117.3   Application of a Velpeau bandage. Direction of the rolled bandage alternates between arm stabilization and chest encirclement.

Gilchrist stockinette-Velpeau sleeve

See Figure 117.4.
1. Cut a piece of 4″-wide stockinette into a 3–4 meter length. Make a horizontal slit halfway across the width of material approximately one-third from the end. Insert the patient's affected arm into the long end of the stockinette until the axilla rests in the slot (Connolly, 1981).
2. Place the injured arm across the chest. Pass the long end of the stockinette around the patient's back, through the space between the injured arm and chest, and loosely drape it over the patient's forearm. Pass the shorter end of the stockinette around the patient's neck, loop it around the wrist, and secure with a safety pin.
3. Pull the loose end of the stockinette tightly, wrap it around the affected arm, and secure with a safety pin.
4. Make a slit in the stockinette over the patient's wrist in order to free the hand. Reinforce the slot with tape to prevent fraying or stretching.

COMPLICATIONS

1. Frozen shoulder or joint stiffness.

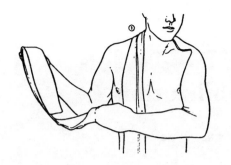
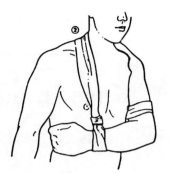
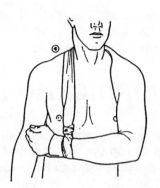

Figure 117.4 The stockinette Velpeau bandage encircles the neck and waist and is secured with safety pins or ties.
(Connolly, 1981, 603–604. Reprinted by permission.)

PATIENT TEACHING

1. Loosen the swathe and reapply it if it becomes too tight or restricts breathing.

REFERENCES

Connolly, J.F. (ed). 1981. *DePalma's the management of fractures and dislocations: An atlas*, 3rd ed. Philadelphia: Saunders.

Tintinalli, J.E., Rothstein, R.J., & Krome, R.L. 1985. *Emergency medicine: A comprehensive study guide.* New York: McGraw-Hill.

SUGGESTED READINGS

Alvero, E.M. 1988. Life on a limb: Management of upper extremity injuries. *Journal of Emergency Medical Services,* 9:42–51.

American Academy of Orthopedic Surgeons. 1987. *Emergency care and transportation of the sick and injured,* 4th ed. Chicago: American Academy of Orthopedic Surgeons.

Hafen, B.Q., & Kerran, K.J. 1989. *Prehospital emergency care and crisis intervention,* 3rd ed. Englewood, CO: Morton.

Hawkins, R.J., & Angelo, R.L. 1987. Displaced proximal humeral fractures: Selecting treatment, avoiding pitfalls. *Orthopedic Clinics of North America,* 18:421–431.

Neviaser, R.J. 1987. Injury to the clavicle and AC joint. *Orthopedic Clinics of North America,* 18:433–438.

Simon, R.R., & Brenner, B.E. 1987. *Emergency procedures and techniques,* 2nd ed. Baltimore: Williams & Wilkins.

Zuidema, G.D., Rutherford, R.B., & Ballinger, W.F. 1985. *The management of trauma,* 4th ed. Philadelphia: Saunders.

118

Knee Immobilization

Ruth L. Schaffler, RN, MA, CEN

The information in this chapter should be used in conjunction with the information in Ch. 112: General Principles of Splinting.

INDICATIONS

1. To immobilize a fracture, dislocation, or soft tissue injury of the knee or adjacent structures.
2. To immobilize an unstable knee joint.

CONTRAINDICATIONS AND CAUTIONS

1. Handle the knee gently and minimize movement of the injured area to decrease pain and the risk of complications.
2. Pad bony prominences and body contours to avoid undue pressure and skin breakdown.
3. Do not force the extremity to fit the splint. You may need to alter the splint to fit the deformity.
4. Assess and document neurovascular status before and after the device is applied. If compromise exists, a physician should be notified immediately. If deterioration occurs after splinting, the device must be readjusted or removed and reapplied.
5. Gross soft tissue swelling may make the application of an immobilizing device difficult or impossible. You may need to apply a plaster splint. (See Ch. 120: General Principles of Plaster Splinting).

EQUIPMENT

Commercial knee immobilizer
or
Plaster splint
    premade plaster splinting
        material or
    12–15 4"-x-30" or 5"-x-30"
        plaster strips

stockinette or rolled cotton
    padding
2–3 rolls of 6" elastic bandage
bucket of lukewarm water
gloves
absorbent pads
pillows

PATIENT PREPARATION

1. Remove constrictive clothing that would lie under the immobilization device. (**Note:** If the immobilizer is to be removed occasionally and swelling is minimal, it may be applied over loose clothing.)
2. Clean and dress all open wounds.
3. Measure the thigh circumference and the length of the leg to determine the correct size of the immobilizing device.
4. Assess and document neurovascular status.

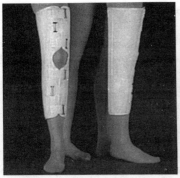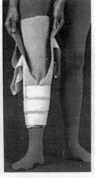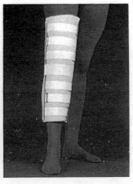

Figure 118.1 Examples of knee immobilizers.
(From Technol, Inc. Copyright 1989 by Technol, Inc. Reprinted by permission.)

PROCEDURAL STEPS

1. Position the immobilizer under the leg while the patient is supine. If the device has a cutout in the front, place it so that the open area is over the patella. If no cutout is present, place the splint with the upper end at midthigh and the lower end at midcalf. (**Note:** splints are available in 16″ and 22″ lengths).
2. Secure the device with the attached buckles or Velcro fasteners. See Figure 118.1.

To apply a plaster long leg posterior splint

1. Splint the knee joint in the position found unless circulatory compromise is present.
2. If possible, place the patient in a prone position on a stretcher.
3. Measure the posterior surface of the unaffected leg from the ball of the foot to midthigh. This measurement determines the length of plaster splinting needed.
4. Wrap the affected leg with rolled cotton bandage or put on stockinette that is cut to the measured length.
5. Moisten the plaster material in the bucket of water and gently pinch to remove the excess water. Do not squeeze or twist.
6. Apply the plaster to the posterior surface of the limb from toes to midthigh. Keep the foot flexed at 90°.
7. Wrap with elastic bandages to cover.
8. Place limb on pillows for support while the plaster dries. Extend the distal leg beyond the edge of the cart to allow the foot to remain in a neutral position. (See Ch. 120: General principles of plaster splinting).
9. Assess and document neurovascular status.

COMPLICATIONS

1. Neurovascular compromise
2. Increased edema
3. Increased pain
4. Joint stiffness due to prolonged immobilization (Connolly, 1981)
5. Joint effusion may occur after 6–12 hours (Tintinalli, 1985)
6. Compartmental syndrome

PATIENT TEACHING

1. Keep plaster splints clean and dry.
2. Apply ice packs to the affected area.

3. Elevate the lower extremity above the level of the heart to reduce swelling and bleeding.
4. Instruct the patient in crutchwalking and weight-bearing limitations if indicated. See Ch. 133: Measuring Crutches and Ch. 134: Teaching Crutch Walking.
5. Notify your physician or return to the emergency department for any numbness, tingling, increased swelling, increased pain, or discoloration of the foot.
6. Review with the patient the length of time to wear the device and when to follow up with the physician or physical therapist. (**Note:** Patients who sustain a knee injury should be referred to an orthopedic specialist.)

REFERENCES

Connolly, J.F. (ed). 1981. *DePalma's the management of fractures and dislocations: An atlas,* 3rd ed. Philadelphia: Saunders.

Tintinalli, J.E., Rothstein, R.J., & Krome, R.L. 1985. *Emergency medicine: A comprehensive study guide.* New York: McGraw-Hill.

SUGGESTED READINGS

American Academy of Orthopedic Surgeons. 1987. *Emergency care and transportation of the sick and injured,* 4th ed. Chicago: American Academy of Orthopedic Surgeons.

Hafen, B.Q., & Kerran, K.J. 1989. *Prehospital emergency care and crisis intervention,* 3rd ed. Englewood, CO: Morton.

Maher, A.B. 1986. Early assessment and management of musculoskeletal injuries. *Nursing Clinics of North America,* 21:717–727.

Redheffer, G.M., & Bailey, M. 1989. Assessing and splinting fractures. *Nursing,* 19, 6:51–59.

Simon, R.R., & Brenner, B.E. 1987. *Emergency procedures and techniques,* 2nd ed. Baltimore: Williams & Wilkins.

119

Finger Immobilization

Linell M. Jones, RN, BSN, CEN, CCRN

Finger immobilization is also known as finger splinting.

The information in this chapter should be used in conjunction with the information in Ch. 112: General Principles of Splinting.

INDICATIONS

1. To relieve pain, provide stability, promote healing, and prevent functional disability in the presence of finger fractures.
2. To protect a repaired tendon, nerve, or vessel from tension.
3. To protect soft tissue injuries from further trauma.

CONTRAINDICATIONS AND CAUTIONS

1. Immobilize in the position of function unless otherwise indicated. Position of function for the hand is 30° wrist extension with the thumb in palmar abduction, 60–90° flexion of the metacarpophalangeal joints, and 10–20° flexion of the interphalangeal joints (Uehara, 1985).
2. The hand performs many intricate maneuvers and even small deficits may cause significant functional limitations.

EQUIPMENT

Dependent upon type of injury

Plaster gutter splint: For stable fractures of the middle and proximal phalanx which do not involve articular surfaces (Simon, 1985). See Ch. 122: Ulnar Gutter Splint and Ch. 123: Radial Gutter Splint.

Dorsal splint of distal phalanx: For mallet type injury of the distal phalanx involving less than 25% of the articular surface or for avulsion of the profundus tendon at the attachment (Simon 1985).

Volar splint (Plaster, unpadded, or padded aluminum splint): For uncomplicated extraarticular fractures, sprains and dislocations (Hossfeld, 1985). See Ch. 125: Volar Splint.

4-Prong or Cage splints: For protection of distal finger injuries such as tuft fractures, fingernail avulsions, or tip amputations.

Fixation pin (K-wire, smooth wire, Riordin pin): For unstable fractures or mallet type fractures involving greater than 25% articular surface, displacement of greater than 3–4 mm, or avulsion fracture of the volar surface attachment of profundus tendon (Simon, 1985).

409

PATIENT PREPARATION

1. Remove rings on all digits of the injured hand.
2. Assess and document neurovascular status.
3. *Assess for rotational malalignment and angulation. With the fingers flexed, lines drawn through the fingernails meet at the scaphoid in the normal hand. See Figure 119.1.
4. *Anesthetize the finger with a digital block prior to manipulation reduction of the fracture. See Ch. 138: Digital Block.

*Indicates portions of the procedure usually performed by a physician.

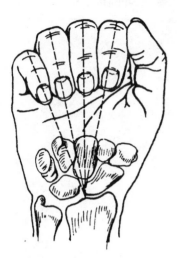

Figure 119.1   Normal alignment of the fingers.
(Simon & Koenigsknecht, 1987: 47. Reprinted by permission.)

PROCEDURE

Dorsal splint of distal phalanx

1. Distal joint is fully extended.
2. Size the splint, apply it to the dorsum of the finger, and tape it to the middle phalanx. Place the splint over any necessary dressings or padding.

4-Prong or cage splint

1. Size splint and mold to fit over dressing.
2. Leave a small gap between the distal end of the digit and the splint to prevent transfer of force if the splint is hit.

K-wire/Riordan fixation pin:

1. Cleanse the affected hand with particular attention to the skin overlying the insertion site with antiseptic solution.
2. *Drill the wire through skin and into the bone.
3. *Test fracture site for stability.
4. Obtain an x-ray to confirm reduction and pin placement.
5. *Cut pin off below the skin line.
6. Apply dressing.
7. Apply an external splint if indicated.

COMPLICATIONS

1. Fracture may deform during splinting.
2. Infection of soft tissue or bone may occur if the skin was broken.
3. Loss of mobility and/or function if the fracture is inadequately reduced or splinted improperly.

PATIENT TEACHING

1. Elevate your arm with your hand above the level of the elbow and the heart.
2. Apply cold packs to fracture site.
3. Report signs of infection such as redness, swelling, draining pus, etc. (for open fractures or pin insertions).
4. Report increasing pain, numbness, or swelling.
5. Wear splint until directed by the physician to remove it.

REFERENCES

Hossfeld, G.E. 1985. Joint injuries of the hand. *Trauma Quarterly*, 1, 2:74–82. Gaithersburg, MD: Aspen Publication.

Simon, R.R. 1985. Phalangeal fractures. *Trauma Quarterly*, 1, 2:55–60. Gaithersburg, MD: Aspen Publication.

Simon, R.R. & Koenigsknecht, S.J. 1987. *Emergency orthopedics: The extremities.* E. Norwalk, CT: Appleton & Lange.

Uehara, D.T. 1985. Principles in the management of acute hand injuries. *Trauma Quarterly*, 1, 2:1–7. Gaithersburg, MD: Aspen Publication.

General Principles of Plaster Splinting

Dawn M. Swimm, RN, CEN

INDICATIONS

To temporarily immobilize fractures or soft tissue injuries. Immobilization aids in healing, pain relief, and helps prevent complications. Unlike circumferential plaster casts, splints allow soft tissue swelling to occur without circulatory compromise.

CONTRAINDICATIONS AND CAUTIONS

1. Assess and document neurovascular status before and after splint application.
2. Protect bony prominences with adequate padding (DePalma, 1970).
3. Never use hot water to wet the plaster. The chemical reaction that sets the plaster is exothermic (heat producing). This heat in combination with the heat of the water may burn the patient. Hot water also acelerates hardening and makes the splint difficult to mold (Rockwood & Green, 1984).
4. The desired position of the extremity should be maintained from the time the first layer of padding is applied. Any movement during the splinting process will weaken the splint.
5. The plaster should never completely encircle an extremity: this allows for postinjury swelling (Schoen, 1986).

EQUIPMENT

Nonsterile gloves
Sheet wadding or padding (SofRoll, Webril, etc.)
Plaster splints or rolls
Scissor or knife (to cut plaster)
Measuring tape
Bucket
Elastic bandages
(**Note:** Preassembled plaster splints with incorporated padding are available in 2″, 3″, or 4″, and 6″ widths in rolls or boxed lengths. Stockingette may be used to provide additional padding under sheet wadding or preassembled splints.)

PATIENT PREPARATION

1. Assess and document neurovascular status and skin integrity prior to splint application. If there is a break in the skin at or near a fracture site,

an open fracture must be considered. Notify the physician before applying the splint. Dress all wounds prior to splint application.

2. If indicated and time permits, cleanse and dry the extremity prior to splint application.
3. Remove all jewelry from the injured extremity. See Ch. 111: Ring Removal.

PROCEDURAL STEPS

1. Prepare bucket of tepid water, 86°F (Tabers, 1977).
2. If possible, when measuring for a splint, use the unaffected side. Accuracy will be increased and discomfort decreased by avoiding movement of the injured extremity.
3. Cut prepared splints, rolls, or loose sheets to measured length. Width is determined by the largest surface to be supported.
4. With loose splint sheets, the number of layers required depends on the size of the extremity to be supported.
5. Pad the entire area to be splinted. One or two layers of sheet wadding will be sufficient unless there is marked edema, friable skin, or bony prominences. These conditions require an extra layer of padding. Padding should be wrapped in circular motion from distal to proximal, seeking conformity and uniform pressure. If padding is too loose, it will wrinkle and pressure sores can develop. If it is too tight, swelling will cause constriction. Place a single layer of padding between any digits to be included in the splint to prevent tissue maceration.
6. Immerse plaster in tepid bath until bubbling stops. Gently squeeze excess moisture out of splint, smooth, and apply. See Figure 120.1. An extra layer of sheet wadding applied to the exterior of the splint prevents the elastic bandage from adhering to the splint and assists with molding and application.

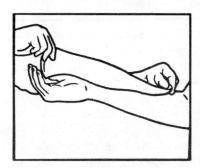 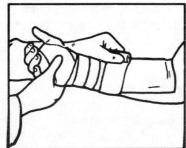 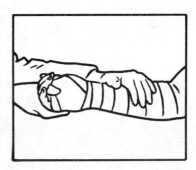

7. Secure the splint with an elastic bandage. Wrap in circular motion from distal to proximal seeking uniform pressure and conformity while molding the splint to the injured extremity. See Figure 120.2.
8. Assess and document neurovascular status after splint application.
9. Elevate the splinted extremity and allow 15 minutes drying time prior to discharge.
10. Apply a sling, if indicated, for upper extremity splints.

Figure 120.1 Submersion, removal, and smoothing of plaster for application.
(Johnson & Johnson Orthopaedics, *Specialists J Splints* (poster). New Brunswick, NJ. Reprinted by permission.)

COMPLICATIONS

1. Pressure sores develop due to wrinkling of the cotton padding or indentations of the plaster. When this pressure continues, compression of the skin and underlying fat can result in tissue necrosis (DePalma, 1970).

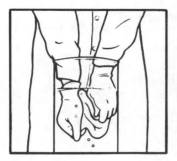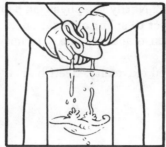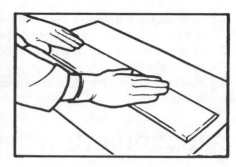

Figure 120.2 Application of plaster, elastic bandage, and molding of plaster to the extremity. (Johnson & Johnson Orthopaedics, *Specialists J Splints* (poster). New Brunswick, NJ. Reprinted by permission.)

2. Plaster burns are related to chemical accelerators, temperature of the water bath, the amount of water in the plaster, thickness of the splint, and padding. Using tepid water to activate the plaster, padding to protect the skin, and adequate air circulation to aid in the drying process will reduce the possibility of plaster burns. If the patient complains that the splint is burning, remove it immediately (Rockwood & Green, 1984).

3. Improper positioning of the splinted extremity can result in misalignment and/or neurovascular compromise. Verify the desired position prior to splint application and check pulses, sensation, and capillary refill prior to and following application of the splint (Schoen, 1986).

4. Compartmental syndrome can develop in conjunction with injury or as a result of plaster application. Neurovascular assessments and patient teaching will assist in rapid recognition and prompt intervention.

PATIENT TEACHING

1. Plaster requires at least 12–24 hours drying time. Care should be taken to prevent impression of the plaster during this first 12–24 hours, which could result in misalignment or pressure sores.

2. Whenever possible, splinted extremities should be elevated with ice packs applied to minimize edema and increase comfort.

3. Watch for swelling, increasing pain, numbness, pale or blue fingers or toes, or tingling in the extremity. If any of these occur, loosen the elastic wrap and elevate the extremity above the level of the heart. If symptoms persist, contact your physician or return to the emergency department.

4. Keep the splint dry. If the plaster gets wet it will crumble and it will not harden again.

5. Do not stick anything into the splint. If itching is a problem, try applying an ice pack to the area.

6. Do not use or walk on the injured extremity. Splints are not strong enough to withstand weight. See Ch. 133: Measuring Crutches and Ch. 134: Teaching Crutch Walking.

REFERENCES

DePalma, A.F. 1970. *Management of fractures and dislocations.* Philadelphia: Saunders.

Rockwood, C.A., & Green, D.P. 1984. *Fractures in adults.* Philadelphia: Lippincott.

Schoen, D.C. 1986. *The nursing process in orthopaedics.* Norwalk, CT: Appleton-Century-Crofts.

Simon, R.R., & Brenner, B.E. 1982. *Procedures and techniques in emergency medicine.* Baltimore: Williams & Wilkins.

Simon, R.R., & Koenigsknecht, S.J. 1987. *Emergency orthopedics: The extremities.* Norwalk, CT: Appleton & Lange.

Tabers Cyclopedic Medical Dictionary, 13th ed. 1977. Philadelphia: Davis.

SUGGESTED READINGS

Shaw, D.C., & Heckman, J.D. 1984. Principles and techniques of splinting musculo-cutaneous injuries. *Emergency Medicine Clinics of North America.* 2, 2:391–407.

Rea, R.E. (ed). 1991. *Trauma nursing core course, (provider) manual,* 3rd ed. Chicago: Award Printing Corporation.

Posterior Short Leg Splint

Dawn M. Swimm, RN, CEN

Posterior short leg splint is also known as posterior boot, posterior slab.

The information in this chapter should be used in conjunction with the information in Ch. 120: General Principles of Plaster Splinting.

INDICATIONS

Fractures or soft tissue injuries of the foot or ankle.

EQUIPMENT

4–6″ Cast padding (SofRoll, Webril, etc.)

4–6″ Plaster splints or rolls (10–15 layers/sheets)

4–6″ Elastic bandages

PROCEDURAL STEPS

1. Measure from the toes to below the knee.
2. Place the foot in 90° angle to the leg.
3. Apply the plaster posteriorly from the metatarsal phalangeal crease of the great toe to just below the knee (Simon & Koenignsknecht, 1987). See Figure 121.1. Knee flexion should not be impeded by the splint.

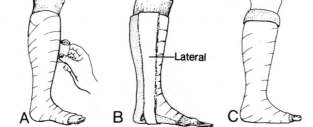

Figure 121.1   Posterior short leg splint application.
(Simon & Brenner, 1982: 26. Reprinted by permission.)

REFERENCES

Simon, R.R., & Brenner, B.E. 1982. *Procedures & techniques in emergency medicine.* Baltimore: Williams & Wilkins.

Simon, R.R., & Koeningsknecht, S.J. 1987. *Emergency orthopedics: The extremities.* Norwalk, CT: Appleton & Lange.

122

Ulnar Gutter Splint

Dawn M. Swimm, RN, CEN

Ulnar gutter splint is also known as phalangeal or metacarpal gutter.

The information in this chapter should be used in conjunction with the information in Ch. 120: General Principles of Plaster Splinting.

INDICATIONS

Fractures or soft tissue injuries of the 4th or 5th metacarpels (e.g., boxer's fractures).

EQUIPMENT

2–3″ Cast padding (SofRoll, Webril, etc.)

3–4″ Plaster splints or rolls (6–8 sheets/layers)

2–3″ Elastic bandage

PROCEDURAL STEPS

1. Measure from fingertips to just below the elbow.
2. Position the hand with the fingers held at a 50° flexion at the metacarpophalangeal joint and 15–20° flexion at the interphalangeal joint with the wrist in a neutral position (Simon & Brenner, 1982). See Figure 122.1.
3. Apply plaster laterally along the ulna and 5th finger from the distal interphalangeal joints to the proximal forearm creating a "gutter" around the arm.

REFERENCE

Simon, R.R., & Brenner, B.E. 1982. *Procedures and techniques in emergency medicine.* Baltimore: Williams & Wilkins.

SUGGESTED READING

Simon, R.R., & Koenigsknecht, S.J. 1987. *Emergency orthopedics: The extremities.* Norwalk, CT: Appleton & Lange.

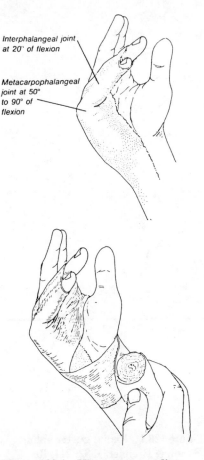

Interphalangeal joint at 20° of flexion

Metacarpophalangeal joint at 50° to 90° of flexion

Figure 122.1 Ulnar gutter splint. (Simon & Brenner, 1982: 211. Reprinted by permission.)

Radial Gutter Splint

Dawn M. Swimm, RN, CEN

Radial gutter splint is also known as phalangeal or metacarpal gutter.

The information in this chapter should be used in conjunction with the information in Ch. 120: General Principles of Plaster Splinting.

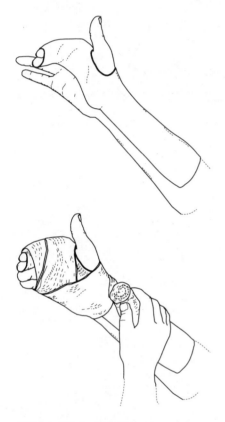

Figure 123.1 Radial gutter splint. (Simon & Brenner, 1982: 211. Reprinted by permission.)

INDICATIONS

Fractures or soft tissue injuries of the 2nd and 3rd fingers.

EQUIPMENT

2–3″ Cast padding (SofRoll, Webril, etc.)
3–4″ Plaster splints or rolls (6–8 sheets/layers)
2–3″ Elastic bandage

PROCEDURAL STEPS

1. Measure from the fingertips to just below the elbow.
2. Cut a hole in the plaster prior to wetting to allow the thumb to protrude and move freely.
3. Position the hand with the fingers held at 50° flexion at the metacarpophalangeal joint and 15–20° flexion at the interphalangeal joint with the wrist in a neutral position (Simon & Brenner, 1982). See Figure 123.1.
4. Apply plaster laterally along the radius and index finger from the distal interphalangeal joints to the proximal forearm creating a "gutter" around the arm.

REFERENCE

Simon, R.R., & Brenner, B.E. 1982. *Procedures and techniques in emergency medicine.* Baltimore: Williams & Wilkins.

SUGGESTED READING

Simon, R.R., & Koenigsknecht, S.J. 1987. *Emergency orthopedics: The extremities.* Norwalk, CT: Appleton & Lange.

124

Thumb Spica

Dawn M. Swimm, RN, CEN

Thumb spica is also known as wrist gauntlet.

The information in this chapter should be used in conjunction with the information in Ch. 120: General Principles of Plaster Splinting.

INDICATIONS

Fractures or soft tissue injuries of the wrist or thumb. Commonly used for navicular (scaphoid) fractures.

EQUIPMENT

2–3″ Cast padding (SofRoll, Webril, etc.)

3–4″ Plaster splints or rolls (8–10 sheets/layers)

3″ Elastic bandage

PROCEDURAL STEPS

1. Measure from the distal tip of the thumb to the midforearm (below elbow allowing flexion, with fingers free allowing full motion of the metacarpophalangeal joints).
2. Position the hand as if the patient is holding a beverage can—(thumb curved toward the fingers, wrist slightly dorsiflexed (Simon & Koenigsknecht, 1987).
3. Apply plaster laterally along the thumb and radial aspect of the forearm. See Figure 124.1.

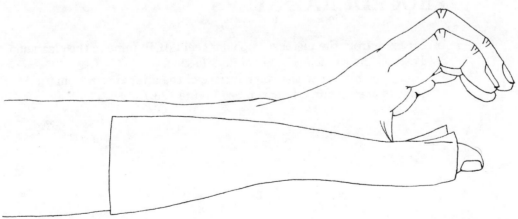

Figure 124.1   Thumb spica.

REFERENCES

Iverson, L.D., & Clawson, D.K. 1982. *Manual of acute orthopedic therapeutics*, 2nd ed. Boston: Little, Brown.

Simon, R.R., & Koenigsknecht, S.J. 1987. *Emergency orthopedics*, S. Norwalk, CT: Appleton & Lange.

Volar Forearm Splint

Dawn M. Swimm, RN, CEN

Volar forearm splint is also known as anterior splint or radial slab.

The information in this chapter should be used in conjunction with the information in Ch. 120: General Principles of Plaster Splinting.

INDICATIONS

Fractures or soft tissue injuries of the wrist.

EQUIPMENT

2–4″ Padding (SofRoll, Webril, etc.)   3–4″ Elastic bandage
3–4″ Plaster splints or rolls (8–10)

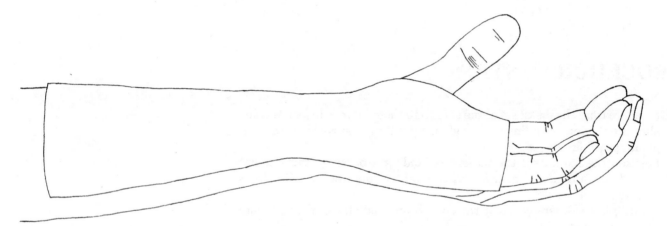

Figure 125.1 Volar forearm splint.

PROCEDURAL STEPS

1. Measure from the metacarpalphalangeal (MCP) joint to the olecranon.
2. Position the wrist in 15–30° of dorsiflexion.
3. Apply the plaster to the volar surface of the injured arm from the MCP joint to the proximal forearm. See Figure 125.1.

126

Sugar Tong Splints: Forearm and Humerus

Dawn M. Swimm, RN, CEN

Sugar tong splints are also known as anterior-posterior splints or sandwich splints.

The information in this chapter should be used in conjunction with the information in Ch. 120: General Principles of Plaster Splinting.

INDICATIONS

Fractures or soft tissue injuries of the forearm and/or the humerus. A forearm sugar tong is most commonly used for distal radius fracture, while the humerus sugar tong is used for initial management of humeral shaft fractures.

EQUIPMENT

3–4″ Cast padding (SofRoll, Webril, etc.)

3–4″ Plaster splints or rolls (8–10 sheets/layers)
3–4″ Elastic bandages

PROCEDURAL STEPS

1. A sugar tong for the forearm requires measurement from the knuckles on the dorsum of the hand over the flexed elbow and on over the volar aspect of the forearm to the midpalmar crease.

   A sugar tong for the humerus requires measurement from the acromion down the humerus encircling the elbow and up to the axilla.
2. Position the forearm in pronation or supination depending on the injury (consult with physician), with 90° flexion of the elbow. See Figure 126.1 for forearm splint and Figure 126.2 for humeral sugar tong.
3. Apply plaster as illustrated in Figure 126.1 or 126.2.

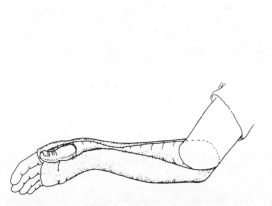

Figure 126.1 Forearm sugar tong splint. (Simon & Brenner, 1987: 224. Reprinted by permission.)

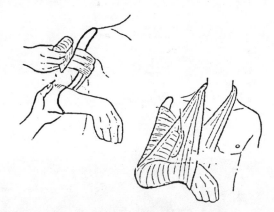

Figure 126.2 Humeral sugar tong splint. (Simon & Brenner, 1982: 217. Reprinted by permission.)

REFERENCES

DePalma, A.F. 1970. *Management of fractures and dislocations.* Philadelphia: Saunders.

Simon, R.R., & Brenner, B.E. 1982. *Procedures & techniques in emergency medicine.* Baltimore: Williams & Wilkins.

SUGGESTED READINGS

Shaw, D.C., & Heckman, J.D. 1984. Principles and techniques of splinting musculocutaneous injuries. *Emergency Medicine Clinics of North America.* 2:391–407.

127

Removal and Bivalving Casts

Dawn M. Swimm, RN, CEN

Bivalving casts is also known as bilateral split.

INDICATIONS

1. To relieve cast pressure resulting in neurovascular impairment.
2. To facilitate care and/or activity when a rigid cast is not needed at all times.
3. To remove a cast when it is no longer required or when a replacement cast is indicated.

CONTRAINDICATIONS AND CAUTIONS

1. Avoid cutting directly over a bony prominence.
2. Cast cutter blades vibrate instead of rotate. Therefore, skin injury is unlikely. However, if excessive pressure is used when cutting the plaster, lacerations or abrasions may occur.

EQUIPMENT

Cover sheet
Cast cutter/saw
Cast spreader
Scissors

Elastic bandages (optional)
Protective eyewear/goggles (to keep plaster dust out the nurse's eyes)

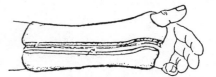

PATIENT PREPARATION

1. Arrange a nonverbal signal so the patient can communicate when excessive heat or pressure is felt. (**Note:** Heat is generated with the movement of the cast blade. A brief pause will relieve the sensation.)
2. Demonstrate the safety of the cutter by touching the blade to your thumb or the stretcher mattress.

PROCEDURAL STEPS

Bivalving

1. Place a sheet under the cast to collect plaster material and cover the patient's clothing.
2. Mark cast lengthwise into two equal parts avoiding bony prominences. (**Note:** Univalving the cast may be sufficient if neurovascular impairment resolves after one side of the cast is cut. See Figure 127.1.
3. Cut with an even up and down motion, releasing when you feel the cutter break through the plaster.

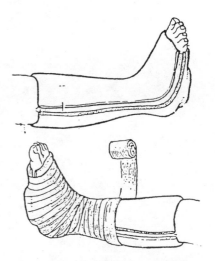

Figure 127.1 a. Split or univalved forearm splint; b. Bivalved lower leg cast; c. Elastic wrapping to bivalved lower leg cast; (DePalma, 1970: 217. Reprinted by permission.)

4. Separate the cast with the cast spreader.
5. Bivalving is now complete. If neurovascular impairment was the indication for the procedure, reassess neurovascular status. If deficits remain, cut the cotton padding to the skin and elevate the extremity. Notify the physician if the neurovascular status does not return to normal.
6. Wrap the cast with an elastic bandage to secure it in place. See Figure 127.1c.

Removal of cast

1. Bivalve cast as directed previously.
2. Separate the cast with the cast spreader.
3. Cut all the way through the padding with scissors.
4. Remove the anterior portion of the cast.
5. Gently remove the posterior portion of the cast while supporting the extremity.
6. Cleanse and dry the skin.
7. Apply splints or other orthopedic devices as ordered by the physician.

COMPLICATIONS

1. Laceration or abrasion of the skin with the cast cutter.
2. Displacement of an unhealed fracture.

PATIENT TEACHING

1. Exercise and weight bearing will be specified by the physician based on the injury and your progress.
2. Continue to use splints, slings, canes, or crutches as directed by the physician.
3. Apply moisturizing lotions if dry skin is a problem. It is normal to have peeling, dry skin where the cast was; this will resolve in a few days.
4. If the cast has been in place several weeks, the muscles in the extremity will probably be smaller. They will gradually return to normal size with exercise.

REFERENCES

DePalma, A.F. 1970. *Management of fractures and dislocations.* Philadelphia: Saunders.

SUGGESTED READINGS

Iverson, L.D., & Clawson, D.K. 1987. *Manual of acute orthopaedic therapeutics,* 3rd ed. Boston: Little, Brown.

128

Skeletal Traction

Linell M. Jones, RN, BSN, CEN, CCRN

Skeletal traction is also known as Steinmann pin, Kirscher wire, K-wire.

INDICATIONS

To maintain alignment of fractured bone ends via continuous pulling on a pin or wire through bone. Skeletal traction may be used when heavier weights and longer periods of immobilization are required than permitted by skin traction (Osborne & DiGiacomo, 1989). It is most frequently used with fractures of the femur, but is also used for fractures of the tibia and humerus.

CONTRAINDICATIONS AND CAUTIONS

Aseptic technique must be maintained to prevent contamination of the pin sites during insertion.

EQUIPMENT

Antiseptic solution
Local anesthetic
#11 Scalpel
Steinmann pin or Kirschner wire
    set (assorted sizes)
    (**Note:** Kirschner wires
    (K-wires) are generally
    smaller in diameter than
    Steinmann pins. Either may
    be smooth or threaded.)
Drill to drive pin
Pin cutter

Cork, tape, or rubber stoppers (such
    as those from blood tubes)
    to place over the cut pin
    ends
Gauze dressings
Antibiotic ointment
Traction bow (Bohler-Steinmann pin
    holder or Kirschner wire
    tractor)
Hospital bed with traction set up
    as indicated
Rope and weights

PATIENT PREPARATION

1. Move the patient onto the hospital bed prior to removal of the temporary splint.
2. Assess and document neurovascular status distal to the injury.

PROCEDURAL STEPS

1. Cleanse the skin at the pin insertion site with antiseptic solution.
2. *Anesthetize the skin, tissue, and periosteum along the intended tract of the pin on both sides.
3. *Make a small incision in the skin at the insertion site in the direction of the pull of traction

*Indicates portions of the procedure usually performed by a physician.

4. *Attach the pin to the drill.
5. *Drive the pin through the bone perpendicular to the long axis of the bone.
6. *Incise the skin over the exit site as it is tented by the exiting pin.
7. *Remove the drill when the pin is sufficiently through the bone to attach the traction bow.
8. *Apply the traction bow and cut off the excess pin.
9. Place cork, tape or rubber stoppers over the cut pin ends.
10. *Attach the rope to the traction bow, run it through the pulley, and attach the weights.
11. *Suspend the extremity as indicated.

   (**Note:** The most common and most versatile traction setup for femur fractures is balanced suspension with Thomas splint and Pearson attachment. The patient is able to move about in bed while the leg remains supported and traction is constant. See Figures 128.1 and 128.2.

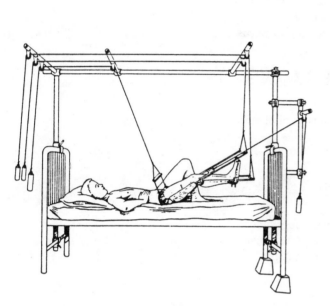

Figure 128.1   Balanced traction.
(Schmeisser, 1963. Reprinted by permission.)

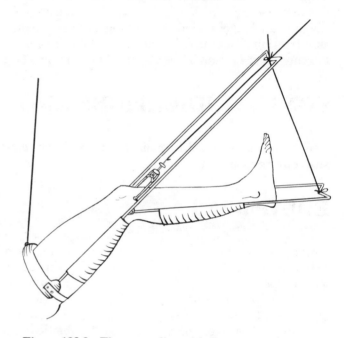

Figure 128.2   Thomas splint with Pearson attachment.
(Schmeisser, 1963. Reprinted by permission.)

12. Assess and document neurovascular status.
13. Pin care as ordered by the physician. Options include:
    a. Gauze dressing around the pin or left uncovered;
    b. With or without antibiotic ointment around the pin entrance and exit;
    c. Pin area cleaned with a specifically ordered solution on a routine basis or not touched (Cardona, 1988).
14. Obtain postreduction x-rays.
15. Secure all rope knots with tape.

COMPLICATIONS

1. Osteomyelitis at the pin insertion site
2. Skin necrosis at the pin site
3. Equipment failure may cause sudden loss of traction and motion of frac-

tured bone ends. Be sure that traction weights hang freely at all times and that knots in traction rope are not caught in the pulleys.

4. Wire or pin migration during insertion or slips after insertion. Both are more common with smooth wires or pins.
5. Compartmental syndrome as a result of excessive traction.

PATIENT TEACHING

1. Do not attempt to adjust traction device. Request help to reposition yourself in bed.
2. Report any signs of infection immediately. These include redness, swelling, increased pain, or pus.
3. Report any signs of compartmental syndrome immediately. These include severe pain, swelling, numbness, or tingling.
4. Report any problems with the pin or traction.

REFERENCES

Cardona, V.D., Hurn, P.D., Mason, P.J.B., Scanlon-Schilpp, A.M., Veise-Berry, S.W. (eds). 1988. *Trauma nursing: From resuscitation through rehabilitation.* Philadelphia: W.B. Saunders.

Osborne, L.J., DiGiacomo, I., 1987. Traction: A review with nursing diagnosis and interventions. *Orthopaedic Nursing,* 6, 4:13–18.

Schmeisser, G. 1963. *A clinical manual of orthopedic traction technique.* Philadelphia: Saunders.

Elastic Bandage Application

Margo E. Layman, RNC, BSN, CEN

Elastic bandage is also known as
Ace wrap.

INDICATIONS

1. To immobilize a fracture in conjunction with a splint.
2. To provide a hemostatic dressing.
3. To anchor dressings and decrease tension on sutures.
4. To provide support, minimize swelling, and prevent further injury in the presence of soft tissue trauma.

CONTRAINDICATIONS AND CAUTIONS

1. Allergy to the sizing in new fabrics.
2. Elastic bandages may decrease peripheral circulation and should be used with caution in the presence of peripheral vascular disease or diabetes.

EQUIPMENT

Elastic bandage (for legs and knees 3–4″ wide; for hands, wrist, and elbows 2–3″ wide)

Tape or pins/clips
Dressings, as indicated
Cast padding (optional)

PATIENT PREPARATION

1. Place the extremity in the position of function. See Ch. 121, 122, 123, 124, 125, and 126 for information on positioning.
2. If possible, before application elevate the extremity for 15–30 minutes to facilitate venous return and help decrease edema.
3. (Optional) Apply 3–4 layers of cast padding under the area to be wrapped. The wrapping configuration is the same as that to be used for the overlying elastic bandage.

PROCEDURAL STEPS

1. Hold the bandage with the roll facing up and anchor the bandage by circling twice around the distal extremity. See Figure 129.1.
2. To assure uniform pressure, unroll the bandage as you wrap the body part. Stretch the bandage only slightly while wrapping.
3. Overlap each layer of the bandage by one-half to two-thirds the width of the bandage.

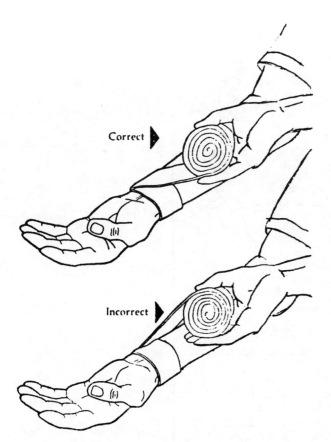

Correct ▶

Incorrect ▶

Figure 129.1 Wrist being wrapped with elastic bandage displaying proper ways to hold bandage and anchor wrap.
(Belland & Wells, 1984: 56. Reprinted by permission.)

4. Wrap firmly but not tightly. You should be able to easily insert a finger under the bandage.
5. Include the wrist when wrapping the hand and the foot when wrapping the ankle.
6. Use a figure-eight wrap on joints. See Figure 129.2. A spiral wrap is used if a joint is not involved. See Figure 129.3.
7. Secure the bandage with tape and/or pins/clips. Do not place pins/clips on posterior or medial surfaces, because they may cause soft tissue injury if pressure is applied to them.
8. Assess and document neurovascular status after bandage application.

COMPLICATIONS

1. Neurovascular impairment or skin irritation may be caused by bandages that are too tight. You should be able to easily insert a finger under the bandage.
2. Distal edema as a result of obstruction of venous return. This can be decreased by including the hand or foot in distal extremity wraps and by elevation of the wrapped extremity.

PATIENT TEACHING

1. Reapply the bandage if it loosens, unless otherwise instructed.
2. Launder the bandage as needed.
3. Watch for numbness, tingling, coldness, swelling, or discoloration of the hand or foot. Loosen the bandage and elevate the extremity if any of

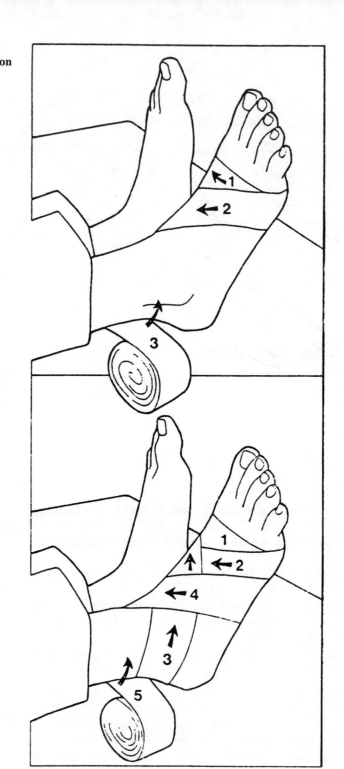

Figure 192.2 Ankle wrapped in a
figure-eight elastic bandage.
(From Belland & Wells, 1984; 57.
Reprinted by permission.)

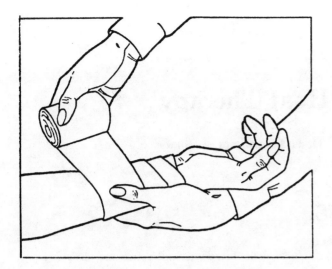

Figure 129.3 Spiral wrap of wrist. (Belland & Wells, 1984; 57. Reprinted by permission.)

these signs or symptoms occur. Report any symptoms not relieved by loosening the bandage or elevating the extremity.

4. Elevate the extremity and apply ice as directed to help prevent and decrease swelling.

SUGGESTED READINGS

Belland, K.H., & Wells, M.A. 1984. *Clinical nursing procedures.* Monterey, CA: Wadsworth.

Guberski, T., & Campbell, M.E. 1970. The effects on leg volume of two methods of wrapping elastic bandage. *Nursing Research,* 19:260–265.

Hamilton, H.K., (ed). 1983. *Procedures.* Springhouse, PA: Springhouse.

130

Heat Therapy

Dawn M. Swimm, RN, CEN

Heat therapy is also known as hot compress, hot pack, warm moist pack.

INDICATIONS

To decrease the pain and stiffness associated with subacute and chronic injuries of soft tissues and joints.

CONTRAINDICATION AND CAUTIONS

1. Heat treatments should be avoided in the patient with severe peripheral vascular disease, venous insufficiency, vasculitis, thromboangiitis obliterans, thrombophlebitis, vasospastic disorders (e.g., Raynaud's), and known sensitivity to heat.
2. Heat treatments should be instituted following the 48-hour acute phase. When started prematurely, increased bleeding and swelling may result and prolong the inflammatory process (Lindsey, 1990).

EQUIPMENT

Hot moist pack
Dry towel
(Note: Moist heat is of greatest benefit. Some dry heating pads can be used in conjunction with a moist pack and there are circulating water heating pads that add the benefit of moist heat and consistent temperature control.)

PROCEDURAL STEPS

1. Place a towel in warm water: 96–103°F, 36–39°C (Lindsey, 1990).
2. Express excess water and place in a dry towel and apply to the injured area. (Note: You may also use a thin plastic wrap to contain the heat and excess moisture.)

COMPLICATIONS

1. Excessive or prolonged heat can burn the skin.
2. Excessive or prolonged contact with the pack can result in maceration of the skin.

Heat treatments applied for 30-minute intervals 2–4 times daily will assist with healing and resumption of normal function. Full trunk and extremity immersion may be used, but do not direct water or air jets toward the injured area for sustained periods, because this can damage tissue.

REFERENCES

Lindsay, B. 1990. Cold and heat applications in musculoskeletal injury. *Journal of Emergency Nursing,* 16:54–57

SUGGESTED READING

Simon, R.R., & Koenigsknecht, S.J. 1987. *Emergency orthopedics: The extremities.* Norwalk, CT: Appleton & Lange.

131

Cold Therapy

Dawn M. Swimm, RN, CEN

Cold therapy is also known as cryotherapy, cold or ice packs.

INDICATIONS

To decrease the edema and pain associated with fractures, soft tissue injuries, sprains, and strains.

CONTRAINDICATIONS AND CAUTIONS

Avoid cryotherapy in patients with a history of severe peripheral vascular disease, venous insufficiency, vasculitis, thromboangiitis obliterans, thrombophlebitis, vasospastic disorders (e.g., Raynaud's), and known sensitivity to cold.

EQUIPMENT

Ice
Ice bag
Cover/towel
(**Note:** Commercial chemical cold packs, or gel packs are also available. Chemical packs should not be used on the face, because puncture of the bag may result in chemical injury to the eyes.)

PROCEDURAL STEPS

1. Place cubed or crushed ice in a container or towel.
2. Wrap in dry towel or icebag cover and apply to injury.
3. Cold packs should be applied for a period of 20 minutes, to reach a skin temperature of 68°F or 20°C (Lindsey, 1990).

COMPLICATIONS

1. Excessive cold or prolonged cold treatments can result in frostbite and vascular damage.
2. Ice bags should have a dry interface with the skin to decrease the risk of damage to the skin.

PATIENT TEACHING

Cold treatment administered for 20 minutes four times daily in conjunction with rest and elevation will assist with lessening pain and edema. The effective period for this treatment is the 48 hours immediately following injury. Complete extremity immersion can be done with caution, limit the exposure time and elevate after therapy.

REFERENCES

Lindsey, B. 1990. Cold and heat application in musculoskeletal injuries. *Journal of Emergency Nursing,* 16:54–57.

SUGGESTED READING

Simon, R.R., & Koenigsknecht, S.J. 1987. *Emergency orthopedics: The extremities.* Norwalk, CT: Appleton & Lange

132

Measuring Compartmental Pressure

Jean A. Proehl, RN, MN, CEN, CCRN

Jean A. Proehl, RN, MN, CEN, CCRN

Compartmental pressure is also known as compartment pressure, intracompartmental pressure, tissue pressure.

Technique A is also known as Whitesides technique;

Technique B is also known as Stryker S.T.I.C.

INDICATIONS

To measure tissue pressure when compartmental syndrome is suspected. Etiologies of compartmental syndrome include, but are not limited to fractures, soft tissue or vascular trauma, crush injuries, exercise, envenomations, tight casts or circumferential dressings, pneumatic antishock garments, automatic blood pressure devices, and burns (Barnes, 1985; Kuska, 1982; Matsen, 1980; Proehl, 1988; Schwartz, 1989).

CONTRAINDICATIONS AND CAUTIONS

1. When compartmental syndrome is clinically evident, there is no need to measure compartmental pressures and the patient should proceed immediately to the operating room for decompression via fasciotomy.
2. Avoid inserting the needle or catheter through infected or contaminated tissue.
3. Insert the needle or catheter as far away from fractured bone ends as possible to prevent conversion of a closed fracture to an open fracture (Allen, 1985).

PATIENT PREPARATION

1. Remove circumferential dressings or casts. See Ch. 127: Removal and Bivalving Casts.
2. Keep the extremity at the level of the heart (**not** elevated) to optimize blood flow to the tissues until compartmental syndrome has been ruled out (Matsen, 1980; Proehl, 1988).
3. Treat systemic hypotension with fluids and/or medications to sustain tissue perfusion (Matsen, 1980; Proehl, 1988).
4. Cleanse the skin overlying the insertion site with antiseptic solution. Multiple insertion sites may be used to measure pressures in different compartments of the same extremity. See Figures 132.1 and 132.2.
5. *Infiltrate the insertion site with local anesthetic (optional). **Note:** This procedure should be no more painful than an intramuscular injection, therefore, local anesthetic is not always necessary or helpful. If local anesthetic is used, care should be taken to infiltrate only the skin, because injection of additional fluid into the compartment could increase the tissue pressure (Whitesides, 1975).
6. Instruct the patient to keep the extremity relaxed during pressure measurements, because movement will cause the pressure to change (Barnes et al., 1985).

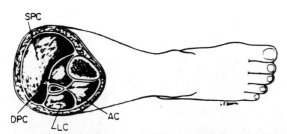

Four compartments of the leg: the anterior compartment (AC), the lateral compartment (LC), the superficial posterior compartment (SPC), and the deep posterior compartment (DPC).

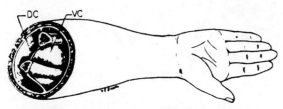

Two compartments of the forearm: the volar compartment (VC) and the dorsal compartment (DC).

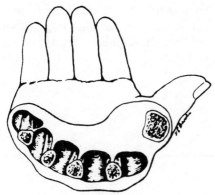

Five interosseous compartments of the hand.

Figure 132.1 Compartments of the lower leg, forearm, and hand. (Matsen, 1980: 82. Reprinted by permission.)

EQUIPMENT FOR TECHNIQUE A

(Whitesides et al., 1975)

Antiseptic solution
Gauze dressings
Local anesthetic, 19 and 27 gauge
    needles, 5-ml syringe
    (optional)
3-way stopcock

2 IV extension tubing sets
30-ml vial of sterile saline for
    injection
20-ml syringe
18 or 19 gauge needles
Mercury manometer

PROCEDURAL STEPS FOR TECHNIQUE A

1. Connect one IV extension set to a side port of the stopcock. Connect an 18 or 19 gauge needle to the distal end of the tubing.
2. Aspirate 15 ml of air into the 20-ml syringe and attach the syringe to the middle stopcock port.

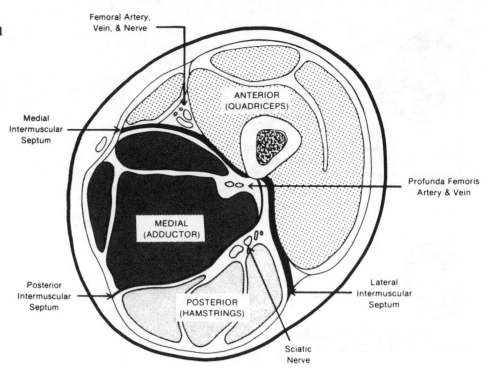

Femoral Artery,
Vein, & Nerve

ANTERIOR
(QUADRICEPS)

Medial
Intermuscular
Septum

Profunda Femoris
Artery & Vein

MEDIAL
(ADDUCTOR)

Posterior
Intermuscular
Septum

POSTERIOR
(HAMSTRINGS)

Lateral
Intermuscular
Septum

Sciatic
Nerve

**Figure 132.2   Compartments of the
thigh.**
(Schwartz, 1989: 394. Reprinted by
permission.)

3.   Insert the needle into the saline vial and inject 1–2 ml of air from the
syringe into the vial. Withdraw saline until the extension tubing is approximately half-filled. It is important that the saline meniscus be easily
visible within the tubing. See Figure 132.3.

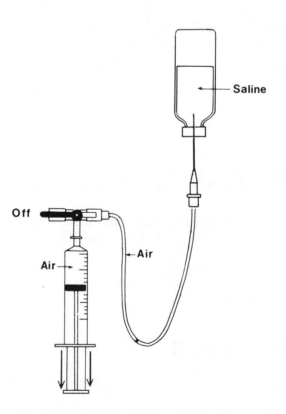

Saline

Off

Air

Air

**Figure 132.3   Fluid meniscus in IV
extension tubing.**
(Kuska, 1982: 77. Reprinted by permission.)

4.   Connect the other IV extension set to the remaining stopcock port. Connect the distal end of the tubing to the mercury manometer. See Figure
132.4.

5.   *Insert the needle into the compartment and open the stopcock so that
all ports are open. See Figure 132.4.

*Indicates portions of the procedure
usually performed by a physician.

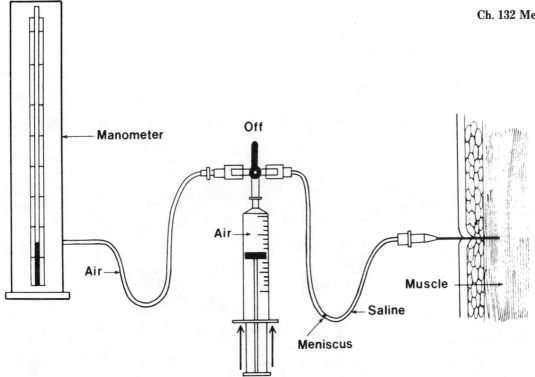

**Figure 132.4   Needle insertion into
the muscle and tissue pressure measurement.
(Kuska, 1982: 78. Reprinted by permission.)**

6.   *Push **gently** on the plunger of the syringe while watching the fluid meniscus and the manometer. (It is helpful to have one person to watch the
meniscus and another to watch the manometer.)

7.   Document the pressure at which the meniscus flattens. Repeat steps 5
through 7 as needed to verify reading.

8.   Change needles and repeat steps 5 through 7 for other compartments.

9.   Tissue pressure is normally 20 mm Hg or less (Whitesides et al., 1975).
Follow-up monitoring is indicated if tissue pressures are between 20–30
mm Hg. Pressures in excess of 30–40 mm Hg in the presence of positive
clinical findings suggest the need for decompression of the compartment
via fasciotomy (Matsen, 1980; Rorabeck, 1984). Metabolically, the difference between mean arterial pressure (MAP) and compartment pressure
may be more important than compartment pressure alone. Research has
indicated that lowest pressure difference normal tissue can withstand is
30 mm Hg (MAP − compartment pressure). However, moderately traumatized tissue can only withstand a minimum pressure difference of 40
mm Hg (Heppenstall, 1986).

EQUIPMENT FOR TECHNIQUE B

Antiseptic solution
Gauze dressings
Local anesthetic
19 and 27 gauge needles
5-ml syringe (optional)
Intracompartmental pressure
     monitor (Stryker,
     Kalamazoo, MI)

Needle, transducer, and syringe
     assembly supplied by
     manufacturer
(**Note:** Through-the-needle slit
     catheters are also available
     for continuous pressure
     monitoring with this unit.)

PROCEDURAL STEPS FOR TECHNIQUE B

1. Turn the pressure monitor on. The pressure should read between 0 and 9 mm Hg (Stryker, 1989).
2. Assemble the needle, transducer, and syringe and place into the pressure monitor with the black side of the transducer down. See Figure 132.5.

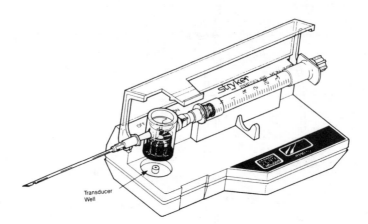

Figure 132.5 Place the needle, transducer, and syringe assembly into the pressure monitor with the black surface of the transducer down in the transducer well. (Stryker Surgical, 1989: 4. Reprinted by permission.)

3. Close the cover of the pressure monitor until latch snaps.
4. Remove the clear end cap of the syringe and attach the plunger to the syringe.
5. Hold the monitor at a 45° angle with needle upright and push on the plunger to purge the unit of air. **Do not** allow fluid to flow back into the transducer well.
6. *Hold the monitor at the intended angle of insertion into the skin, press and release the zero button. The digital display should read 00 after a few seconds. The display must read 00 before continuing. See Figure 132.6.

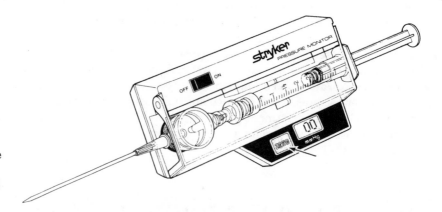

Figure 132.6 Zero the pressure monitor prior to inserting the needle into the compartment. (Stryker Surgical, 1989: 4. Reprinted by permission.)

7. *Insert the needle into the compartment. Slowly inject less than 0.3 ml of saline into the compartment to equilibrate the monitor with the interstitial fluids (Stryker, 1989).
8. Wait for the digital display to reach equilibrium and note the pressure. For additional readings repeat steps 8 and 9.
9. Tissue pressure is normally 20 mm Hg or less (Whitesides, 1975). Follow-up monitoring is indicated if tissue pressures are between 20–30 mm Hg. Pressures in excess of 30–40 mm Hg in the presence of positive clinical

findings suggest the need for decompression of the compartment via fasciotomy (Matsen, 1980; Rorabeck, 1984). Metabolically, the difference between mean arterial pressure (MAP) and compartment pressure may be more important than compartment pressure alone. Research has indicated that lowest pressure difference normal tissue can withstand is 30 mm Hg (MAP − compartment pressure). However, moderately traumatized tissue can only withstand a minimum pressure difference of 40 mm Hg (Heppenstall, 1986).

(Note: Other equipment setups may include pressure monitoring systems of the type used for arterial lines, continuous infusion devices, and wick or slit catheters. The techniques presented here are the most easily implemented in the emergency department setting, but are not be suitable for continuous pressure monitoring. Several sources provide information on other monitoring setups (Barnes, 1985; Larson, 1986; Matsen, 1980; McDermott, 1983; Russell, 1985; Stryker, 1989).

COMPLICATIONS

1. Inaccurate pressures will be obtained if the needle is inserted into a tendon or occluded with tissue (Kuska, 1982; Whitesides et al., 1975). Needle function can be tested by squeezing the extremity; immediate pressure fluctuations should be noted if the needle is patent (Barnes, 1985; Larson, 1986; Russell, 1985).
2. Infection (late)

PATIENT TEACHING

1. Report the following symptoms immediately:
      pain of increasing severity;
      pain that does not respond to prescribed pain medications;
      pain on passive movement;
      numbness or tingling;
      weakness;
      tenseness of the injured extremity in comparison to the noninjured
         extremity;
      pallor, mottling, cyanosis, or coldness of the extremity.
2. Position the injured extremity as instructed. (Note: If an early compartmental syndrome is suspected, the patient will be instructed to keep the extremity at the level of the heart to optimize blood flow to the tissue.)

REFERENCES

Allen, M.J., Stirling, A.J., Crawshaw, C.V., & Barnes, M.R. 1985. Intracompartmental pressure monitoring of leg injuries. *Journal of Bone & Joint Surgery*, 67B:53–57.

Barnes, M.R., Gibson, M.J., Scott, J., Bentley, S., & Allen, M.J. 1985. A technique for the long term measurement of intra-compartmental pressure in the lower leg. *Journal of Biomedical Engineering*, 7:35–39.

Heppenstall, R.B., Sapega, A.A., Scott, R., Shenton, D., Park, Y.S., Maris, J., & Chance, B. 1986. The compartment syndrome: An experimental and clinical study of muscular energy metabolism using phosphorus nuclear magnetic resonance spectroscopy. *Clinical Orthopedics and Related Research*, 226:138–155.

Kuska, B.M. 1982. Acute onset of compartment syndrome. *Journal of Emergency Nursing*, 8, 2:75–79.

Larson, M., Leigh, J., & Wilson, L.R. 1986. Detecting compartmental syndrome using continuous pressure monitoring. *Focus on Critical Care*, 13, 5:51-56.

Matsen, F.A., III. 1980. *Compartmental syndromes*. New York: Grune & Stratton.

McDermott, A.G.P., Marble, A.E., & Yabsley, R.H. 1984. Monitoring acute compartment pressures with the S.T.I.C. catheter. *Clinical Orthopedics and Related Research*, 190:192-198.

Proehl, J.A. 1988. Compartment syndrome. *Journal of Emergency Nursing*, 14:283-292.

Rorabeck, C.H. 1984. The treatment of compartment syndromes of the leg. *Journal of Bone and Joint Surgery*, 66B:93-97.

Russell, W.L., Apyan, P.M. & Burns, R.P. 1985. An electronic technique for compartment pressure measurement using the wick catheter. *Surgery, Gynecology, & Obstetrics*, 161:173-175.

Schwartz, J.T., Jr., Brumback, R.J., Lakatos, R., Poka, A., Bathon, G.H., & Burgess, A.R. 1989. Acute compartment syndrome of the thigh: A spectrum of injury. *Journal of Bone and Joint Surgery*, 71A:394.

Stryker Surgical 1989. 295 Intra-compartmental pressure monitor system: *Maintenance manual and operating instructions*. Kalamazoo, MI: Stryker.

Whitesides, T.E., Jr., Haney, T.C., Morimoto, K., & Harada, H. 1975. Tissue pressure measurements as a determinant for the need of fasciotomy. *Clinical Orthopedics and Related Research*, 113:43-51.

133

Measuring for Crutches

Dawn M. Swimm, RN, CEN

INDICATIONS

Inability to bear weight on a lower extremity requiring use of crutches.

CONTRAINDICATIONS AND CAUTIONS

The energy consumption associated with nonweight bearing crutch walking is substantial. Elderly, debilitated, or sedentary patients could be at risk for severe exercise challenge and pronounced fatigue (Walters, 1987).

EQUIPMENT

Measuring tape   Adjustable crutches

PROCEDURAL STEPS

Standing measurement

1. With the patient balancing on the unaffected extremity, measure from 3.75–5.0 cm, 1.5–2.0 in.) below the axillary fold to a point on the floor 10 cm (4 in.) in front of the patient and 15 cm (6 in.) laterally from the small toe (Schoen, 1986; Bruno, 1984).
2. Crutch tips should be 10 cm (4 in.) in front and 15 cm (6 in.) to the side of the lower extremities. See Figure 133.1.
3. There should be two finger breadths of space between the axillary fold and the armpiece of the crutch.
4. With the patient erect, shoulders and back straight, there should be a 30° flexion of the elbow when the hands are gripping the handbars.

Bed Measurement

1. While the patient is supine in bed, measure from the anterior fold of the axilla to the sole of the foot and add 5 cm (2 in.).
2. Once the patient is measured, have him stand and assume a tripod position with crutches under each arm and unaffected extremity bearing weight.
3. Crutch tips should be 10 cm (4 in.) in front and 15 cm (6 in.) to the side of the lower extremities. See Figure 133.1.
4. There should be two finger breadths of space between the axillary fold and the armpiece of the crutch.
5. With the patient erect, shoulders and back straight, there should be a 30° flexion of the elbow when the hands are gripping the handbars.

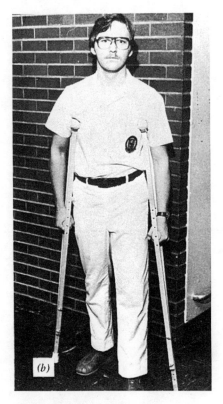

Figure 133.1 Standing measurement position for crutches. (Mourad & Droste, 1988: 438. Reprinted by permission.)

443

COMPLICATIONS

If bearing weight is inappropriately applied to the axilla, damage to the brachial plexus can occur.

REFERENCES

Bruno, J. 1984. Some considerations and guidelines for crutch walking. *Clinics in Podiatry,* 1:291–294.

Mourad, L., & Droste, M. 1988. *The nursing process in the care of adults with orthopaedic conditions,* 2nd ed. New York: Wiley, 438.

Schoen, D.C. 1986. *The Nursing Process in Orthopaedics.* Norwalk, CT: Appleton-Century-Crofts.

Walters, R.L., Campbell, J., & Perry, J. 1987. Energy cost of three point crutch ambulation in fracture patients. *Journal of Orthopedic Trauma,* 1:170–173.

134

Teaching Crutch Walking

Dawn M. Swimm, RN, CEN

INDICATIONS

To facilitate unilateral, nonweight-bearing ambulation.

CONTRAINDICATIONS AND CAUTIONS

The energy consumption associated with nonweight-bearing crutch walking is considerable. Elderly, debilitated, or sedentary patients could be at risk for severe exercise challenge and pronounced fatigue. The three point gait requires the most strength and balance (Waters, 1987).

PATIENT PREPARATION

Measure and adjust the crutches to the proper size. See Ch. 133: Measuring for Crutches.

PROCEDURAL STEPS

1. Begin in tripod position, balanced on unaffected leg with crutches on either side of body.
2. Simultaneously move the affected leg and crutches forward. Bear your weight on the palms at the handgrips, not the underarm pads/axillary bar. Straighten and lock your elbow to increase endurance. Look forward, not at your feet.
3. Move the unaffected leg forward and through to a position slightly ahead of the crutches. See Figure 134.1.
4. To go up stairs, hold both crutches in the hand opposite the handrail. Push down on the crutches and the handrail while stepping up with the affected leg. Straighten your back and lift the crutches and affected leg up to the same step. See Figure 134.2.
5. To go down stairs, hold both crutches in the hand opposite the handrail. Bend the unaffected leg (to assist with balance) and lower both crutches and the affected leg one step. Leaning on the crutches and the handrail, step down to the same step with the unaffected leg (Bruno, 1984).
6. If there are no handrails, bend the unaffected leg (to assist with balance) and lower both of the crutches and the affected leg to the step. See Figure 134.3.

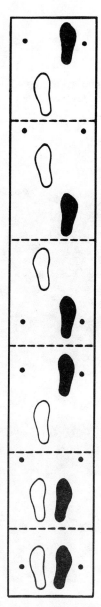

Figure 134.1 Diagram of foot and crutch position for the three-point nonweight-bearing gait. (From Kitt & Kaiser, 1990: 382. Reprinted by permission.)

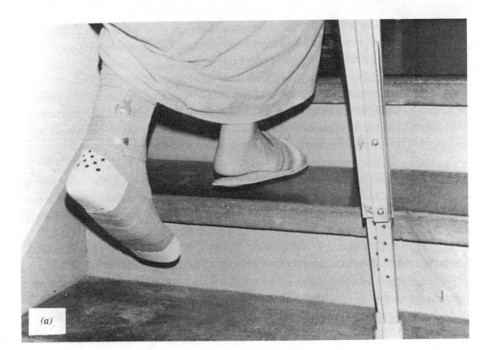

Figure 134.2 Patient walking up the stairs with both crutches in one hand.
(Mourad & Droste, 1988: 439. Reprinted by permission.)

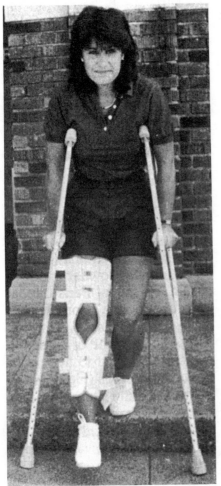

Figure 134.3 Patient descending a step without the aid of a rail.
(Luckmann & Sorensen, 1987: 1501. Reprinted by permission.)

PATIENT TEACHING

1. Wear sturdy, low-heeled shoes
2. Remove trip hazards such as throw rugs, toys, etc. from the walking environment.
3. Be extremely cautious when taking medications or alcohol, because perception and judgment will be affected.

COMPLICATIONS

If weight bearing is inappropriately placed with pressure to the axilla, damage to the brachial plexus can occur. Crutch walking takes skill and practice. Falls, with the potential for additional injury, are not uncommon.

REFERENCES

Bruno, J. 1984. Some considerations and guidelines for crutch walking. *Clinics in Podiatry*, 1: 291–294.

Kitt, S., & Kaiser, J. 1990. *Emergency nursing: A physiological and clinical perspective*. Philadelphia: Saunders.

Luckmann, J., & Sorensen, K.C. 1987. *Medical-surgical nursing: A psychophysiologic approach*, 3rd ed. Philadelphia: Saunders.

Mourad, L.A., & Droste, M.M. 1988. *The nursing process in the care of adults with orthopaedic conditions*, 2nd ed. New York: Wiley.

Walters, R.L., Campbell, J., & Perry, J. 1987. Energy costs of three-point crutch ambulation in fracture patients. *Journal of Orthopedic Trauma*, 1:170–173.

SUGGESTED READINGS

Oliver, M. 1983. Have crutch will travel. *American Journal of Nursing*, 15, 2:73–75.

135

Arthrocentesis/Intra-articular Injection

Jean A. Proehl, RN, MN, CEN, CCRN

Arthrocentesis is also known as joint aspiration, joint tap.

INDICATIONS

1. To relieve the pain and distention associated with intra-articular fluid accumulation.
2. To determine the etiology of acute joint swelling. Joint swelling may be due to traumatic, gouty, infectious, or rheumatoid arthritis (Simon & Brenner, 1987).
3. To inject medications, usually steroids, into the joint space.

CONTRAINDICATIONS AND CAUTIONS

1. Local cellulitis overlying the joint and bacteremia are relative contraindications.
2. Caution should be exercised with patients who have bleeding disorders or who are on anticoagulant medications (Wolf, 1978).

EQUIPMENT

Antiseptic solution
Gauze dressings
Local or topical anesthetic
Syringes and needles for local
    anesthesia administration
Sterile towels or drapes
20-ml syringe

20-gauge 1 1/2″ needle
Elastic bandage (optional)
Sample tubes for laboratory
    specimens, as indicated
Medications for intraarticular
    injection, as ordered

PROCEDURAL STEPS

1. Cleanse the skin at the puncture site with an antiseptic solution. The needle is usually introduced on the extensor surface of the joint to decrease the risk of neurovascular injury (Simon & Brenner, 1987; Suruda, 1988). Also, the synovial pouch is closer to the skin on the extensor surface (Simon & Brenner, 1987).
2. *Anesthetize the skin at the puncture site.
3. Position the joint. Placing the joint in 20–30° of flexion and gently applying longitudinal traction to the bone distal to the joint will help to open the joint space (Simon & Brenner, 1987).
4. *Insert the needle into the joint space and aspirate until synovial fluid is obtained. See Figure 135.1.
5. For removal of synovial fluid,
   a. Apply manual pressure to the opposite side of the joint to help force

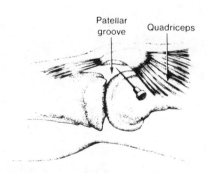

Figure 135.1 Arthrocentesis of the knee.
(Simon & Brenner, 1987: 201. Reprinted by permission.)

*Indicates portions of the procedure usually performed by a physician.

fluid over to the needle (Suruda, 1988). The joint may also be wrapped with an elastic bandage, leaving the puncture site exposed, to help compress the fluid into the puncture area (Berkowitz, 1983; Simon & Brenner, 1987).

b. *Aspirate all readily accessible fluid (Simon & Brenner, 1987).

c. Place fluid in appropriate specimen containers to send to the laboratory. Commonly performed laboratory tests include viscosity, cell count, mucin clot, protein, glucose, culture, and gram stain. Synovial fluid requires special handling; package per laboratory protocol.

6. For injection of medications,

a. *Taking care not to displace the needle, remove the syringe from the needle and attach the syringe containing the medication (Berkowitz, 1983).

b. *Inject the medication into the joint space.

7. *Remove the needle.

8. Apply direct pressure to the puncture site for 2 minutes and then apply a sterile dressing.

9. Apply an elastic bandage to help stabilize the joint if a large amount of fluid was aspirated (Berkowitz, 1983). See Ch. 129: Elastic Bandage Application.

COMPLICATIONS

1. Joint infection. This is a rare occurrence if the skin has been properly cleansed (Wolf, 1978).

2. Hemarthrosis as a result of bleeding into the joint.

PATIENT TEACHING

1. Report any fever, increased pain, redness, or recurrent swelling, which could indicate infection.

2. Avoid excessive use of the joint for the next few days.

3. Apply ice to the joint and elevate it above the level of your heart to help prevent recurrent swelling.

4. Change dressings as indicated if the joint is draining.

5. Wear the elastic bandage as instructed to help stabilize the joint.

REFERENCES

Berkowitz, D.M. 1983. Synovial fluid analysis. *Nursing,* 13, 5:24AA–24OO.

Suruda, A.J. 1988. Arthritis. In P. Rosen, F.J. Baker, II, R.M. Barkin, G.R. Braen, R.H. Dailey, & R.C. Levy (eds). *Emergency medicine: Concepts and clinical practice,* 2nd ed. St. Louis: Mosby; 1685–1702.

Simon, R.R., & Brenner, B.E. 1987. *Emergency procedures and techniques,* 2nd ed. Baltimore: Williams & Wilkins.

Wolf, A.W., Benson, D.R., Shoji, H., Riggins, R.S., Shapiro, R.F., Castles, J.J., & Wild, J. 1978. Current concepts in synovial fluid analysis. *Clinical Orthopedics and Related Research,* 134:261–265.

136

Wound Cleansing and Irrigation

Christine A. Miller, RN, MS

Wound cleansing and irrigation is also known as wound prep.

INDICATIONS

1. To cleanse any disruption in skin integrity.
2. To cleanse the skin prior to incision and drainage, invasive procedures, and removal of foreign bodies.

CONTRAINDICATIONS AND CAUTIONS

1. Injuries that require special care include

   Eyelids: Assess the eye itself for trauma and check visual acuity. Suturing of the eyelid may require specialty consultation.

   Neck: Wounds of the neck can appear superficial. Care should be taken not to underestimate a penetrating injury that could quickly compromise the patient's airway.

   Spray gun injuries: Extensive tissue destruction may be present in spite of a benign-appearing entrance wound. Injected chemicals or embedded foreign bodies may necessitate surgical exploration.

   Scalp: Lacerations may disguise skull fractures and the patient may lose a significant amount of blood because of the scalp's extensive vascularity. The extent of a scalp laceration can be easily overlooked because of hair matting, the patient lying supine on a backboard, etc.

   Crush or avulsion injuries: Wounds with extensive tissue damage or loss of tissue are at increased risk for infection and delayed healing.

   Tendon and nerve injuries: Injuries involving nerves and tendons may result in permanent disability.

   Facial: Meticulous care of facial wounds is required for optimal cosmetic results.

   Hand: Impairment of hand function, especially the dominant hand, may result in permanent disability.

   Associated fractures: Open fractures are at high risk for infection. Specialty consultation is indicated.
2. Puncture wounds require special evaluation. The type and condition (e.g., rusty or dirty) of the penetrating object is important. If the puncture occurred through clothing or a shoe, a foreign body should be suspected.
3. Soaking macerates the skin. There is no evidence that it is of any benefit (Verdile, 1987).
4. Excessive scrubbing and powerful irrigation can damage healthy tissue.
5. Wound cleansing agents:

   Hydrogen peroxide should be used with caution. It is painful and ineffective against anaerobes, absorbs oxygen in the wound and destroys cells. If used, it should always be diluted with equal parts normal saline (Westaby, 1982).

Povodine-iodine solutions effectively kill gram positive and negative rods, bacilli, fungi, viruses, protozoa, and yeast. They can also harm healthy tissue and cause burning and allergic reactions. Diluted solutions (1%) appear safe (Humphreys & Barthel, 1983; Gravett, 1987; Simon, 1988).

Nontoxic agents such as *pluronic F-68 (Shur Clens)* are nontoxic to open wounds and eyes. They appear to be safe and effective but have no antimicrobial activity (Simon, 1988).

A *baby shampoo scrub* of facial lacerations provides gentle cleansing of fragile tissue but is nonsterile and is not antimicrobial.

EQUIPMENT

Wound cleansing agent (See Cautions.)
Sterile sponges or gauze dressings
Cotton swabs
Sterile drapes or towels
For wound irrigation: 16- or 18-gauge needle or plastic cannula, sterile basin and normal saline or other irrigating agents of choice (See Cautions.)
For contaminated wounds and wounds with embedded

foreign bodies: sterile toothbrush or surgical brush, #11 blade, Adson forceps
For tar wounds: petroleum jelly, topical antibiotic ointment, or mineral oil
(**Note:** Commercial kits are available that contain gloves, drapes, sponges, cotton swabs, and cleansing agents.)

PATIENT PREPARATION

1. Obtain a history including time of injury, mechanism of injury, location and extent of injury, and the potential for the wound to be contaminated with soil or dirt.

    If it is a missile injury (e.g., gunshot wound) or puncture (e.g., nail through a shoe), assess for foreign objects such as clothing or missile fragments.
2. Assess and document neurovascular status. Assess for adjacent bony injury and/or open fractures. Suspect damage to muscle and tendons if deep fascia is involved.
3. Obtain radiologic studies to rule out presence of foreign bodies, fractures, and air in a joint space.
4. Anesthetize the area as indicated. See Ch. 137: Local Infiltration and Topical Agents, Ch. 138: Digital Block, and Ch. 138: Bier Block.
5. Drape the patient to protect clothing if extensive irrigation is planned.

PROCEDURAL STEPS

*Indicates portion of procedure usually performed by a physician.

1. Maintain hemostasis by direct pressure. *Clamping and ligation of vessels may also be necessary. A pneumatic tourniquet or blood pressure cuff may also be used to help control bleeding during wound cleansing and repair, if ordered by a physician.
2. Shaving is not usually indicated. Skin nicks can increase the chance of infection. If necessary, clip hair close to a wound edge (Edlich, 1988). Never shave eyebrows, because realignment is difficult without anatomical landmarks.

3. Wound cleansing is begun using sponges or brushes and a cleansing agent. The prep should start at the wound and move distally encompassing a large area of skin surrounding the wound. For example, when cleaning a hand laceration, prep the hand and arm to the elbow. Continue cleansing until the wound appears clean.

4. Wounds that are contaminated or those containing foreign bodies must be irrigated. Wound irrigation helps to remove foreign bodies and also dilutes bacteria. To be effective, high pressure irrigation is necessary and can be accomplished with an 18-gauge needle or plastic cannula and a 35-cc syringe (Simon & Brenner, 1987). See Figure 136.1. Other options include a needle attached to a pressurized IV bag/tubing or a commercially available irrigation setup. Normal saline or diluted provodine-iodine solution can be used. One guide for adequate irrigation is the Kirz rule: irrigate with 50-cc normal saline per inch of wound per hour of age of wound (Lanros, 1988). Low-pressure irrigation (i.e., with a bulb syringe) is not effective.

5. Abrasions with embedded foreign bodies require careful wound preparation to remove the foreign bodies and prevent traumatic tattooing. Surgical scrub brushes, sterile toothbrushes, forceps, and the point of a #11 blade can be used for foreign body removal (Simon & Brenner, 1987). See Figure 136.2.

6. Tar removal is facilitated by use of petroleum jelly, antibiotic ointment, or mineral oil. After application, allow tar to dissolve for 10–15 minutes prior to attempting removal. Repeat applications may be necessary.

Figure 136.1 Irrigation of a wound. An 18-gauge needle or plastic cannula attached to a 35-cc syringe is ideal for providing proper irrigation pressures.
(Simon & Brenner, 1987: 289. Reprinted by permission.)

COMPLICATIONS

1. Infection, including cellulitis, soft tissue abscess, or osteomyelitis is higher with wounds to the hands and feet (due to poor circulation), with dirty wounds, and with old wounds (bacterial growth begins in wounds after 3 hours) (Edlich, 1986).

2. Medications such as steroids and hormones may impair wound healing (Simon & Brenner, 1987).

3. Other medical conditions may impair wound healing. Diabetics, patients with infection, associated trauma, hypoxia, uremia, circulatory impairment, and the elderly are all at increased risk for infection and delayed healing (Simon & Brenner, 1987).

PATIENT TEACHING

1. High-risk patients should return for wound evaluation and dressing change in 24–48 hours.

2. Keep the wound dry. Change wet dressings as soon as possible.

3. Clean the wound 4 times a day with 1/2 strength hydrogen peroxide or mild soapy water. Remove crusted material gently with cotton swabs. Use a light layer of topical antibiotic ointment after wound care prior to dressing application.

4. Report bleeding, a wound that reopens, signs of circulatory compromise, or signs of infection such as wound edge tenderness, redness. Some erythema occurs at wound edges with normal healing or wound drainage (Verdile, 1987).

5. Elevate the injured area as much as possible.

6. Avoid exposing new wounds to the sun for 6 months. Permanent hyperpigmentation may result (Edlich et al., 1988). Sunblock is advisable, especially for facial wounds.

Figure 136.2 Removal of embedded particles from a traumatic abrasion with a sterile toothbrush. The tip of a #11 blade can be used to remove deeply embedded or larger particles. (Simon & Brenner, 1987: 289. Reprinted by permission.)

REFERENCES

Edlich, R., Kenney, J., Morgan, R., Nichter, L., Freidman, H., & Rodeheaver, G., 1986. Antimicrobial treatment of minor soft tissue lacerations: A critical review. *Emergency Medicine Clinics of North America,* 4:561–580.

Gravatt, A., Sterner, S., Clinton, J., & Ruiz, E. 1987. A trial of povodine-iodine in the prevention of infection in sutured lacerations. *Annals of Emergency Medicine,* 16:167–171.

Humphreys, P., & Barthel, C. 1983. Power spray cleaning for those hard-to-clean wounds. *Nursing,* 13:42–43.

Lanros, N. 1988. *Assessment and Intervention in Emergency Nursing,* 3rd ed. S. Norwalk, CT: Appleton & Lange.

Simon, B. 1988. Treatment of wounds. In Rosen, P., Baker, T., Barkin, R., Braen, G., Dailey, R., Levy, R. *Emergency Medicine: Concepts and Clinical Practice,* 2nd ed. St. Louis: Mosby; 363–373.

Simon, R., & Brenner, B.E. 1987. *Emergency Procedures and Techniques,* 2nd ed. Baltimore: Williams & Wilkins.

Verdile, V., Freed, H., Gerard, J. 1989. Puncture wounds to the foot. *Emergency Medicine in Review,* 7:193–199.

Westaby, S. 1982. Wound Care: No 6 – wound closure. *Nursing Times,* 78:21–24.

SUGGESTED READINGS

Humby, M. 1988. Suturing and wound care. *The Practitioner,* 232:247–252.

Trott, A., DeChatelet, J., & Levy, R., 1982. Suture and wound training program for emergency nurses. *Journal of Emergency Nursing,* 8:221–224.

137

Wound Anesthesia: Local Infiltration and Topical Agents

Christine A. Miller, RN, MS

INDICATIONS

To provide local anesthesia prior to
1. suturing a laceration,
2. removing an imbedded foreign body,
3. incision and drainage of an abscess,
4. invasive procedures (chest tube insertion, lumbar puncture, endotracheal intubation, etc.),
5. wound debridement and cleansing,
6. insertion of nasal packing or nasal tubes.

CONTRAINDICATIONS AND CAUTIONS

1. Known sensitivity or history of allergic reaction to local anesthetics.
2. The use of agents containing epinephrine may be contraindicated in patients with known peripheral vascular disease. Because of epinephrine's vasoconstrictive action, it may delay healing and increase the patient's risk of infection.
3. The use of epinephrine may be helpful in vascular areas (i.e., face, scalp) to slow absorption and lower peak blood levels of anesthesia. Epinephrine also decreases bleeding at the site.
4. The use of epinephrine preparations is contraindicated in cartilaginous areas (ear, nares) and in areas served by end arteries (fingers, toes, and the penis). Epinephrine will also distort and discolor the vermillion border of the lip and is contraindicated in lip lacerations that extend through the lip border. Epinephrine preparations should be used with caution in patients with history of heart disease.
5. Injection of anesthetic agents can distort wound margins, which may increase the complexity of plastics repair. Care should be used in flap-type lacerations to preserve vascularity of the flap by not injecting directly into the flap and avoiding the use of epinephrine preparations.
6. Use amide preparations cautiously in patients with liver disease. (See discussion under Background Information.)
7. Patient reported allergic reactions to amide preparations are rare. (See discussion under Background Information.)
8. Cocaine is very vasoconstrictive and absorption can continue for up to 4 hours. It should be used topically only and with caution in the pediatric and elderly population. One death has been reported as a result of tetracaine-adrenalin-cocaine (TAC) use in a 7½ month old girl after application to nasal mucosa (Dailey, 1988).
9. The use of tetracaine-adrenalin-cocaine solutions on mucosal surfaces is contraindicated. Because mucosal surfaces are very vascular, the potential for systemic absorption of cocaine and tetracaine is high. TAC, be-

Table 137.1 Local Anesthetic Agents: Concentrations and Clinical Uses. See text for further discussion. (Simon & Brenner, 1982. Reprinted by permission.)

Agent	Concentration and Clinical Use	Onset and Duration of Action	Maximum Single Dose (mg)	Comments
AMIDES				
Lidocaine (Xylocaine)	0.5–1.0% for infiltration or IV 1.0–1.5% for peripheral nerve 4.0% for topical	Rapid onset; short to intermediate duration (60–120 min)	300 plain 500 adrenalin	Excellent spreading ability. Wide range of applications.
Prilocaine	0.5–1.0% for infiltration or IV block 1.0% for peripheral nerve	Slower onset; short to intermediate duration (60–120 min)	400 plain 600 adrenalin	0.5% is choice for intravenous block. Most rapidly metabolized and safest of all amide-type agents. Doses in excess of 600 mg produce significant amounts of methemoglobin. Therefore, avoid doses above 600 mg and repeated doses. Good choice in outpatient block. Not suitable for obstetrics.
Mepivacaine (Carbocaine)	1.0% for infiltration 1.0–1.5% for peripheral nerve	Slower onset; intermediate to longer duration (90–180 min)	300 plain 500 adrenalin	Duration slightly longer than equal dose of lidocaine, and blood levels not as sensitive to inclusion of adrenalin as lidocaine; thus may be useful if adrenalin not desirable.
Etidocaine	0.5% for infiltration 0.5–1.0% for peripheral nerve	Rapid onset; long duration (4–8 hrs)	200 plain 300 adrenalin	Capable of producing profound motor block. Useful in postoperative pain management by peripheral blocks.
Bupivacaine (Marcaine)	0.25–0.5% for infiltration 0.25–0.5% for peripheral nerve	Slow onset; long duration (4–8 hrs)	175 plain 250 adrenalin	Favored for obstetric nerve blocks because of minimal fetal effects. Excellent for postoperative analgesia because of minimal motor block.

cause it contains epinephrine, is also contraindicated in areas served by end arteries. See 4 above. (Schaffer, 1985).

10. Benzocaine is found in a wide variety of over-the-counter preparations for sunburn and abrasions. Allergic reactions are common (Altman, 1985).

11. Cetacaine spray has two principal ingredients: benzocaine (14%) and tetracaine (2%). Tetracaine is rapidly absorbed by the pharynx and tracheobronchial tree and is long-acting. Spray application greater than 2 seconds is contraindicated because of rapid mucosal absorption and potential toxicity (Altman, 1985).

EQUIPMENT

Gloves
Alcohol or povidone-iodine wipes
Local or topical anesthetic of choice (Table 137.1)

3-cc, 5-cc, and 10-cc syringes, 18-G, 25-G, and 27-G needles (for infiltration)

Table 137.1   (Continued)

Agent	Concentration and Clinical Use	Onset and Duration of Action	Maximum Single Dose (mg)	Comments
ESTERS				
Procaine (Novocain)	1.0% for infiltration	Slow onset; short duration (30–45 min)	500 plain 600 adrenalin	Indicated with history of malignant hyperpyrexia (MH). Ideal for skin infiltration. Very rapidly metabolized.
Chloroprocaine	1.0–2.0% as for procaine	Rapid onset; short duration	600 plain 750 adrenalin	Drug of choice for obstetric and outpatient neural blockade. Metabolized four times more rapidly than procaine.
Amethocaine (Tetracaine)	0.5–1.0% for topical 0.1–0.2% for infiltration and peripheral nerve	Slow onset; long duration	100 approx.	May be useful alternative if amides contraindicated (e.g., MH). Metabolized four times more slowly than procaine.
Cocaine	4.0–10.0% for topical	Slow onset; medium duration	150 approx. (1.5 ml of 10% or 4 ml of 4%)	Topical use only. Addictive. Indirect adrenoceptor stimulation. No evidence that 10% solution more effective than 4%. Patients sensitive to exogenous catecholamines should receive topical lidocaine rather than cocaine.
Benzocaine	0.4–5.0% for topical only. Usually dispensed in admixture with other therapeutic ingredients related to site of application.	Rapid onset; short duration	No information	Occasionally dispensed in urethane solution. Urethane is a suspect carcinogen and should not be used.

BACKGROUND INFORMATION

Prior to the use of local anesthetic agents, the practitioner must understand the principles of agents and mechanisms of their action.

1. The actual mechanism of anesthesia is unclear. Agents probably act by stabilizing nerve cell membranes and preventing depolarization of pain transmitting fibers (Pollack, 1989).
2. Nerve fibers are classified by their conduction velocity. Smaller fibers responsible for pain, temperature, and autonomic activity are affected rapidly by anesthetic. Local infiltration provides pain reduction without blockage of motor function (Altman, 1985).
3. Anesthetic agents act as vasodilators because of their relaxant effect on smooth muscles. Vasoconstrictors, such as epinephrine may be added to aid in hemostasis when vascular areas have been injured (Simon & Brenner, 1987).
4. Two different anesthetic structures have been identified, esters and amides.

Esters (cocaine, procaine, chloroprocaine, tetracaine, benzocaine) are hydrolyzed by pseudocholinesterase in serum (Simon & Brenner, 1987). All ester agents except cocaine share a common degradation pathway via serum to para-aminobenzoic acid (PABA), which can produce allergic or sensitizing reactions. (Altman, 1985). Cocaine is the only agent excreted unchanged in the liver (Simon & Brenner, 1987).

Amides (lidocaine, prilocaine, mepivicaine, bupivacaine) are structurally different than the esters and are metabolized in the liver. Amide-type agents are believed to be incapable of stimulating antibody formation and so are noteworthy for their low evidence of sensitivity reactions. Reactions probably are toxic in nature, rather than allergic (Altman, 1985). However, patients may be allergic to the preservatives found in multiple dose vials.

5. Diphenhydramine (benadryl) may be used for local infiltration in patients with a history of allergic reaction to other local anesthetics. Dilute 50 mg (1 ml) with 4 ml normal saline to make 5 ml of a 1% solution. Duration of anesthesia is about 30 minutes (Pollack, 1989).

PATIENT PREPARATION

Carefully question patient about medication allergies. Patients may confuse vagal response with allergy history. True allergy is rare but does occur and may include urticaria, bronchospasm, and fatal cardiac collapse. Allergic reaction is more common with ester preparations. See Table 137.1.

PROCEDURAL STEPS

Topical anesthetics

1. Lidocaine (xylocaine) can be applied topically as a liquid, jelly, or viscous fluid. Absorption is rapid. Care should be taken not to exceed recommended dosage, because total absorption cannot be calculated.

2. Cetacaine spray is a benzocaine and tetracaine preparation used primarily for oral procedures. Refer to Table 137.1. Spray application should not exceed 2 seconds (Altman, 1985).

3. Tetracaine-adrenalin-cocaine (TAC) solution
   a. Solutions of TAC are commonly available with a solution of Tetracaine 0.5% (slow onset, long duration anesthetic), adrenalin 1:2000 (vasoconstrictor), and cocaine 11.8% (anesthetic, potent vasoconstrictor) in normal saline. Other mixtures with less tetracaine and cocaine have been shown to be equally effective and have less potential for dangerous side effects (Smith, 1988; Bonadio, 1989).
   b. TAC is primarily used for minor facial and scalp lacerations in lieu of injectable anesthetic, especially in children (Schaffer, 1985).
   c. TAC is applied by saturating sterile gauze and applying it to the wound with firm pressure for several minutes, by dripping into a wound with a syringe, or by application to a wound with sterile cotton swabs.
   d. Gloves should be worn during TAC application by the caregiver to prevent inadvert absorption. Care should be taken to ensure TAC does not run or drip into the eyes, nasal passages, or mouth. Observe the patient carefully during administration.
   e. The maximum dose of TAC applied to each wound in a child is 3 cc (Schaffer, 1985; Bonadio, 1988).
   f. Assess sharp-dull sensation to ensure adequate anesthesia prior to beginning the procedure.

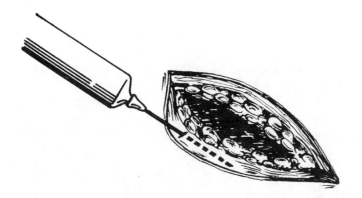

Figure 137.1 Injection of local anesthetic into dermal layer of a wound margin. See text for discussion. (Warner, 1983: 265. Reprinted by permission.)

Wound Infiltration

1. Use the smallest possible needle (a 27-G needle is usually adequate except for digital blocks, the scalp, or callused areas when a 25-G needle may be required). The pain of infiltration is related to needle size, strength of anesthetic, and amount and rate of infiltration (Lanros, 1988).
2. Infiltrate wound edges through the dermis and not through the skin. Approaching the dermal layer directly from the cut margin of the wound is less painful. See Figure 137.1. Continue to infiltrate as the needle passes through the dermis, injecting as you go.
3. As additional needle entry is needed, reenter through infiltrated areas where anesthesia is already accomplished.
4. Assess sharp-dull sensation to ensure adequate anesthesia prior to beginning the procedure.

COMPLICATIONS

1. Local reactions may include local irritation, burning, erythema, and skin sloughing.
2. One death has been reported following improper TAC application (Dailey, 1988).
3. The major cause of systemic reactions is high serum levels. This is most common after topical applications to the trachea and upper airway passages due to very rapid bronchial tree absorption (Klippel, 1979).
4. Resistance to injection or patient complaint of paraesthesia may indicate intraneural injection. Withdraw the needle 1–2 mm and reinject to avoid disruption of nerve fibers.
5. Signs of CNS toxicity include tremor, lightheadedness, muscle twitching, incoherent speech, and seizures. As toxicity increases, the anesthesia may interfere with the electrical and mechanical function of the myocardium. Symptoms include a prolonged PR and QRS, bradycardia, hypotension, and asystole. Factors influencing toxicity include quantity; concentration of solution; presence/absence of epinephrine; vascularity of injection site; rate of absorption of drug; rate of destruction of drug; hypersensitivity of patient; patient age, physical status, and weight (Klippel, 1979).
6. Avoid reactions by not exceeding recommended dosages and avoid intravenous administration by injecting with a moving needle and aspirating frequently (Klippel, 1979).
7. True allergic reactions are rare and may occur in response to the preservatives found in multiple dose vials. Symptoms include bronchospasm

and urticaria. If epinephrine has been used, patients may experience pallor, anxiety, palpations, tachycardia, hypertension, and tachypnea.

PATIENT TEACHING

1. Instruct patient when to expect return of sensation. (See Table 137.1.)
2. Protect the area until sensation returns.
3. Begin analgesia when anesthesia wears off.

REFERENCES

Altman, R., Smith-Coggins, R., & Ampel, L. 1985. Local anesthetics. *Annals of Emergency Medicine,* 14:1209–1217.

Bonadio, W., & Wagner, V. 1989. TAC: A review. *Pediatric emergency care,* 5:128–130.

Dailey, R. 1988. Fatality secondary to misuse of TAC solution. *Annals of Emergency Medicine,* 14:1077–1080.

Klippel, A., & Anderson, C. 1979. *Manual of Emergency and Outpatient Techniques.* Boston: Little, Brown.

Lanros, N. 1988. *Assessment & Intervention in Emergency Nursing,* 3rd ed. S. Norwalk, CT: Appleton & Lange.

Pollack, C., & Swindle, M. 1989. Use of diphenhydramine for local anesthesia in "caine"-sensitive patients. *Clinical Communications,* 611–614.

Schaffer, D. 1985. Clinical comparison of TAC anesthetic solutions with and without cocaine. *Annals of Emergency Medicine,* 14:1077–1080.

Simon, R., & Brenner, B.E. 1987. *Emergency Procedures and Techniques,* 2nd ed. Baltimore: Williams & Wilkins.

Smith, S. 1988. Summarized in *Convention Reporter,* read before American Society of Hospital Pharmacists, 1–4.

Warner, C. (ed). 1983. *Emergency Case Assessment and Intervention,* 3rd ed. St. Louis: Mosby.

SUGGESTED READINGS

P. Rosen, F. Baker, R. Barkin, G. Braen, R. Dailey, & R. Levy, (eds). 1988. *Emergency Medicine: Concepts and Clinical Practice,* 2nd ed. St. Louis: Mosby.

Schwartz, G., Safar, P., Stone, J., Storey, P., and Wagner, D. 1986. *Principles and Practice of Emergency Medicine,* 2nd ed. Philadelphia: Saunders.

White, W., Iserson, K., & Criss, E. 1986. Topical anesthesia for laceration repair: Tetracaine versus TAC. *American Journal of Emergency Medicine,* 4:319–322.

138

Digital Block

Christine A. Miller, RN, MS

INDICATIONS

To provide digital anesthesia for patients
1. with isolated finger lacerations or fingertip amputations;
2. requiring removal of a fingernail or repair of a nailbed;
3. for reduction of interphalangeal joint dislocation;
4. to obtain a satisfactory examination of the finger if pain prevents patient cooperation.

(**Note:** Regional nerve block of the toes is beyond the scope of this chapter.)

CONTRAINDICATIONS AND CAUTIONS

1. Known sensitivity or history of allergic reaction to local anesthetics.
2. Do not perform digital blocks on the stumps of digits under consideration for replantation (O'Hara, 1987).
3. Monitor the vascular status of the finger during and after injection.
4. **Never** use preparations containing epinephrine for digital blocks, because gangrene may result (Ervin, 1986).
5. Circumferential ring block (placing a "ring" of anesthesia in a circle around a finger) generally is contraindicated because of the risk of vasospasm and ischemia, except in the thumb (Melone, 1985).

EQUIPMENT

Local anesthetic without epinephrine (usually lidocaine 1.0–2.0% or bupivacaine 0.25–0.5%)

3-ml or 5-ml syringe
18-G and 25-G needles

BACKGROUND INFORMATION

1. Basic review and knowledge of anatomy of the hand and fingers are essential for successful digital blocks. See Figure 138.1.
2. The primary nerve supply of the hand is received from the radial, ulnar, and median nerves. See Figure 138.2. Anatomic variation of the radial nerve can be significant making the thumb difficult to block.
3. Each digit is supplied by 4 nerve branches that are the terminal branches of the radial, ulnar, and median nerves (2 dorsal and 2 palmar). Thus, the digital nerves lie in pairs on either side of the phalanges (Adriani, 1985).

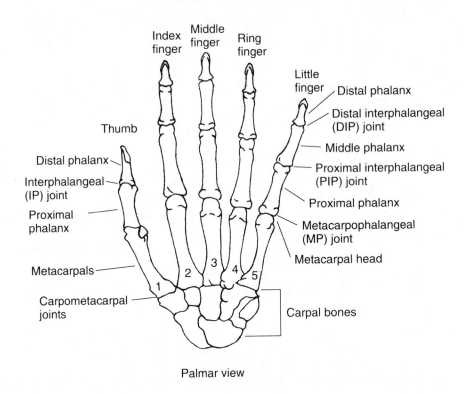

Figure 138.1 Bony anatomy of the hand.

Palmar view

PATIENT PREPARATION

1. Place patient in a supine position with hand extended on a firm surface.
2. Assess and document the patient's distal sensation, circulation and mobility. Mobility can be tested by testing grip, opposition of thumb and fingers, and function of the interphalangeal and metacarpophalangeal joints. Sensation can be effectively evaluated by the use of 2-point discrimination using 2 blunt ends of a paper clip.
3. Suspect nerve injury if a digital artery laceration is present, because of the nerve's proximity to the artery. **Do not attempt to clamp a digital artery,** because of the risk of damaging a digital nerve. Digital nerve laceration will cause hemisensory loss to the finger (Melone, 1985).

PROCEDURAL STEPS

General remarks for any technique

1. After infiltration of local anesthesia, gently massage the tissue to facilitate spread of anesthetic and increase absorption.
2. Anesthesia will not be effective if the periosteum has not been anesthetized. Introduce the needle down to the periosteum and infiltrate closely to the bone (Nardi, 1982).

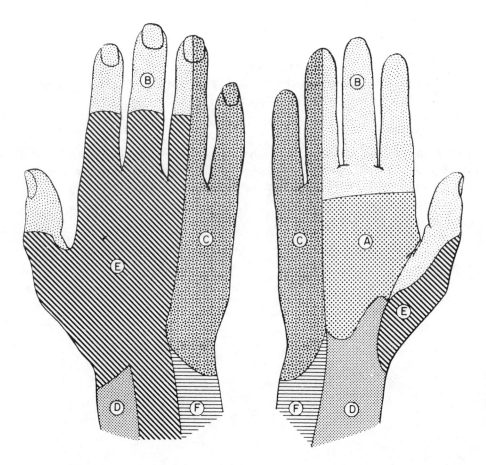

Figure 138.2 Sensory distribution in the hand. Diagram of normal sensory distribution of the hand indicates areas supplied by A, palmar cutaneous branch of the median nerve; B, digital branches of the median nerve; C, superficial branches of the ulnar nerve; D, lateral antebrachial cutaneous branch of the musculocutaneous nerve; E, superficial branches of the radial nerve; and F, medial antebrachial cutaneous nerve.
(Wilkins, 1989: 808. Reprinted by permission.)

3. It is difficult to reach the nerves on both sides of a finger with a single injection, separate injections on either side of the digit are usually needed.
4. Determine anesthesia of choice; see Table 137.1, Ch. 137: Topical Anesthesia and Local Infiltration. Patients who may require lengthy procedures or additional evaluation will benefit from the use of bupivacaine.

Two approaches may be used to block the common digital nerves, metacarpal and dorsal.

Metacarpal approach

1. Palpate the metacarpal head approximately at level of distal palmar crease.
2. Cleanse volar surface with alcohol or povidone-iodine solution.
3. Insert a 25-gauge needle perpendicular to skin just medial or lateral to metacarpal head. See Figure 138.3.

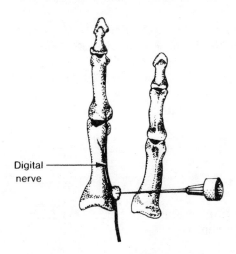

Digital nerve

Figure 138.3 Digital nerve block. (Simon & Brenner, 1982: 109. Reprinted by permission.)

4. After aspirating to ensure vascular penetration has not occurred, inject 1–2 ml as needle is advanced to the periosteum.
5. Repeat step 4 on the opposite side of the metacarpal head. See Figure 138.2. In total, 3–4 ml of anesthesia is required for effective anesthesia, 1.5–2 ml on each side of the digit.

Dorsal approach

1. Cleanse dorsal surface with alcohol or povidone-iodine solution.
2. Inject anesthetic to raise a wheal of anesthesia on the dorsum of the finger near the base, with a 25-gauge needle. See Figure 138.4.

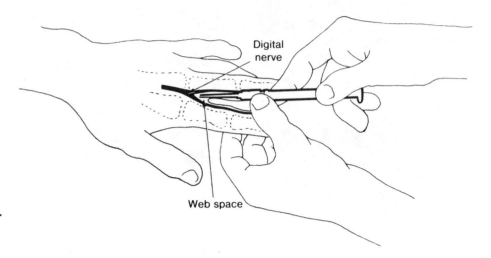

Figure 138.4 Dorsal approach for digital nerve block in the web space. (Simon & Brenner, 1982: 109. Reprinted by permission.)

3. Inject a total of 3–5 cc anesthetic through the wheal by passing the needle downward until the needle is felt on the palmar surface (do not pierce the palmar skin).
4. Subcutaneous infiltration is now accomplished at the base of the finger into the intraosseous spaces (Adriani, 1985).
5. For the index and little finger, the appropriate digital nerve is located in subcutaneous fatty tissue just anterior to the metacarpal head. Injection of anesthesia will produce a half-ring wheal on the radial border of the index finger and on the ulnar border of the little finger (Ervin, 1986; Melone, 1985).

Infiltration of the thumb

1. Circumferential block is completed by placing a ring of anesthetic around the thumb. Block of the thumb is more difficult to attain because it is supplied by multiple branches of the radial and median nerves (Melone, 1985).
2. Insert the needle at the base of the thumb on the dorsal surface and angle it toward the web space while injecting the anesthetic. Then reverse needle direction and inject toward the opposite side of the thumb.
3. Next, inject on the palmar side at the base of the thumb while angling needle toward the web space. Then, reverse the needle direction while injecting toward the opposite side of the thumb, thus completing the ring (Melone, 1985).

COMPLICATIONS

1. Avoid repeated jabbing while injecting to minimize hematoma formation and to decrease post anesthesia neuritis.

2. Position the needle adjacent to the nerve. Intraneural infiltration should be suspected if excessive injection force is required. Reposition the needle to avoid nerve injury.
3. Frequent aspiration will help avoid intravascular infiltration.
4. Vascular compromise may result if too large a volume of anesthesia is used. The amount required varies with each patient. An effective block can usually be accomplished with 3–4 ml.
5. Digital block is used with even minor finger injuries or infections. Local wound infiltration of the finger is contraindicated because of the risk of circulatory impairment (Flynn, 1982; Ervin, 1986).

PATIENT TEACHING

1. Report any signs of circulatory compromise or nerve/motor impairment. (Be sure the patient understands how to assess motor or nerve impairment.)
2. Adjacent fingers may also be numb because the nerve pathways are close together.
3. Begin analgesia when anesthesia wears off if needed. Instruct patient when to expect return of sensation if lidocaine (60–120 minutes) or bupivacaine (4–8 hours) was used (Simon & Brenner, 1987). If numbness persists more than 24 hours, contact your physician.
4. Wound or fracture care as indicated.

REFERENCES

Adriani, J. 1985. *Labat's Regional Anesthesia Techniques and Clinical Applications* 4th ed. St. Louis: Warren H. Green.

Ervin, M.E. 1986. Minor Surgical Procedures. In G. Schwartz, P. Safar, J. Stone, P. Storey, & D. Wagner, (eds). *Principles and Practice of Emergency Medicine*, 2nd ed. Philadelphia: Saunders; 465–475.

Flynn, J. 1982. *Hand Surgery*, 3rd ed. Baltimore: Williams & Wilkins.

Melone, C. 1985. Anesthesia for hand injuries. *Emergency Medicine Clinics of North America*, 3:235–243.

Nardi, G., & Zuidema, G. 1982. *Surgery Essentials of Clinical Practice*, 14th ed. Boston: Little, Brown.

O'Hara, M. 1987. Emergency care of the patient with traumatic amputation. *Journal of Emergency Nursing*, 13:272–277.

Simon, R., & Brenner, B. eds. (1987). *Emergency Procedures and Techniques*, 2nd ed. Baltimore: Williams & Wilkins.

SUGGESTED READINGS

Green, D. 1988. *Operative Hand Surgery*. New York: Churchill Livingston.

Klippel, A., & Anderson, C. 1979. *Manual of emergency and outpatient techniques.* Boston: Little, Brown.

Schwartz, S. 1989. *Principles of Surgery*, 5th ed. New York: McGraw-Hill.

Spinner, M. 1984. *Kaplan's functional and surgical anatomy of the hand*, 3rd ed. Philadelphia: Lippincott.

139

Bier Block

Christine A. Miller, RN, MS

Bier block is also known as intravenous regional anesthesia.

A Bier block is a regional block that employs local anesthesia to cause a temporary block of nerve conduction. Venous blood of the extremity (usually upper extremity) is drained by gravity or bandaging and filled with local anesthetic held in place by a tourniquet. This type of regional anesthesia provides a bloodless field and anesthesia for injured extremities.

INDICATIONS

1. To provide regional anesthesia for patients who require evaluation of soft tissue injuries, for fracture reduction, for repair of nerves and tendons, and for complex suturing in an extremity. Bier block anesthesia is rapid, reliable, and low risk. It provides good muscle relaxation and a bloodless field.
2. To permit patient cooperation when constant evaluation of nerve and motor function is required. Bier block decreases the patient's pain and anxiety.

CONTRAINDICATIONS AND CAUTIONS

1. Sensitivity or history of allergic reaction to local anesthetics.
2. Peripheral vascular disease or blood coagulation disorders.
3. If the patient exhibits excessive fear or anxiety that prevents cooperation, a Bier block may not be appropriate.
4. Close attention must be paid to proper maintenance of equipment with detailed check of equipment prior to use.
5. Bier block can be used only when adequate monitoring and resuscitation equipment are available.

EQUIPMENT

Local anesthesia without preservative (usually lidocaine or 0.25% Bupivacaine)
Alcohol wipes
60-cc syringe, 18-G needle, 21-G needle for anesthesia
Equipment to start an IV or heparin lock
Cardiac monitor/defibrillator
Resuscitation equipment
3–4″ Elastic bandage
Pneumatic tourniquet (The use of a standard blood pressure cuff is not acceptable due to the risk of air leakage and release of anesthesia systemically)
Cast padding

PATIENT PREPARATION

1. Establish intravenous access distal to site of injury (either with an over-the-needle-catheter or butterfly. You may use a heparin lock or continuous infusion).
2. Establish second intravenous site in uninjured extremity for emergency access, if needed.
3. Place patient on cardiac monitor.
4. Apply 2–3 layers of cast padding at the tourniquet site to protect the skin.
5. Assess and document vital signs.
6. Place the patient in a supine position.

PROCEDURAL STEPS

1. Test pneumatic tourniquet by inflating it to 250 mm Hg and ensure that there is no air leakage.
2. *Place the pneumatic tourniquet proximally on the injured extremity.
3. *Exsanguinate the extremity by either wrapping with an elastic bandage and/or elevating it to allow gravity drainage. Proper exsanguination is important to evenly distribute anesthesia, to ensure a bloodless field, and to decrease early tourniquet pain. See Figure 139.1.

*Indicates portions of the procedure usually performed by a physician.

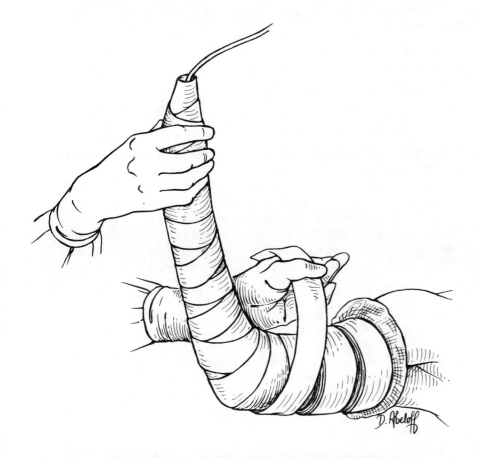

Figure 139.1 Exsanguinate the extremity by wrapping with an elastic bandage and/or elevating the extremity.
(Rosen & Sternbach, 1983: 209. Reprinted by permission.)

4. *Inflate the tourniquet to 250 mm Hg to assure absence of radial artery pulsation. Patients who are hypo/hypertensive may require less/more tourniquet inflation. Inflate the cuff to 100 mm Hg above patient's systolic blood pressure. (Brown, 1989)

5. *The use of a double tourniquet system is advocated for procedures lasting over 30 minutes to decrease tourniquet pain. The proximal cuff is inflated first. When the patient begins to develop tourniquet pain, the distal cuff is inflated and the proximal cuff is deflated. The area under the distal cuff is already anesthetized thus, the patient does not experience tourniquet pain. Many emergency departments use a single cuff system. A double tourniquet system has narrower cuffs that require higher pressure to occlude arteries. See Figure 139.2.

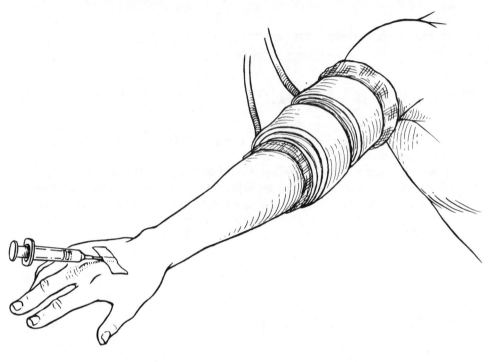

Figure 139.2   A double tourniquet system.
(Rosen & Sternbach, 1983: 209. Baltimore: Williams & Wilkins. Reprinted by permission.)

6. *With the tourniquet inflated, inject the anesthetic into the intravenous line of injured extremity. The agent of choice depends on physician preference, rapidity of onset required, duration and degree of motor block needed, relative toxicity of agent and spreading power of agent. Dose should be individualized with patient weight.

Anesthetic agents should not contain preservatives. Medications used include:

Lidocaine (Xylocaine)

Onset: rapid onset 5–15 minutes with good distribution
Duration: 60–90 minutes duration
Dosage: 8–11 mg/kg maximum dose (Green, 1988)
Comments: most commonly used; low incidence of patient sensitivity; 1% strength ensures loss of sensation, 1.5%–2% necessary for complete sensory and motor block when muscle relaxation needed.

Bupivacaine (Marcaine)

Onset: onset begins in 2–5 minutes, complete in 10 minutes
Duration: duration 4–8 hours
Dosage: dosage 2.5–3.5 mg/kg maximum dose (Green, 1988)
Comments: used if lengthy anesthesia required after release of tourniquet; decreases need for postoperative analgesia; potentially lethal if equipment malfunction causes systemic absorption.

Duration: 30–60 minutes

Dose: 12–15 mg/kg maximum dose (Simon & Brenner, 1987)

Comments: should be ideal because of rapid biotransformation but has increased risk of thrombophlebitis

7. After injection of anesthesia, continue to monitor patient's vital signs, cardiac rhythm, and level of consciousness. Discontinue the IV in the injured extremity.

8. If the patient has a fracture, casting or splinting and postreduction films are done prior to tourniquet release.

9. *At completion of the procedure, tourniquet release is begun (see complications).

      If total tourniquet time is 20–30 minutes, use cycled deflation technique:

   a. deflate tourniquet totally for 2–3 seconds, reinflate for 1 minute.

   b. Deflate again for 2–3 seconds and reinflate for 1 minute, then deflate totally (Brown, 1989).

   If total tourniquet time is over 40 minutes, deflate without cycling (Brown, 1989). If tourniquet is inflated over 30 minutes, 50% of the anesthetic is bound to tissue and systemic reactions are rare (Green, 1988).

10. After release of the tourniquet, continue to monitor the patient's vital signs, cardiac rhythm, and level of consciousness for symptoms of anesthetic toxicity.

11. Continue to monitor circulation, sensation, and mobility of patient's injured extremity for 30–60 minutes after release of tourniquet.

COMPLICATIONS

1. Severe toxicity is rare and is usually due to a faulty tourniquet. High blood concentrations of anesthetic as a result of rapid release into the systemic circulation may be life threatening.

2. Systemic toxicity is dose dependent and is related to the effects of anesthesia on the cardiovascular or central nervous systems.

      CNS effects include perioral numbness, dizziness, visual disturbances (blurred vision), light-headedness, near syncope, seizure, and coma.

      Cardiovascular effects (extremely uncommon) include hypotension and arrhythmias: conduction disturbances, bradycardia, asystole (Green, 1988).

3. Reactions are more common if the tourniquet is released in less than 30 minutes, if the tourniquet is released too rapidly, or if the anesthetic dosage is too high.

4. Tourniquet pain if a single tourniquet is used for procedures lasting longer than 30 minutes. Even with use of a double cuff, tourniquet pain limits the use of this procedure to 1 hour (Green, 1988).

5. True allergic reactions are rare and are usually caused by ester derivative anesthetics such as novocain, nesacaine, cocaine, and benzocaine.

PATIENT TEACHING

1. Report any signs of circulatory compromise, nerve or motor impairment. (Be sure that the patient understands how to assess nerve or motor impairment.)

2. Begin analgesia when anesthetic begins to wear off. (Instruct patient when to expect return of sensation, etc.)

REFERENCES

Brown, E., McGriff, J., & Malinowsky, R. 1989. Intravenous regional anaesthesia (Bier block): Review of 20 years experience. *Canadian Journal of Anaesthesia*, 36:307–310.

Green, D. 1988. *Operative Hand Surgery*, 2nd ed. New York: Churchill Livingston.

Rosen, R., & Sternbach, G. 1983. *Atlas of emergency medicine*, 2nd ed. Baltimore: Williams & Wilkins.

Simon, R., & Brenner, B.E. 1987. *Emergency procedures and techniques*, 2nd ed. Baltimore: Williams & Wilkins.

SUGGESTED READINGS

Flynn, J. 1982. *Hand Surgery*, 3rd ed. Baltimore: Williams & Wilkins.

Luce, E.A., & Mangubat, E. 1983. Loss of hand and forearm following Bier block: A case report. *The Journal of Hand Surgery*, 8:280–283.

Maneksha, F. 1987. Techniques and drugs for regional anesthesia in surgery of the hand. *Orthopaedic Review*, 16:98–105.

Rosenberg, P., Kalso, E., Tuominen, M., & Linden, H. 1983. Acute bupivacaine toxicity as a result of venous leakage under the tourniquet cuff during a Bier block. *Anesthesiology*, 58:95–98.

Vatashsky, E., Aronson, H., Wexler, M., & Rousso, M. 1980. Anesthesia in a hand surgery unit. *The Journal of Hand Surgery*, 5:495–497.

140

Wound Care for Amputations

Jean A. Proehl, RN, MN, CEN, CCRN

INDICATIONS

To preserve amputated tissue or appendages for possible replantation.

CONTRAINDICATIONS AND CAUTIONS

1. Amputations are only addressed after life-threatening problems are resolved.
2. Consult your referral replantation team as soon as possible to determine if a replantation attempt is indicated.
3. The method of preserving amputated parts is controversial: consult your referral replantation team to determine which method is preferred.
4. Regardless of the preservation method used, the part should not be permitted to freeze. Freezing causes cell membrane rupture and irreversibly damages the tissue. A temperature of 4°C is optimal (Van Giesen, 1983).
5. Do not use dry ice, because it will result in temperatures that are too cold (O'Hara, 1987).
6. Avoid tourniquets, tying, or clamping vessels in the stump, because these maneuvers may damage the structures that will be reanastomosed during replantation. Control bleeding with direct pressure if possible (Epifanio, 1989; Hing, 1986; O'Hara, 1987).
7. Avoid digital block anesthesia of the stump, because it may damage and constrict the vessels needed for replantation (O'Hara, 1987).

EQUIPMENT

Gauze dressings
Plastic bag or watertight container
Ice
Sterile normal saline or lactated
        Ringer's solution (not used
        for all methods)

Insulated container (for prolonged
        storage or transport to
        another facility)

PATIENT PREPARATION

1. Consult with your referral replantation team as soon as possible to determine the feasibility of replantation and receive specific instructions regarding care of the part and patient preparation.
2. Apply a soft-pressure dressing and elevate the stump. Splint the stump as indicated (Hing, 1986; O'Hara, 1987).

3. Administer parenteral antibiotics as prescribed (Hing, 1986; O'Hara, 1987).
4. Administer tetanus prophylaxis as indicated (Hing, 1986; O'Hara, 1987).
5. To begin the anticoagulation process essential for the survival of the replanted part, administer an aspirin suppository if prescribed (Hing, 1986; O'Hara, 1987).
6. Administer analgesia as prescribed.
7. Obtain x-rays of the stump and the amputated part (Hing, 1986; O'Hara, 1987).
8. Prepare the patient for transport if indicated.

PROCEDURAL STEPS FOR A COMPLETE AMPUTATION

1. Cleanse the part by gently rinsing with normal saline or lactated Ringer's solution to remove gross contamination (Hing, 1986; O'Hara, 1987).
2. Protect the part with one of the following techniques according to the preference of your referral replantation team.

   Technique A
   a. Wrap the amputated tissue in dry, sterile dressings and seal in plastic bag or watertight container (Epifanio, 1989; O'Hara, 1987).
   b. Place the plastic bag or watertight container on ice or in an insulated container with ice.

   Technique B
   a. Wrap the amputated part in gauze moistened with saline or lactated Ringer's and seal it in a plastic bag or watertight container. Be sure to wrap the part well so that it is protected from freezing (Hing, 1986; Van Giesen, 1983).
   b. Place the plastic bag or watertight container on ice or in an insulated container with ice.

   Technique C
   a. Immerse the amputated part in saline or lactated Ringer's solution in a plastic bag or watertight container (Van Giesen, 1983).
   b. Place the plastic bag or watertight container on ice or in an insulated container with ice.
3. Label the bag or container containing the amputated part so that it is not inadvertently discarded.

PROCEDURAL STEPS FOR PARTIAL AMPUTATION

1. Wrap the entire extremity in moist or dry dressings per replantation team orders.
2. Splint and elevate the extremity.
3. Cooling the extremity is usually not possible because it is very painful (O'Hara, 1987).

COMPLICATIONS

1. Cellular damage or death as a result of freezing or inadequate cooling.
2. Cellular damage or death as a result of excess time between injury and

replantation. Time limits vary with the type of injury, the body part involved, how the part is stored, etc. Every effort should be made to replant the part as soon as possible.

PATIENT TEACHING

1. No smoking, eating, or drinking until after surgery.
2. Keep the injured part elevated.
3. The replantation surgeon is the most qualified person to discuss your prognosis with you.

REFERENCES

Epifanio, P.C., Hixon, J.D., & Cross, N.K. 1989. Nursing interventions for the patient with acute hand trauma. *Operating Room Nursing Forum*, 3, 3:1–8.

Hing, D.N., Buncke, H.J., Alpert, B.S., & Gordon, L. 1986. Preparing the amputated part for transfer. *Hospital Physician*, 22, 3:36–37, 40.

O'Hara, M.M. 1987. Emergency care of the patient with a traumatic amputation. *Journal of Emergency Nursing*, 13:272–277.

Van Giesen, P.J., Seaber, A.V., & Urbaniak, J.R. 1983. Storage of amputated parts prior to replantation: An experimental study with rabbit ears. *Journal of Hand Surgery*, 8:60–65.

141

Suture Removal

Stephanie Kitt, RN, MSN

INDICATIONS

For removal of nonabsorbable suture material inserted for the purpose of wound approximation and primary healing. Adequate epithelialization of the wound is evidenced by a sturdy wound appearance, approximated edges, and evidence of healing.

Timely suture removal is important in minimizing scar formation. The dense vascularity and lack of tension on the face allows for quick, early healing and permits removal of sutures in only 3–5 days. Sutures on the trunk are left in place 6–7 days and extremity sutures may remain for longer periods. See Table 141.1.

CONTRAINDICATIONS AND CAUTIONS

1. Suture removal should be timely in order to attain optimal cosmetic and functional results. Leaving sutures in too long increases the risk of stitch abscess, scar formation, and subsequent deformity (Rosen & Sternbach, 1983). Premature suture removal predisposes the patient to wound disruption, delayed healing, and scar formation.
2. When the suture line is located in an area exposed to tensile stretch (i.e., joints), the sutures may be kept in place for up to 2 weeks, and thereafter, the wound may require superficial support with skin tapes for an additional 5–7 days. Skin tapes prevent disruption of the wound and more importantly may minimize tension to help reduce ultimate scar widening (Finley, 1984).

EQUIPMENT

Scissors or #11 scalpel blade
Forceps
Gauze sponges
Normal saline irrigation solution

(**Note:** Prepackaged kits containing the listed items are available.)

PROCEDURAL STEPS

1. Grasp the knot of the suture with forceps and raise away from the skin.
2. Cut the suture distal to the knot and near the skin. This assures that contaminated suture is not drawn through the suture tract as the suture is withdrawn. See Figure 141.1.

    If a vertical or horizontal mattress suture is in place, the suture must be cut on the side opposite the knot at a skin orifice. See Figure

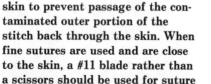

Figure 141.1 Correct method of removing a suture. The suture should be removed by cutting the end away from the knot near the skin to prevent passage of the contaminated outer portion of the stitch back through the skin. When fine sutures are used and are close to the skin, a #11 blade rather than a scissors should be used for suture removal. The tip of the blade is inserted under the suture loop, and the suture is cut.
(Simon & Brenner, 1987: 334. Reprinted by permission.)

Table 141.1 Removal times for sutures

Location	Time of Removal (days)
Face	3– 4 (adult)
	2– 3 (children)
Lower extremity	8–10
Upper extremity	7–10
Extensor surface of joints	10–14
Delayed closure	8–12

(Simon & Brenner, 1987: 334. Reprinted by permission.)

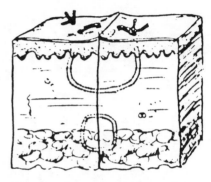

141.2a and 141.2b. Because it is impossible to avoid pulling a small portion of suture that has been outside the skin through the suture tract, the area should be cleansed with an antiseptic solution prior to suture removal.

Running or continuous sutures (Figure 141.3) should be cut at each skin orifice on one side and removed through the other. The objective in each instance is to remove the suture without pulling through the skin any portion of the suture that has been outside the skin (Nealon, 1979).

3. Pull the suture out of the wound and discard.
4. Cleanse the wound with normal saline or an antiseptic solution to rid the area of crusted secretions.
5. Leave the suture line open to air or apply dressing per physician's orders.

A

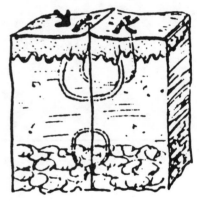

COMPLICATIONS

1. Wound infection
2. Scar formation
3. Wound dehiscence

PATIENT TEACHING

1. Keep your wound clean and dry. Any crusted areas should simply be allowed to come off with usual soap and water cleansing. Do not pick at crusts or scabs.
2. Report any of the following signs and symptoms: fever, increasing redness around the wound or on the extremity involved, swelling, drainage of pus, increased pain or tenderness, or opening of the wound.

B

Figure 141.2 Examples of A. vertical mattress suture; B. horizontal mattress suture. Arrow indicates point where suture should be cut. (Schwartz et al., 19: 2084. Reprinted by permission.)

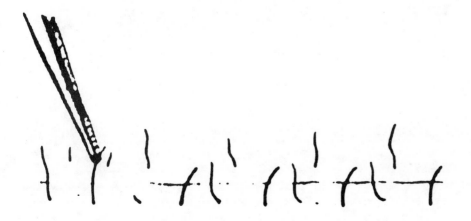

Figure 141.3 Alternative loops of a continuous suture are cut, each piece being removed by lifting the intervening loop.
(Rob et al., 1981: 14. Reprinted by permission.)

REFERENCES

Nealon, T.F. 1979. *Fundamental skills in surgery,* 3rd ed. Philadelphia: Saunders.

Rosen, P., & Sternbach, G. 1983. *Atlas of emergency medicine,* 2nd ed. Baltimore: Williams & Wilkins.

Rob, C., Smith, R., & Dudley, H. (eds). 1981. *Atlas of surgery.* London: Butterworth.

Schwartz, S.I., Shires, G.T., & Spencer, F.C. (eds). 1989. *Principles of surgery,* 5th ed. New York: McGraw-Hill.

SUGGESTED READINGS

Deane, M. 1981. General care of wounds and techniques of suturing. In Rob, C., Smith, R., & Dudley, H. (eds). *Atlas of general surgery,* London: Butterworth; 14.

Peacock, E.E. Jr., 1989. Wound healing and wound care. In Schwartz, S.I., Shires, G.T., & Spencer, F.C. (eds). *Principles of surgery,* 5th ed. New York: McGraw-Hill; 321–23.

Rosen, J. 1989. Emergency wound management. *Topics in Emergency Medicine,* 11:1.

Simon, R.R., & Brenner, B.E., 1987. *Emergency procedures and techniques,* 2nd ed. Baltimore: Williams & Wilkins.

142

Staple Removal

Stephanie Kitt, RN, MSN

INDICATIONS

For removal of skin staples inserted for the purpose of wound approximation and primary healing. Adequate epithelialization of the wound is evidenced by a sturdy wound appearance, approximated edges, and evidence of healing. Timely staple removal is important to minimize scar formation. Generally, staples are removed in 7–10 days.

CONTRAINDICATIONS AND CAUTIONS

Staple removal should be timely in order to attain optimal cosmetic and functional results. Leaving staples in too long increases the risk of stable abscess, scar formation, and subsequent deformity (Rosen, 1984). Premature staple removal predisposes the patient to wound disruption, delayed healing, and scar formation.

EQUIPMENT

Staple extractor (There are a variety of disposable skin stapler devices on the market. Each device has its own specific staple extractor.)
Gauze dressings
Normal saline irrigation solution

PROCEDURAL STEPS

1. Position the nose of the extractor centrally beneath the staple span. See Figure 142.1.
2. Squeeze down with the thumb to reform the staple until the motion of the extractor is halted making sure the staple is totally reformed. See Figure 142.2.
3. Lift the extractor from the skin. Never pull up before the extractor is fully closed. See Figure 142.3.

COMPLICATIONS

1. Wound infection
2. Scar formation
3. Wound dehiscence

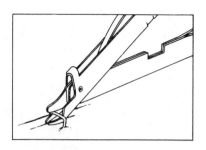
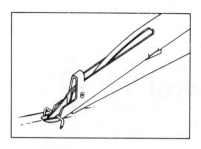
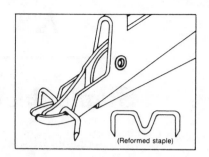

142.1 Placing the extractor beneath the staple.

Figure 142.2 Reformation of the staple.

Figure 142.3 Removal of the staple from the skin.

(Figures 142.1, 142.2, and 142.3 are from Ethicon, Inc. (1987). *Proximate III disposable skin stapler and staple extractor.* Somerville, NJ: Ethicon, Inc. Reprinted by permission.)

PATIENT TEACHING

1. Keep your wound clean and dry. Any crusted areas should simply be allowed to come off with usual soap and water cleansing. Do not pick at crusts or scabs.
2. Report any of the following signs and symptoms: fever, increasing redness around the wound or on the extremity involved, swelling, drainage of pus, increased pain or tenderness, or opening of the wound.

REFERENCE

Rosen, P., & Sternbach, G. 1984. *Atlas of emergency medicine*, 2nd ed. Baltimore: Williams & Wilkins.

SUGGESTED READINGS

Phung, D., Abidin, M.R., Thacker, J.G., Rodeheaver, G.T., Westwater, B.A., Doctor, A., & Edlich, R.F. 1988. Evaluation of automatic disposable rotating cartridge skin staplers. *Journal of Burn Care and Rehabilitation*, 9:538–546.
Rubio, P.A. 1986. *Atlas of stapling techniques.* Rockville, MD: Aspen.

143

Minor Burn Care

Marilyn K. Bourn, RN, MSN, REMTP

This chapter discusses the debridement and dressings of minor burns only. Minor burns, as defined by the American Burn Association, include burns with

1. less than 10% of the total body surface area (TBSA) involved;
2. in a patient <35 years old or >4 years old;
3. with no significant previous medical history;
4. no burns to the hands, face, feet or perineum;
5. no circumferential burns;
6. no concomitant injuries (e.g., inhalation, electrical, fractures, etc.) (Archambeault-Jones & Feller, 1983).

The majority of burn units request that, in the case of major burns that require admission, no debridement of the wound be done in the emergency department. Initially, the major burns should be cooled with sterile normal saline. During the transfer, a dry sterile gauze dressing should be applied. If moist dressings are used during transfer, extreme caution should be exercised to prevent hypothermia.

INDICATIONS

Debridement and dressing of minor burn wounds

1. minimize the potential for bacterial infection;
2. prevent the conversion of partial-thickness burn to full-thickness burn;
3. promote spontaneous healing;
4. maximize patient comfort;
5. minimize cosmetic changes (Kuehn, Ahrenholz, & Solem, 1989).

These procedures are indicated for any minor burn which will be managed on an outpatient basis.

CONTRAINDICATIONS AND CAUTIONS

1. The burn wound must be thoroughly cleaned and debrided prior to applying ointments or dressing. If not, infection may be encouraged rather than avoided.
2. Be sure the patient and/or family has the financial, mental, and physical capabilities to follow aftercare instructions. If not, other arrangements or admission may be required.
3. Careful assessment must be made to determine if, for any reason, admission of the patient is warranted.

EQUIPMENT

Sterile gown, mask, and gloves
Sterile basin
Sterile towels
Sterile surgical instruments such as
fine tipped scissors and
forceps (with or without
teeth)
Sterile normal saline for irrigation
(warmed to body
temperature, if possible)
(**Note:** Many institutions
use warm tap water.)
Mild soap, germicidal soap,
chlorhexidine or
povidone-iodone
Safety razor
Mineral oil or petroleum ointments
(for tar removal)

Sterile gauze dressings
Sterile (soft) surgical brush
Sterile gauze bandages
Adhesive tape
Burn dressing options (See Table
143.1.):
Sterile, fine-mesh gauze
1% silver sulfadiazine
(Silvadine)
Antibiotic ointment (Neosporin,
Bacitracin, Polysporin)
Nonadhering dressing (Adaptic)
Transparent wound dressing
(Opsite, Tegaderm, etc.)
Xeroform petroleum gauze
Biobrane

Table 143.1 Antibiotic ointments and creams.

	Silver Sulfadiazine	Mafenide Cream	Gentamycin Cream or Ointment	Povidone-Iodine Ointment	Bacitracin Ointment	Nystatin Cream	Nitrofurazone Ointment
Antimicrobial Spectrum	Good gr−.* Fair gr+ Fair fungi	Excellent gr− Good fungi Fair gr+	Mostly gr− No fungi	Good gr−, gr+, and fungi	Mostly gr+ No fungi	Fungi	Good gr+ Some gr−
Eschar penetration	Good	Excellent	Good	Fair	Fair	Fair	Fair
Local tissue toxicity	Low	Some	Low	Some	Low	Low	Low
Systemic toxicity	Low transient marrow suppressor	High† metabolic acidosis	Low† ototoxicity and renal	Low† Iodine toxicity	Low† Renal	Low	Low† Renal
Pain	Rare	Yes	Rare	Yes	No	No	Yes
Skin allergy	Rare	5–10%	Rare	Rare	Rare	Rare	Rare

*gr−: gram-negative; gr+: gram positive
†All agents if used in excess amounts will lead to significant systemic toxicity.

(Demling & LaLonde, 1989: 304. Reprinted by permission.)

PATIENT PREPARATION

1. Apply a moist room temperature, sterile dressing to wound as soon as possible to stop the burning process. Do not apply ice to the wound.
2. If chemicals are involved, consult appropriate resources (Poison Control, Chemtrec, Poisindex) prior to initiating wound debridement. Most chemicals require a minimum of 20 minutes fluid irrigation; additional therapy may also be necessary.
3. Administer tetanus toxoid as indicated.
4. Administer analgesia as prescribed.

PROCEDURAL STEPS

Wound debridement

1. On a sterile towel arrange and organize all supplies, instruments, and medications prior to initiating wound care.
2. Don sterile gown, mask, and gloves.
3. Using sterile saline and a cleansing solution, gently begin to wash the injured area. It may be less painful to begin in the center of the burn and work toward the margin. Use sterile gauze dressings or a soft, sterile surgical brush. Maintain a circular motion and attempt to create a moderate amount of suds or foam.
4. Rinse with sterile saline and repeat as often as necessary until the wound is thoroughly cleaned.
5. If the blister is ruptured, debride the tissue. Management of intact blisters remains very controversial and research remains inconclusive. It is important to know the protocol for your department or receiving burn unit. Blisters may be managed in several ways:
   a. The blister may be left intact and the underlying wound allowed to heal in the fluid (Demling & LaLonde, 1989).
   b. The blister may be punctured and fluid evacuated, (Artz & Moncrief, 1969) but the overlying tissue (roof) left.
   c. Small blisters may be debrided, while large ones remain intact (Kuehn, 1989).
6. Shave the affected area.
7. Using fine-tipped scissors and forceps, elevate loose, devitalized tissue and remove it.
8. Remove tar with mineral oil or petroleum ointments.
9. Continue the above procedures until the area is clean, moist, and pink.
10. Reassess the wound depth as necessary.
11. Apply a wound dressing
12. Monitor vital signs, especially temperature.

Wound dressings

Topical agents may be applied to the burn wound in an open (open to the environment) or closed method (dressing and bandage placed over the topical agent). The open method is easy to apply, decreases risk of infection and avoids difficult dressing. The open method, however, may increase discomfort and heat loss, increase cross contamination, and not be practical for a working or active individual. The closed method may be more practical and comfortable, aid in debridement, and help prevent infection. The closed method may require ingenious application of the dressing and bandage in awkward areas (Demling & LaLonde, 1989).

1% Silver sulfadiazine (Silvadine). The most commonly used cream is Silvadine.

1. Using a sterile, gloved hand or sterile tongue blade, apply a thin ($^1/_8''$ or thickness of a nickel, per manufacturer), smooth layer of cream over the area. Fine-mesh gauze may also be impregnated with the silver sulfadiazine. The gauze is then cut to the appropriate size and placed over the wound.
2. If using the closed method, cover with a sterile gauze dressing and bandage. Anchor as necessary.
3. Silver sulfadiazine applied to the face may become dry, cakey, and turn gray in color. To provide greater patient comfort and avoid the cream running in the eyes, nares, and mouth, the impregnated, fine-mesh gauze method is preferred.

Antibiotic ointment (Neosporin, Bacitracin, Polysporin).

1. Apply a thin layer of ointment to the wound and place a piece of non-adhering dressing (Adaptic) over the area.
2. Cover with a sterile gauze dressing and bandage. Anchor as necessary.

Transparent wound dressing (Opsite, Tegaderm, others). Such dressings may be applied directly over the burn wound.
1. Using sterile technique apply the appropriate size dressing.
2. Leave a ¹/₂″ margin that can adhere to the nonburned skin.
3. Apply a gauze pressure dressing and bandage.

Xeroform petroleum gauze. Apply in the same manner as transparent wound dressing.
1. A gauze bandage should be placed over the xeroform gauze.
2. Wrap with gauze for protection, absorption of exudate, and increased adherence.

Biobrane Biobrane is a synthetic skin substitute that consists of a flexible silicone-nylon membrane and bonded collagen peptides.
1. Apply Biobrane directly over the clean wound.
2. Use sterile strips or a gauze bandage to hold the Biobrane in place.

COMPLICATIONS

1. Infection
2. Loss of function
3. Remove a dressing too vigorously may damage newly formed epithelium and slow healing (Warden, 1987).

PATIENT TEACHING

1. Keep bandage clean and dry. (Do not wash dishes, swim, or shower.)
2. If the bandage requires changing, remove it carefully and reapply. If it sticks to the skin, soak it in lukewarm water. Remove and pat dry with a clean towel.
3. Do not break any blisters.
4. Clean the area once or twice a day with warm soapy water. Reapply a thin layer of antibiotic cream or ointment.
5. Dress and bandage as instructed.
6. If Opsite or Biobrane is used, trim the edges as they loosen.
7. Return for followup appointments as instructed (usually within 24 hours).
8. Report the following signs or symptoms:
   a. Increased pain, swelling, redness, foul odor, or red streaks from the wound.
   b. Fever over 100.4°F.
   c. Numbness or swelling distal to a joint or inability to move the joint.

REFERENCES

Archambeault-Jones, C., & Feller, I. 1983. Burn nursing is nursing. In T.L. Wachtel, V. Kahn, & H.A. Frank (eds). *Current topics in burn care.* Rockville, MD: Aspen; 187–202.

Artz, C.P., & Moncrief, J.A. 1969. Office treatment of burns. In C.P. Artz, & J.A. Moncrief (eds). *The treatment of burns.* Philadelphia: Saunders.

Demling, R.H., & LaLonde, C. 1989. *Burn trauma.* New York: Theime; 53–61.

Kuehn, C.N., Ahrenholz, D.H., & Solem, L.D. 1989. Care of the burn wound. In J.B. Johnston, & E.D. Deitch (eds). *Trauma Quarterly,* 5, 4:33–55.

Warden, G.D. 1987. Outpatient management of thermal injuries. In J.A. Boswick (ed). *The art and science of burn care.* Rockville, MD.: Aspen.

144

Escharotomy and Fasciotomy

Marilyn K. Bourn, RN, MSN, REMTP

Escharotomies and fasciotomies are not considered routine emergency department procedures. However, some emergency departments perform these procedures in the management of seriously burned patients. For this reason these procedures are included for your reference. An escharotomy is a surgical incision through burned tissue (eschar). A fasciotomy extends through the fascia.

INDICATIONS

To decrease elevated tissue pressures in the presence of
1. Circumferential or electrical burns to the extremities causing loss of distal pulses; impaired capillary filling; paresthesias or motor weakness; cyanosis of distal, uninjured skin; and/or tense edema with rigid muscle compartments (Monafo & Freedman, 1987; Braen, 1988). See Figure 144.1.
2. Circumferential burns to the chest with constricting eschar that may compromise respirations (Braen, 1988).
3. Other injuries of the extremities causing significant compartmental syndrome (e.g., snake bite).

CONTRAINDICATIONS AND CAUTIONS

1. Failure to perform emergency escharotomy and/or fasciotomy may result in loss of neuromuscular function, loss of a portion of the limb (Monafo & Freedman, 1987), or inability to ventilate lung parenchyma.
2. This procedure may cause significant blood loss in the patient already predisposed to hypovolemic shock (Braen, 1988) and/or altered coagulation.
3. The open wounds may further predispose the patient to sepsis.
4. Underlying tissues may be damaged if procedures are incorrectly performed.
5. If compartmental pressures do not decrease after escharotomy, a fasciotomy must be performed as well (Monafo & Freedman, 1987). Tissue pressure exceeding 30 mm Hg indicates a need for surgical escharotomies (Demling & Lalonde, 1989). See Ch. 132: Measuring Compartmental Pressure.

EQUIPMENT

Sterile gown, mask, and gloves
Local anesthetic for infiltration
    (optional in deep, insensate
    burns)

Intracompartmental pressure
    monitor (may not be used in
    emergency situations)
Doppler to assess pulses

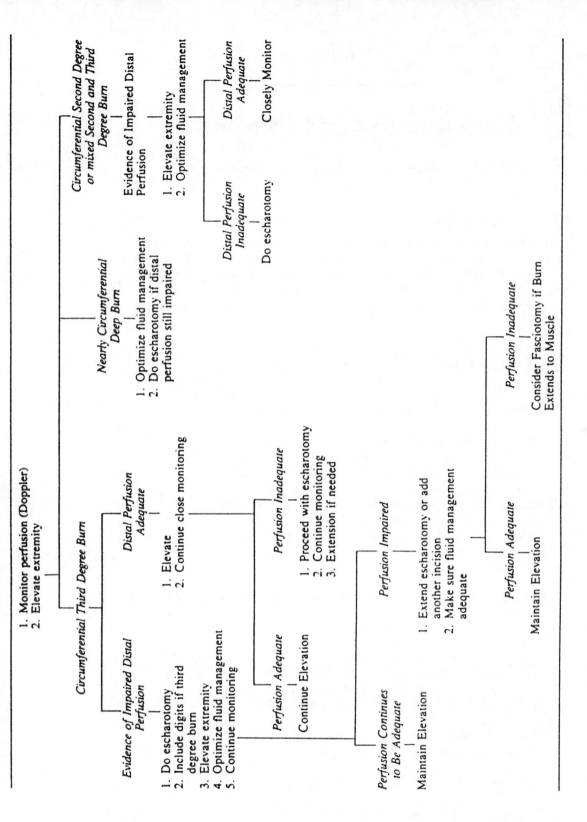

Figure 144.1 Algorithm for escharotomies of extremity burns (Demling & Lalonde, 1989: 63. Reprinted by permission.)

Sterile drapes
Sterile scalpel (coagulating/cutting
  device may be preferable)

Sterile dressing and bandages
Antibacterial creams

483
**Ch. 144 Escharotomy and
Fasciotomy**

PATIENT PREPARATION

1. Remove all constricting clothing and jewelry.
2. Elevate the burned extremity slightly above the level of the heart.
3. Administer pain medications as prescribed.
4. Place patient (unless contraindicated) in a supine anatomical position.
   See Figure 144.2.

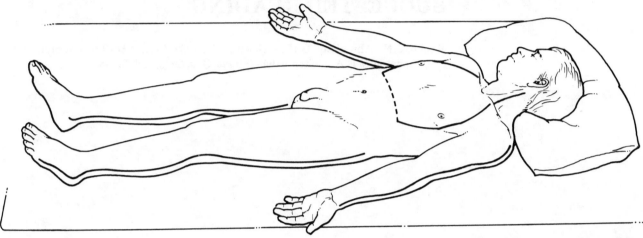

**Figure 144.2   Correct anatomical
positioning of escharotomy sites.
(Adapted from McDougal et al.,
1978. Reprinted by permission.)**

PROCEDURAL STEPS

1. Drape below and around the surgical area.
2. *Anesthetize with local infiltration of anesthesia, regional nerve block,
   or general anesthesia.
3. *Incise indicated areas. See Figure 144.2.
   Chest: Along the lateral aspects of the chest and across the chest
   wall at the level of the diaphragm.
   Digits & Extremities: Medial and lateral aspects of digit and extremity.
   Hands: Dorsal aspect of the hands.
4. Reassess respiratory function and distal circulatory status.
5. Apply direct pressure, cautery, or thrombate to all bleeding areas. Significant bleeding may occur and must be managed rapidly!
6. Reassess hematocrit and consider transfusion of blood if necessary.
7. Apply dressings impregnated with antibacterial creams to reduce infection (Monafo & Freedman, 1987).

*Indicates those portions of the
procedure usually performed by a
physician.

COMPLICATIONS

1. Wound infection
2. Sepsis
3. Blood loss
4. Nerve or vessel damage

REFERENCES

Braen, G.R. 1988. Thermal injury (burns). In P. Rosen, F.J. Baker, G.R. Braen, R.H.
Dailey, & R.C. Levy (eds). *Emergency medicine: Concepts and clinical practice,*
2nd ed. St. Louis: Mosby; 573–584.

Demling, R.H., & Lalonde, C. 1989. *Burn trauma.* New York: Thieme Medical Publishers; 42–65.

McDougal, W.S., Slade, C.L., & Pruitt, B.A. 1978. *Manual of burns.* New York:
Springer-Verlag.

Monafo, W.W., & Freedman, B.M. 1989. Electrical and lightning injury. In J.A.
Boswick (ed). *The art and science of burns care.* Rockville, MD: Aspen Publications, 241–253.

SUGGESTED READING

Kuehn, C.N., Ahrenholz, D.H., & Solem, L.D. 1989. Care of the burn wound. In J.B.
Johnston & E.A. Deitch (eds). *Trauma Quarterly,* 5, 4:33–55.

145

Incision and Drainage

Margo E. Layman, RNC, BSN, CEN

*Incision and drainage is also known as I&D.

INDICATIONS

1. To drain localized infections such as, sebaceous cysts, carbuncles, etc.
2. To remove foreign objects from soft tissue.

CONTRAINDICATIONS AND CAUTIONS

1. Patients with poor hygiene, malnutrition, diabetes, and immune deficiencies require careful techniques and followup.
2. Patients with bleeding disorders should be referred to a surgeon.
3. Abscesses on the hands, feet, or eye should be referred to the appropriate specialist.

EQUIPMENT

Antiseptic solution
Local anesthetic
Syringes and needles for local
    anesthesia
1/4- or 1/2-inch iodoform or plain
    sterile gauze packing
4-x-4-inch gauze dressings
Tape

Hydrogen peroxide (optional)
Scalpel with #11 blade
Hemostat (curved or straight)
Plain forceps
Surgical scissors
Cotton swabs
Culture swabs for aerobic and
    anaerobic specimens

PATIENT PREPARATION

1. Drape the area with waterproof drapes.
2. Clip hair or shave the area as indicated.
3. Cleanse the area with antiseptic solution with firm circular scrubbing motions from the abscess outward.
4. *Anesthetize the area with local anesthetic. See Ch. 137: Local Infiltration and Topical Agents.

PROCEDURAL STEPS

1. *Incise the periphery of the abscess cavity with the scalpel, purulent material will be expressed immediately. See Figure 145.1.
2. *Disrupt adhesions with a hemostat.
3. Obtain cultures (anaerobic and aerobic) from the drainage.

*Indicates portions of the procedure usually performed by a physician.

4. Cleanse the cavity with cotton swabs, then irrigate the cavity with peroxide or sterile saline. See Ch. 136: Wound Cleansing and Irrigation. Irrigation.
5. Pack the wound loosely with plain or iodoform gauze. This keeps the wound open and permits drainage. See Figure 145.2.
6. Apply a sterile dressing and secure with tape.

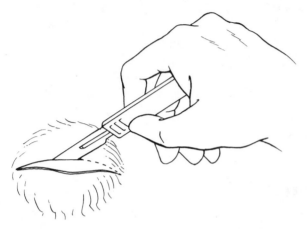

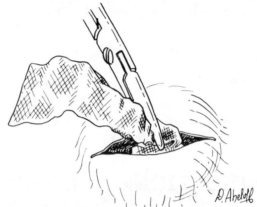

Figure 145.1 Incision of peripheral area with scalpel.
(Rosen & Sternbach, 1983: 185. Reprinted by permission.)

Figure 145.2 Gauze packing loosely placed into incised wound using a hemostat.
(Rosen & Sternbach, 1983: 185. Reprinted by permission.)

COMPLICATIONS

1. Reoccurrence of the abscess
2. Spread of the infection especially in perineal and rectal area
3. Systemic infection or sepsis

PATIENT TEACHING

1. Leave dressing in place for 24 hours unless it becomes soiled with excessive drainage; then it can be changed.
2. In 24 hours, remove the external dressing, and leave the packing in place.
3. Follow up with the physician in 2 days to have packing removed.
4. After the packing is removed, soak the site for 20–30 minutes in warm water 3 to 4 times a day.
5. Continue the soaks for 5 to 7 days or until the incision has healed. Redress the incision with clean dressing after each soaking.
6. Watch for signs of ongoing or worsening infection such as redness, swelling, draining pus, fever.

SUGGESTED READINGS

Mayhew, H.E., Rodgers, L.A. (eds). 1984. *Basic procedures in family practice.* Toronto: Fleschner.
Rosen, P., & Sternbach, G. (eds). 1983. *Atlas of emergency medicine,* 2nd ed. Baltimore: Williams & Wilkins.

146

Measures to Reverse Hypothermia

Dorothy Schulte, RN, MS
Jean A. Proehl, RN, MN, CEN, CCRN

INDICATIONS

To increase the core temperature in patients with temperatures less than 35°C (95°F) due to a decrease in heat production, an increase in heat loss, a combination of both, or an impaired thermoregulatory system. The goal of rewarming in hypothermia is to increase the core temperature between 0.5 to 2.0°C (1.0–3.0°F) per hour (Danzl, 1988).

CONTRAINDICATIONS AND CAUTIONS

1. Hypothermia creates myocardial irritability, so patients must be handled gently and procedures performed cautiously, because stimulation may precipitate ventricular fibrillation.
2. With active external rewarming, patients may experience rewarming shock, which is evidenced by a decrease in blood pressure due to vasodilation in previously vasoconstricted extremities.
3. With active external rewarming, patients may experience a temperature afterdrop, which results from the shunting of cold blood from extremities to the core which further chills the myocardium and increases the potential for ventricular fibrillation.
4. Use medications judiciously, because most drugs will have little effect on the hypothermic patient and may cause complications upon rewarming due to delayed metabolism of drugs (e.g., metabolic alkalosis with sodium bicarbonate, hypoglycemia with insulin).
5. Do not massage or rub skin and do not use alcohol on the skin of hypothermic patients, because these techniques will increase vasodilation and move cold blood from the extremities to the core.
6. Attempts at defibrillation are usually unsuccessful until core temperature is above 28–30°C (82–86°F) (Danzl, 1988).

EQUIPMENT

Warm IV solution (37.7°C) (100°F)
IV tubing
Warm normal saline for irrigation
Warm blankets
Heating pads
Hot water bottles
Cascade nebulizer or similar
    equipment to administer
    heated, humidified oxygen

Peritoneal lavage equipment
Foley catheter
Hemodialysis equipment
Cardiac bypass equipment
Gastric lavage equipment
Hypothermia thermometer
    (capability to measure
    temperatures of less than
    34.4°C (94°F))

PATIENT PREPARATION

1. Initiate resuscitation as indicated for the patient in cardiac arrest. Endotracheal intubation is necessary unless the patient is alert and has intact protective airway reflexes. Preoxygenate the patient prior to intubation to avoid dysrhythmias. Factors precipitating dysrhythmias during intubation are rough technique, hypoxia, and acid-base abnormalities (Danzl, 1988).
2. Check the rectum for stool before placement of the thermometer probe, if the probe is placed in feces, the reading will be inaccurate.
3. Apply the cardiac monitor for ongoing assessment during the rewarming procedures. See Ch. 57.
4. Obtain a baseline 12-lead ECG. See Ch. 58: 12-Lead ECG.
5. Obtain blood for CBC, ABG, K+, glucose, and cardiac enzymes determinations.

PROCEDURAL STEPS

There are three methods of rewarming: passive external, active external, and active core. The method chosen is determined by the duration and degree of hypothermia, the available resources, and the time needed to mobilize them and the specific contraindications to use of that procedure (Rueller, 1978). Core rewarming must precede or accompany peripheral rewarming to prevent afterdrop.

Methods of passive external rewarming

(For mild hypothermia)
1. Remove the patient from the cold or wet environment. Remove all clothing, dry the patient, and place the patient on a stretcher covered with sheets or blankets to prevent heat loss via conduction.
2. Cover the patient with blankets to prevent heat loss from radiation and convection.

Methods for active external rewarming

(Used in combination with active core rewarming for moderate to severe hypothermia).
1. Immerse the patient in water heated to 40°C (104°F), if possible.
2. Cover the patient with warm or electric blankets.
3. Place heated objects (heating pads, hot water bottles) in the groin, or axilla or on the trunk.
(Note: The current recommendation is to heat only the thorax during active external rewarming and leave the extremities unheated to allow for the maintenance or peripheral vasoconstriction, thus preventing afterdrop and rewarming shock (Danzl, 1988).

Methods of active core rewarming

(For moderate to severe hypothermia)
1. Initiate an IV line with fluid warmed to 37.7°C (100°F). Administer 300 ml as rapidly as possible and the remainder in one hour (Bangs & Hamlet, 1980).
2. Administer warm, humidified oxygen via a cascade nebulizer or similar device.
3. Peritoneal lavage with fluid warmed to 40.5–42.5°C (105–108.5°F) to conduct heat directly through the intraperitoneal structures, posterior

parietal peritoneum to the kidneys, and through the diaphragm to the heart and lungs. (Danzl, 1988). See Ch. 97.

4. Gastric lavage with warm fluid. See Ch. 100.
5. High colonic infusions of warm water.
6. Bladder irrigation with warm fluid.
7. Warmed mediastinal irrigation via thoracotomy (usually performed in the operating room).
8. Hemodialysis with warm fluid.
9. Extracorporeal blood rewarming (requires cardiac bypass equipment and an operating room).

COMPLICATIONS

1. Precipitation of ventricular fibrillation resulting from stimulation associated with procedures.
2. Rewarming shock and afterdrop associated with active, external rewarming.
3. Burns as a result of heating devices in direct contact with the skin.

PATIENT TEACHING

Following the reversal of mild hypothermia in the emergency department, patients should be instructed in the early signs of hypothermia (lethargy, incoordination, confusion) and the necessity to wear adequate clothing for weather.

REFERENCES

Auerbach, P., & Geehr, E. 1983. *Management of wilderness and environmental emergencies.* New York: MacMillan.

Bangs, C., & Hamlet, M. 1980. Out in the cold – Management of hypothermia, immersion, and frostbite. *Aspen;* 19–37.

Danzl, D.F. 1988. Accidental hypothermia. In P. Rosen, F. Baker, G.R. Braen, R. Dailey, & R. Levy, *Emergency Medicine: Concepts and Clinical Practice,* 2nd ed. St. Louis: Mosby; 663–692.

Rueller, J.B. 1978. Hypothermia: Pathophysiology, clinical settings, and management. *Annals of Internal Medicine,* 89:519–527.

147

Measures to Reverse Hyperthermia

Dorothy Schulte, RN, MS
Jean Proehl, RN, MN, CEN, CCRN

INDICATIONS

To lower body temperature to 39°C (102°F) or less through rapid cooling in patients whose temperatures are greater than 40.5°C (105°F). Hyperthermia may result from fever, heat stroke, metabolic disorders, thermoregulatory dysfunction, or medications (malignant hyperthermia).

CONTRAINDICATIONS AND CAUTIONS

1. Cooling must be initiated immediately upon the discovery of a hyperthermic state and must proceed rapidly. For a successful outcome, temperatures must be decreased to 39°C (102°F) or below within 1 hour of initiating treatment (Stine, 1979).
2. The use of antipyretic medications is controversial, because they will not correct thermoregulatory abnormalities and may have a negative effect on hemostasis, which is already compromised by the hyperthermic state (McElroy, 1980).

EQUIPMENT

Ice packs
Ice water
Large circulating fans
Bathtub or wash basin

Cooling blanket
Peritoneal lavage equipment
Thermometer

PATIENT PREPARATION

1. Place the patient on high-flow oxygen, because oxygen demand is increased in the hyperthermic state. Initiate resuscitation as indicated for the patient in cardiac arrest.
2. Place the patient on a cardiac monitor, because nonspecific ST segment changes, conduction disturbances, and ventricular arrhythmias have been reported during cooling. See Ch. 57.
3. Initiate an IV to restore intravascular fluid.
4. Draw blood for CBC, K^+, Na^+, Phosphorus, Ca^{++}, PT, PTT, ABG, Platelet, BUN, Glucose, Creatinine, SGOT, LDH, and CPK determinations.
5. Monitor temperature continually (if possible) using a rectal or esophageal thermometer.
6. Obtain baseline 12-lead ECG. See Ch. 58.
7. Insert a urinary bladder catheter. See Ch. 103: Urinary Bladder Catheter Insertion.

PROCEDURAL STEPS

A variety of modalities may be used for rapid cooling depending on the patient's condition, availability of resources, and institutional protocol. Modalities include:
1. Remove all clothing.
2. Immerse the patient in cold water. Massage the extremities to help counteract vasoconstriction, which will decrease heat loss.
3. Sponge the patient with ice water.
4. Cover the patient with cooling blanket.
5. Cover the patient with wet towels or spray patient with warm water while circulating air around patient with large fans to promote heat loss through evaporation.
6. Apply ice packs to neck, axilla, and inguinal area.
7. Administer dantrolene as ordered for malignant hyperthermia.

COMPLICATIONS

1. Violent shivering may develop with rapid cooling and may result in further heat production. This can be controlled with chlorpromazine 25–50 mg IVP (Danzl, 1988).
2. Hypotension
3. Acute renal failure
4. Metabolic acidosis
5. Increased serum K^+
6. Frostbite secondary to ice packs

PATIENT TEACHING

Patients who have experienced hyperthermic episodes are predisposed to future recurrences. Instruct the patient on prevention strategies as indicated by the etiology of this episode.

REFERENCES

Danzl, D.F. 1988. Accidental hypothermia. In P. Rosen, F. Baker, G.R. Braen, R. Dailey, & R. Levy. *Emergency medicine: Concepts and clinical practice*, 2nd ed. St. Louis: Mosby; 663–692.

McElroy, C. 1980. Update on heat illness. *Environmental Medical Emergencies*. Baltimore: Aspen.

Stine, R. 1979. Heat illness. *Journal of the American College of Emergency Physicians*, 8:154–159.

148

Heat Shield

Barbara E. Gamrath, RN, MN, CEN

Heat shield is also known as radiant heat warmer.

INDICATIONS

To minimize heat dissipation that may occur through convection, conduction, and evaporation. Use of a heat shield combines active and passive external rewarming techniques that may be especially useful when other sources of rewarming may not be appropriate. Heat shields may be used on burn patients that cannot tolerate insulative material directly on the skin, or on patients exposed to chemicals or chemotherapy resulting in skin sloughing.

CONTRAINDICATIONS AND CAUTIONS

1. Frequent temperature assessment is necessary to identify advancing hypothermia or hyperthermia that adversely affects oxygen consumption and metabolic function (McKenzie, 1988).

EQUIPMENT

Heat shield

PROCEDURAL STEPS

1. Remove wet or heavy clothing from the patient.
2. Place a light blanket or sheet over the patient (if appropriate).
3. Place the heat shield over the patient allowing enough space for continued patient assessment and intervention.

COMPLICATIONS

1. Hyperthermia due to inappropriate setting or placement of the heat shield.
2. See Ch. 149: Heat Lamp.

PATIENT TEACHING

1. Explain to the patient the effect of the heat shield in reducing heat loss. Explain that when the air is stationary, less heat is lost to conduction, convection, and radiation (Danzl, 1983).

Danzl, D. 1988. Accidental hypothermia. In P. Rosen, F.J. Baker, R.M. Barkin, G.R. Braen, R.H. Dailey, R.C. Levy (eds). *Emergency Medicine: Concepts and Clinical Practice,* 2nd ed. St. Louis: Mosby; 663–692.

McKenzie, C.A.M. Perinatal crisis. *AACN's Reference for Critical Care Nursing.* New York: McGraw-Hill; 867.

149

Heat Lamp

Barbara E. Gamrath, RN, MN, CEN

INDICATIONS

To provide direct transfer of exogenous heat (active external rewarming) to a patient who is hypothermic due to environmental exposure, cerebrovascular accidents with impaired thermogenesis, etc.

CONTRAINDICATIONS AND CAUTIONS

1. Frequent temperature assessment is necessary to identify hypothermia or hyperthermia that adversely affects oxygen consumption and metabolic function (McKenzie, 1988).
2. Caution must be exercised to avoid thermal burns when using heat lamps (Danzl, 1983).
3. External rewarming measures (i.e., heat lamps, warming blankets, water bottles, and heating pads) should be combined with core rewarming measures (i.e., peritoneal lavage, warm IV fluids, etc.) to help prevent afterdrop and rewarming shock in patients with core temperatures less than 30°C (86°F) (Danzl, 1988).

EQUIPMENT

Heat lamp   Light sheet or blanket
Yard stick

PATIENT PREPARATION

1. Remove any wet, frozen, or heavy clothing from the patient. Cover the patient with a light sheet or blanket for privacy.
2. Initiate cardiac monitoring, because hypothermia may lower the threshold for ventricular fibrillation. See Ch. 57.

PROCEDURAL STEPS

1. Place the heat lamp over the thorax. If the heat lamp is focused only on the extremities, active external rewarming will not be as effective (Harnett, 1980).
2. Place the heat lamp at least 3 feet from the patient to avoid burns and skin irritation.
3. Duration of patient exposure to the heat lamp should be kept to a maximum of 5 minute intervals to avoid burns and skin irritation. Many lamps have a timer for this purpose.

COMPLICATIONS

1. Afterdrop may occur during use of external active rewarming measures such as heat lamps (Harnett, 1980).
2. Active external rewarming causes a decrease in shivering thermogenesis (Collis, 1977). When the core temperature is greater than 30°C (86°F), active external rewarming suppresses shivering and rewarming may be impeded (Danzl, 1983).
3. Shock due to peripheral vasodilatation may occur with active external rewarming.
4. Burns, skin irritation.

PATIENT TEACHING

Sudden movements of the hypothermic patient may induce ventricular fibrillation. Extra care in handling the patient by family and healthcare deliverers must be exercised.

REFERENCES

Collis, M. 1977. Accidental hypothermia: An experimental study of practical rewarming methods. *Aviation, Space, and Environmental Medicine,* 48:625.

Danzl, D. 1988. Accidental hypothermia. In P. Rosen, F.J. Baker, R.M. Barkin, G.R. Braen, R.H. Dailey, R.C. Levy (eds). *Emergency Medicine: Concepts and Clinical Practice,* 2nd ed. St. Louis: Mosby; 663–692.

Harnett, R. 1980. Initial treatment of profound accidental hypothermia. *Aviation, Space, and Environmental Medicine,* 51:680.

McKenzie, C.A.M. 1988. Perinatal crisis. *AACN's Reference for Critical Care Nursing,* New York: McGraw-Hill; 867.

Assessing Visual Acuity

Marijane Smallwood, RN, BSN

INDICATIONS

To assess the vision of patients presenting with ocular complaints.

CONTRAINDICATIONS AND CAUTIONS

With the exception of chemical exposures to the eye, visual acuity testing should precede treatment. Copious irrigation with saline should be performed immediately for all chemical exposures. See Ch. 152: Eye Irrigation. Visual acuity testing follows irrigation in this instance.

EQUIPMENT

Snellen chart
or
Symbol chart (for illiterate patients or preschool children)
Eye spoon/patch/opaque card to cover eye not being tested (optional)

Penlight (optional)
Marked distance of 20 feet for testing
Topical ophthalmic anesthetic (optional)

PATIENT PREPARATION

1. Instruct the patient how to occlude one eye during the acuity test. If using a cupped hand, remind the patient to keep fingers together to prevent a false reading by using binocular vision. Instruct the patient not to apply excessive pressure on the eye being occluded, as blurred vision may result.
2. Instill prescribed topical ophthalmic anesthetic to increase patient comfort level during the exam (optional).
3. Leave glasses or contact lenses in place during the exam.

PROCEDURAL STEPS

1. Seat or stand the patient at a marked distance of 20 feet from the standard Snellen chart with the chart at the patient's eye level. Visual acuity is recorded as a fraction: the numerator represents the distance to the chart and the denominator represents the distance from which a normal eye can read the lines. For example, 20/50 means that the patient can

read what a person with 20/20 vision can read at 50 feet. If the patient is unable to read the first line of the Snellen chart at 20 feet, he or she may be placed at a distance of 10 feet from the chart and asked to read the lines. The acuity is then recorded as 10/50, etc.

2. Test the vision of one eye at a time. Test the unaffected eye first to serve as a control.

3. Place the eye spoon, patch, or patient's hand over the eye not being tested.

4. Ask the patient to read the Snellen chart starting with the top line and working downward until the letters are no longer legible.

5. Record the lowest line the patient is able to read including the number of mistakes made on that line. For example, OD (ocular dexter or right eye) 20/20 means the patient can read the 20/20 line with no mistakes. OS (ocular sinister or left eye) 20/25-1 means the patient can read the 20/25 line with 1 mistake.

6. Repeat steps 3–5 for the opposite eye.

7. If the patient is unable to read the top line of the Snellen chart, the following visual tests are acceptable for documentation:
   a. counts fingers at a measured distance;
   b. recognizes hand motions at a measured distance;

8. If the patient is unable to recognize hand motions, light perception is tested. Use a penlight and record whether the patient can determine the direction from which the light is coming.

9. If unable to recognize light perception, record visual acuity as "no light perception."

10. Use the Symbol Chart for illiterate patients or preschool children. The patient is asked to point his or her fingers in the direction of the E bars. Follow the same procedure as for the Snellen chart.

11. Handheld visual acuity cards are commercially available when distance testing is not possible (Kitt & Kaiser, 1990). The card is held 14 inches away from the patient. Attaching a 14-inch string to the card will facilitate correct usage. The procedure is the same as for the Snellen chart testing.

12. If commercially prepared charts are unavailable, have the patient read a newspaper or similar print and record the distance at which the patient is able to read the print.

13. Occasionally, patients with glasses or contact lenses carry the prescription in their wallet. This may serve as a gross baseline prior to injury.

Alternative methods

1. When the patient's glasses or contact lenses are not available, testing should be documented as "uncorrected visual acuity."

2. The pinhole method may be used to assess a refractive error when the patient's glasses or contact lenses are not available. The patient reads the Snellen chart while looking through a pinhole in an opaque card. If the visual acuity is improved, the decreased visual acuity may be attributed to a refractive error. If no improvement is noted, other etiologies should be explored (Powers & Meador, 1986).

3. Another alternative suggested by Powers & Meador (1986) is the use of a handheld ophthalmoscope to aid in obtaining a corrected visual acuity in the emergency department. The patient is instructed to dial the ophthalmoscope to the lens that provides the clearest view of the Snellen chart. The procedure and documentation is the same as outlined above for Snellen testing with the addition of recording the lens that provides the clearest view. "O.S.: correctable to 20/20 with a −10 lens" is an acceptable method to record visual acuity when using this technique.

COMPLICATIONS

1. Injury causing edema or blepharospasm may prevent the patient from keeping eyes open without manual assistance or medications to decrease the pain/spasm.
2. Excessive tearing may blur vision and affect test results.

REFERENCES

Fortin, S. 1990. Ocular emergencies. In S. Kitt, & J. Kaiser (eds). *Emergency nursing: A physiologic and clinical perspective.* Philadelphia: Saunders.

Powers, D. & Meador, S. 1986. Testing visual acuity in the emergency department: A simple method of correcting refractive error by using the hand-held ophthalmoscope. *Annals of emergency medicine,* 15:818–819.

SUGGESTED READINGS

Fincke, M., & Lanros, N. 1986. *Emergency nursing: A comprehensive review.* Rockville, MD: Aspen.

Havener, W.A. 1984. *Synopsis of ophthalmology.* St. Louis: Mosby.

151

Contact Lens Removal

Margo E. Layman, RNC, BSN, CEN

INDICATIONS

1. To assist a patient who is unable to remove lenses.
2. To remove contact lenses in the presence of chemical irritants or foreign bodies.
3. To remove contact lenses from a patient with an altered level of consciousness.

CONTRAINDICATIONS AND CAUTIONS

1. Never use force to remove a lens. If you have difficulty, slide the lens onto the sclera and notify the physician.
2. Look for any "lost" lenses in the upper cul-de-sac of the eye. This is their most common hiding place.
3. Do not replace the lens until a physician examines the patient's eyes.
4. If you suspect your patient has a penetrating injury to the eye, do not manipulate the eye in any way.
5. If the eyes appear dry, instill several drops of sterile saline solution and wait a few minutes before removing the lens to help prevent corneal damage.
6. Do not instill medications while the patient is wearing contact lenses. Contact lenses can combine chemically with the medication and cause eye irritation or lens damage.
7. Do not use saline with preservatives because it may damage the lenses.

EQUIPMENT

Contact lens storage case or 2 plastic specimen containers with lids
Contact lens soaking solution or sterile saline without preservative
Suction cup (optional)
Towel

PATIENT PREPARATION

1. Place patient in semi-Fowler's or supine position.
2. Place a clean towel around the neck and across the chest.
3. Remove any glass particles with cellophane tape. Roll the adhesive to the outside and gently touch the adhesive against the patient's closed eyes to remove glass particles.
4. Gently remove blood, dirt, or makeup from eyelids with a cotton ball moistened with saline.

5. Place several milliliters of sterile saline in each specimen container and label containers "left" and "right." If a contact lens case is used, place a few drops of saline in each compartment.

PROCEDURAL STEPS

Hard lenses

1. Use one thumb to pull the patient's upper eyelid toward the orbital rim.
2. With your other thumb on the lower lid, gently move the lids toward each other to trap the lens edge and break the suction. See Figure 151.1.

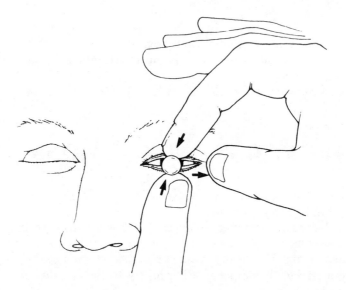

Figure 151.1   Removal of hard contact lens.
(Kitt & Kaiser, 1990: 141. Reprinted by permission.)

3. Cup your hand below the eye to catch the lens when it pops out.
4. Place the lens in an appropriate specimen container or contact lens case compartment.
5. Remove and care for the opposite lens using the same technique.
6. Examine the patient's eyes for redness or irritation.

Soft lenses

1. Raise the upper eyelid with your index finger and hold it against the orbital rim.
2. Lightly place your thumb on lower lid and pull it down.
3. Have the patient look up and slide the lens down gently with the index finger of your other hand.
4. Pinch the lens together with your thumb and index finger and lift it out of the patient's eye. See Figure 151.2
5. Place the lens in the appropriate specimen container or contact lens case compartment.
6. Remove and care for the opposite lens using the same technique.
7. Examine the patient's eyes for redness or irritation.

SUCTION CUP REMOVAL OF HARD AND SOFT LENSES

1. Wet the suction cup with a drop of sterile saline.
2. Gently pull up the patient's upper eyelid with your index finger and pull the lower lid down with your thumb.

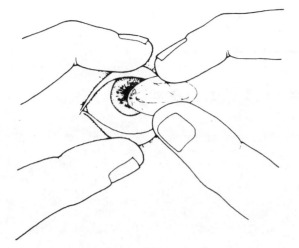

Figure 151.2 Removal of soft contact lens.
(Kitt & Kaiser, 1990: 142. Reprinted by permission.)

3. Press the suction cup gently to the center of the lens. See Figure 151.3.
4. Pull the suction cup and lens away from the eye in a straight line.
5. Place the lens in the appropriate specimen container or contact lens case compartment.
6. Remove and care for the opposite lens using the same technique.
7. Examine the patient's eyes for redness or irritation.

COMPLICATIONS

1. Corneal damage as a result of touching the cornea with the suction cup or attempting to remove dry lenses.
2. Corneal damage could occur if the lens is replaced in the wrong eye. Always label the containers and place the lenses in the proper containers or compartments.

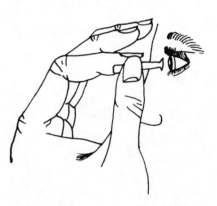

Figure 151.3 Suction cup removal of contact lens.

PATIENT TEACHING

1. Watch for signs of eye irritation such as purulent drainage, redness, swelling, etc.
2. Follow usual cleaning procedures for lenses.

SUGGESTED READINGS

Boyd-Monk, H. 1978. Taking a closer look at contact lenses. *Nursing,* 8:39–43.
Ford, E., (ed). 1985. *Emergency care handbook.* Springhouse, PA: Springhouse Corporation.
Hamilton, H.K., (ed). 1983. *Procedures.* Springhouse, PA: Springhouse Corporation.
Kitt, S., & Kaiser, J. (eds). (1990). *Emergency nursing: A Physiologic and clinical perspective.* Philadelphia: Saunders.
Sutton, A.L. (1969). *Bedside nursing techniques in medicine and surgery.* Philadelphia: Saunders.
1986. How to remove contact lenses. *Nursing Life,* 14–15.

152

Eye Irrigation

Marijane Smallwood, RN, BSN

Eye irrigation is also known as eye flushing.

INDICATIONS

1. To remove chemicals from the eye and restore a normal pH.
2. To remove foreign objects from the eye and help prevent ocular damage and vision loss following eye injury.
3. To relieve pain or burning that is usually associated with a foreign body or chemical injury to the eye.

CONTRAINDICATIONS AND CAUTIONS

Caution is required when a penetrating injury is present or suspected.

EQUIPMENT

Topical ophthalmic anesthetic
Sterile normal saline
    1000 ml IV bag
    or
    3000 ml bladder irrigation bag
IV macrodrip tubing
18- or 20-G over-the-needle catheter
    with stylet removed.
    irrigation (Morgan) lens, or
        syringe irrigating device

Basin
Gauze dressings
Towels or patient gown
Tissues
Cotton-tipped applicators
Shampoo board (optional)
Desmarres retractor or paperclip
    fashioned retractor (See
    Figure 152.1.)
pH paper

PATIENT PREPARATION

1. Instill prescribed topical anesthetic into affected eye(s).
2. If a chemical exposure occurred, obtain a baseline pH measurement of the eye by placing pH paper in the conjunctival sac.
3. Another person may be necessary to hold the eyelids open manually or with retractors if an irrigating lens is not used.
4. Inform the patient that the eye irrigation may cause postnasal drip.
5. Use a gown to protect the patient from excessive dampness during the procedure.
6. Position a basin or large plastic bag to catch irrigant or position the patient over a sink. Using a shampoo board under the patient's head is another method to facilitate collection of the irrigant. Place patient in supine position. Pad under patient's neck with towels to increase comfort.

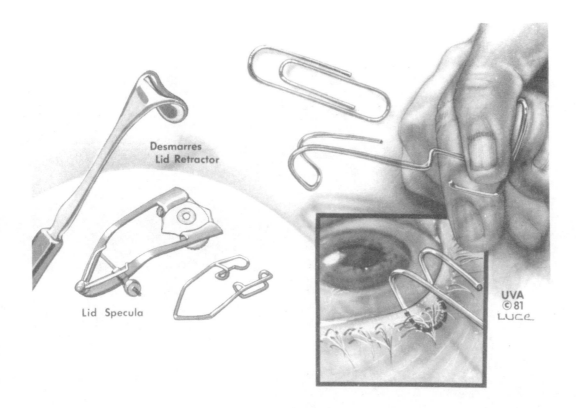

Figure 152.1 Devices for separating eyelids. Desmarres Ltd. Retractor and improvised paperclip. (Haddad & Winchester, 1983. Reprinted by permission.)

PROCEDURAL STEPS

Technique A

1. Attach IV tubing to IV fluid and catheter or irrigating syringe.
2. Use gauze pads to hold eyelids open if necessary.
3. Direct flow of irrigant from inner to outer canthus. See Figure 152.2.
4. Instruct patient to roll eyes in all directions to ensure total eye irrigation.
5. For acidic exposure, irrigate with a minimum of 1000 ml of normal saline per eye. Acids are quickly neutralized by the proteins of the eye surface. When irrigated out, acids cause no further damage (Barr & Hedges, 1985).
6. Irrigate alkaline injuries with a minimum of 2 liters of normal saline per eye over 1 hour. Because alkaline substances, hydrofluoric and heavy metal acids can penetrate the cornea rapidly and continue to produce damage for days, extensive irrigation is required (Barr & Hedges, 1985).
7. Measure the pH of the eye at intervals during irrigation by placing pH paper in the conjunctival sac. Continue the irrigation until the pH is restored to normal or near normal. Normal tear pH is 7.4.
8. *Evert the eyelid and use a wet cotton-tipped applicator to swab the fornices to remove traces of alkali. See Figure 152.3.
9. Determine the patient's comfort level at intervals. Instill additional topical ophthalmic anesthetic as necessary.
10. Recheck the eye pH 20–30 minutes following the irrigation to ensure it remains normal. Delayed pH changes often result from inadequate irrigation techniques (Barr & Hedges, 1985).
11. Prepare the patient for a corneal examination to determine the extent of injury. See Ch. 153: Fluorescein Staining.

*Indicates portions of procedure usually performed by a physician.

503

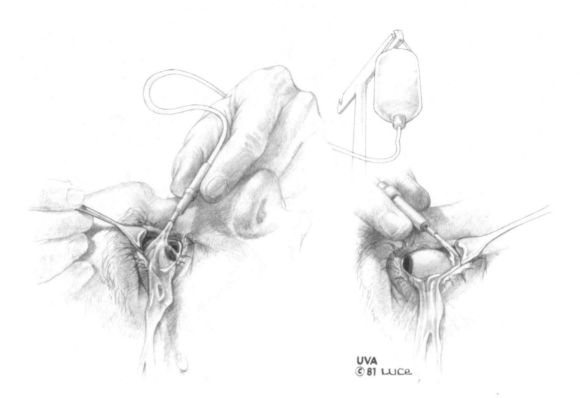

UVA
© 81 LUCE

Figure 152.2 Irrigation technique using Desmarres Retractor.
(Haddad & Winchester, 1983. Reprinted by permission.)

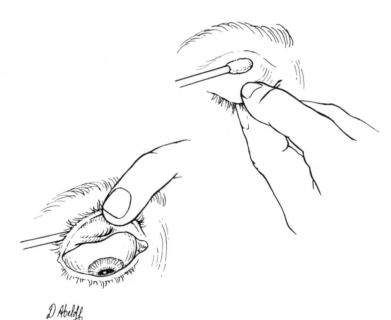

Figure 152.3 Eyelid eversion: A. Have patient look downward and grasp eyelashes and pull downward. B. Place cotton-tipped applicator midpoint of eyelid and pull eyelid over applicator. Lid eversion is complete.
(Rosen & Sternbach, 1983: 157. Reprinted by permission.)

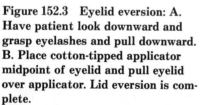
D. Abeloff

Technique B: Irrigating or Morgan therapeutic lens

1. The irrigating lens fits onto the cornea like a soft contact lens and provides optimal, continuous irrigation of the corneal surface while providing increased patient comfort. The lens allows the patient to close his or her eyelids and decreases the risk of iatrogenic trauma often encountered during a difficult irrigation. See Figure 152.4.

2. Attach the IV tubing to the lens device, open the clamp and adjust the flow to a level tolerated well by the patient, and proceed with continuous irrigation. A wide open flow may create too much pressure and actually create more discomfort for the patient.

3. See Steps 4–10 of Technique A for remainder of procedure.

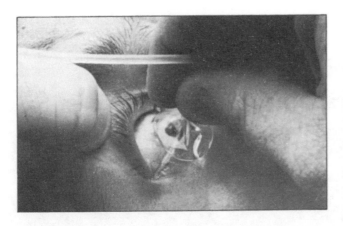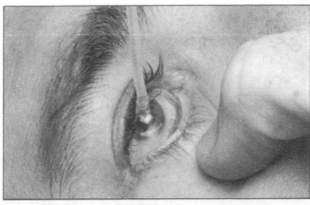

Figure 152.4 Placement of the Morgan lens for eye irrigation.
A. Have patient look downward, insert lens under upper lid. Have patient look up, retract lower lid.
B. For removal, have patient look up, retract lower lid, hold position and slid lens out.
(From *Instructional Chart for Morgan Lens,* MorTan, Inc., 1988. Copyright 1988 by MorTan, Inc. Reprinted by permission.)

COMPLICATIONS

1. Corneal or conjunctival abrasions may result from holding the eyelids open during the irrigation process.
2. Swelling or periorbital edema may occur following irrigation.
3. A fine punctate keratitis may result from the irrigation itself (Barr & Hedges, 1985).

PATIENT TEACHING

Ophthalmologic followup is essential.

REFERENCES

Barr, D., & Hedges, J. 1985. Ophthalmologic procedures. In J. Roberts, & J. Hedges, (eds). *Clinical procedures in emergency medicine,* Philadelphia: Saunders; 890–893.

Haddad, L.M., & Winchester, J.F. (1983). *Clinical management of poisoning and drug overdose.* Philadelphia: Saunders.

Rosen, P., & Sternbach, G.L. (1983). *Atlas of Emergency Medicine,* 2nd ed. Baltimore: Williams & Wilkins.

SUGGESTED READINGS

Bourg, P., Sherer, C., & Rosen, P. 1986. *Standardized nursing care plans for emergency departments.* St. Louis: Mosby.

Fincke, M., & Lanros, N. 1986. *Emergency nursing: A comprehensive review.* Rockville, MD: Aspen.

Rea, R.E. (ed). 1991. *Trauma nursing core course (provider) manual,* 3rd ed. Chicago: Award Printing Corporation.

153

Fluorescein Staining of Eyes

Marijane Smallwood, RN, BSN

Fluorescein staining of the eye is also known as ultraviolet exam, Woods lamp exam, black light exam.

INDICATIONS

1. To diagnose blunt or penetrating eye injuries.
2. To evaluate suspected corneal abrasions, foreign bodies, or infections of the eye.
3. To prepare the corneal surface for applanation tonometry to measure intraocular pressure with the slit lamp (Barr & Hedges, 1985). (This is not commonly done in the emergency department except by a consulting ophthalmologist.)
4. To test for epiphoria, a condition displayed by the overflow of tears due to blockage of the lacrimal drainage system. If the drainage system is patent, traces of fluorescein will be present in oral and nasal secretions (Havener, 1984).
5. To perform the Seidel test, which is used for detection of a perforated eye. On examination, a perforation is present when the fluorescein solution presents as a greenish stream in contrast to the orange color over the rest of the sclera (Cain, 1981).

CONTRAINDICATIONS AND CAUTIONS

1. Soft contact lens should be removed because the fluorescein stain may cause permanent tinting of the lens. See Ch. 151: Contact Lens Removal. Recently a high molecular density fluorescein solution has been developed which can be used with soft lenses in place (Stein, 1988). However, it is not commonly available in the emergency department. Hard contact lenses are not affected by the dye.
2. With deep corneal disruption, the dye may enter the anterior chamber of the eye (Barr & Hedges, 1985). While the dye is nontoxic, it is difficult to completely flush out.
3. Multiple dose bottles of fluorescein stain are easily contaminated and pseudomonas aeruginosa flourishes in fluorescein solution. Therefore, sterile fluorescein impregnated strips are safer (Stein, 1988). If fluorescein solution is used, individual dosettes are preferred.

EQUIPMENT

Saline 0.9%, artificial tears, or dextrose solution for irrigant
Sterile fluorescein impregnated strips
Light source: Cobalt blue penlight, blue filter of slit lamp, or Woods lamp

Patient gown or towel
Tissues
Emesis basin
Topical ophthalmic anesthetic (optional)

PATIENT PREPARATION

1. Remove glasses and contact lens. See Ch. 151: Contact Lens Removal.
2. Cover the patient's clothing with a gown or towel. Fluorescein is a dye and may permanently stain clothing.
3. Place the patient in either a seated or supine position.
4. Provide tissues and instruct patient to gently blot tears. This is especially important if the physician uses a topical anesthetic for the procedure because additional corneal irritation may result.

PROCEDURAL STEPS

1. Instill 2 drops of the prescribed topical anesthetic in the affected eye or eyes (optional).
2. Grasp sterile fluorescein strip by the white end. Wet the orange end with one drop of saline, artificial tear, dextrose solution, or topical anesthetic.
3. Depress the lower eye lid and gently place the fluorescein strip into the conjunctival sac. Placement of a nonmoistened fluorescein strip may cause additional epithelial damage. See Figure 153.1.
4. Instruct the patient to blink once. An alternative method to having the patient blink is to touch the fluorescein strip to the conjunctival sac and observe the flow of dye into the sac until an adequate amount is present to coat the corneal surface. Remove the strip.
5. Instruct the patient to close his or her eyes for approximately 30–60 seconds. This promotes maximal distribution of the dye over the cornea by retaining tears within the eyelids.
6. Use irrigant to remove excessive fluorescein dye. This enhances the contrast between the injured and normal ares.
7. Dim the lights in the exam room.
8. *Use a cobalt blue penlight or light source of choice to inspect the corneal surface for epithelial defects, foreign bodies, or abrasions. Disrupted corneal surfaces are visualized as bright green under the blue light.
9. Following the exam, irrigate the eye with saline or other irrigant to remove the fluorescein dye and prevent staining of clothing and face. An emesis basin can be held close to the patients cheek to catch the irrigant solution. Step 9 is optional and performed for aesthetics only.

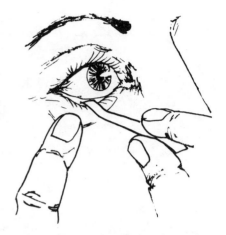

Figure 153.1 Placement of fluorescein strip into conjunctival sac. (Sheehy, 1990: 429. Reprinted by permission.)

*Indicates portions of the procedure usually performed by a physician.

COMPLICATIONS

1. While topical fluorescein is considered nontoxic, rare reactions such as redness or swelling have been noted when fluorescein solution was used. These reactions are usually caused by contaminants in the solution rather than the solution itself (Stein, 1988).
2. Barr & Hedges (1985) cite two reports that describe vasovagal reactions and a generalized convulsion following the use of a solution containing fluorescein. They note that the reactions were probably due to another factor, but caution should be used if using the fluorescein solution rather than the impregnated strips.

PATIENT TEACHING

1. Yellowish/orange tinged fluid may drain from your eyes or nose.
2. Do not wear soft contact lenses for 3–5 hours following fluorescein staining to prevent permanent staining of the lens.
3. Hard contact lens wearers require no special instructions.

REFERENCES

Barr, D., & Hedges, J. 1985. Ophthalmologic procedures. In J. Roberts, & J. Hedges (eds). *Clinical procedures in emergency medicine.* Philadelphia: Saunders; 888–890.

Cain, W. 1981. Detection of anterior chamber leakage with Seidel's test. *Archives of Ophthalmology,* 99:2013.

Havener, W.A. 1984. *Synopsis of ophthalmology.* St. Louis: Mosby.

Sheehy, S. 1990. *Mosby's manual of emergency care,* 3rd ed. St. Louis: Mosby.

Stein, H. 1988. *The ophthalmic assistant: fundamentals and clinical practice.* St. Louis: Mosby.

154

Ophthalmic Foreign Body Removal

Marijane Smallwood, RN, BSN

INDICATIONS

To remove a foreign body in a timely manner, thus preventing further ocular damage. Foreign bodies usually result from trauma or acts of nature such as wind blown objects or insects.

CONTRAINDICATIONS AND CAUTIONS

1. If a foreign body is impaled in the eye, immobilize the object and patch the opposite eye to decrease ocular movement. See Ch. 156: Eye Patching, and Ch. 158: Foreign Body Immobilization.
2. Contact lenses should be removed immediately in the presence of a foreign body. See Ch. 151: Contact Lens Removal.
3. Chemical injuries are considered penetrating and require immediate copious irrigation to prevent irreversible damage. See Ch. 152: Eye Irrigation.
4. If you are unable to locate an external foreign body and the patient still complains of a foreign body sensation, consider the possibility of an intraocular or intraorbital foreign body. Symptoms suggestive of a penetrating injury include an irregular pupil, hyphema, lens opacification, hemorrhage, or prolapsed iris. Tonometry should not be performed if a penetrating injury is suspected (Barr & Hedges, 1985).

   If nothing is visualized during the direct/indirect ophthalmoscopic exam, a computerized tomography scan may be used to locate the presence of an intraocular foreign body. While magnetic resonance imaging is useful, it may cause additional damage to an eye injured by a ferromagnetic object, because iron-based objects tend to move during the procedure (Lagouros, 1987).
5. Abrasions or actinic injuries often mimic the sensation of an ocular foreign body, but are easily diagnosed with the fluorescein exam. See Ch. 153: Fluorescein Staining.

EQUIPMENT

Topical ophthalmic anesthetic
Sterile fluorescein strip
Irrigation solution
Sterile cotton swabs
25- or 27-G needle or eye spud
3-ml syringe (or any size that is comfortable to hold)
Ophthalmoscope
Ultraviolet light
Penlight
Magnification source: Loupes or slit lamp
Eye patches
Adhesive tape
Cycloplegic ophthalmic drops
Antibiotic ophthalmic drops or ointment
Lid retractor/paperclip devised as retractor (See Figure 152.1.)
Eye drill with drill bits (optional)

PATIENT PREPARATION

1. Position the patient in a sitting or high Fowler's position.
2. Assess and document visual acuity. See Ch. 150: Assessing Visual Acuity.
3. Remove contact lens if present. See Ch. 151: Contact Lens Removal.
4. Anesthetize the affected eye(s) with 1–2 drops of topical ophthalmic anesthetic, as prescribed.
5. Apply fluorescein stain. See Ch. 153: Fluorescein Staining.

PROCEDURAL STEPS

*Indicates portions of procedure usually performed by a physician.

1. Use a penlight to examine the anesthetized corneal surface, lower fornix, conjunctiva, and upper lid conjunctiva. Ask the patient to look in all directions. Vertical scratches suggest a foreign body trapped under the lid.
2. *Evert the upper eye lid using a cotton swab. Place the applicator in the middle of the upper lid and instruct the patient to gaze downward. Grasp the patient's eye lashes, pull downward, and then fold upward over the swab. Laying the swab shaft across the bridge of the nose adds support when everting the eyelid. While the eyelid is everted, use a moist cotton swab to sweep the upper fornix area and remove any debris.
3. Removal techniques vary once the foreign body is located. Options include
   a. Gently irrigate the eye to dislodge the foreign body into the lower conjunctival sac. Remove the foreign body with a moist cotton swab.
   b. *Attempt to remove the foreign body by gently touching it with a moist cotton swab. Do not use a dry applicator or attempt prolonged dislodgement of the object, because additional epithelial damage may result.
   c. *Under slit lamp or loupe magnification, embedded foreign bodies may be removed with a 27 or 25 gauge needle attached to a syringe or a cotton swab. The syringe or cotton swab acts as a handle. See Figure 154.1. If available, a commercial eye spud may also be used. The needle or eye spud is held tangentially to the cornea to gently scrape the foreign body off of the cornea (Barr 1985). See Figure 154.2. Ideally, use a slip lamp that has a chin rest to secure the head, adequate illumination, magnification, and a light focus point. The patient may also be asked to focus on the practitioner's ear to steady the eye. In the event a slit lamp is unavailable, instruct the patient to fix his or her gaze on a stationary object. Secure the patient's head against the exam chair headrest with your fingers, steadying your hand against the patient's face. Dim the room lights. Use a penlight to provide increased illumination to the eye. Head supported magnification (loupes) may be used.
4. *When these methods are unsuccessful, an eye drill may also be used.
5. *Completely remove any rust ring with the eye drill. Patients may be referred to an ophthalmologist for rust ring removal. If removal is incomplete, the rust ring softens within 24–48 hours facilitating easy removal (Barr, 1985).
6. *Magnetic removal is a recent approach for removal of ferromagnetic foreign bodies. A magnet is placed on the handle of sterile jeweler's forceps, the magnet attracts the foreign body, which is lifted or grasped from the cornea (Arnold & Erie, 1988).
7. Following foreign body removal, irrigate the eye with at least 10 cc of

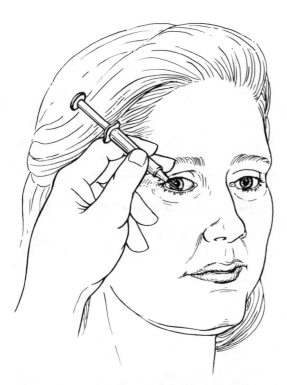

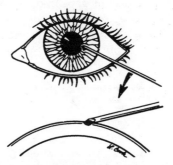

Figure 154.1 Removal of foreign body using a syringe as a handle and a small gauge needle. (Rosen & Sternbach, 1983: 157. Reprinted by permission.)

Figure 154.2 Removal of a foreign body from the cornea. Hold the syringe tangential to the foreign body and gently scrape from the cornea. The side view demonstrates the thickness of the cornea relative to the beveled needle edge. (Barr & Hedges, 1985: 895. Reprinted by permission.)

saline to remove remaining traces of fluorescein or other particulate matter.

8. Apply prophylactic antibiotic ophthalmic drops or ointment as ordered to prevent bacterial or fungal corneal ulceration. Cycloplegics may be ordered to decrease ciliary muscle spasms and increase patient comfort.
9. Patch the eye. See Ch. 156: Eye Patching.

COMPLICATIONS

1. Incomplete removal of a foreign body causes inflammation and retardation of healing. Due to oxidation of iron, metallic foreign bodies create rust rings within hours. Unremoved rust rings cause continuing irritation of the eye.
2. Conjunctivitis may occur following removal of a foreign body, usually this is the result of the patient rubbing the injured eye (Barr, 1985).
3. Use of a cotton swab, especially when dry, may cause additional epithelial damage.
4. Insect parts should be completely removed to prevent a prolonged inflammatory response that mimics an infectious keratitis (Lawton, 1988).

PATIENT TEACHING

1. Leave the patch in place as directed, usually 24–48 hours.
2. Rest the uninjured eye, thus preventing involuntary movement of the injured eye.
3. Television viewing is permitted at a distance of 10 feet or more. Fixed gaze television watching limits movement of the eye as opposed to reading, which necessitates eye movement (Barr, 1985).
4. The sensation of having a foreign body in the eye may return after the topical anesthetic wears off.
5. No driving or operating machinery with a patch in place, because there is loss of depth perception.

    (Never give the patient topical anesthetic to take home for pain relief. Continued use retards healing and may mask pain associated with complications.)

REFERENCES

Arnold, R.W., & Erie, J. 1988. Magnetized forceps for metallic corneal foreign bodies. *Archives of Ophthalmology,* 106:1502.

Barr, D., & Hedges, J. 1985. Ophthalmologic procedures. In J. Roberts, & J. Hedges (eds). *Clinical procedures in emergency medicine,* Philadelphia: Saunders; 893–897.

Lagouros, A., Langer, B., Peyman, G., Mafee, M., Spigos, D., & Grisolano, J. 1987. Magnetic resonance imaging and intraocular foreign bodies. *Archives of Ophthalmology,* 105:551–553.

Lawton, A. 1988. Insect foreign body in the cornea. *Archives of Ophthalmology,* 106:1171.

Newell, S. 1985. Management of corneal foreign bodies. *American Family Physician,* 31:149–156.

Rosen, P., & Sternbach, G.L. 1983. *Atlas of emergency medicine,* 2nd ed. Baltimore: Williams & Wilkins.

SUGGESTED READINGS

Deutsch, T., & Feller, D. 1985. *Management of ocular injuries.* Philadelphia: Saunders.

Havener, W.A. 1984. *Synopsis of ophthalmology.* St. Louis: Mosby.

155

Instillation of Eye Medications

Valerie Novotny-Dinsdale, RN, MSN, CEN

INDICATIONS

1. To reduce the potential for infection related to eye injury.
2. To decrease pain related to eye irritation or injury.
3. To provide treatment for an existing problem or infection.
4. To assist in the examination of the eyes by anesthetizing the cornea and/or paralyzing the ciliary muscles.

CONTRAINDICATIONS AND CAUTIONS

1. Do not instill medications in the presence of penetrating injuries to the globe without a physician's order.
2. Local ocular steroids can promote bacterial, viral, and yeast infections and should be used only on the order of an opthamologist (Cosgriff & Anderson, 1984; Shingleton, Frederick, & Hutchinson, 1989).
3. Caution should be used in instillation of cycloplegic or steroid drops in the elderly, because angle-closure glaucoma can be induced (Brinkley, 1984).

EQUIPMENT

Sterile gauze or tissues (if sterility is not indicated)   Prescribed ophthalmic medication

PATIENT PREPARATION

1. Assess visual acuity. See Ch. 150: Assessing Visual Acuity. This should be done prior to instillation of medications. Medicolegally this will document that any decreased vision is not a result of medications or management (Barr & Hedges, 1985).
2. Place the patient in a supine position or with head tilted back while sitting.
3. Determine patient medication allergies.
4. Determine significant past ocular history.

PROCEDURAL STEPS

Instillation of eye drops

1. Instruct the patient to look up toward the top of his or her head.
2. Gently pull the lower eyelid down or evert the lower lid using a piece of gauze or a cotton swab.

3. Instill a single drop into the conjunctival sac at the center of lower lid. More than one drop at a time is not recommended because this will increase tearing and decrease the concentration of the medication (Barr & Hedges, 1985).
4. Have the patient gently close his or her eyes or blink to spread the medication.

Instillation of eye ointment

1. Instruct the patient to look up toward the top of his or her head.
2. Gently pull the lower eyelid down or evert the lower lid using a piece of gauze or a cotton swab.
3. Spread a 1/2-inch ribbon of ointment in a thin line from the inner to outer canthus of the conjunctival sac (Karash & Keyes, 1988).
4. Have the patient gently close or blink his or her eyes a few times to spread the medication.
5. The eyes should remain closed until an eye patch is applied. See Ch. 156: Eye Patching.

COMPLICATIONS

1. Introduction of contaminated medication may result in an infection.
2. Trauma to the eye from movement of the patient's head during instillation.
3. Precipitation of an attack of angle-closure glaucoma.
4. Prolonged use of topical anesthetics can result in epithelial damage to the cornea.
5. Blurred vision (temporary) from the effects of the medication or from the presence of ointment in the eye.

PATIENT TEACHING

1. Do not rub your eyes or squeeze the lids together.
2. Some medications will make your eyes sensitive to light, you may need to wear sunglasses.
3. Report any increase in eye pain, purulent drainage, or visual problems immediately.

REFERENCES

Barr, D., & Hedges, J. 1985. Opthamalogic procedures. In J. Roberts, & J. Hedges (eds). *Clinical procedures in emergency medicine.* Philadelphia: Saunders; 886–914.

Brinkley, J. 1984. Emergency management of ocular trauma. *Topics in emergency medicine*, 6, 1:35–45.

Cosgriff, J., & Anderson, D. 1984. *The practice of emergency care,* 2nd ed. Philadelphia: Lippincott.

Karash, J., & Keyes, B.J. 1988. Ocular trauma. In V.D. Cardona, P.D. Hurn, P.J. Bastnagel Mason, A.M. Scanlon-Schilpp, & S.W. Veise-Berry, (eds). *Trauma Nursing: From resuscitation through rehabilitation.* Philadelphia: Saunders; 598–619.

Shingleton, B.J., Frederick, A.R., & Hutchinson, B.T. 1989. Ocular emergencies. In E.W. Wilkins, Jr. (ed). *Emergency medicine: Scientific foundations and current practice.* Baltimore: Williams and Wilkins; 876–891.

SUGGESTED READINGS

Budassi, S., & Barber, J. 1984. *Mosby's manual of emergency care: Practices and procedures.* St. Louis: Mosby.

Fortin, S. 1990. Ocular emergencies. In S. Kitt & J. Kaiser (eds). *Emergency nursing: A physiologic and clinical perspective.* Philadelphia: Saunders; 137–161.

Lawler, M. 1989. Common ocular injuries and disorders. Part I: Acute loss of vision. *Journal of Emergency Nursing,* 15, 1:32–36.

Lawler, M. 1989. Common ocular injuries and disorders. Part II: Red eye. *Journal of Emergency Nursing,* 15, 1:36–41.

156

Eye Patching

Valerie Novotny-Dinsdale, RN, MSN, CEN

INDICATIONS

1. To avoid further injury after trauma to the eye(s) such as in corneal abrasion.
2. To protect the eye following administration of an anesthetic.
3. To aid in resting the eye(s).
4. To protect an injured globe without applying any pressure to the eye, a metal eye shield or paper cup may be used. Injuries that require this type of protection include hyphema, globe perforation, and protruding foreign objects imbedded in the globe such as fish hooks, knives, etc.

CONTRAINDICATIONS AND CAUTIONS

1. Patching is contraindicated when corneal epithelial loss is the result of an infection. Patching an infected eye, provides a dark, moist environment for bacterial growth. Additionally, if epithelial loss is all the way through the cornea, the bacteria has access to the anterior chamber of the eye (Barr, & Hedges, 1985).
2. A pressure patch should never be applied in a penetrating injury. Pressure applied to a globe that has anterior or posterior penetration can cause extrusion of aqueous or vitreous humor, resulting in further injury to the eye (Barr & Hedges, 1985).
3. The patch must be firm enough to keep the eyelid closed. A corneal abrasion may result if the patient is able to open his or her eye(s) under the patch, thereby scraping off new cells and further irritating the abraded area.
4. Eye irrigation or eye medications should not be used for penetrating injuries to the globe, without an opthamology consult (Vaughn & Asbury, 1986).

EQUIPMENT

Eye patches (minimum of two per eye to be patched)

Metal eye shield (for selected injuries as noted above)

Tapeless eye shield (for long-term use)

Tape

PATIENT PREPARATION

1. Place the patient in a supine position or seated with the head tilted back.
2. Cleanse the skin around the eye to remove dirt, fluids, drainage, or residual eye medications.

3. Beards may need to be partially shaved in order to securely anchor the tape.

PROCEDURAL STEPS

Eye patches

1. Determine the number of eye pads needed according to the depth of the patient's eye socket:
   a. Ask the patient to gently close his or her eyes.
   b. Fold the first eye patch in half and place it over the closed lid.
   c. Cover that patch with one or more flat eye patches to fill the eye socket.
2. Tape from the cheek to the forehead to anchor the eye patches and apply firm pressure to the lid (Brinkley, 1984). Several strips of tape will be needed. Placing the tape as horizontally as possible will help reduce discomfort from the tape during facial movements, such as smiling and talking.
3. The tape should cover the entire eye patch to prevent slipping of the patch and movement of the eye lid. See Figure 156.1.

Metal eye shield

1. Stabilize any protruding objects with gauze dressings and tape.
2. Place a metal shield or paper cup over the affected eye. The eye shield or cup may need to be cut to accommodate a protruding object. See Ch. 158: Foreign Body Immobilization.
3. Apply strips of tape to secure the shield so that movement or irritation from a foreign object is eliminated.
4. The uninjured eye is often patched to minimize movement of the injured eye.

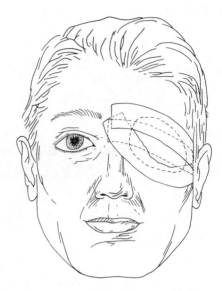

Figure 156.1 Eye patch taped in place.

COMPLICATIONS

1. Eye patches applied too tightly can result in increased ocular damage (such as central retinal artery occlusion).
2. Further trauma may occur to the injured eye from excessive lid motion under a loose eye patch.
3. Corneal abrasion from eyelashes trapped between the lids.

PATIENT TEACHING

1. Report any increase in eye pain or signs of infection (redness, swelling, drainage, etc.)
2. Limit reading and television viewing to help rest the injured eye, because both eyes move together.
3. Patching affects depth perception. Driving or operating dangerous machinery should be avoided. You may have difficulty walking up and down stairs.

REFERENCES

Barr, D., & Hedges, J. 1985. Ophthalmologic procedures. In J. Roberts, & J. Hedges (eds). *Clinical procedures in emergency medicine*. Philadelphia: Saunders.

Brinkley, J. 1984. Emergency management of ocular trauma. *Topics in Emergency Medicine,* 6, 1:35–45.

Vaughan, D., & Asbury, T. 1986. *General Opthamology,* 11th ed. E. Norwalk, CT: Appleton-Century-Crofts.

SUGGESTED READINGS

Budassi, S., & Barber, J. 1984. *Mosby's manual of emergency care: Practices and procedures,* 2nd ed. St. Louis: Mosby.

Cosgriff, J., & Anderson, D. 1984. *The practice of emergency care,* 2nd ed. Philadelphia: Lippincott.

Kitt, S., & Kaiser, J. 1990. *Emergency nursing: A physiologic and clinical perspective.* Philadelphia: Saunders.

Lawler, M. 1989. Common ocular injuries and disorders. Part II: Red eye. *Journal of Emergency Nursing,* 15:36–41.

157

Tonometry

Sharon Gavin Fought, PHD, RN
Jean A. Proehl, RN, MN, CEN, CCRN

Tonometry is also known as Schiotz tonometry.

INDICATIONS

To assess intraocular pressure (IOP) in patients:

1. At risk for having increased intraocular pressure, including elderly patients, elderly patients with glaucoma who are hypertensive, children and adult patients with glaucoma who are normotensive, patients with diabetes or history of retinal detachment.
2. Suspected of having acute glaucoma. These individuals may have an optic nerve that is cupped or atrophic (Shingleton, Frederick, & Hutchinson, 1989). Up to 2% of the population older than 40 years may have increased IOP. Increased IOP can occur if the patient has a shallow anterior chamber, with physiologic or pharmacologic mydriasis precipitated by a number of situations, including stress, a darkened environment, or belladonna-like drugs.
3. With a history of eye or periorbital pain that may be related to increased IOP, frequently seen with concurrent signs and symptoms of hazy cornea, sinusitis, headache, decreased visual acuity or "hazy vision," midrange nonreactive pupil unilaterally.
4. Schiotz tonometry is preferred when the patient is unable to sit upright for applanation tonometry, which requires a slit lamp.

CONTRAINDICATIONS AND CAUTIONS

1. Suspected or confirmed penetration of the globe; tonometry should not be performed if there is any question about the integrity of the globe. Application of pressure to the eye will likely result in extrusion of contents and loss of vision.

EQUIPMENT

Topical ophthalmic anesthetic
Schiotz tonometer with 5.5-gram
     weight

PATIENT PREPARATION

1. Place the patient in a darkened room to help decrease ocular pain.
2. Place the patient in a supine position, or in a chair that can be reclined.
3. Instruct the patient to **not** rub or touch his or her eyes at any time for at least 30 minutes after the procedure.

PROCEDURAL STEPS

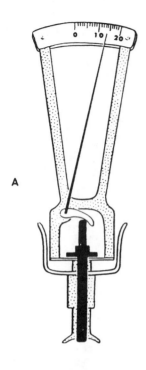

A

(**Note:** A rough estimate of IOP can be obtained by applying light, gentle digital pressure to the lids when there is no perforation of the globe. If in the comparison of the two eyes, one feels firmer or fuller, the patient may have unilateral increased IOP.

1. Instill topical anesthetics/cycloplegics as prescribed. Anesthetics should be administered before cycloplegics.
2. Place the patient in a supine position and ask him or her to look up at the ceiling.
3. *Place your thumb on the orbital rim to lift and secure the upper lid while the forefinger is used to open the lower lid. Remind the patient to "look up" at a fixed point on the ceiling.
4. *Place the footplate of the tonometer on the mid or central cornea.
5. Read the value (to the nearest 0.5 value) indicated by the needle placement on the scale of the tonometer. See Figure 157.1.

    Translate the value obtained to the IOP by using a standard IOP table (Karesh & Keys, 1988). See Figure 157.2.

    Normal IOP values are 12–21 mm Hg; a significant increase in IOP exists when the pressure is greater than 30 mm Hg. If the pressure is less than 10, it is likely that perforation of the globe has occurred; the procedure should be halted and an ophthalmology consult initiated (Karesh & Keyes, 1988).

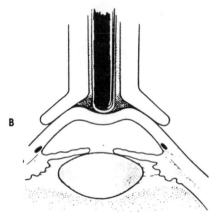

B

Figure 157.1 A. Schiotz tonometer. The plunger (in black) measures the pressure required to indent the cornea. B. Ocular pressure measured by indentation of the cornea by the plunger.
(Newell, 1982: 342. Reprinted by permission.)

Figure 157.2 Intraocular pressure table for use with Schiotz tonometer.
(Reprinted by permission of J. Sklar Manufacturing Co., Inc. Long Island City, NY 11101.)

Scale Reading	Plunger Load (In gms.)			
	5.5	7.5	10.0	15.0
0	41	59	82	127
.5	38	54	75	118
1.0	35	50	70	109
1.5	32	46	64	101
2.0	29	42	59	94
2.5	27	39	55	88
3.0	24	36	51	82
3.5	22	33	47	76
4.0	21	30	43	71
4.5	19	28	40	66
5.0	17	26	37	62
5.5	16	24	34	58
6.0	15	22	32	54
6.5	13	20	29	50
7.0	12	19	27	46
7.5	11	17	25	43
8.0	10	16	23	40
8.5	9	14	21	38
9.0	9	13	20	35
9.5	8	12	18	32
10.0	7	11	16	30
10.5	6	10	15	27
11.0	6	9	14	25
11.5	5	8	13	23
12.0		8	11	21
12.5		7	10	20
13.0		6	10	18
13.5		6	9	17
14.0		5	8	15
14.5			7	14
15.0			6	13
15.5			6	11
16.0			5	10
16.5				9
17.0				8
17.5				8
18.0				7

COMPLICATIONS

1. Extrusion of the globe contents can occur during the exam if there is a penetrating injury to the globe.
2. Transient increases in IOP can occur if the patient coughs, sneezes, or gags during the procedure.

PATIENT EDUCATION

1. Do not blink or touch your eyes during the exam.
2. Do not rub your eyes after the exam.
3. Do not bend over, cough, blow nose, or strain at stool (if IOP is elevated).

REFERENCES

Boyd-Monk, H., & Steinmetz, C.G. 1987. *Nursing care of the eye* Norwalk, CT: Appleton & Lange.

Karesh, J., & Keyes, B.J. 1988. In V.D. Cardona, P.D. Hurn, P.J.B. Mason, A.M. Scanlon-Schlipp, & S.B. Veise-Gerry, (eds). *Trauma nursing resuscitation through rehabilitation.* Philadelphia: Saunders; 600–607.

Newell, F.W. 1982. *Ophthalomolgy: Principles and Concepts,* 5th ed. St. Louis: Mosby.

Shingleton, B.J., Frederick, A.R., & Hutchison, B.T. 1989. In Wilkins, E.W. (ed). *Emergency medicine: Scientific foundations and current practice,* 3rd ed. Baltimore: Williams and Wilkins; 878–885.

SUGGESTED READING

Boyd-Monk, H. 1988. In E. Howell, L. Widra, & M.G. Hill, (eds). *Comprehensive trauma nursing.* Boston: Scott, Foresman, 507–517.

158

Immobilization of Ophthalmic Foreign Body

Sharon Gavin Fought, PHD, RN

INDICATIONS

To immobilize a foreign object penetrating the eye or periorbital region.

CONTRAINDICATIONS AND CAUTIONS

1. Ophthalmic injuries are treated immediately after life-threatening conditions are stabilized.
2. Special caution is required in foreign objects that are irritating metal or might result in additional adverse consequences for the eye; such elements include: aluminum, copper, iron, lead, and vegetation. These elements can result in additional corrosion of the globe or, in the case of vegetation, fungal infections (Boyd-Monk, 1988).
3. Do not apply pressure to the eye. Direct pressure should not be used to stop bleeding from or around the eye when a penetrating object is suspected or evident.
4. The use of ophthalmic ointments is contraindicated, because they may enter the globe and, in the case of anesthetic ointments, may have a prolonged effect.

EQUIPMENT

Rigid eye shields
Gauze eye patches
4-x-4″ gauze dressings
Fluffs
Roller bandages

Paper cups
Adhesive tape
Skin prep material such as alcohol
    or acetone

PATIENT PREPARATION

1. Instruct the patient to not touch or rub the eye.
2. Unless contraindicated by other injuries, elevate the head of the bed to decrease intraocular pressure.

PROCEDURAL STEPS

1. Obtain the description and composition of the foreign body, distance it traveled to the eye, direction of travel, and direction in which the eye was gazing or looking at the time of the injury.

2. Use a thick dressing to immobilize the foreign object. A variety of materials can be used, including gauze dressings, fluffs, paper drinking cup, or paper cone.
3. Place the dressing around the foreign object to immobilize it and prevent further injury to the eye and surrounding structures. A hole may be cut in the center of the dressing or the dressing can be arranged around the penetrating object to further immobilize it; the penetrating object should be in the center of the bandage.
4. Place a paper cup or other solid, lightweight object over the penetrating object. The paper cup should rest on the dressing. It should not place pressure on the eye or touch the penetrating object. With larger penetrating objects, it may be difficult or impossible to cover the end of the penetrating object with this type of protective bandage.
5. Tape or bandage the paper cup securely to further immobilize the penetrating object.
6. Patch or shield the uninjured eye to prevent movement in the injured eye. See Ch. 156: Eye Patching.

COMPLICATIONS

1. Bacterial or fungal infection
2. Loss of vision or visual acuity
3. Penetration of sinuses or brain with concurrent risk of meningitis

PATIENT EDUCATION

1. Do not touch the injured eye.
2. Do not strain, cough, bend over, touch or rub eye.
3. Do not move either eye.

REFERENCES

Boyd-Monk, H. 1988. Ocular trauma. In E. Howell, L. Widra, & M.G. Hill (eds). *Comprehensive Trauma Nursing*. Boston: Scott, Foresman; 513–520.

SUGGESTED READINGS

Carbal, J. 1987. Ocular emergencies. In T.C. Kravis, & C.G. Warner, (eds). *Emergency medicine: A Comprehensive review*, 2nd ed. Rockville, MD: Aspen; 1213–1248.

Fought, S.G. 1986. Eye trauma. In R. Rea, (ed). *Trauma Nursing Core Course (provider) Manual*, 2nd ed. Chicago: Award Printing Corporation; ix01–ix10.

Karesh, J.W., & Keyes, B.J. 1988. In V.D. Cardona, P.D. Hurn, P.J.B. Mason, A.M. Scanlon-Schlipp, & S.B. Veise-Berry, (eds). *Trauma nursing from resuscitation through rehabilitation*. Philadelphia: Saunders; 610–617.

Wilkins, E.W. (ed). 1989. *Emergency medicine: Scientific foundations and current practice*, 3rd ed. Baltimore: Williams & Wilkins.

159

Instillation of Ear Medications

Barbara E. Gamrath, RN, MN, CEN

INDICATIONS

To apply medicated solutions/suspensions (antibiotics, steroids, analgesics, or ceruminolytic agents) into the external auditory canal for otitis externa (swimmer's ear), otitis media, or cerumen accumulation.

CONTRAINDICATIONS AND CAUTIONS

1. Caution should be exercised to identify any perforation of the tympanic membrane before instilling medications into the external auditory canal, because inadvertent introduction of foreign material into the middle ear may result in a bacterial infection.
2. Medications in suspension (oil based) do not absorb into ear wicks. Use ear wicks with medications in solution form only.

EQUIPMENT

Otoscope
Ear wick or cotton ball
Ear medication (antibiotic,

analgesic, ceruminolytic
agent) as ordered

PROCEDURAL STEPS

1. Place the patient on his or her side with the affected ear up.
2. Examine the external auditory canal. In adults, pull the helix of the ear up and back to straighten the external canal. In pediatric patients, pull the lobule of the ear down and forward to straighten the canal.
3. Clear any debris from the ear canal. See Ch. 162: Ear Foreign Body Removal or Ch. 163: Cerumen Removal.
4. For antibiotic and steroid application, gently place a cotton wick in the ear canal. See Ch. 160: Ear Wick Insertion. Saturate the wick with a topical otic medication.

COMPLICATIONS

1. If cotton balls are used instead of an ear wick, disintegration may occur and removal may be difficult. To avoid retention of pieces of cotton balls, they should be placed only at the meatus.
2. Without an ear wick or cotton ball, solutions or suspensions may extravasate from the canal.

3. Otic *solutions* frequently cause a burning or stinging sensation; *suspensions* are less painful.

PATIENT TEACHING

1. Ear pain, an edematous canal, tender ear cartilage, purulent drainage, or hearing loss may result from an accumulation of debris in the ear (Sheehy, 1985). Any of these signs should be evaluated promptly.
2. Leave wick in place for 48 to 72 hours. Repeat instillation of medication onto the ear wick three or four times per day or as directed (Sheehy, 1985). Moisten the ear wick prior to removal to decrease trauma to the ear canal.
3. Continuation of medication may be necessary after ear wick removal (approximately 10 days for antibiotics).
4. If an ear wick is not used, a cotton ball may be placed at the meatus of the ear canal after instillation of medication to prevent extravasation of the medication.

REFERENCES

Sheehy, S.B. 1985. Ear, nose, throat, and dental emergencies. *Emergency nursing: Principles and practice,* 2nd ed. St. Louis: Mosby.

160

Ear Wick Insertion

Margo E. Layman, RNC, BSN, CEN

INDICATIONS

To apply medication to the external ear canal in the presence of otitis externa.

CONTRAINDICATIONS AND CAUTIONS

1. Lacerations of the ear canal.
2. A ruptured tympanic membrane could allow the wick to slip into the hole in the tympanic membrane.
3. Alcohol or acidic medications may cause a burning or stinging sensation.

EQUIPMENT

Cotton, 1/2-x-1/2″ selvedged gauze, or compressed hydroxycellulose manufactured ear wick
Prescribed ear drops
Cerumen spoon
Small metal suction tip
Miniature alligator forceps
Otoscope

PATIENT PREPARATION

1. Place the adult patient in semi-Fowlers position.
2. Place the small child in a supine position, restrain the knees, and hold arms firmly against the head with the face turned to the left or right.

PROCEDURAL STEPS

1. Using an otoscope, check the external ear for redness or drainage.
2. Examine the internal ear with an otoscope.
3. Suction debris from the ear with small metal suction tip or gently use a cerumen spoon to remove debris.
4. Use a miniature alligator forcep to place the ear wick in the canal. Prepare cotton or selvedged gauze by wrapping tightly around tip of alligator forcep and then grasp cotton or gauze with forcep and place in ear canal.
5. Place the prescribed ear drops in the ear canal, taking care not to touch dropper to the ear canal. Place the drops along the side of the canal so

that air is displaced as they flow in. Cold drops may cause vertigo; this can be avoided by warming them slightly before administration.
6. Place 1–2 additional drops on ear wick to saturate it.

COMPLICATIONS

1. The ear wick may adhere to the ear canal if not kept moist.
2. The ear wick may slip deeper into the canal. This could cause irritation of the tympanic membrane.

PATIENT TEACHING

1. Remove the ear wick in forty-eight hours. Make sure the wick is moist prior to removal. Have someone assist by using clean tweezers to remove the ear wick.
2. Instill ear drops as instructed. Cold ear drops may cause dizziness. Warm the bottle between your hands or in a cup of warm (not hot) water prior to instillation of drops.
3. Symptoms should subside in 1–2 days. If no improvement or if symptoms worsen, contact your physician.
4. To prevent the ear wick from slipping, do not touch ear and remove ear wick as instructed.

SUGGESTED READINGS

Marcy, M.S. 1985. Infections of the external ear. *Pediatric Infectious Disease,* 4:192–201.
Pope, T.H., & Michel, R.C. 1973. External otitis: treatment using an improved expandable wick. *Oto-Rhino-Laryngology,* 37:16–17.
Upchurch, D.T. (ed). 1989. *Otolaryngology problems in primary care.* Oradell, NJ: Medical Economics, Inc.
Wilkins, E.W. (ed). 1983. *MGH Textbook of emergency medicine,* 2nd ed. Baltimore: Williams & Wilkins.

161

Ear Irrigation

Dean M. Kelly, RN, BSN, CEN

INDICATIONS

1. To remove drainage, cerumen, or foreign bodies from the external auditory canal.
2. To irrigate the external auditory canal with antiseptic solution.
3. To apply heat or cold to the external auditory canal.

CONTRAINDICATIONS AND CAUTIONS

1. Irrigation is contraindicated if the tympanic membrane is not intact (secondary to injury, myringotomy tubes, recent surgery, etc.)
2. The patient may experience sudden vertigo during irrigation and, therefore, should be seated in a reclining chair or lying on a stretcher to prevent injury due to a fall.
3. The temperature of the solution should be 37–40°C (100–105°F) to prevent triggering of the vestibular reflex, which produces vertigo, nausea, and vomiting (Graber, 1986).
4. To prevent injury to the canal or tympanic membrane, the solution should not be administered with excessive force.

EQUIPMENT

Metal ear syringe
or
60-cc plastic syringe with a
      19-gauge IV butterfly,
      attached to syringe, with
      end of tubing cut off
      approximately 1½″ from
      hub end (See Figure 162.3.)
or

Oral hygiene appliance (Water Pik)
Basin with irrigant
Thermometer to measure the
      solution temperature
Emesis basin
Towels
Otoscope
Cotton balls or gauze dressings

PATIENT PREPARATION

1. Position the patient with the head tilted toward the affected ear.
2. Protect the patient's clothing by draping the neck and shoulders with towels.
3. Cleanse the outer ear of any discharge.

PROCEDURAL STEPS

1. Examine the ear with an otoscope before and after every irrigation attempt to determine progress.
2. Draw up approximately 50 ml of irrigation solution in the syringe.
3. Direct the patient to hold the emesis basin directly under the ear against the neck.
4. Grasp the auricle and gently pull upward and outward. See Figure 161.1.
5. Introduce the syringe or catheter ¼″ into ear canal. Aim at the side or the top of ear canal and gently inject the solution. Assess for foreign bodies or cerumen as the solution drains out into the emesis basin.
6. Examine the canal with the otoscope and repeat irrigation if necessary. Allow the patient to rest as needed between irrigations.
7. For the patient with impacted hard cerumen, the physician may order a cerumen softening agent prior to irrigation.
8. When removing foreign bodies that may absorb water, (e.g., beans, vegetable matter, etc.) use warmed isopropyl alcohol to prevent the object from swelling while in ear (Campbell, 1984).

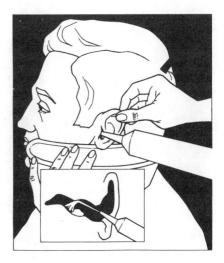

Figure 161.1 Direct the irrigating solution toward the top of the ear canal.
(Belland & Wells, 1984: 334. Reprinted by permission.)

COMPLICATIONS

1. Vertigo or nausea during and/or after procedure.
2. Injury to the external canal or tympanic membrane.

PATIENT TEACHING

Report any pain or dizziness.

REFERENCES

Campbell, C. 1984. *Nursing diagnosis and intervention in nursing practice,* 2nd ed. New York: Wiley.

Belland, K.H., & Wells, M.A. 1984. Clinical nursing procedures. Belmont, CA: Wadsworth.

Graber, R.F. 1986. Procedures for your practice: removing impacted cerumen. *Patient care,* 20, 1:151–153.

162

Otic Foreign Body Removal

Barbara E. Gamrath, RN, MN, CEN

INDICATIONS

To remove a foreign body from the ear by water irrigation, suction, direct instrumentation, or magnet, when digital removal has failed.

CONTRAINDICATIONS AND CAUTIONS

1. Anatomic narrowing occurs at two separate points in the external auditory canal. See Figure 162.1. Many objects become lodged at these points. Avoid pushing the foreign body beyond these narrowings during extrication attempts, because damage to the ear may result (Pons, 1988).

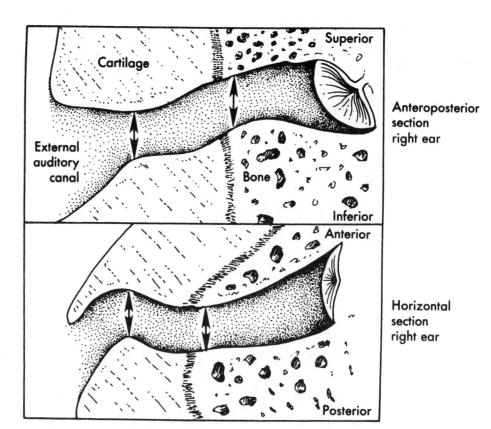

Figure 162.1 Horizontal and vertical cross-sections of external ear canal showing points of anatomic narrowing.
(Pons, 1983: 650. Reprinted by permission.)

2. Local anesthesia of the external auditory canal involves subcutaneous injection. Injection at this site can be quite painful and difficult to achieve in the unsedated patient. Systemic sedation may be necessary to achieve patient cooperation (Brownstein, 1988). Some patients may re-

quire general anesthesia. Topical anesthesia is generally ineffective due to the impermeable membranes of the ear (Abramson, 1969).

3. If patient history or physical examination suggests tympanic membrane disruption, irrigation is contraindicated for foreign body removal.

4. Irrigation of foreign bodies that have the potential to swell and become more firmly impacted when hydrated (such as vegetable matter) should be avoided.

5. Live insects should be killed before removal is attempted. Instill mineral oil or alcohol in the ear to kill the insect. Another method is to irrigate with 2% lidocaine solution (Schittek, 1980), which quickly kills the insect.

6. Miniature batteries lodged in the ear canal pose a special problem. In addition to the mechanical trauma that may occur with miniature batteries, a chemical reaction may occur due to leakage of the battery contents. Tympanic membrane perforation, facial nerve paralysis, or ossicular chain damage may result. Prompt removal of the battery using a right angle hook followed by water irrigation is imperative to avoid these complications (Cannon, 1988).

7. Contralateral ear examination should be done to rule out bilateral ear foreign bodies (Das, 1984).

8. Instrumentation or direct irrigation onto the foreign body may cause it to move deeper into the canal toward the tympanic membrane.

EQUIPMENT

Various procedures may be used for ear foreign body removal some or all of the following equipment may be needed:

Adequate light source (operating otoscope, diagnostic otoscope head with magnifying lens or head lamp)

Ear speculum

Magnetized speculum (used for removal of ferromagnetic metallic batteries)

Blunt right angle hook, wire loops, cerumen curette, alligator forceps or bayonet forceps (See Figure 162.2).

Suction catheter (Frazier)

Suction

Schuknecht foreign body remover—a suction catheter that works well on smooth, round foreign bodies (Hodge, 1989)

Irrigation equipment (20-cc syringe with flexible 18-G intravenous catheter or the tubing of a butterfly catheter with the needle removed) (See Figure 162.3.)

Fogarty biliary catheter

Papoose board or sheet for restraint of children

PATIENT PREPARATION

1. Sedate or restrain as indicated.
2. Emphasize the importance of not moving during the procedure.
3. For irrigation, drape the patient with towels and place an emesis basin for collection of irrigation fluid.

PROCEDURAL STEPS

One or more of the following procedures may be necessary to remove a foreign body from the external auditory canal:

1. *Place the tip of the suction catheter on the foreign body and gently

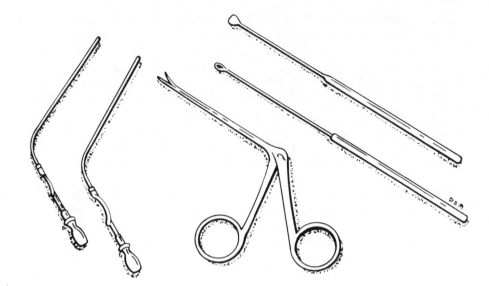

Figure 162.2 Instruments used for removal of foreign bodies from the external auditory canal: (left to right) Frazier suction catheters, alligator forceps, wire loop, and ear curette.
(Votey & Dudley, 1989: 124. Reprinted by permission.)

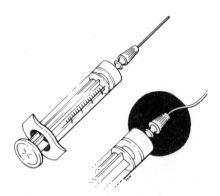

Figure 162.3 A flexible gauge intravenous catheter attached to a 20-cc syringe (left), and a butterfly catheter with the needle cut off attached to a 20-cc syringe (right).
(Votey & Dudley, 1989: 124. Reprinted by permission.)

*Indicates portions of the procedure usually performed by a physician.

retract. See Figure 162.4. If using a Schuknecht foreign body remover, apply suction only after the catheter has conformed to the shape of the foreign body.

2. Irrigate the ear canal with lukewarm water, to avoid stimulation of the labyrinths (Politzer, 1883), normal saline (Buttaravoli, 1985), or alcohol (Ballantyne, 1971), directing the stream of fluid to the edge of the foreign body in an attempt to gently force fluid behind the foreign body and out the ear canal.

3. *Pass a right angle hook (blunt ended) beyond the foreign body and gently retract.

4. *If removing a battery, directly visualize the battery and insert as solid ferromagnetic metallic speculum in the external auditory meatus. The object should move toward the speculum and can then be withdrawn (Mattucci, 1987).

5. *Insert a Fogarty biliary catheter past the foreign body, inflate the balloon and retract the catheter dislodging the foreign body.

6. *Once the foreign body can be visualized in the external ear canal, it may be removed with forceps, a curette, or loop.

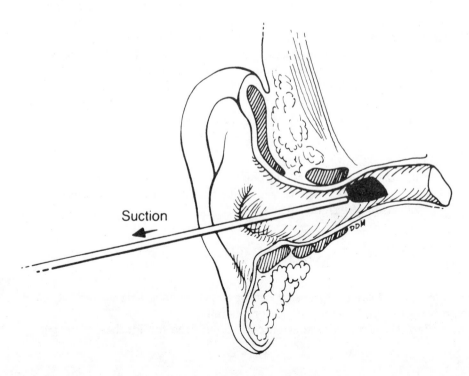

Suction

Figure 162.4 Use of Frazier suction catheter for removal of a foreign body in the external auditory canal.
(Votey & Dudley, 1989: 124. Reprinted by permission.)

COMPLICATIONS

1. Blind attempts at foreign body removal may lead to complications such as tissue trauma or pushing the foreign body further into the ear canal. Direct visualization should always be used to remove foreign bodies in the ear (Brownstein, 1988).
2. Perforation of the tympanic membrane may occur as a complication of instrumentation of the ear canal.
3. Topical antimicrobial therapy may be indicated if trauma to the epithelial tissue of the external canal was sustained during the procedure.
4. Part of the foreign body may be retained. Repeat direct visualization once the foreign body has been removed.

PATIENT TEACHING

1. Do not attempt to remove future foreign objects not readily visible or not capable of being easily grasped (Baker, 1987).
2. Uncomplicated foreign body removal does not routinely require followup care unless there is evidence of otitis externa, injury to the external auditory canal or tympanic membrane, or possible retained foreign body (Fritz, 1987). If drainage from the ear, fever, pain, or swelling occurs, seek medical attention.
3. Bleeding may occur due to damage caused by instrumentation.

REFERENCES

Abramson, M. 1969. Topical anesthesia of the tympanic membrane. *Archives of Otolaryngology*, 90:147–149.

Baker, M.D. 1987. Foreign bodies of the ears and nose in childhood. *Pediatric Emergency Care*, 3:67–70.

Ballantyne, J., & Grove, J. 1971. *Scott-Brown's Diseases of the ear, nose and throat*, 3rd ed. Philadelphia: Lippincott.

Brownstein, D. 1988. Foreign bodies of the eye, ear, and nose. *Pediatric Emergency Care*, 4:215–218.

Buttaravoli, P., & Stair, T., 1985. *Common Simple Emergencies*, Harrisburg, Virginia: Donnelley.

Cannon, C.R. 1988. The miniature battery: A new foreign body hazard. *Journal Mississippi State Medical Association*, 29:41–42.

Das, S. 1984. Aetiological evaluation of foreign bodies in the ear and nose. *Journal of Laryngology Otolaryngology*, 98:989–991.

Fritz, S. 1987. Foreign bodies of the external auditory canal. *Emergency Medical Clinics of North America*, 5:183–193.

Hodge, D., & Brownstein, D. 1989. Letters. *Pediatric Emergency Care*, 5:73.

Mattucci, W. 1987. Removal of metallic foreign bodies of the external auditory canal. *International Surgery*, 65.

Politzer, A. 1883. *A Textbook of the Diseases of the Ear and Adjacent Organs*. Philadelphia: Leas.

Pons, P. 1983. Foreign Bodies. In P. Rosen et al. (eds.) *Emergency medicine: Concepts and clinical practice*, St. Louis: Mosby; 647–650.

Schittek, A. 1980. Insect in the external auditory canal: A new way out. *Journal of the American Medical Association*, 243: 331.

Votey, S., & Dudley, J.P. 1989. Emergency ear, nose and throat procedures. *Emergency Medical Clinics of North America*, 7:117–155.

163

Cerumen Removal

Barbara E. Gamrath, RN, MN, CEN

INDICATIONS

To remove cerumen accumulation (partial occlusion of the ear canal) and/or impaction (complete occlusion of the ear canal with no visualization of the tympanic membrane) from the external auditory canal.

CONTRAINDICATIONS AND CAUTIONS

1. If an intact tympanic membrane cannot be visualized, irrigation for treatment of cerumen accumulation or impaction is contraindicated, because of the potential for bacterial contamination of the middle ear. An accurate history should be taken to identify signs of infection or past problems with the ears that may indicate perforation.
2. Irrigation is contraindicated in the presence of any of the following: tympanic membrane perforation, tympanotomy tubes, or an intact tympanic membrane that has an atrophic region after perforation and suboptimal spontaneous healing (Bailey, 1984).
3. Hearing loss, tinnitus, and head noise have been linked to impacted cerumen, along with the potential for psychosocial disturbances. Conductive hearing loss may be caused by cerumen impaction and is frequently overlooked (Mahoney, 1987).

EQUIPMENT

Otoscope
Ceruminolytic agent (optional)
Low pressure water irrigation
    equipment (including: ear
    syringe, tubing and basin)
or
High pressure water irrigation
    equipment (including:

Water-Pic instrument,
    tubing and basin)
Cerumen loop (either metal or
    plastic)
Suction tip (optional)
Suction setup (optional)
Mirror

PATIENT PREPARATION

1. Drape the patient with towels to absorb excess irrigation fluid.
2. Advise the patient that during irrigation, sensations of dizziness are commonly experienced.
3. The patient should be placed in a sitting or semi-Fowler's position with the head tilted toward the affected ear.

PROCEDURAL STEPS

1. Perform an otoscopic examination before and after cerumen removal. Gently pull the helix of the pinna in a posterior-superior direction in adults prior to inserting the otoscope. Identify the cerumen plug and ascertain the integrity of the tympanic membrane.
2. If the tympanic membrane is intact, ceruminolytic agents may be used to penetrate the keratin of the cerumen accumulation and loosen the plug to allow easy and less irritating removal (Mahoney, 1987). See Ch. 159: Instillation of Ear Medications.
3. For irrigation tilt the head 15 degrees toward the affected ear and position a basin to collect the fluid as it drains (Bradley, 1986). Use lukewarm water to avoid dizziness and nystagmus.
4. Direct the flow of water to the edge of the cerumen, not directly onto the tympanic membrane.
5. Removal of cerumen can also be done with various sizes and shapes of suction tips (Ruggles, 1983). See Figure 163.1. Wall or portable suction can then be applied through the suction tip which is placed directly on the cerumen plug.

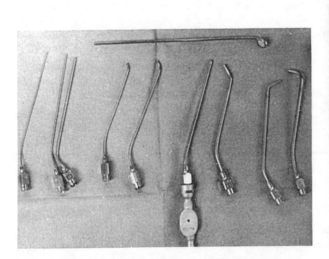

Figure 163.1   Various sizes and shapes of suction tips.
(Ruggles, 1983: 566–567. Reprinted by permission.)

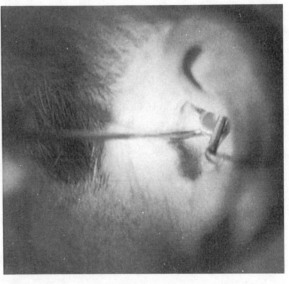

Figure 163.2   Mirror and aspirator.
(Ruggles, 1983: 567. Reprinted by permission.)

6. When using suction for cerumen removal, use of a mirror may help in visualization of the plug. See Figure 163.2.
7. A cerumen loop (either metal or plastic) may be used to gently scrape and remove cerumen from the external auditory canal.

COMPLICATIONS

1. Otitis media may result from irrigation in the presence of a tympanic membrane perforation.
2. If cold water is used with irrigation, dizziness and nystagmus may result.

PATIENT TEACHING

1. Cerumen accumulation may cause a hearing loss. Hearing loss may also be caused by sensorineural problems that result from damage to the eighth cranial nerve. A combination of conductive and sensorineural hearing loss may occur (Mahoney, 1987). Seek medical care promptly in the presence of hearing loss.
2. Cerumen impaction, dermatitis, and skin infections may result from self-treatment with cotton swabs or other objects. Use of cotton-tipped ear swabs may be harmful due to the rubbing away of protective keratin layers leaving the living skin cells exposed to minor trauma and infection. Swabs may also lead to wax impaction in the bony meatus of the external auditory canal (Warwick-Brown, 1986). Avoid introducing objects into your ears.
3. Excessive ear hair may cause difficulty in manual removal of earwax and may require special attention to prevent cerumen buildup.
4. Hearing aids may increase wax production and prevent the normal propelling action of the ear cilia.

REFERENCES

Bailey, B. 1984. Removal of cerumen. *Journal of the American Medical Association*, 251:1681.

Bradley, M.E. 1986. A new ear syringe model. *The Journal of Laryngology and Otology*, 100:635–636.

Mahoney, D.F. 1987. One simple solution to hearing impairment. *Geriatric Nursing*, Sept./Oct.: 242–245.

Ruggles, R. 1983. Care of the ear canal and mastoid. *Annals of Otology, Rhinology and Laryngology*, 92:566–567.

Warwick-Brown, N.P. 1986. Wax impaction in the ear. *The Practitioner*, 230:301.

164

Topical Vasoconstrictors for Epistaxis

Margo E. Layman, RNC, BSN, CEN

INDICATIONS

To stop or slow anterior or posterior epistaxis.

CONTRAINDICATIONS AND CAUTIONS

Topical vasoconstrictors may cause blood pressure elevations and tachycardia and should be used with caution in patients with cardiopulmonary problems or hypertension.

EQUIPMENT

Headlamp
Nasal speculum
Topical vasoconstrictor and/or
     anesthetic (phenylephrine
     HCL, ephedrine,
epinephrine, cocaine,
     oxymetazoline)
Cotton swabs
Tissues

PATIENT PREPARATION

1. Place the patient in a semi-Fowler's position or seated in a dental chair.
2. Have the patient blow his or her nose to expel clots and apply firm direct pressure by pinching the nares for a full 10 minutes.

PROCEDURAL STEPS

1. Place cotton swabs soaked with the topical vasoconstrictor in the nose for 5–10 minutes. Alternatively, have patient spray the medication into each nare twice while inhaling through the nose. Spray application maybe repeated if bleeding does not stop within a few minutes. Do not exceed the maximum safe dose of the medication.
2. *Examine both nares using a headlamp and nasal speculum.

*Indicates portions of the procedure usually performed by a physician.

COMPLICATIONS

1. Dizziness, tachycardia, dysrhythmias, or hypertension.
2. Topical therapy may fail to control bleeding.
3. Continued blood loss may result in hypovolemia and shock.

PATIENT TEACHING

1. Apply petroleum jelly or antibiotic ointment to the nares, to decrease drying and scab formation.
2. Use a humidifier at home, especially in your bedroom at night.
3. Avoid bending over, coughing, heavy lifting, sneezing, or blowing your nose for 4–5 days. If you must sneeze, open your mouth to relieve pressure.
4. Report any recurrence of bleeding.

SUGGESTED READINGS

Fairbanks, D.N.F. 1986. Complications of nasal packing. *Otolaryngology-Head and Neck Surgery,* 94:412–415.

Petruzzelli, G.J., & Johnson, J.T. 1989. How to stop a nosebleed. *Postgraduate Medicine,* 86:44–56.

Rosen, P., Baker, II, F.Z., Barkin, R.M., Braen, G.R., Dailey, R.H., & Levy, R.C. 1988. *Emergency Medicine: Concepts and Clinical Practice.* 2nd ed. St. Louis: Mosby.

Silfen, E.Z., & Stair, T. 1984. Nasal emergencies. *Topics in emergency medicine,* 74:40–47.

165

Electrical and Chemical Cautery for Epistaxis

Margo E. Layman, RNC, BSN, CEN

INDICATIONS

To stop anterior epistaxis.

EQUIPMENT

Headlamp
Nasal speculum
Frazier nasal suction tip
Silver nitrate sticks

or

Electrocautery
Cotton swabs
Topical or local anesthetic

PATIENT PREPARATION

1. Seat patient in a dental chair or in a semi-Fowler's position on a stretcher.
2. Have the patient blow his or her nose to clear it of clots.
3. Attach grounding pad to patient if using electrocautery.

PROCEDURAL STEPS

1. *Locate the bleeding site.
2. Suction the area until the site is visualized and dry. The bleeding site must be dry for silver nitrate sticks to be effective.
3. *Anesthetize the nasal mucosa with a topical anesthetic for use of silver nitrate or via infiltration of a local anesthetic for electrocautery. See Ch. 137.
4. *The silver nitrate sticks or electrocautery coagulate the bleeding site.
   Silver nitrate: Hold the stick in place for only 20–30 seconds.
   Electrocautery: Coagulate only a 1 mm. area. The cautery damages and weakens tissue and may cause additional bleeding (Taylor, 1983).
5. *After application of silver nitrate, dry the cautery site with cotton swabs to prevent the silver nitrate from spreading.
6. Apply antibiotic ointment to the cautery site to soften the crust formed by the cautery.

*Indicates portions of the procedure usually performed by a physician.

COMPLICATIONS

1. If cautery is unsuccessful, anterior or posterior packing will be required (Petruzzelli, 1989).
2. Cauterization can weaken the tissue and make future cauterization more harmful (Taylor, 1983).
3. Bilateral electrocautery can cause septal perforation.
4. Continued blood loss may result in hypovolemia and shock.

PATIENT TEACHING

1. Avoid activities that might dislodge the cautery crust such as sneezing and blowing or picking nose. If you must sneeze, do so with your mouth open.
2. Report any recurrence of bleeding.

REFERENCES

Petruzzelli, J. & Johnson, J.T. 1989. How to stop a nosebleed. *Postgraduate Medicine,* 86:44–56.

Taylor, R.B., Buckingham, J.L., Donatelle, E.P., Jacott, W.E., & Rosen, M.G. 1983. *Family Medicine: principles & practices,* 2nd ed. New York: Springer-Verlag.

SUGGESTED READINGS

Erwin, A. 1987. Epistaxis. *Postgraduate Medicine,* 82:59–65.

Rosen, P., Baker, II, F.J., Barkin, R.M., Braen, G.R., Dailey, R.H., & Levy, R.C. 1988. *Emergency Medicine: Concepts and Clinical Practice.* 2nd ed. St. Louis: Mosby.

Sheeny, S.B., & Barber, J. 1985. *Emergency Nursing: Principles and Practice,* 2nd ed. St. Louis: Mosby.

166

Anterior Packing for Epistaxis

Margo E. Layman, RNC, BSN, CEN

INDICATIONS

To tamponade bleeding from the anterior nasal cavity.

CONTRAINDICATIONS AND CAUTIONS

1. People age 50 to 80 with histories of cardiac and pulmonary disorders may develop problems due to already compromised cardiac and pulmonary systems.
2. Establish baseline oxygenation with ABGs or pulse oximetry for patients with cardiopulmonary disease, because hypoxia may result from anterior nasal packing.
3. Patients with bilateral packs may require admission to the hospital (Rosen & Sternbach, 1983).

EQUIPMENT

Headlamp
Topical anesthetic agent (e.g., cocaine, etc.)
Topical vasoconstricting agent (e.g., phenylephrine, etc.)
Intravenous sedation (e.g., diazepam, etc.)
Silver nitrate sticks
1-inch-wide strips of plain gauze impregnated with antibiotic ointment or petroleum jelly

Frazier nasal suction tip
Long bayonet forceps
Nasal speculum
2-x-2″ gauze pads
4-x-4″ gauze pads
Tape
Cotton tipped applicators
(Note: Commercially prepared surgical sponges are also available for nasal packing.)

PATIENT PREPARATION

1. Seat the patient in a dental chair or in a semi-Fowler's position on a stretcher.
2. Administer sedation as ordered.

PROCEDURAL STEPS

1. *With a headlamp, introduce a nasal speculum into the naris and suction clotted blood from the nose. See Figure 166.1.
2. *Determine the locus of the hemorrhage and anesthetize the area with cotton tipped applicators soaked in a topical anesthetic.

*Indicates portions of the procedure usually performed by a physician.

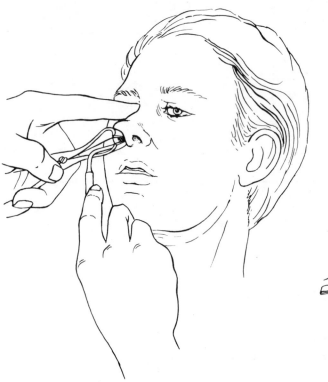

Figure 166.1   Nasal speculum in nose, while clots are suctioned out.
(Rosen & Sternbach, 1983: 163. Reprinted by permission.)

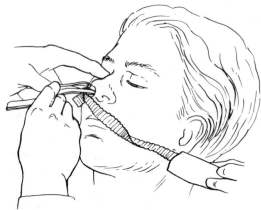

Figure 166.2   Long bayonet forceps packing lubricated 1-inch gauze into nose.
(Rosen & Sternbach, 1983: 163. Reprinted by permission.)

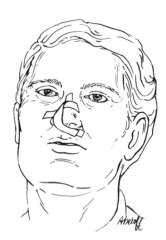

Figure 166.3   Packing taped in place with 4-x-4″ gauze under nose.
(Rosen & Sternbach, 1983: 163. Reprinted by permission.)

3.   *Apply silver nitrate to cauterize the bleeding site.
4.   *Pack anterior nose loosely with gauze impregnated with antibiotic ointment or petroleum jelly, using bayonet forceps and allowing both ends to protrude. See Figure 166.2
5.   The pack can then be held in place with a gauze dressing taped under the nose. See Figure 166.3.

COMPLICATIONS

1.   Hypovolemia from blood loss
2.   Inadequate hemostasis with recurrent hemorrhage
3.   Airway obstruction from swelling or dislodgment of the packing
4.   Hypoxia (Nasal packing can cause a decreased PaO_2 as a result of naso-pulmonary reflexes.)
5.   Sinusitis
6.   Toxic shock syndrome

PATIENT TEACHING

1.   Use a humidifier at home especially in your bedroom at night.
2.   Avoid bending over, coughing, heavy lifting, sneezing, or blowing your nose for 4–5 days.
3.   After the packing is removed, lubricate the nose with antibiotic ointment or petroleum jelly daily.

4. Do not remove the packing, see your physician for removal in 48 hours.
5. Watch for recurrent bleeding, difficulty breathing, blood draining down the back of your throat, fever, malaise, or rash.

REFERENCE

Rosen, P., & Sternbach, G. (eds). 1983. *Atlas of emergency medicine,* 2nd ed. Baltimore: Williams & Wilkins.

SUGGESTED READINGS

Erwin, S.A. 1987. Epistaxis: How to control the persistent nosebleed. *Postgraduate Medicine,* 82, 4:59–65.

Fairbanks, D.N.F. 1986. Complications of nasal packing. *Otolaryngology-Head and Neck Surgery,* 94, 3:412–415.

Lockhart, J.S., & Griffin, C. 1986. Epistaxis. *Nursing,* 16:69.

167

Posterior Packing for Epistaxis

Margo E. Layman, RNC, BSN, CEN

INDICATIONS

To tamponade bleeding from posterior nasal cavity.

CONTRAINDICATIONS AND CAUTIONS

1. People age 50 to 80 with histories of cardiac and pulmonary disorders may develop problems due to already compromised cardiac and pulmonary systems.
2. Establish baseline oxygenation with ABGs or pulse oximetry for patients with cardiopulmonary disease, because hypoxia may result from posterior nasal packing.
3. Patients with posterior packs should be admitted to the hospital (Rosen & Sternbach, 1983).

EQUIPMENT

Headlamp
Topical anesthetic agent (e.g., cocaine, etc.)
Topical vasoconstricting agent (e.g., phenylephrine, etc.)
Intravenous sedation (e.g., diazepam, etc.)
Silver nitrate sticks
1-inch-wide strips of plain gauze lubricated with antibiotic ointment or petroleum jelly
Frazier nasal suction tip
Long bayonet forceps

Nasal speculum
2-x-2″ gauze pads
4-x-4″ gauze pads
0 silk suture
Red rubber catheter size 8–10
Straight medium hemostat
Tape
Cotton tipped applicators
Umbilical clamp
(Note: Commercially prepared surgical sponge posterior packs are also available.)

PATIENT PREPARATION

1. Seat the patient in a dental chair or in a semi-Fowler's position on a stretcher.
2. Administer sedation as ordered.

PROCEDURAL STEPS

1. Roll and cut to 1¾ inch length, a 4-x-4-inch gauze and then tie silk suture around the pack.
2. Using cotton tipped applicators, apply topical anesthetic and/or vasoconstrictor to the interior of the nose.
3. *With a headlamp, introduce a nasal speculum into the naris and suction clotted blood from the nose. See Figure 167.1

*Indicates portions of the procedure usually performed by a physician.

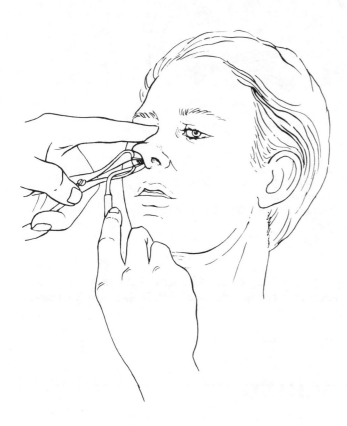

Figure 167.1 Nasal speculum in nose, while clots are suctioned out. (Rosen & Sternbach, 1983: 165. Reprinted by permission.)

4. *Insert a red rubber catheter through the nose into the oropharynx. Then, with a hemostat pull it out through the mouth. See Figure 167.2.
5. *Tie the postnasal pack to the catheter and pull the pack with the catheter through the mouth into the posterior nasopharynx. A bulge of the postnasal pack should be visible above the soft palate. See Figure 167.3.
6. *If necessary, push the postnasal pack into place manually. A tongue blade or bite block will help prevent the uncooperative patient from biting you.
7. *Remove the catheter and tie the suture ends protruding from the nose
8. *Pack the anterior nose with gauze coated with antibiotic ointment or petroleum jelly using bayonet forceps and allowing both ends to protrude. See Ch. 166.
9. Tape a drip pad in place below rolled gauze.

COMPLICATIONS

1. Hypovolemia from blood loss
2. Inadequate hemostasis with recurrent hemorrhage

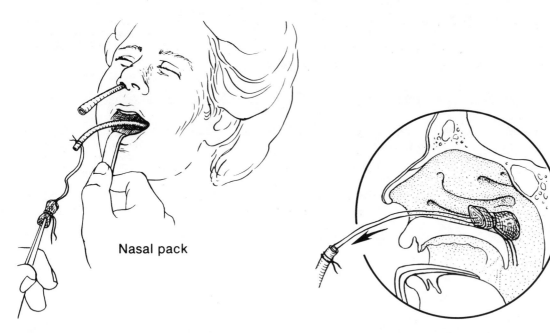

Nasal pack

Figure 167.2 Foley catheter threaded through nose and gauze packing anchored to end of the catheter ready to pull into place.
(Rosen & Sternbach, 1983: 165. Reprinted by permission.)

Figure 167.3 Gauze packing in place in posterior nasopharynx.
(Rosen & Sternbach, 1983: 165. Reprinted by permission.)

3. Airway obstruction from swelling or dislodgment of the postnasal pack
4. Hypoxia (Nasal packing can cause a decreased PaO_2 as a result of naso-pulmonary reflexes.)
5. Sinusitis
6. Toxic shock syndrome

PATIENT TEACHING

1. Avoid bending over, coughing, sneezing, heavy lifting, coughing, or blowing your nose. If you must sneeze, do so with your mouth open.
2. Call for assistance for any shortness of breath or if bleeding resumes.
3. Report any fever, malaise, or rash.

REFERENCE

Rosen, P., & Sternbach, G.L. 1983. *Atlas of Emergency Medicine*, 2nd ed. Baltimore: Williams & Wilkins.

SUGGESTED READINGS

Erwin, S.A. 1987. Epistaxis: How to control the persistent nosebleed. *Postgraduate Medicine*, 82, 4:59–65.

Fairbanks, D.N.F. 1986. Complications of nasal packing. *Otolaryngology–Head and Neck Surgery*, 94, 3:412–415.

Lockhart, J.S., & Griffin, C. 1986. Epistaxis. *Nursing*, 16:69.

Silfen, E.Z., & Stair, T. 1984. Nasal emergencies. *Topics in emergency medicine*, 74:40–47.

168

Balloon Catheters for Epistaxis

Margo E. Layman, RNC, BSN, CEN

INDICATIONS

1. To tamponade anterior epistaxis
2. To tamponade posterior epistaxis

CONTRAINDICATIONS AND CAUTIONS

1. People age 50 to 80 with histories of cardiac and pulmonary disorders already have compromised cardiac and pulmonary systems.
2. Establish baseline oxygenation with ABGs or pulse oximetry for patients with cardiopulmonary disease, because hypoxia may result from balloon catheter packing.
3. Patients with posterior packs should be admitted to the hospital (Rosen & Sternbach, 1983).
4. Inflate the balloons with air instead of water to prevent aspiration if the balloon ruptures.

EQUIPMENT

Headlamp
Topical anesthetic (e.g., cocaine, etc.)
Topical vasoconstrictor (e.g., phenylephrine, etc.)
Intravenous sedation (e.g., diazepam, etc.)
Silver nitrate sticks
Antibiotic ointment or petroleum jelly
Frazier nasal suction tip

Long bayonet forceps
Nasal speculum
4-x-4″ gauze dressings
Cotton tipped applicators
Intranasal balloon (See Figure 168.1).
(Foley catheters may also be used instead of commercial balloons.)
Umbilical clamp, for use with Foley catheter

PATIENT PREPARATION

1. Seat the patient in a dental chair or in semi-Fowler's position on a stretcher.
2. Administer sedation as prescribed.

PROCEDURAL STEPS

1. *With a headlamp, introduce a nasal speculum into the naris and suction clotted blood from the nose.

*Indicates portions of the procedure usually performed by a physician.

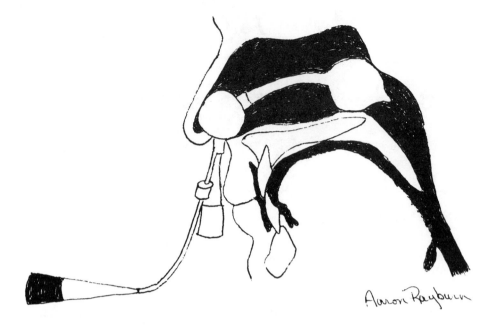

Figure 168.1   Nasal cavity with commercially prepared epistaxis balloon in place and inflated with air.

2.   *Apply local anesthetic with cotton tipped applicators.
3.   Coat the intranasal balloon with antibiotic ointment or petroleum jelly.
4.   *Insert the intranasal balloon under direct vision with a headlamp.
5.   Instill 3–6 ml of air into the posterior port and pull the balloon taut. See Figure 168.2.
6.   Instill 6–9 ml of air into the anterior balloon port.
7.   Immobilize the balloon by looping rubber strap around ear and taping in place for commercially prepared product. For the foley catheter, use an umbilical clamp and pad the nose. See Figure 168.3.
8.   Bilateral balloons may be used if indicated. The patient may require hospital admission (Rosen & Sternbach, 1983).

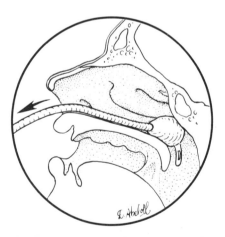

Figure 168.2   Foley catheter is placed in nasopharynx and inflated with 5–6 ml of air. (Rosen & Sternbach, 1983: 165. Reprinted by permission.)

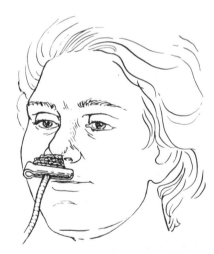

Figure 168.3   Umbilical clamp holding Foley catheter balloon in place in nasopharynx. (Rosen & Sternbach, 1983: 165. Reprinted by permission.)

COMPLICATIONS

1. Hypovolemia from blood loss
2. Inadequate hemostasis with recurrent hemorrhage
3. Airway obstruction from swelling, balloon dislodgment, or balloon over-inflation
4. Hypoxia (Nasal balloons can cause a decreased PaO_2 as a result of naso-pulmonary reflexes.)
5. Sinusitis
6. Pressure necrosis of nasopharyngeal structures (Rosen & Sternbach, 1983)

PATIENT TEACHING

1. Avoid bending over, coughing, sneezing, heavy lifting, or blowing your nose. If you must sneeze, do so with your mouth open.
2. Call for assistance for any shortness of breath or if bleeding resumes.
3. Do not remove or manipulate the balloon.

REFERENCE

Rosen, P., & Sternbach, G.L. 1983. *Atlas of Emergency Medicine*, 2nd ed. Baltimore: Williams & Wilkins.

SUGGESTED READINGS

Cook, P.R., Renner, G., & Williams, F. 1985. A comparison of nasal balloons and posterior gauze packs for posterior epistaxis. *Ear, Nose and Throat Journal,* 64:78–82.

Erwin, S.A. 1987. Epistaxis, How to control the persistent nosebleed. *Postgraduate Medicine,* 82, 4:59–65.

Fairbanks, D.N.F. 1986. Complications of nasal packing. *Otolaryngology – Head and Neck Surgery,* 94:412–415.

Harvey, M. 1987. Controlling nasal haemorrhage. *Nursing Times,* 83:48–49.

Jastremski, M.S. 1985. *The whole emergency medicine catalog.* Philadelphia: Saunders.

Keene, M.S., & Moran, W.J. 1985. Control of epistaxis in the multiple trauma patient. *Laryngoscope,* 95:874–875.

Lockhart, J.S., & Griffin, C. 1986. Epistaxis. *Nursing,* 16:69.

Silfen, E.Z., & Stair, T. 1984. Nasal Emergencies, *Topics in emergency medicine,* 74:40–47.

169

Nasal Foreign Body Removal

Margo E. Layman, RNC, BSN, CEN

INDICATIONS

1. To remove known nasal foreign body.
2. To rule out foreign body in children or mentally compromised patients with foul, purulent nasal discharge or epistaxis. Unilateral nasal drainage is especially suspicious for foreign body.

CONTRAINDICATIONS AND CAUTIONS

1. Beans or other vegetable matter should be removed as rapidly as possible because they will swell as they absorb fluid.
2. If pushed further into the nose, the object could be aspirated.
3. The patient may need to be restrained to prevent injury while the foreign object is removed.

EQUIPMENT

Headlamp
Nasal speculum
Topical vasoconstrictor (e.g., cocaine, neosynephrine, etc.)
Topical anesthetic (e.g., lidocaine, etc.)

Cotton tipped applicators
Miniature alligator forceps
Suction with #5 or #7 neurosuction tip (Frazier suction tip)
Nasal packing
Bayonet forceps

PATIENT PREPARATION

1. Place patient in Trendelenburg position.
2. Restrain or sedate patient as indicated.

PROCEDURAL STEPS

*Indicates portions of the procedure usually performed by a physician.

1. *Attempt to reach foreign object with miniature alligator forceps.
2. If nasal swelling prevents visualization, the turbinates should be sprayed with topical vasoconstrictor or use cotton applicators to apply the vasoconstrictor.
3. *Using a headlamp and nasal speculum, attempt to visualize of the foreign body.
4. *Remove mucous and debris to facilitate visualization, with a small suction tip.

5. *After the swelling has decreased and the nasal debris is removed, then the bayonet forceps, the miniature alligator forceps, or suction is used to retrieve the foreign body.
6. Nasal packing may be needed to control bleeding caused by irritation or manipulation.
7. Antibiotic ointment or petroleum jelly may be applied to the interior of the nose with cotton tipped applicators.

COMPLICATIONS

1. Irritations and infection (including sinus infections) as a result of prolonged retention of a nasal foreign body.
2. Perforation of the nasal canal as a result of manipulation of the foreign object.
3. Airway obstruction if the foreign body is aspirated.

PATIENT TEACHING

1. Use a humidifier in your bedroom at night.
2. Do not place foreign objects in the nose.
3. Use antibiotic ointment or petroleum jelly in the interior of the nose for 2–3 days after foreign body removal.

SUGGESTED READINGS

Barber, J., & Sheehy, S.B. 1985. *Emergency nursing principles and practice*, 2nd ed. St. Louis: Mosby.

Rund, D.A. 1986. *Essentials of emergency medicine.* Toronto: Appleton-Century-Crofts.

Upchurch, D.T. (ed). 1989. *Otolaryngology problems in primary care.* Oradell, NJ: Medical Economics.

170

Indirect Laryngoscopy

Linell M. Jones, RN, BSN, CEN, CCRN

INDICATIONS

1. To evaluate foreign body sensation or locate a foreign body in the posterior pharynx and larynx.
2. To evaluate hoarseness.

CONTRAINDICATIONS AND CAUTIONS

Attempt to rule out epiglottitis prior to attempting indirect laryngoscopy.

EQUIPMENT

Laryngeal mirror (size 3–6)
Gauze to grip tongue and pad the
    lower teeth
Light source such as a headlamp or
    headmirror
Method to warm mirror and
    prevent fogging, such as
    alcohol lamp, warm water,
    electric light bulb, or a light
    coating of a liquid soap

Topical anesthetic (e.g., cocaine,
    lidocaine, or cetacaine)
Sedation (rarely needed)
(Note: Indirect laryngopharyngeal
    scopes with light source as
    well as fiber optic larynx
    and pharynx illuminators
    that are compatible with
    Welch Allyn handles are
    also available.)

PATIENT PREPARATION

*Indicates portions of the procedure usually performed by a physician.

1. Place patient in high-Fowler's position with head slightly forward.
2. Place emesis basin in patient's hands.
3. *Anesthetize the pharynx. See Ch. 137: Local Infiltration and Topical Agents.

PROCEDURE

1. Have patient protrude the tongue out as far as possible.
2. *Lay gauze over the tongue then wrap it under the tongue.
3. *Grip the gauze-wrapped tongue between the thumb and middle finger of the nondominant hand and brace the index finger against the upper lip or teeth.
4. *Warm the mirror and test the temperature on your hand.
5. *Place the mirror with the back side against the uvula.
6. *Elevate the uvula and soft palate using one motion.

7. *Avoid touching the posterior tongue, because this will induce gagging.
8. Have the patient breath normally through the mouth.
9. *Direct the light onto the mirror.
10. *Examine structures, look for pathology or foreign body.
11. *Ask patient to say "E" and "A." Observe the vocal cords as the epiglottis moves out of the way.

COMPLICATIONS

1. Inability to perform the exam due to uncontrollable gagging
2. Burns from the laryngeal mirror
3. Contusing the lips or the underside of the tongue by utilizing too much pressure against the teeth

PATIENT TEACHING

1. Have nothing to eat or drink until topical anesthetic is no longer active (approximately one hour).
2. Use caution when resuming oral intake. Begin slowly with sips of water.

SUGGESTED READING

DeWeese, D.D., & Saunders, W.M., 1973. *Textbook of otolaryngology,* 4th ed. Saint Louis: Mosby.

171

Esophageal Foreign Body Removal

Linell M. Jones, RN, BSN, CEN, CCRN

INDICATIONS

To remove documented foreign bodies from the esophagus.

Technique A: Endoscopy

This is the procedure of choice, because it provides direct visualization of the foreign body, the ability to evaluate the esophagus for pathology, and provides for greater control of the object during removal (Webb, 1988).

CONTRAINDICATIONS AND CAUTIONS

Esophageal perforation (rare)

EQUIPMENT

Intravenous access equipment   Endoscopic equipment
Sedative (as prescribed)   Pulse oximeter
Topical anesthetic

PATIENT PREPARATION

1. Establish venous access for medication administration.
2. *Consider endotracheal intubation if airway is at risk for compromise.
3. Place the patient in a Trendelenburg, lateral decubitus position.

PROCEDURAL STEPS

1. Assess vital signs and oxygen saturation and continue to monitor them frequently throughout the procedure.

*Indicates portions of the procedure usually performed by a physician.

2. Administer local anesthetic to control gag as prescribed.
3. Administer sedative as prescribed.
4. *Intubate the esophagus with the endoscope.
5. *Visualize the foreign body.
6. *Push the foreign body into the stomach, grasp it and remove it through the scope, or grasp it and remove it with the scope as a unit.
7. *Evaluate the esophagus for preexisting pathology and/or foreign body induced trauma.
8. *Dilate the esophagus as necessary.

Technique B: Foley Catheter

This technique is used for removal of coins and other nonobstructing, blunt foreign bodies in very cooperative patients with ingestions of only a few hours duration.

CONTRAINDICATIONS AND CAUTIONS

1. Esophageal perforation or aspiration may occur.
2. There is no direct visualization of either the object or the esophagus.
3. There is no direct control of the object.

EQUIPMENT

Fluoroscopy equipment
Foley catheters, 8–12-French

Suction equipment
Laryngoscope with Magill forceps

PATIENT PREPARATION

Place the patient in deep Trendelenberg (30°) position on fluoroscopy table.

PROCEDURAL STEPS

1. Inflate the Foley catheter balloon to insure that it expands evenly.
2. *Under continuous fluoroscopy, insert the catheter through the mouth until the balloon is distal to the foreign body.
3. *Inflate the balloon with air.
4. *With smooth, steady traction withdraw the catheter until the foreign body enters the patient's mouth. Grasp the object with forceps if it is not expelled by the patient.

Technique C: Glucagon

The technique has been used to treat meat impactions of the distal esophagus by relaxing the smooth muscle of the stomach and reducing distal esophageal sphincter pressure. It does not directly effect esophageal motor function (Gilman, 1985). Success rates with the use of glucagon are approximately 50% (Webb, 1988).

PATIENT PREPARATION

Establish intravenous access.

PROCEDURAL STEPS

1. Administer glucagon as ordered. The usual dose is 0.5–1.0 mg IV or 2.0 mg IM
2. Observe the patient for relief of symptoms as the bolus passes.

3. Observe the patient for adverse glucagon effects such as generalized allergic reaction, nausea and/or vomiting, marked increase of blood pressure, or hypoglycemia.

Technique D: Papain and gas forming agents

Papain (enzymatic meat tenderizer) and gas forming agents may be used but have very poor success rates and higher complication rates (Zimmers, 1988). Esophageal rupture is the most common complication. For these reasons, this technique will not be discussed further in this text.

COMPLICATIONS

1. Esophageal rupture may be caused by erosion of the foreign body, puncture by foreign body, tears from violent vomiting, or iatrogenic trauma from the procedures used to remove the foreign body.
2. Development of esophageal fistula (Webb, 1988)
3. Aspiration of saliva, vomit, or the foreign body during removal

PATIENT TEACHING

1. Avoid future occurrences by
   a. avoiding alcohol while eating;
   b. taking smaller bites and chewing food well;
   c. place nothing but food in the mouth.
2. Report fever, difficulty swallowing, shortness of breath, chest pain, abdominal pain, or swelling of neck (subcutaneous emphysema) immediately (Webb, 1988).
3. Advance diet slowly as tolerated or directed by the physician.

REFERENCES

Gilman, A.G., Goodman, L.S., Rall, T.W., & Murad, F. 1985. *Goodman and Gilman's The pharmacological basis of therapeutics,* 7th ed. New York: Macmillan.
Webb, W.A. 1988. Management of foreign bodies of the upper gastrointestinal tract. *Gastroenterology,* 94:204–216.

172

Tooth Replantation and Preservation

Sharon Gavin Fought, PHD, RN

INDICATIONS

To preserve and/or replant an avulsed tooth.

CONTRAINDICATIONS AND CAUTIONS

1. Patients who are unresponsive, combative, or have compromised airways are unable to facilitate preservation of teeth by replacing them in the socket. Replantation should not be attempted due to risk of aspiration.
2. Fractures of the tooth below alveolar bone require extraction of the tooth and root (Kelly, 1987).
3. If the bone and soft tissue are too traumatized to support the tooth, replantation should not be attempted.
4. Teeth should be replanted as quickly as possible. Handle the tooth gently, without touching the soft tissue or root portion.
5. Deciduous (baby) teeth may not be replanted. Even when partially in place, these teeth are usually extracted. Conversely, deciduous teeth can be retained if properly replanted (Krasner, 1990).
6. Teeth should not be debrided, because this procedure can destroy the periodontal fibers essential for successful replantation (Cosgriff & Anderson, 1984).

EQUIPMENT

Solution for tooth storage. Options, listed in order of preference, (Krasner, 1990) include
1. Hank's solution (available from medical research supply laboratories)
2. Sterile saline
3. Milk
4. Saliva

Sterile container with lid for tooth and solution
2-x-2″ gauze or dental pads
emesis basin
Optional equipment
    Local anesthetic
    Peridontal packing
    Dental mirror
    Methyl methacrylate

PATIENT PREPARATION

1. Cleanse the mouth with gentle rinse of normal saline to remove debris, blood, and dirt.
2. Elevate the head of the bed, unless contraindicated, to help prevent the patient from swallowing blood, which may precipitate nausea.

PROCEDURAL STEPS

1. Control hemorrhage in the mouth. An oral surgery consult is indicated if there is significant bleeding from the pulp (Sheehy, 1989).
2. If the tooth is obviously dirty (particles of dirt attached), soak it gently in preservation fluid to loosen particles. Do not scrub the tooth.
3. Replace the avulsed tooth into the socket in anatomical position.
4. Have the patient bite on a piece of gauze or padded tongue blade to seat the tooth in its socket and maintain its position.
5. If the patient is not able to cooperate with the above procedure, store the tooth in one of the following solutions:
   a. Hank's solution—for up to 12 hours (Krasner, 1990).
   b. sterile saline—for up to 1–2 hours only;
   c. cold whole milk—for very short periods of time;
   d. saliva—for up to 1 hour only;
6. If the tooth has been placed in a fluid other than Hank's solution, place the tooth in Hank's solution for 30 minutes prior to replantation to support viability of the periodontal ligament cells (Krasner, 1990; Matsson, 1982).
7. *Inject local anesthesia.
8. *Insert the tooth into the socket.
9. *If methyl methacrylate is available and the method of choice, stir the powder and liquid per manufacturer's instructions until it reaches a chewing gum texture and surround the tooth with this mixture (Gruber, 1989).
10. *Stabilize the tooth with suture, periodontal packing, or wire to the adjacent teeth.

*Indicates portions of the procedure usually performed by a physician.

COMPLICATIONS

1. Pain from reinsertion of tooth
2. Infection
3. 50% rate of loss of tooth (Gruber, 1989)
4. Need for root canal to remove pulp if damaged beyond its ability to recover.

PATIENT EDUCATION

A soft diet is indicated for 7–10 days to 3 weeks.

REFERENCES

Cardona, V.D., Hurn, P.D., Mason, P.J., Scanlon-Schlipp, A.M., & Veise-Berry, S.W. (eds). 1988. *Trauma Nursing: Resuscitation Through Rehabilitation*. Philadelphia: Saunders; 570–796.

Cosgriff, J.H., & Anderson, D.L. 1984. *The Practice of Emergency Care*, 2nd ed. Philadelphia: Lippincott.

Gruber, R.P. 1989. Maxillofacial trauma. *Topics in Emergency Medicine*, 11: 65–76.

Kelly, J.P. 1987. Dental emergencies. In T.C. Kravis, & C.G. Warner, (eds). *Emergency Medicine: A Comprehensive Review*, 2nd ed. Rockville, MD: Aspen; 1283–1290.

Krasner, P.R. 1990. *Journal of Emergency Nursing*, 16:29–33.

Matsson, L., Andreason, J.O., Cvek, M., & Granath, L. 1982. Ankylosis of experimentally reimplanted teeth related to extra alveolar period and storage environment. *Pediatric Dentistry,* 4:327–329.

Sheehy, S.B., Marvin, J.A., & Jimmerson, C.L. 1989. *Manual of Clinical Trauma Care.* St. Louis: Mosby.

SUGGESTED READINGS

Guralnick, W., Donoff, R.B., & Kelly, J.P. 1989. In E.D. Wilkins, (ed). *Emergency Medicine: Scientific Foundations and Current Practice,* 3rd ed. Baltimore: Williams and Wilkins; 795–798.

Howell, E., Shere, C., & Leydon, A. (1988). Face and neck trauma. In E. Howell, L. Widra, & M.G. Hill, (eds). *Comprehensive Trauma Nursing.* Glenview, IL: Scott, Foresman; 470–478.

173

Nitrous Oxide Administration

Jean A. Proehl, RN, MN, CEN, CCRN

Nitrous oxide is also known as laughing gas.

INDICATIONS

1. To provide rapid onset (2–6 minutes), quickly reversible (2–5 minutes) analgesia for 30 minutes or less. Nitrous oxide may be used to relieve the pain associated with trauma, renal colic, myocardial infarction, minor surgical procedures, wound care, diagnostic procedures, reduction of fractures and dislocations, etc. (Baskett, 1977; Flomenbaum, 1979; Moore, 1983; Nieto & Rosen, 1980; Pons, 1988; Proehl, 1985; Stewart, 1986).
2. To relieve the anxiety associated with painful conditions and procedures (Sundin, 1981).

CONTRAINDICATIONS AND CAUTIONS

1. When used for analgesia in the emergency setting (versus anesthesia in the operative setting), the gas mixture should be fixed at 50% nitrous oxide to 50% oxygen. For altitudes above 3,500 feet, a 65% nitrous oxide to 35% oxygen mixture is recommended, because the lower partial pressure of the nitrous oxide at higher altitudes does not provide adequate analgesia (Miller, 1989; Nieto & Rosen, 1980).
2. The patient should always self-administer the gas to prevent oversedation. Therefore, the patient must be cooperative and able to follow instructions. The mask or mouthpiece should **never** be strapped to the patient's face.
3. Nitrous oxide causes drowsiness and should not be used in patients with altered levels of consciousness, head injuries, or those who are heavily sedated or intoxicated (Pons, 1988; Proehl, 1985). Patients who have received narcotics should be individually evaluated for suitability to receive nitrous oxide (Nieto & Rosen, 1980).
4. The gas mixture contains 50% oxygen (35% at high altitude); therefore, it will not supply enough oxygen for patients in pulmonary edema and may suppress the hypoxic respiratory drive in a patient with chronic obstructive pulmonary disease (Miller, 1989; Pons, 1988, Proehl, 1985).
5. Nitrous oxide collects in dead air spaces and can expand the pre-existing pockets of air associated with pneumothorax, otitis media, perforated viscous, bowel obstruction, air embolism, and decompression sickness (McKinnon, 1981; Miller, 1989; Pons, 1988).
6. Nitrous oxide should not be used during early pregnancy, because it has been associated with fetal defects and spontaneous abortion (Pons, 1988; Proehl, 1985).
7. A scavenger system to dispose of exhaled gas is recommended to protect healthcare providers who administer nitrous oxide. Studies involving operating room and dental personnel have associated chronic exposure to nitrous oxide with psychomotor impairment, congenital malforma-

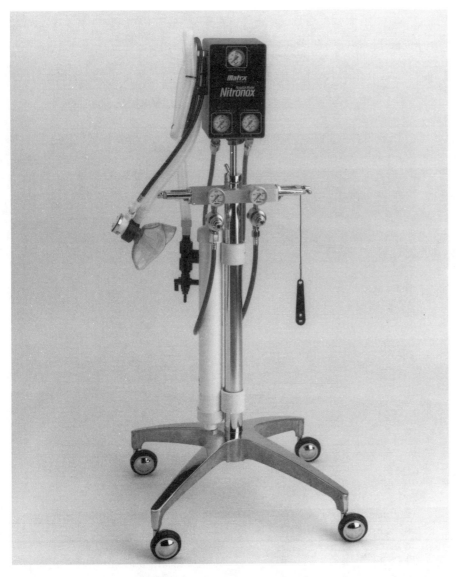

Figure 173.1 Nitronox nitrous oxide unit with demand valve and scavenger system. (Nitrous oxide and oxygen tanks are not show.) (Photo courtesy of Matrx Medical, Inc., Orchard Park, NY.)

tions, and spontaneous abortion in exposed women and sexual partners of exposed men. Possible association with bone marrow suppression, cancer, liver, and renal disease has also been reported (Bruce & Bach, 1975).

8. A mask is preferred to facilitate disposal of exhaled gas. If the patient is unable to use a mask due to facial trauma, etc.; a mouthpiece may be used in place of a mask (Proehl, 1985).

9. Nitrous oxide has abuse potential. The unit should be kept in a secure area.

10. A failsafe valve should be incorporated into the system to prevent administration of 100% nitrous oxide if the oxygen supply is interrupted.

11. A nurse or physician should be present at all times during nitrous oxide administration.

EQUIPMENT

Nitrous oxide and oxygen tanks connected by a blender preset to deliver 50% nitrous oxide and 50% oxygen (65% nitrous oxide and 35% oxygen at altitudes above 3,500 feet) with demand valve (see Figure 173.1) and scavenger (if a scavenger is not

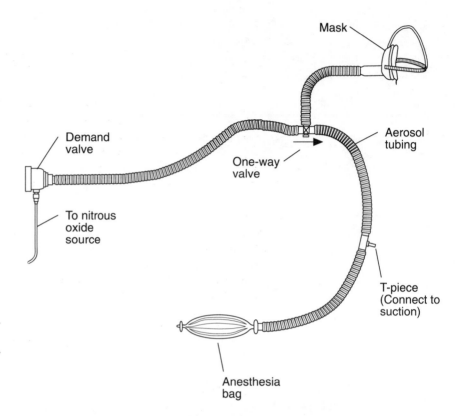

Figure 173.2 Nitrous oxide scavenger setup constructed of commonly available respiratory therapy equipment. The suction should be just high enough to keep the anesthesia bag deflated.

included as part of the system one may be constructed per Figure 173.2.).
(**Note:** Units are also available for use with pipeline supplied nitrous oxide.
Mask or mouthpiece
Wall suction and suction connection tubing

PATIENT PREPARATION

1. Assess and document vital signs.
2. Instruct the patient to
   a. form a tight seal with the mask or mouthpiece and take slow, deep breaths;
   b. exhale into the mask/mouthpiece so that the exhaled gas is removed by the scavenger;
   c. avoid unnecessary conversation to limit exhalation of nitrous oxide into the room;
   d. discontinue use if nausea, lightheadedness, or other side effects occur.

PROCEDURAL STEPS

1. Turn on the nitrous oxide and oxygen tanks. Check that the mixture pressure is within the safe level per manufacturer's specifications (>30 psi for Nitronox by Matrx Medical, Inc.).

2. Connect the scavenger to wall suction and turn the suction on. Turn ball valve lever on scavenger tube to the on position. Adjust the suction to 30–60 lpm.
3. Attach mask/mouthpiece to the demand valve.
4. Allow the patient to inhale the gas for 3–4 minutes before beginning any procedures. Some patients may require up to 6 minutes for adequate induction (Proehl, 1985).
5. As the patient becomes relaxed, he or she will be unable to create an adequate amount of negative pressure to trip the demand valve. This prevents excessive sedation.
6. When the patient drops the mask/mouthpiece, position or hold it so that the exhaled gas can be taken up by the scavenger.
7. Allow the patient to resume gas inhalation when he or she is able to hold the mask/mouthpiece.
8. Nitrous oxide administration is usually limited to a maximum of 30 minutes. Side effects are unusual but may require termination of nitrous oxide administration. Side effects may include vomiting (however some patients credit nitrous oxide with relieving nausea (Thal, 1979)), shortness of breath, excitement, drowsiness, confusion, and light-headedness (Nieto & Rosen, 1980, Pons, 1988; Proehl, 1985).
9. (Optional) When the procedure is completed, turn off the nitrous tank and have the patient continue breathing oxygen and exhaling into the mask for 5 minutes. This allows the scavenger to dispose of the exhaled gas.

   Note: Some sources recommend that the patient be placed on supplemental oxygen for a period of time after receiving nitrous oxide to counteract the effects of diffusion hypoxia caused by the diffusion of nitrous oxide from the arterial blood into the alveoli which dilutes alveolar oxygen levels. Research has demonstrated that diffusion hypoxia does not occur in healthy subjects after self-administration of nitrous oxide analgesia (Holcombe, 1976; Nieto & Rosen, 1980; Stewart, 1986).
10. Assess and document vital signs.

COMPLICATIONS

1. Side effects are unusual but may include vomiting, excitement, shortness of breath, light-headedness, drowsiness, or confusion (Proehl, 1985). However, nitrous oxide has been credited with relieving nausea (Thal, 1979). It may be necessary to discontinue nitrous oxide use in these cases.
2. Propping or holding the mask against the patient's face may result in excessive sedation. The patient must hold the mask to prevent overdosage.
3. Aspiration may occur if the patient vomits with the mask in place.

PATIENT TEACHING

1. Immediately report any uncomfortable sensations during nitrous oxide use.
2. Keep conversation to a minimum and exhale into the mask/mouthpiece.

REFERENCES

Baskett, P. 1977. Nitrous oxide and its uses today in the emergency patient. ACEP EDNA Scientific Assembly, San Francisco.

Flomenbaum, N., Gallagher, E.J., Eagen, K., & Jacobson, S. 1979. Self-administered nitrous oxide: An adjunct analgesic. *Journal of the American College of Emergency Physicians,* 8, 3:95–97.

Holcomb, C., Erdmann, W., & Corssen, G. 1976. The significance of diffusion hypoxemia. *Southern Medical Journal,* 69:1282–1284.

McKinnon, K.D.L. 1981. Prehospital analgesia with nitrous oxide/oxygen. *Canadian Medical Association Journal,* 125:836–840.

Miller, K. 1989. Analgesia: Issues and options. *Emergency,* 16–21.

Moore, M. 1983. The potential use of Entonox by nurses in A & E Departments . . . a pre-mixed gas containing 50% nitrous oxide and 50% oxygen. *Nursing Times,* 79:29–32.

Nieto, J., & Rosen, P. 1980. Nitrous oxide at higher elevations. *Annals of Emergency Medicine,* 9:610–612.

Pons, P. 1988. Nitrous oxide analgesia. *Emergency Medicine Clinics of North America,* 6:777–782.

Proehl, J.A. 1985. Nitrous oxide for pain control in the emergency department. *Journal of Emergency Nursing,* 11:191–194.

Stewart, R.D., Gorayeb, M.J., & Pelton, G.H. 1986. Arterial blood gases before, during, and after nitrous oxide administration. *Annals of Emergency Medicine,* 15:1177–1180.

Sundin, R.H., Adriani, J., Alam, S., Butler, J., Hatrel, P., Hyde, P., Mangum, F., Nicoletti, J., & Wallace, C.J. 1981. Anxiolytic effects of low-dosage nitrous oxide-oxygen mixtures administered continuously in apprehensive subjects. *Southern Medical Journal,* 74:1489–1492.

Thal, E.R., Montgomery, S.J., Atkins, J.M., Roberts, B.G. 1979. Self-administered analgesia with nitrous oxide. *Journal of the American Medical Association,* 242:2418–2419.

174

Calculating IV Medication Drips

Ruth A. Slabach, MSN, SCN, RN

INDICATIONS

1. To individualize medication administration.
2. To change dosage of medications as a patient's condition changes.
3. To calculate with accuracy the administration of potent drugs.
4. To validate accuracy of a dosage chosen from an administration chart.

CONTRAINDICATIONS AND CAUTIONS

1. Basic math skills needed to calculate IV medication drips include: knowledge of fractions, cancellation of units, ratio and proportion, and converting to the metric system.
2. Potent medications should always be administered with infusion pumps and must be closely monitored.
3. To save time and to improve accuracy, use a pocket calculator.
4. Ask a coworker to validate your calculations.

PROCEDURAL STEPS

Several basic calculations must be performed first.
1. Convert the patient's weight to kilograms. (Divide pounds by 2.2.)
2. Convert grams (g) to milligrams (mg). (Multiply grams by 1,000).
3. Convert milligrams to micrograms (mcg). (Multiply mg by 1,000).
4. Remember, if using microdrip tubing, 60 microdrops (mcgtts) equal 1 milliliter (ml). Therefore, the rate of microdrops per minute corresponds to the infusion rate per hour (i.e., 50 microdrops/min = 50 ml/hr).

A. Calculating IV flow rate

A variety of infusion sets exist with different drop factors. The number of drops per milliliter is printed on the package. Macrodrip sets deliver large drops per milliliter (10–20 gtts/ml). Those with small drops (60 gtts/ml) are called microdrip or minidrip sets. Several different methods may be used to calculate IV flow rate.

Formula 1

$$\frac{\text{ml/hr} \times \text{gtts/ml (IV set)} = \text{gtts/min}}{60 \text{ min/hr}}$$

Example: Macrodrip tubing labeled 10 gtts/ml. Infuse 1000ml of D_5W at 125 ml/hr.

$$\frac{125 \text{ ml} \times 10 \text{ gtts/ml}}{60 \text{ min/hr}} = 20.8 \text{ or } 21 \text{ gtts/min}$$

Formula 2

$$\frac{\text{ml of fluid} \times \text{gtts per ml (IV set)}}{\text{hrs to administer} \times 60 \text{ min/hr}} = \text{gtts/min}$$

Example Macrodrip tubing labeled 15 gtts/ml. Infuse 1000 ml of normal saline over 10 hours.

$$\frac{1000 \text{ ml} \times 15 \text{ gtts/ml}}{10 \text{ hours} \times 60 \text{ min}} = \frac{15000}{600} = 25 \text{ gtts/min}$$

B. Calculating dilution/concentration

The following formula describes how to determine amount of drug in each ml of solution.

Formula Amount of drug added, divided by amount of solution, equals the concentration.

$$\frac{\text{amount of drug}}{\text{amount of solution}} = \text{concentration}$$

Ratio/Proportion may also be used.

Example 1. units/ml
Heparin 5000 units (U) in D_5W 500 ml.
What is the concentration of drug per ml of solution?

Formula

$$\frac{5000 \text{ U}}{500 \text{ ml}} = 10 \text{ U/ml}$$

Ratio/proportion Solve for x.

$$5{,}000 \text{ U} : 500 \text{ ml} = x \text{ units} : \text{ml}$$

(The means are the two inside numbers.
The extremes are the 2 outside numbers. Multiply means and extremes).

$$500x = 5000$$
$$x = 10 \text{ U/ml}$$

Example 2. mg/ml
Lidocaine 2 gm in D_5W 500 ml.
What is the concentration of drug (in mg) per ml of solution?
Convert grams to milligrams.

$$2 \text{ g} \times 1000 \text{ mg} = 2000 \text{ mg}$$

Formula

$$\frac{2000 \text{ mg}}{500 \text{ ml}} = 4 \text{ mg/ml}$$

Ratio/proportion Solve for X.

$$2000 \text{ mg} : 500 \text{ ml} = x \text{ mg} : \text{ml}$$
$$500x = 2000$$
$$x = 4 \text{ mg/ml}$$

Example 3. mcg/ml
Isuprel 2 mg in D_5W 250 ml.
What is the concentration of drug (in mcgs) per ml of solution?
Convert mg to mcg.

$$2 \text{ mg} \times 1000 \text{ mcg} = 2000 \text{ mcg}$$

Formula

$$\frac{2000 \text{ mcg}}{250 \text{ ml}} = 8 \text{ mcg/ml}$$

Ratio/proportion

$$2000 \text{ mcg} : 250 \text{ ml} = x : \text{ml}$$
$$250x = 2000$$
$$x = 8 \text{ mcg/ml}$$

C. Calculating infusion rate

1. Infusion rate may be calculated per unit time, or microdrops per minute.
2. Infusion rate may be either the rate of *volume* given or the rate of *concentration* given.
3. Potent drugs are frequently ordered by concentration per unit time (e.g., 3 mcg/min).
4. Unit time may be per hour or per minute.

Example 1. Drug in units.
Heparin 5000 U in D_5W 500 ml to infuse at 45 ml per hour.
Concentration of solution is 10 U/ml. Note that rate is given as volume/hr.

a. Volume per minute

Formula Rate per hour divided by 60 equals rate per minute.

$$\frac{45 \text{ ml}}{60 \text{ min}} = .75 \text{ ml/min}$$

Ratio/proportion

$$45 \text{ ml} : 60 \text{ min} = x \text{ ml} : \text{min}$$
$$60x = 45$$
$$x = .75 \text{ ml/min}$$

b. Concentration per minute

Formula Concentration of solution multiplied by the volume per minute equals the concentration per minute.

$$10 \text{ U/ml} \times .75 \text{ ml/min} = 7.5 \text{ U/min}$$

c. Concentration per hour

Formula Volume per hour multiplied by concentration per ml equals concentration per hour.

$$45 \text{ ml/hr} \times \text{U/ml} = 450 \text{ U/hr}$$

Example 2. Drug in milligrams
Lidocaine 2 g in D_5W 500 cc at 3 mg/min.

a. Concentration per hour

Formula Concentration per minute multiplied times 60 equals concentration per hour.

$$3 \text{ mg/min} \times 60 \text{ min} = 180 \text{ mg/hr}$$

b. Volume (milliliters) per hour
Concentration is 4 mg/ml (see calculating dilution and concentration).
Formula Divide the concentration per hour by the concentration per ml.

$$\frac{180 \text{ mg/hr}}{4 \text{ mg/ml}} = 45 \text{ ml/hr}$$

c. Rate per minute

Formula Divide rate per hour by 60.

$$\frac{45 \text{ ml/hr}}{60 \text{ min}} = .75 \text{ ml/min}$$

Remember, microdrops per minute corresponds to ml/hr (i.e., 45 ml/hr equals 45 microdrops per minute)

Example 3 Drug in micrograms

Isuprel 4 mg in D_5W 500 ml to infuse at 10 mcg/min.

Convert mg to mcg.

$$4 \text{ mg} \times 1000 = 4000 \text{ mcg}$$

a. Concentration (micrograms) per hour. Concentration per minute is given at 10 mcg/min.

Formula Concentration per minute multiplied by 60 min equals concentration per hour.

$$10 \text{ mcg/min} \times 60 = 600 \text{ mcg/hr}$$

b. Volume (ml) per hour

Concentration of drug in solution is 8 mcg/ml (see section on calculating dilution and concentration).

Formula Concentration per hour divided by concentration of solution equals volume per hour.

$$\frac{600 \text{ mcg/hr}}{8 \text{ mcg/ml}} = 75 \text{ ml/hr}$$

Remember, microdrops per minute corresponds to ml per hr infusion rate.

D. Calculating infusion rates per kilogram of body weight per unit time

Preliminary steps

1. Calculate concentration of solution.
2. Calculate patient's body weight in kilograms (divide pounds by 2.2).
3. Convert mg to mcg (if needed).

Formula 1

$$\frac{\text{Desired dose} \times \text{Weight} \times 60}{\text{Concentration of solution}} = \text{rate}$$

Formula 2

Calculate drop factor.

$$\frac{60 \text{ min/hr} \times \text{wt in kg}}{\text{Concentration in mcg}} = \text{Drop factor}$$

Multiply drop factor by concentration desired to equal rate.

Whenever the desired concentration changes, you need only to multiply the drop factor by the new concentration desired to calculate the new rate.

Formula 3

Desired dose times weight (in kg) equals total minute dose.

Total minute dose divided by drug concentration equals ml per min.

Mls per min times drop factor (60) equals microdrops per minute to infuse (or mls per hour on infusion pump).

Example 1. Drug in mcg/kg

Infuse dobutamine 500 mg in D_5W 250 ml at 10 mcg/kg/min. Patient weighs 165 lbs (75 kg). Concentration of solution in mcg is 2000 mcg/ml.

Formula 1

$$\frac{10 \text{ mcg} \times 75 \text{ kg} \times 60}{2000 \text{ mcg}} = 22.5 \text{ mcgtts/min}$$

Formula 2

$$\frac{60 \text{ min/hr} \times 75 \text{ kg}}{2000 \text{ mcg/ml}} = 2.25 \text{ drop factor}$$

$$2.25 \times 10 \text{ mcg} = 22.5 \text{ mcgtts/min}$$

If the desired dosage changed to 12 mcg/kg/min you would only need to multiply the drop factor of 2.25 × 12 to calculate the new rate.

$$2.25 \times 12 = 27 \text{ mcgtts/min}$$

Formula 3

$$10 \text{ mcg} \times 75 \text{ kg} = 750 \text{ mcg/min}$$

$$\frac{750 \text{ mcg}}{2000 \text{ mcg/ml}} = .375 \text{ ml/min}$$

$.375 \text{ mls/min} \times 60 = 22.5 \text{ mcgtts/min (or 22.5 ml/hr)}$

E. Calculating dose of medication currently infusing

Preliminary steps
1. Calculate drug concentration per ml.
2. Check drop rate or infusion rate of pump.
3. Calculate patient's weight in kilograms.

Formula 1

$$\frac{\text{Total amount of med} \times \text{drip rate}}{\text{Total ml of IV} \times \text{kg} \times 60 \text{ min}} = \text{amt/kg/min}$$

Formula 2
Calculate drop factor (see section on calculating infusion rates per kilogram of body weight per unit time, formula 2).
Divide infusion rate per hr by drop factor.

Formula 3
1. Microdrops per minute divided by 60 equals mls per min infusing.
2. Mls per min multiplied by concentration per ml equals concentration per min infusing.
3. Concentration per min divided by patient weight (in kg) equals concentration per kilogram per minute dose.

Example 1. Calculate units/kg/min. Infusion of heparin 5,000 units in D5W 500 ml is infusing at 50 ml/hr (or 50 microdrops per minute). Patient weighs 60 kg.

Formula 1

$$\frac{5,000 \text{ U} \times 50 \text{ mcgtt}}{500 \text{ ml} \times 60 \text{ kg} \times 60 \text{ min}} = .14 \text{ U/kg/min}$$

Formula 2 Drop factor is 360

$$\frac{50 \text{ ml/hr}}{360} = .14 \text{ U/kg/min}$$

Formula 3

$$\frac{50 \text{ cc/hr}}{60 \text{ min}} = .83 \text{ ml/min infusing}$$

$$.83 \text{ ml/min} \times 10 \text{ U/ml} = 8.3 \text{ U/min}$$

$$\frac{8.3 \text{ U/min}}{60 \text{ kg}} = .14 \text{ U/kg/min infusing}$$

Example 2 Calculate mcg/kg/min. Infusion of dopamine 800 mg in D5W 250 ml is infusing at 15 microdrops per minute (or 15 ml/hr). Patient weighs 70 kg. (Concentration is 3200 mcg/ml.)

Formula 1

$$\frac{800{,}000 \text{ mcg} \times 15 \text{ mcgtt}}{250 \text{ ml} \times 70 \text{ kg} \times 60} = 11.4 \text{ mcg/kg/min}$$

Formula 2 Drop factor is 1.312.

$$\frac{15 \text{ ml/hr}}{1.312} = 11.4 \text{ mcg/kg/min}$$

Formula 3

$$\frac{15 \text{ mcgtts/min}}{60} = .25 \text{ ml/min infusing}$$

$$.25 \text{ ml/min} \times 3200 \text{ mcg/ml} = 800 \text{ mcg/min infusing}$$

$$\frac{800 \text{ mcg/min}}{70 \text{ kg}} = 11.4 \text{ mcg/kg/min}$$

Ratio proportion method

Example 3 Calculate mcg/kg/min. Nitroprusside 100 mg in D_5W 250 ml infusing at 30 ml per hour. The patient weighs 80 kg. How many mcg/kg/min of nitroprusside is the patient receiving? 100 mg = 100,000 mcg

1. Determine mcg/ml.

$$100{,}000 \text{ mcg} : 250 \text{ ml} = x \text{ mcg} : \text{ml}$$
$$250x = 100{,}000$$
$$x = 400 \text{ mcg/ml}$$

2. Determine mcg/kg/ml.

$$400 \text{ mcg} : 80 \text{ kg} = x \text{ mcg} : \text{kg}$$
$$80x = 400$$
$$x = 5 \text{ mcg/kg/ml}$$

3. Determine mcg/kg/min.

$$5 \text{ mcg} : 60 \text{ mcgtt} = x \text{ mcg} : 30 \text{ mcgtt}$$
$$60x = 150$$
$$x = 2.5 \text{ mcg/kg/min}$$

F. Calculating total amount of drug infused

To determine total amount of drug infused over a period of time, the concentration of the drug must be known, and the exact time the drug was started.

Example Dobutamine 250 mg in D_5W 250 ml at 10 ml per hour has been infusing at this rate for 2 hours. How much total medication has the patient received?

Concentration is 1 mg/ml.

1. Calculate concentration per hour.

$$1 \text{ mg/ml} \times 10 \text{ ml per hour} = 10 \text{ mg/hr}$$

2. Calculate total amount of drug infused.

$$10 \text{ mg/hr} \times 2 \text{ hr} = 20 \text{ mg}$$

Total amount of dobutamine infused over two hours was 20 mg.

G. Adjusting infusion rate for titration of drugs.

Example Isuprel 1 mg in D_5W 250 ml to infuse at 2–5 mcg/min to maintain blood pressure at 100. (1 mg = 1,000 mcg.)

1. Determine concentration. Concentration of solution is 4 mcg/ml.
2. Concentration per minute is given (2–5 mcg/min).
3. Determine upper dose of infusion rate and lower dose of infusion rate. Divide concentration per minute by concentration per ml.

Lower dose

$$\frac{2 \text{ mcg/min}}{2 \text{ mcg/ml}} = 0.5 \text{ ml/min}$$

Higher dose

$$\frac{5 \text{ mcg/min}}{4 \text{ mcg/ml}} = 1.25 \text{ ml/min}$$

4. Determine infusion rates

    Lower dose

    Multiply volume per min by 60.

    $$.5 \text{ ml/min} \times 60 = 30 \text{ ml/hr (or 30 mcgtt/min)}$$

    Higher dose

    $$1.25 \text{ ml/min} \times 60 = 75 \text{ ml/hr}$$

SUGGESTED READINGS

Kee, J.L., & Marshall, S.M. 1988. *Clinical calculations.* Philadelphia: Saunders.
Northridge, J.A. 1987. Calculating IV medications with confidence. *Nursing,* 9:55–57.

175

Intravenous Streptokinase Administration

Ruth Altherr Giebel, MS, RN

Streptokinase is also known as STK, SK, Streptase, Kabikinase.

INDICATIONS

To lyse thromboses in the presence of
1. Acute myocardial infarction (MI) diagnosed by
   a. Typical ischemic chest pain lasting for at least 30 minutes and less than 6 hours duration, which is unresponsive to sublingual nitroglycerin. Time limit may be extended if severe pain persists beyond 6 hours.
   b. And ST segment elevation of greater than 0.1 mV (measured 0.25 sec from the J point) in one of the following locations.
      i. Two of 3 inferior leads (II, III, AVF)
      ii. Two of 6 precordial leads (V1 through V6)
      iii. Lateral leads I and AVL
2. Pulmonary embolism
3. Deep vein thrombosis
4. Arterial thrombosis or embolism
5. Occlusion of arteriovenous cannulae

ABSOLUTE CONTRAINDICATIONS

1. Active internal bleeding
2. Recent (within 2 months) cerebrovascular accident, intracranial, or intraspinal surgery
3. Intracranial neoplasm
4. Severe, uncontrolled hypertension
5. History of allergic reactions to streptokinase (Streptase, 1988)

RELATIVE CONTRAINDICATIONS AND WARNINGS

Relative contraindications to the use of streptokinase are those events or conditions that either in isolation or combination may increase the potential risk of streptokinase therapy and include
1. Prior treatment with streptokinase or exposure to streptococcus infections in past 6 months (this could result in formation of antibodies and create resistance to the drug).
2. Recent (within 10 days) major surgery, obstetrical delivery, organ biopsy.
3. Recent (within 10 days) gastrointestinal bleeding.
4. Recent (within 10 days) trauma including cardiopulmonary resuscitation.

5. Recent (within 10 days) puncture of subclavian or internal jugular vessel.
6. Hypertension: systolic BP >180 mm Hg and/or diastolic BP >110 mm Hg.
7. High likelihood of left heart thrombus, e.g., mitral stenosis with atrial fibrillation.
8. Subacute bacterial endocarditis
9. Hemostatic defects including those secondary to severe hepatic or renal disease
10. Pregnancy
11. Age >75 years
12. Cerebrovascular disease
13. Diabetic hemorrhagic retinopathy
14. Septic thrombophlebitis or occluded AV cannula at seriously infected site
15. Current treatment with oral anticoagulants (e.g., warfarin sodium.)
16. Any other condition in which bleeding constitutes a significant hazard or would be particularly difficult to manage because of its location

EQUIPMENT

IV starting equipment
Streptokinase vial
Sodium chloride injection, USP or dextrose (5%) injection, USP for reconstitution, 5 ml
Sodium chloride injection, USP or dextrose (5%) injection, USP for further dilution, 40 to 90 ml
Syringes
    2–5-ml
    1–50-ml

18-G needles
Catheter plug (also known as click, lock, PRN adaptor, heparin lock, buffalo cap)
Volumetric infusion pump for IV solutions
Pump tubing
Lidocaine 100 mg for IV administration (if indicated)
Atropine 1 mg for IV administration (if indicated)

PATIENT PREPARATION

1. Thorough assessment to include
   a. Complete history and physical exam including time of chest pain onset;
   b. 12-lead ECG;
   c. Review of selection criteria for streptokinase therapy.
2. Establish continuous cardiac monitoring. See Ch. 57.
3. Establish IV access with a minimum of three sites. An 18–20-gauge catheter is preferred. The double-lumen peripheral IV catheter may be useful to limit the number of needed venous punctures.
4. Provide routine acute MI care as ordered, which may include but is not limited to
   a. Oxygen therapy
   b. Intravenous nitroglycerin
   c. Prophylactic lidocaine bolus and infusion
   d. Intravenous narcotic analgesia
   e. Aspirin
   f. Intravenous beta blocker therapy
   g. Calcium channel blocker therapy
   h. Pretreatment with corticosteriods or diphenhydramine

5. Obtain initial laboratory studies to include
   a. CPK with MB fraction
   b. Chemistry profile
   c. Electrolyte profile
   d. PT, PTT
   e. CBC with platelets

PROCEDURAL STEPS

Streptokinase reconstitution

1. Mix streptokinase for administration as directed below. In some institutions the pharmacy prepares the streptokinase solution.
   a. Slowly add 5 ml NS D_5W to the streptokinase vial, directing the fluid stream against the side of the vial rather than into the drug powder. Foaming may occur during mixing but it does not affect the drug's potency.
   b. Roll and tilt the vial gently to mix contents. To prevent foaming; **do not shake vial.**
   c. Withdraw the reconstituted solution from the vial slowly and carefully dilute to total volume as listed in Table 175.1.

Table 175.1 Recommended dosages of streptokinase. (Streptase, 1988).

Indication	Loading Dose/Duration	Maintenance Dose/Duration
Acute MI	1,500,000 IU within 60 min	Not applicable
Pulmonary embolism	250,000 IU over 30 min	100,000 IU per hr for 24 hr
Deep vein thrombosis	250,000 IU over 30 min	100,000 IU per hr for 72 hr
Arterial thrombosis or	250,000 IU over 30 min	100,00 IU per hr for 24–72 hr
Arteriovenous cannulae occlusion embolism	250,000 IU inserted in limb(s) of occluded cannula and then clamp off cannula limb(s) for 2 hr. After 2 hr, aspirate contents of infused cannula limb(s), flush with saline, and reconnect cannula.	

2. When diluting the 1,500,000 IU infusion bottle (50 ml), as in acute MI, you follow the same procedure as in step a, but after initial reconstitution the drug can be further diluted in the same vial with an additional 40 ml of diluent.
3. Assemble IV tubing. An inline IV filter size 0.8 um or larger may be used.
4. Because streptokinase contains no preservatives, it must be reconstituted just prior to use. It may be stored up to 8 hours at 2–8°C if necessary.
5. Due to the limited availability of compatibility information, no other medications should be added to the container of streptokinase.
6. Administer the loading dose and initiate the maintenance dose as outlined in Table 175.1.
7. Anticoagulation with heparin sodium has been recommended following streptokinase administration. A bolus dose is not administered and the

continuous heparin infusion is begun only after the PTT falls to 2 times the normal control value. It is important to note that this can take several hours to occur following the conclusion of the streptokinase infusion. The PTT should therefore be monitored every 2 hours to determine when it falls in that range.

PATIENT MANAGEMENT

1. Continuously monitor cardiac rhythm and neurologic status.
2. Monitor for signs of allergic response which can vary from a low grade fever to an anaphylactic reaction. For a mild to moderate reaction, the physician may order a corticosteroid and antihistamine, but the streptokinase infusion can be continued. For a severe allergic reaction, the streptokinase infusion should be stopped and emergency measures initiated.
3. Assess and document vital signs every 5 to 10 minutes during streptokinase infusion. Be alert for a precipitous drop in blood pressure. Decrease the rate of the streptokinase infusion if hypotension occurs. Hypotension may require pressor therapy. (Lew, 1985).
4. Monitor and document clinical signs of reperfusion which include cardiac arrhythmias, resolution of chest pain, and normalization of ST segments. The arrhythmias seen are the same as those seen in many MI patients and may include: ventricular tachycardia, ventricular fibrillation, sinus bradycardia, accelerated idioventricular rhythm, and heart block. Any arrhythmias that occur are treated following advanced cardiac life support (ACLS) guidelines.
5. Assess for signs of bleeding complications and coronary artery reocclusion every 15 minutes during the infusion and every 2 hours thereafter until 2 hours after heparin is discontinued.
6. Document the time the chest pain resolves and the time the streptokinase infusion ends.
7. Monitor PTT every 2 hours. When PTT falls to less than 2 times the normal control, a continuous heparin infusion should be initiated.
8. Institute thrombolytic bleeding precautions which should include
   a. Avoid the use of automatic inflatable blood pressure cuffs if possible.
   b. Avoid unnecessary arterial and venous punctures. All punctures sites should be compressed manually for a minimum of 10 minutes for venous punctures and 20 minutes for arterial punctures. Apply pressure dressings after discontinuation of lines and following vessel punctures.
   c. Use a heparin/saline lock for blood draws and consolidate blood draws when possible.
   d. Monitor all puncture sites and gingivae for evidence of bleeding.
   e. Use draw sheet to move and position patient to avoid contusions. Instruct patient to request assistance when changing positions.
   f. Observe for frank blood and test urine, stools, emesis for occult blood.
   g. Avoid IM injections.
   h. Monitor hemoglobin and hemacrit for evidence of acute blood loss.

COMPLICATIONS

1. Bleeding should be expected to occur following streptokinase therapy. The goal is to prevent significant bleeding through careful screening and

observation of thrombolytic bleeding precautions. Careful monitoring and prompt treatment are critical to minimize the effects of bleeding if it does occur. Types of bleeding seen with streptokinase therapy include

   a. Intracranial
   b. Gastrointestinal
   c. Genitourinary
   d. Epistaxis
   e. Retroperitoneal
   f. Venous and arterial puncture sites
   g. Femoral artery catheter site
   h. Gingival bleeding
   i. Ecchymosis
2. Allergic reaction
3. Fever

PATIENT TEACHING

1. Request assistance when moving.
2. Report any bleeding. Some minor bleeding and bruising is normal.
3. Report any change in chest pain or other symptoms immediately.

REFERENCES

Lew, A.S., Laramee, P., Cercek, B., Shah, P.K., & Ganz, W. 1985. The hypotensive effect of intravenous streptokinase in patients with acute myocardial infarction. *Circulation,* 72:1321–1326.

Streptase (streptokinase) Prescribing Information. 1988. Somerville, NJ: Hoechst-Roussel Pharmaceuticals, Inc.

SUGGESTED READINGS

Belle-Isle, C. 1989. Patient selection and administration of thrombolytic therapy. *Journal of Emergency Nursing,* 15:155–164.

Blakeley, W.P., Hollis, J., Larson, K., Novak, J., & Sherer, B.K., 1983. Standard care plan for systemic administration of streptokinase. *Critical Care Nurse,* July/August, 86–89.

Brewer, C.C. & Markis, J.E. 1986. Streptokinase and tissue plasminogen activator in acute myocardial infarction. *Heart and Lung,* 15:552–558.

Kabikinase (streptokinase) Prescribing Information. 1987. Alameda, CA: Kabivitrum, Inc.

tPA Administration

Ruth Altherr Giebel, MS, RN

tPA is also known as tissue plasminogen activator, TPA, rt-PA, alteplase, and activase.

INDICATIONS

To lyse thromboses in the presence of
1. Acute myocardial infarction (MI) diagnosed by
   a. Typical ischemic chest pain lasting for at least 30 minutes and less than 6 hours duration which is unresponsive to sublingual nitroglycerin. Time limit may be extended if severe ischemic pain persists beyond 6 hours.
   b. And ST segment elevation of more than 0.1 mV in one of the following three locations:
      Two of 3 inferior leads (II, III, AVF)
      Two of 6 precordial leads (V1 through V6)
      Lateral leads I and AVL
   Caution should be exercised in the presence of left bundle branch block or previous MI in same location.
2. Pulmonary embolism

ABSOLUTE CONTRAINDICATIONS

1. Active internal bleeding
2. Any history of cerebrovascular accident
3. Recent (within 2 months) intracranial or intraspinal surgery or trauma
4. Intracranial neoplasm, arteriovenous malformation or aneurysm
5. Known bleeding disorder
6. Severe uncontrolled hypertension (Activase, 1988)

RELATIVE CONTRAINDICATIONS AND CAUTIONS

Relative contraindications to the use of tPA are those events or conditions that either in isolation or combination may increase the potential risk of tPA therapy.
1. Recent (within 10 days) major surgery
2. Cerebrovascular disease
3. Recent (within 10 days) gastrointestinal or genitourinary bleeding
4. Recent (within 10 days) trauma including CPR
5. Recent (within 10 days) puncture of subclavian or internal jugular vessel
6. Hypertension: systolic BP greater than or equal to 180 mm Hg and/or diastolic BP greater than or equal to 110 mm Hg
7. High likelihood of left heart thrombus (e.g., mitral stenosis with atrial fibrillation)
8. Acute pericarditis

9. Subacute bacterial endocarditis
10. Hemostatic disorders including those secondary to severe hepatic and renal disease.
11. Pregnancy
12. Diabetic hemorrhagic retinopathy or other hemorrhagic ophthalmic conditions
13. Septic thrombophlebitis or occluded AV cannula at seriously infected site
14. Advanced age (i.e., >75 years)
15. Current treatment with oral anticoagulants (e.g., warfarin sodium).
16. Any condition in which bleeding constitutes a significant hazard or would be particularly difficult to manage because of its location.

EQUIPMENT

Two 50-mg tPA kits (each contains one 50-mg vial of tPA powder and one 50-ml vial of sterile water) and
150-ml empty IV bag or bottle or soluset
or
One 100-mg tPA kit (contains one 100-mg vial of tPA powder, one 100-ml vial of sterile water, and one double-sided transfer device)
Syringes
Two 20–30-ml
One 10-ml

18-G needles
25 ml NaCl or D_5W
IV starting equipment
IV catheter plug (also known as click lock, PRN adaptor, heparin lock, buffalo cap)
Lidocaine, 100 mg for IV administration (if indicated)
Atropine, 1 mg for IV administration (if indicated)
Volumetric pump for IV solution administration (vented if using 100-mg vial)
Pump tubing

PATIENT PREPARATION

1. Thorough assessment to include
   a. Complete history and physical exam including time of chest pain onset;
   b. 12-lead ECG;
   c. Review of selection criteria for tPA therapy.
2. Establish continuous cardiac monitoring. See Ch. 57.
3. Establish IV access with a minimum of three sites using an 18–20-gauge catheter. The use of a double-lumen peripheral IV catheter may reduce the number of IV punctures.
4. Provide routine acute myocardial infarction care as ordered which may include but is not limited to
   a. Oxygen therapy
   b. Intravenous nitroglycerin
   c. Prophylactic lidocaine bolus and infusion
   d. Intravenous narcotic analgesia
   e. Aspirin
   f. Intravenous beta blocker therapy
   g. Calcium channel blocker therapy
5. Obtain initial laboratory studies to include
   a. CPK with MB fraction
   b. Chemistry profile
   c. Electrolyte profile
   d. PT, PTT
   e. CBC with platelets

PROCEDURAL STEPS

tPA reconstitution

Mix tPA solution for administration as directed below. In some institutions the pharmacy prepares the tPA solution.

1. 50-mg vials: Add 50 ml of sterile water to each of two vials of 50 mg tPA lyophilized powder. Never use bacteriostatic water since the preservatives may inactivate the tPA, It is best to use a 20–30-ml syringe and an 18-gauge needle to promote powder dissolution without stimulating foaming and to aid in the fluid aspiration. The sterile water should be injected with the fluid stream directed at the lyophilized powder to facilitate dissolution.

   100-mg vial: Insert one end of transfer device into vial containing diluent. Hold tPA vial upside-down and insert the other end of the transfer device into the center of the stopper. Invert the vials.

2. After injecting the sterile water, gently swirl or invert the vial to mix the contents. **Do not shake.** If foaming occurs, allow the vial to stand for 2–5 minutes for the foam to dissipate.

3 Assemble IV tubing without the use of an inline IV filter. An inline filter is not used because it can trap the tPA molecule and prevent it from reaching the patient. Vented tubing must be used to administer the solution directly from the 100-mg vial.

4. Once reconstituted, the tPA solution (1 mg/cc) may be used for direct administration. Although it may be further diluted with either 0.9% sodium chloride (NS) or 5% dextrose in water for injection (D_5W), most institutions prefer the 1:1 dilution for ease of calculation and to conserve fluids.

5. 50-mg vials: Place the tPA solution into an empty IV bag, bottle, or soluset and label the bag clearly, indicating the time the infusion is started.

   100-mg vial: Hang the vial for direct infusion or transfer the contents of the vial to an IV bag, bottle, or soluset.

6. Set up infusion pump with the IV tubing and prime the tubing with the tPA solution.

7. Once reconstituted, the tPA solution may be stored for 8 hours at 2–30°C. After 8 hours, any unused portion should be discarded.

8. The reconstituted tPA is not light sensitive and no special handling is required. However, unreconstituted tPA may be sensitive to light and, therefore, it should be stored in its carton until use.

9. tPA is not compatible with other medications; use a separate IV line for tPA administration.

tPA dosing and administration for acute myocardial infarction

1. Withdraw 10 mg from the tPA bag/vial to be given as the tPA loading dose.

2. Set infusion pump at 50 cc/hr to deliver the remaining 50 mg of first hour's dose.

3. Inject 10 mg tPA bolus over 1–2 minutes and then immediately start infusion pump at 50 mg/hr.

4. At the end of one hour decrease IV rate to 20 mg/hr and continue until the infusion is complete. **Remember to decrease the rate at end of the first hour.**

5. When the pump alarms indicating infusion is complete, place 20 cc of NS or D_5W injection into the tPA bag or soluset and continue to infuse at the same rate until bag is empty. This step ensures that the complete dose has been administered. After the full dose has been infused, the

tPA IV line can be converted to a heparin/saline lock to use for blood draws.

6. The tPA dosing described here is based on the Food and Drug Administration (FDA) recommended dose of 100 mg which is given over a 3-hour period. The dosing schedule is based on the following format:

Total dose = 100 mg

Hour one = 60 mg	Give 60% of total dose with 10% of first hour's infusion as a bolus over 1–2 minutes.
Hour two = 20 mg	Give remaining 40% equally
Hour three = 20 mg	divided over last two hours.

7. If a patient weighs less than 65 kg, it may be beneficial to dose the patient based on a mg/kg schedule. The total dose as approved by the FDA should be 1.25 mg/kg over 3 hours following the same format described above (Activase, 1990).

8. It is generally recommended to administer a loading dose of heparin and then begin a continuous infusion before the end of the tPA administration period. The PTT is then maintained at one and one-half times control to prevent reocclusion. Table 176.1 summarizes some of the dosage and administration guidelines for tPA.

Table 177.1 Activase dosage: Key steps in successful administration. (From Ramsden, 1988: 16. Adapted with permission.)

Dilution	1:1	
Concentration = 1.0 mg/ml	50 mg tPA + 50 ml sterile water + No further dilution.	50 mg tPA + 50 ml sterile water

	Dose	Flow rate
	Lytic dose	
	10 mg	10 ml IV Push
	Hour 1, 50 mg	50 ml/hr
	Maintenance dose	
	Hour 2, 20 mg	20 ml/hr
	Hour 3, 20 mg	20 ml/hr

Total recommended dose = 100 mg

For Patients < 65 kg: 1.25 mg/kg

Dose by Weight

Weight (kg)	Dose (mg)	Weight (kg)	Dose (mg)
64	80	50	62.5
60	75	45	56.25
55	68.75	40	50

A dose of 150 mg of tPA should not be used.

tPA Dosing and Administration for pulmonary embolism

1. The recommended dose of tPA for pulmonary embolism is 100 mg over 2 hours.

2. Heparin therapy should be instituted near the end or immediately following the tPA infusion when the PTT returns to twice normal or less (Activase, 1990).

Patient management

1. Continuously monitor cardiac rhythm and neurologic status.
2. Assess and document vital signs and status for clinical signs of reperfusion, bleeding complications (e.g., neuro checks), and signs of coronary artery reocclusion every 15 minutes during tPA infusion and every 2 hours thereafter until 2 hours after heparin is discontinued. Clinical signs of reperfusion may include cardiac arrhythmias, resolution of chest pain, and resolution of ST segment elevation. These signs may indicate the tPA has been successful, however, their absence does not indicate tPA has failed. The arrhythmias seen are the same as those seen in many MI patients and may include ventricular tachycardia, ventricular fibrillation, sinus bradycardia, accelerated ventricular rhythm, and heart block. Any arrhythmias that occur are treated following advanced cardiac life support guidelines.
3. Document the time the chest pain resolves.
4. Be sure to turn down the tPA infusion and document the time at exactly 1 hour into the infusion.
5. Monitor tPA infusion closely to ensure it is infusing at the correct rate.
6. Maintain heparin infusion and monitor PTT every 6 hours. Obtain order and adjust heparin infusion to keep PTT one and one-half to two times control. Patient may be on heparin several days until time of cardiac catheterization or other diagnostic tests.
7. Institute thrombolytic bleeding precautions, which should include
   a. Avoid the use of automatic inflatable blood pressure cuffs if possible.
   b. Avoid unnecessary arterial and venous punctures. All puncture sites should be compressed manually for a minimum of 10 minutes for venous punctures and 20 minutes for arterial punctures. Apply pressure dressings after discontinuation of lines and vessel punctures.
   c. Use a saline/heparin lock for blood draws and consolidate blood draws when possible.
   d. Monitor all puncture sites and gingivae for evidence of bleeding.
   e. Use draw sheet to move and position patient to avoid contusions. Instruct patient to request assistance when changing positions.
   f. Observe for frank blood and test urine, stools, and emesis for occult blood.
   g. Avoid IM injections
   h. Monitor hemoglobin and hematocrit for evidence of acute blood loss.
   i. Suggest use of antecubital or femoral sites for placement of central lines if needed.

COMPLICATIONS

The only adverse reactions attributable to tPA therapy are due to the bleeding that occurs following tPA therapy. Bleeding should be expected to occur during and following the tPA infusion. The goal is to prevent serious bleeding through careful screening and by observation of thrombolytic bleeding precautions. Thorough assessment and prompt treatment are also critical to minimize the effects of bleeding when it does occur. Most bleeding can be divided into two categories: surface bleeding and internal bleeding. Examples of the types of bleeding seen with TPA include

1. Intracranial
2. Gastrointestinal
3. Genitourinary
4. Epistaxis
5. Retroperitoneal

6. Venous, arterial puncture sites
7. Femoral artery catheter sites
8. Gingival bleeding
9. Ecchymosis

Intracranial bleeding (ICB) is the most serious form of bleeding that can occur following thrombolytic therapy. While ICB is rare (less than 1%), it is so potentially devastating that care must be taken to exclude patients at risk for intracranial hemorrhage and to recognize and treat changes in neurologic status without delay (Data on file, 1988, Genentech, Inc.)

PATIENT TEACHING

1. Ask for assistance before moving.
2. Report any bleeding.
3. Report any change in chest pain or other symptoms immediately.

REFERENCES

Activase, Alteplase, recombinant Prescribing Information, 1988. S. San Francisco: Genentech, Inc.

Ramsden, C.S. 1988. *Management of the acute myocardial infarction patient receiving fibrinolytic therapy with Activase.* S. San Francisco: Genentech, Inc.

Data on file. 1988. S. San Francisco: Genentech, Inc.

SUGGESTED READINGS

Dillon, J., Philbrook, P., Klementowizc, V., Masek, R., & Hankins, T. 1989. Rapid initiation of thrombolytic therapy for acute MI. *Critical Care Nurse* 9:55–61.

Giebel, R.A., Pavey, S.S., & Bryant, P.P. 1988. Clinical articles: tPA therapy in acute myocardial infarction. *Journal of Emergency Nursing,* 14:206–213.

Hammond, B.B. (ed). 1989. Thrombolytic therapy for acute myocardial infarction: Implications for emergency nursing. *Journal of Emergency Nursing,* 15:145–210.

Rafter, R.H. 1988. Thrombolytic therapy orders and record sheets: Nursing care made easier. *Journal of Emergency Nursing,* 14:237–239.

177

Intravenous APSAC Administration

Ruth Altherr Giebel, MS, RN

APSAC is also known as anisoylated plasminogen streptokinase activator complex, anistreplase, Eminase.

INDICATIONS

To lyse coronary artery thromboses in the presence of acute myocardial infarction (MI) diagnosed by

1. Typical ischemic chest pain lasting for at least 30 minutes and less than 6 hours duration which is unresponsive to sublingual nitroglycerin. Time limit may be extended if evidence of ongoing injury persists beyond 6 hours.
2. And ST segment elevation of greater than 0.1 mV (measured 0.25 sec from the J point) in one of the following locations and in the absence of left bundle branch block or previous MI in the same location:
   a. Two of 3 inferior leads (II, III, AVF)
   b. Two of 6 precordial leads (V1 through V6)
   c. Lateral leads I and AVL

ABSOLUTE CONTRAINDICATIONS

1. Active internal bleeding
2. History of cerebrovascular accident
3. Recent (within 2 months) intracranial or intraspinal surgery or trauma
4. Intracranial neoplasm, arteriovenous malformation, or aneurysm
5. Known bleeding disorder
6. Severe uncontrolled hypertension
7. History of allergic reactions to streptokinase or APSAC (Eminase, 1990)

RELATIVE CONTRAINDICATIONS AND CAUTIONS

Relative contraindications to the use of APSAC are those events or conditions that either in isolation or in combination may increase the potential risk of APSAC therapy.

1. Prior treatment with streptokinase or APSAC or exposure to streptococcus infections in the past 6 months (this could result in formation of antibodies and create resistance to the drug).
2. Recent (within 10 days) major surgery, obstetrical delivery, organ biopsy.
3. Recent (within 10 days) serious gastrointestinal bleeding.
4. Recent (within 10 days) trauma including cardiopulmonary resusitation.
5. Recent (within 10 days) puncture of subclavian or internal jugular vessel.
6. Hypertension: systolic BP > 180 mm Hg and/or diastolic BP > 110 mm Hg.

7. High likelihood of left heart thrombus (e.g., mitral stenosis with atrial fibrillation).
8. Subacute bacterial endocarditis
9. Acute pericarditis
10. Hemostatic defects including those secondary to severe hepatic or renal disease.
11. Pregnancy
12. Age > 75 years
13. Cerebrovascular diseases
14. Diabetic hemorrhagic retinopathy or other hemorrhagic ophthalmic conditions
15. Septic thrombophlebitis or occluded AV cannula at seriously infected site.
16. Current treatment with oral anticoagulants (e.g., warfarin sodium.)
17. Any other condition in which bleeding constitutes a significant hazard or would be particularly difficult to manage because of its location.
18. Hypotension, which is unrelated to bleeding or anaphylaxis, may occur following APSAC administration. While the hypotension is usually not severe, careful monitoring and prompt treatment with fluids and/or pressor therapy should be available (Eminase, 1990).

EQUIPMENT

IV starting equipment
APSAC vial, 30 units
    (**Note:** APSAC must be refrigerated between 2–8°C (36°–46°F) at all times
Sterile water (nonbacteriostatic) for reconstitution, 5 ml
One 5-ml syringe
One 18-gauge needle

One 21-gauge needle
Catheter plug (also known as PRN adaptor, click lock, heparin lock, buffalo cap) or IV bag and tubing
Lidocaine, 100 mg for IV administration (if indicated)
Atropine, 1 mg for IV administration (if indicated)

PATIENT PREPARATION

1. Thorough assessment to include
   a. complete history and physical exam including time of chest pain onset;
   b. 12-lead ECG;
   c. review of selection criteria for APSAC therapy.
2. Establish continuous cardiac monitoring. See Ch. 57.
3. Establish IV access with a minimum of three sites. An 18–20-gauge catheter is preferred. The double-lumen peripheral IV catheter may be useful to limit the number of needed venous punctures.
4. Provide routine acute MI care as ordered which may include but is not limited to
   a. Oxygen therapy
   b. Intravenous nitroglycerin
   c. Prophylactic lidocaine bolus and infusion
   d. Intravenous narcotic analgesia
   e. Aspirin
   f. Intravenous beta blocker therapy
   g. Calcium channel blocker therapy
   h. Pretreatment with corticosteriods or diphenhydramine
5. Obtain initial laboratory studies to include

a. CPK with MB fraction
b. Chemistry profile
c. Electrolyte profile
d. PT, PTT
e. CBC with platelets

PROCEDURAL STEPS

APSAC reconstitution

Prepare APSAC for administration as directed below. It is recommended that the solution be prepared by the nurse on the unit just prior to administration.

1. Slowly add 5 ml sterile water without preservatives to the APSAC vial using an 18-gauge needle and by directing the fluid stream against the side of the vial rather than into the drug powder.
2. Roll and tilt the vial gently to mix contents. To prevent foaming, **do not shake vial.**
3. Withdraw the reconstituted APSAC from the vial slowly using the 18-gauge needle. Change to the 21-gauge needle prior to administration if desired.
4. Because APSAC begins to breakdown as soon as it is reconstituted, it must be used within 30 minutes of the time it is reconstituted. If it is not used in that time interval, the unused portion should be discarded.
5. No other medication should be added to the vial or syringe containing APSAC.
6. Administer the APSAC intravenously. The recommended dose of APSAC is 30 units given slowly IV over 2–5 minutes (Eminase, 1990).
7. Anticoagulation with heparin sodium has been recommended following APSAC administration. A bolus dose is not administered and the continuous heparin infusion is begun only after the PTT falls to 2 times the normal control value. It is important to note that this can take several hours following the administration of APSAC. The PTT should therefore be monitored every 2 hours to determine when it falls in that range. However, heparin may be empirically started 4–8 hours after administration of APSAC (Anderson, 1989).

Patient management

1. Continuously monitor patient's cardiac rhythm and neurologic status.
2. Monitor patient for signs of allergic reaction which can vary from a low grade fever to an anaphylactic reaction. For a mild to moderate reaction, the physician may order a corticosteroid and antihistamine. For a severe allergic reaction, the APSAC infusion should be stopped if possible and emergency measures initiated.
3. Monitor and document patient's vital signs every 15 minutes immediately following the APSAC administration for one hour then every 30 minutes for 5 hours. Be alert for a precipitous drop in blood pressure, which may require pressor therapy (Lew, 1985).
4. Assess and document clinical signs of reperfusion which might include cardiac arrhythmias, resolution of chest pain, and resolution of ST segments. These signs may indicate APSAC has been successful, however, their absence does not indicate APSAC has failed. The arrhythmias seen are the same as those seen in many MI patients and may include ventricular tachycardia, ventricular fibrillation, sinus bradycardia, accelerated idioventricular rhythm, and heart block. Any arrhythmias that occur are treated following ACLS guidelines.
5. Monitor and document any signs of bleeding complications or coronary

artery reocclusion every 15 minutes during the infusion and every 2 hours thereafter until 2 hours after heparin is discontinued.
6. Document the time the chest pain resolves.
7. Monitor PTT every 2 hours. When PTT falls to less than two times the normal control, a continuous heparin infusion should be initiated.
8. Institute thrombolytic bleeding precautions which should include
   a. Avoid the use of automatic inflatable blood pressure cuffs if possible.
   b. Avoid unnecessary arterial and venous punctures. All puncture sites should be compressed manually for a minimum of 10 minutes for venous punctures and for a minimum of 20 minutes for arterial punctures. Apply pressure dressings after discontinuation of lines and following vessel punctures.
   c. Use a heparin/saline lock for blood draws and consolidate blood draws when possible.
   d. Monitor all puncture sites and gingivae for evidence of bleeding.
   e. Use draw sheet to move and position patient to avoid contusions. Instruct patient to request assistance when changing positions.
   f. Observe for frank blood and test urine, stools, and emesis for occult blood.
   g. Avoid IM injections
   h. Monitor hemoglobin and hematocrit for evidence of acute blood loss.
   i. Suggest use of antecubital or femoral sites for placement of central lines if needed.

COMPLICATIONS

1. Bleeding should be expected to occur following APSAC therapy. The goal is to prevent significant bleeding through careful screening and by observation of thrombolytic bleeding precautions. Thorough assessment and prompt treatment are critical to minimize the effects of bleeding when it does occur. Types of bleeding seen with APSAC therapy include
   a. Intracranial
   b. Gastrointestinal
   c. Genitourinary
   d. Epistaxis
   e. Retroperitoneal
   f. Venous and arterial puncture sites
   g. Femoral artery catheter site
   h. Gingival
   i. Ecchymosis
2. Hypotension; a 5–10 mm Hg decrease in blood pressure should be expected in most patients. Some patients may have a profound decrease in BP and may require pressor therapy. The decrease in BP may be exacerbated by concomitant nitroglycerin and morphine sulfate administration (Angel, 1989).
3. Allergic reaction
4. Fever

PATIENT TEACHING

1. Request assistance when moving.
2. Report any bleeding immediately.
3. Report any change in chest pain or other symptoms immediately.

REFERENCES

Anderson, J.A. 1989. Optimal thrombolytic therapy: For whom, when, how. *Hospital Practice* 24, Suppl: 13–17.

Angel, J.A. 1990. *Thrombolytic therapy: The nursing perspective.* Bristol, TN: SmithKline Beecham Pharmaceuticals.

Eminase (Anistreplase) *Full Prescribing Information.* 1990. Bristol, TN: SmithKline Beecham Pharmaceuticals.

Lew, A.S., Laramee, P., Cercek, B., Shah, P.K., & Ganz, W. 1985. The hypotensive effect of intravenous venous streptokinase in patients with acute myocardial infarction. *Circulation,* 72:1321–1326.

SUGGESTED READINGS

Anderson, J.A. 1988. Uses of APSAC in the management of acute myocardial infarction: Current status. *Practical Cardiology,* 14:37–48.

178

Application of Restraints

Christine A. Miller, RN, MS

INDICATIONS

Partial or full patient restraint may be indicated under the following circumstances when less restrictive forms of patient therapy have been unsuccessful.

1. If the patient exhibits violent behavior that may be harmful to himself or herself, to other patients, or to staff.
2. If the patient is legally in police custody.
3. If the patient is being detained under court order or mental health hold.
4. If it is determined the patient is incapable of making an informed decision due to being under the influence of drugs or alcohol.
5. If the patient is expressing suicidal or homicidal ideation.
6. If the patient's disease process has rendered him or her incapable of making appropriate treatment choices (Jacobs, 1983).
7. If the patient's incapacity will last a significant time and treatment must be initiated involuntarily to avoid patient compromise (Mills, 1983).

CONTRAINDICATIONS AND CAUTIONS

1. Carefully consider the patient's right to refuse treatment.
2. Restraint should be used as a last resort, when all other means of control have failed.
3. Restraints should not be utilized for convenience, because staffing is inadequate.
4. The least restrictive restraint should be utilized after careful evaluation of the patient. The patient should be frequently reassessed to determine if restraints are still indicated.
5. The use of gauze rolls for limb restraints should be utilized only as an emergency measure. Soft limb restraints are preferable to prevent circulatory compromise.
6. Be aware of your verbal techniques in dealing with combative or violent patients. Patients may be hostile and paranoid. Avoiding direct verbal confrontation may prevent combative or violent patients from accelerating further (Jacobs, 1983).
7. Assume a nonthreatening stance when approaching patients in need of restraint.
8. Always be aware of the potential mechanics of a violent patient. Paranoia and hostility are common reactions when patients are being evaluated against their will.
9. Position yourself cautiously when dealing with a combative or violent patient.

a. Stand on the side of the patient (never in front) to protect your vulnerable zone.
b. Stand more than an arm's length from the patient to protect yourself from the patient who lunges or kicks.
c. Never turn your back on the patient.
d. Never precede a patient into a room.
d. Always place yourself (not the patient) closest to the door (Jacobs, 1983).

10. Case law has restricted the use of involuntary restraints. The Rogers v. Okin decision of 1979 established that restraints could only be utilized in cases of emergency or serious threat. Although this court decision dealt with the committed psychiatric patient, it advanced the rights of the mentally ill. The restrictions challenge the rights of all healthcare workers to restrain patients (Shindul, 1981).

11. Thoroughly search the patient and remove all objects from his or her pockets after applying restraints.

12. After restraints are discontinued, remove the belts from the room or lock them to the stretcher so they cannot be used as weapons.

13. Have a clear policy and procedure regarding restraint application. The policy should include
    a. indications for restraint application,
    b. personnel who may place restraints,
    c. development of emergency codes to notify security for assistance,
    d. communication guidelines for patients prior to and during restraint,
    e. how to monitor a patient in restraints,
    f. guidelines for removal of restraints

14. If the patient is in locked restraints, the key should be readily accessible in case of emergency.

EQUIPMENT

A variety of soft and locked restraints are commercially available. In the emergency department setting, limb restraints are most commonly utilized. For patients who require less restrictive restraint methods (i.e., the confused patient), a vest restraint may be adequate to gently remind the patient to not get out of bed unattended. Locked leather restraints should be utilized for patients who are combative; violent; or on police, alcohol, or mental health holds.

PATIENT PREPARATION

1. If possible, undress the patient. At a minimum, attempt to remove the patient's belt and shoes to prevent the patient from harming himself or herself or others.

2. Attempt voluntary restraint application, but do not bargain with the patient.

3. The patient should receive a thorough medical exam. This may need to be deferred until restraint application has been completed if the patient is violent or combative.

4. Consider obtaining alcohol and toxicology panels. Also consider the need to rule out organic and neurologic disorders, especially in the elderly. Patient history is critical (Jacobs, 1983).

Swedish Medical Center

EMERGENCY DEPARTMENT
Restraint Flow Sheet

Name: _____

Hospital No: _____

DATE: TIME:	RESTRAINTS APPLIED NEURO-VASCULAR STATUS INTACT				CARE/ACTIVITY			MENTAL STATUS						COMMENTS/OTHER
	RA	RL	LA	LL	Fluids Meal	BR B. Pan Urinal	Ambul. ROM	Asleep	Awake Approp.	Awake Inappr.	Agitat.	Combat.	Initial	
0000														
0015														
0030														
0045														
0100														
0115														
0130														
0145														
0200														
0215														
0230														
0245														
0300														
0315														
0330														
0345														
0400														
0415														
0430														
0445														
0500														
0515														
0530														
0545														
0600														
0615														
0630														
0645														
0700														
0715														
0730														
0745														
0800														
0815														
0830														
0845														
0900														
0915														
0930														
0945														
1000														
1015														
1030														
1045														
1100														
1115														
1130														
1145														

Initials/Signature:

_____

Behavior justifying use of restraints: _____

_____

Alternative to restraints attempted: _____

_____

NI-0965

Figure 178.1 Emergency department restraint flow sheet.
(Swedish Medical Center Emergency Department, Englewood, CO. Reprinted by permission.)

1. Establish a treatment plan that protects the patient's rights. Consider pharmacological therapy if necessary.
2. Ideally 4–5 people should assist in the application of restraints. One person should be assigned to the head and each extremity. Holding the patient's head to the side with pressure on the forehead and mandible will help decrease movement of the patient's body.
3. Use the least restrictive (soft versus locked leather or locked metal) restraints possible. Avoid 4-point limb restraint unless the patient is violent.
4. If time permits, pad the patient's extremities when using locked leathers. Apply cuffs snugly to prevent escape. Secure the restraints to the stretcher frame (never the siderails) and leave only enough slack to position the extremity safely.
5. If not using 4-point restraints, use at least 2-point restraints utilizing an upper and lower extremity on opposite sides. This prevents the patient from removing restraints, flipping off the stretcher, or tipping the stretcher over in an attempt to stand.
6. Consider a vest restraint in addition to 4-point restraints to protect a patient from injury if the patient is thrashing about.
7. The restrained patient should be positioned prone, side-lying, or supine with the head of the bed slightly elevated. Because restrained patients often are intoxicated, suction and airway equipment should be readily available.
8. If necessary, restraints may be applied while the patient is on the floor. In this case, carry the patient to the stretcher in the prone position to decrease his or her ability to struggle effectively.
9. Documentation is critical and should include:
    a. why a patient is restrained,
    b. type of restraints,
    c. frequency restraints are checked and reassessed to ensure safety and avoid circulatory compromise,
    d. frequency vital signs are checked,
    e. patient status including level of consciousness and activity.
10. A restraint checklist is a useful tool and includes provision for ensuring a patient is offered food, water, and bathroom privileges if appropriate. See Figure 178.1.

COMPLICATIONS

1. Circulatory compromise of restrained extremities.
2. Injury to staff or patient during application of restraints.

REFERENCES

Jacobs, D. 1983. Evaluation and management of the violent patient in emergency settings. *Psychiatric Clinics of North America*, 6:259–269.

Mills, M., Yesavage, J., & Gutheil, T. 1983. Continuing case law development in the right to refuse treatment. *American Journal of Psychiatry*, 140:715–719.

Shindul, J, & Snyder, M. 1981. Legal restraints on restraints. *American Journal of Nursing*, 81:393–394.

SUGGESTED READINGS

Applebaum, P., & Roth, L. 1984. Involuntary treatment in medicine and psychiatry. *American Journal of Psychiatry,* 141:202–205.

Calfee, B. 1988. Are You Restraining Your Patient's Rights? *Nursing* 18, 5:148–149.

Sheridan, G. 1989. Baffle locks: In whose best interest? *Nursing Times,* 85, 22:69–70.

Silver, M. 1987. Using restraint. *American Journal of Nursing,* 87:1414–1415.

179

Preparation for Interfacility Air Transport

Wendy R. Reeves, RN, BSN, CCRN

INDICATIONS

To prepare a critically ill or injured patient for air transport to another facility for medical care and/or diagnostic testing.

CONTRAINDICATIONS AND CAUTIONS

1. Hemodynamically unstable patient with impending cardiac or respiratory collapse.
2. Cardiac or respiratory arrest in progress
3. Inability to maintain life sustaining therapies enroute
4. Irrational or combative patient
5. Weather prohibiting flight at either origination or destination
6. Patients with extreme fear of flying
7. Any patient with a condition that might be exacerbated by altitude and pressure changes and which cannot be managed enroute

EQUIPMENT

The equipment required depends on the patient's injuries and diagnosis. All air transports of critical patients should be accomplished with advanced life support equipment and medications.

PROCEDURAL STEPS

1. Obtain informed consent from patient and/or significant others (**Note:** Per COBRA/OBRA legislation, all transports of patients with emergency medical conditions are subject to specific requirements. Refer to your institution's specific transfer policy.)
2. Obtain flight orders from referring physician.
3. Obtain flight orders from receiving physician as indicated.
4. Obtain flight orders from air ambulance company as indicated.
5. Report patient information and estimated time of arrival to receiving nurse.
6. Copy the patient's medical records, laboratory reports, advance directives for care, and x-rays.
7. Undress patient, provide a dry warm gown and blankets.
8. Remove all jewelry that could interfere with monitoring.
9. Place patient on backboard with securing straps or follow air ambulance's protocol for mode of immobilization for transport.

10. Position for comfort, unless otherwise indicated.
11. Intervene to provide physiologic stability prior to transport. Maintain patent airway, provide high flow supplemental oxygen, and intravenous access.
12. Have patient void or empty urine collection bag.
13. Attach one-way flutter valve with vented collection bag to chest tubes. Open gastric tubes and surgical drains to atmospheric pressure to prevent gas expansion at altitude. See Ch. 44.
14. Medicate with analgesics as indicated/ordered.

HELIPAD SAFETY

1. Always approach and leave the helicopter in a crouched position in view of the pilot. See Figure 179.1.

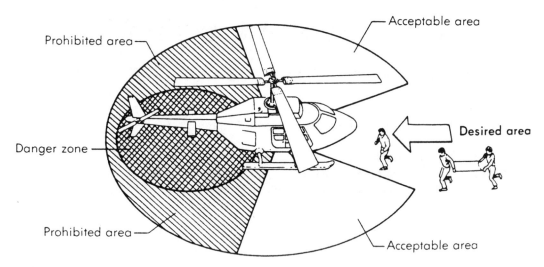

Safe approach zones

Prohibited area

Acceptable area

Desired area

Danger zone

Prohibited area

Acceptable area

Figure 179.1 Safe approach zones. (Lee, 1991: 600. Reprinted by permission.)

2. High-speed tail rotor blades are difficult to see, therefore, never approach from the rear unless otherwise instructed by the air crew members.
3. On slopes or uneven ground, always approach or leave from the downhill side.
4. Due to strong winds that are produced during landings and departures (rotor wash), all lightweight items must be secured. Sheets need to be taped down to the stretcher. Tall items such as IV poles should be lowered.
5. Earplugs may be used to protect you from loud noise.
6. Goggles or eye protection are indicated to protect you from loose objects such as gravel.

PATIENT TEACHING

1. Instruct patient on importance of not moving about during transport. Ask patient to request assistance if repositioning is necessary.
2. Have patient report any changes in symptoms during transport.
3. Explain loading and unloading procedures, and the noise levels associated with air ambulance.

REFERENCES

ASHBEAMS. 1988. *Air-Medical Crew National Standard Curriculum*. Pasadena, CA: Ashbeams.

Groves, M. 1988. Intrahospital transport of shock trauma patients. In J.M. Strange, (ed). *Shock trauma care plans*. Springhouse, PA: Springhouse Corporation.

Harahill, M. 1990. Preparing the trauma patient for transfer. *Journal of Emergency Nursing*, 16:25–27.

Lee, G. 1991. *Flight Nursing: Principles and Practice*. St. Louis: Mosby.

Sheehy, S.B., Marvin, J.A., & Jimmerson, C.L. 1989. *Manual of Clinical Trauma Care*. St. Louis: Mosby.

180

Collection of Bite Mark Evidence

Ruth L. Schaffler, RN, MA, CEN

Special thanks to Peter F. Hampl, DDS, Forensic Odontologist, of Tacoma, WA for his assistance and contribution to the preparation of this material. His expertise is invaluable to the fields of medicine, nursing, law enforcement, and forensics.

INDICATIONS

1. To obtain samples of saliva residue remaining on the patient's skin. (**Note:** It is nearly impossible to bite without leaving traces of saliva. Over 80% of the general population secrete substances in body fluids (e.g., perspiration, semen, vaginal secretions, and saliva) that establishes their major blood type (Hampl, 1980; Sperber, 1981) as well as other factors that are detectable by laboratory analysis.
2. To obtain a sample of the patient's saliva as a control for comparison to skin samples.
3. To obtain blood samples from the patient as a comparison to samples obtained from the skin if appropriate.
4. To photograph wounds identified or suspected of being bite marks.
5. To collect, preserve, and surrender specimens according to local chain-of-custody protocols.
6. To document the original appearance of the patient and all history, interventions, or pertinent observations. (**Note:** Law enforcement personnel and a forensic odontologist should be involved as soon as possible. Contact the American Academy of Forensic Sciences. 225 South Academy Boulevard, Suite 201, Colorado Springs, CO 80910; (303) 596-6006, for names and locations of forensic odontologists).

CONTRAINDICATIONS AND CAUTIONS

1. Life-saving interventions may destroy or alter potential evidence.
2. Early identification of medicolegal cases is necessary to minimize the loss of evidence through cleaning of wounds.
3. Improper collection, preservation, and/or labeling of specimens may result in the evidence being inadmissable in a court of law. Maintain chain-of-custody protocols for all evidence and film.
4. Bite marks may be misinterpreted as contusions, abrasions, or dermatologic lesions.
5. Bites can be located on any part of the body, so thorough inspection is necessary. If one bite is present, suspect others as well.
6. Deceased persons should be refrigerated but not embalmed. (Hampl, 1980).

EQUIPMENT

Sterile gloves
Distilled water or normal saline solution
Sterile cotton swabs for collecting samples and controls

One sterile test tube for each area swabbed
Lavender topped blood collection tubes
1"-x-1" gauze squares

Sterile specimen containers
Nonflexible metric ruler or scale
Camera with black-and-white and
    color film
      35 mm or other nondistorting

model for close-up views
    and precision enlargement
(Note: Polaroid cameras are of
    limited value.)

PATIENT PREPARATION

1. Document interventions that may interfere with evidence or produce other wounds such as venipuncture or defibrillation.
2. Obtain and document a thorough history. Ask conscious patients if they were bitten or if they bit anyone. A suspect may have been bitten by the victim as well and may have identifiable bite marks that can be examined for evidence.
3. Do not clean wounds until after photographs and samples are taken.
4. Obtain a written consent for photographs as necessary according to hospital policy.

PROCEDURAL STEPS

Photographing bite marks

(**Note:** Forensic photography is a specialty. The information supplied here is offered to assist with evidence collection when a specially trained photographer is not available. Law enforcement personnel should be involved with these cases as soon as possible and can determine the need for photography. Nurses who take evidentiary photographs may be required to testify in court and have their photography skills and training questioned by the defense attorney).

1. Place the area to be photographed on a firm flat surface.
2. Place the ruler as close to the bite mark as possible. (**Note:** A flexible ruler such as a tape measure conforms to the contours of the body and may distort the appearance of the bite in the photograph).
3. Position the camera so that it is perpendicular to the bite mark. This is especially important if the bite is on a rounded surface such as an extremity, shoulder, or breast. See Figure 180.1.
4. Take photos with and without the ruler from a close distance to show that there are no wound areas under the ruler.
5. Photograph wounds from several angles both before and after cleaning the area. Include close-up views from several angles as well as orienting photographs to show the relationship of the bite area to the rest of the body.

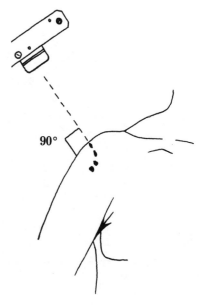

Figure 180.1 The camera is held perpendicular (at 90° angle) to the bite mark when taking the photograph.

Collecting swab samples

1. Moisten swabs in distilled water or saline solution.
2. Swab the bite area in a circular motion **from the periphery toward the center** using sterile technique. Rotate the swab so the sample is equally distributed on its surface.
3. Collect a similar sample from an unbitten area to use as a control.
4. Air dry the swabs thoroughly.
5. Place the sample and control swabs in separate sterile test tubes that are appropriately labeled.
6. Collect a sample of saliva by having the patient chew on a 1″-x-1″ square of gauze for 1 minute (Hampl, 1980).
7. Air dry the gauze, place it in an appropriately labeled sterile specimen container, and refrigerate it.
8. Collect blood samples as needed. (**Note:** This may include skin samples as well as venipuncture).

COMPLICATIONS

1. Failure to recognize a bite mark.
2. Incisions, punctures, or other wounds made in close proximity to the bite mark during medical treatment may alter or destroy evidence.
3. Improper collection or preservation of evidence or a break in the chain of custody may result in the evidence being declared inadmissible during legal proceedings.

PATIENT TEACHING

Follow up with law enforcement regarding legal proceedings and the possible need for additional photographs at a later date (i.e., after bruising is well developed).

REFERENCES

Hampl, P.F. 1980. *A training booklet on bite mark evidence in crimes against persons.* Tacoma, WA: Author.

Sperber, N.D. 1981. Bite mark evidence in crimes against persons. *FBI Law Enforcement Bulletin,* 7:16–19.

SUGGESTED READINGS

Beckstead, J.W., Rawson, R.D., & Giles, W.S. 1979. Review of bite mark evidence. *Journal of the American Dental Association,* 99, 1:69–74.

Bernstein, M.L. 1983. The application of photography in forensic dentistry. *Dental Clinics of North America,* 27:151–171.

Carmona, R. & Prince, K. 1989. Trauma and forensic medicine. *Journal of Trauma,* 29:1222–1225.

Gold, M.H., Roenigk, H.H., Smith, E.S., & Pierce, L.J. 1989. Evaluation and treatment of patients with human bite marks. *American Journal of Forensic Medicine and Pathology,* 10, 2:140–143.

Johnson, L.T., & Cadle, D. 1989. Bite mark evidence: Recognition, preservation, analysis and courtroom presentation. *New York State Dental Journal,* 3:38–41.

Levine, L.J. 1977. Bite mark evidence. *Dental Clinics of North America,* 21:145–158.

Mittleman, R.E., Goldberg, H.S., & Waksman, D.M. 1983. Preserving evidence in the emergency department. *American Journal of Nursing,* 12:1653–1656.

181

Evidence Collection for Sexual Assault Victims

Evidence collection for sexual assault is also known as alleged sexual assault (ASA) or rape exam.

Linell M. Jones, RN, BSN, CEN, CCRN

INDICATIONS

1. To obtain specimens from the sexual assault victim for examination by the crime laboratory when the assault occurred less than 48 hours prior to presentation.
2. To obtain control specimens from the victim.
3. To aid in the investigation and prosecution of the assailant.

CONTRAINDICATIONS AND CAUTIONS

1. Each jurisdiction has specific requirements. Check with the local law enforcement agency and crime laboratory for specific specimen collection and handling requirements.
2. Patient refuses exam for other than medical reasons and understands the consequences of such refusal (i.e., inability to prosecute).
3. The assault occurred more than 48 hours prior to examination. While the exam for trauma and prophylaxis is still valuable, there is no remaining evidence to be collected if there has been no contact for 48 hours or more. Each case needs to be evaluated individually and the physician may feel that an attempt at evidence collection would be valuable.
4. Place clothing in plastic bags to prevent leakage of blood/body fluids. If the clothing is wet, notify the receiving law enforcement agency that it will need to be dried as soon as possible to prevent the formation of mold and mildew.
5. Care should be taken not to be judgmental. Avoid any assumptions about guilt, innocence, or contributing factors.
6. These procedures may also be used for male victims.

PATIENT PREPARATION

1. Provide immediate privacy and emotional support for the victim.
2. Immediately assign the victim a primary nurse.
3. Initiate referrals to a rape relief agency or victim's advocate, social worker, law enforcement and/or anyone else the patient requests.
4. Obtain consent for treatment, evidence collection, law enforcement involvement, photographs (if needed), and release of information.
5. Obtain a brief history of the assault and post assault period to determine what care is needed and what samples are required. A detailed description of the assault is not necessary and should be left to law enforcement personnel.
6. Obtain a brief medical history and vital signs and assess the victim for physical trauma. Using a standardized sexual assault form (see Figure 181.1) facilitates consistent information collection and documentation.

AUTHORIZATION FOR COLLECTION AND RELEASE OF INFORMATION AND EVIDENCE

I hereby authorize Valley Medical Center to collect any specimens and photographs and to supply the specimens, photographs and copies of all medical reports to appropriate law enforcement agencies.

Patient/Guardian Signature	Witness Signature and Title

GYN HISTORY

LMP:_____

Contraceptives:_____

Menstrual Duration:_____

Gravida___ Para___

Last Voluntary coitus

within 7 days:_____

MISC:

Photographs taken? _____

Photographer:_____

Woods Lamp:_____

Labs:

Thayer Martin:_____

Chlamydia:_____

Gram Stain:_____

Wet Mount:_____

RPR:_____

HCG:_____

DISCHARGED:

MAT:

ANTIEMETIC:

VD PROPHYLAXIS:

OTHER MEDICATIONS:

MAT INFO SHEET:

PT INFO SHEET:

REFERRAL MD:

ASSAULT HISTORY

Approximate-

TIME OF ASSAULT:_____

DATE OF ASSAULT:_____

NUMBER OF ASSAILANTS:_____

TYPE OF ASSAULT: (1) penis (2) finger (3) object

    Vaginal:(_____) Oral:(_____)

    Rectal:(_____) Other:(_____)

ARE YOU INJURED OR HURT? _____

_____

_____

_____

_____

_____

_____

POST ASSAULT

Wiped genitals_____	Brushed teeth _____
Urinated _____	Changed clothes_____
Bathed _____	Eaten _____
Douched _____	Gargled _____
Vomited _____	
Defecated _____	

NOTES:

RN SIGNATURE:	DATE:

VALLEY MEDICAL CENTER
SEXUAL ASSAULT FORM

Figure 181.1 Sample of a sexual assault form.
(Courtesy of Valley Medical Center, Renton, WA.)

PHYSICAL EXAMINATION

(Describe or mark any abrasions, lacerations, tears, edema, erythema, ecchymosis, foreign bodies or fluorescence with woods lamp.)

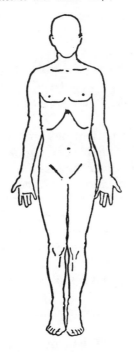

HEENT _____

NECK _____

BACK _____

CHEST _____

ABDOMEN _____

ARMS _____

LEGS _____

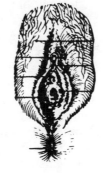

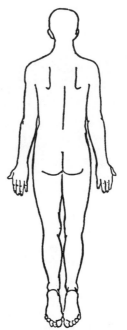

GENITALS _____

PELVIC EXAMINATION

VULVA _____

HYMEN _____

CERVIX _____

FUNDUS _____

ADNEXAE _____

RECTAL _____

** INCLUDE ALL SIGNS OF TRAUMA (size and development of sex organs if child or adolescent).

ASSESSMENT: (somatic complaints relevant to assault and/or current problems impacted by assault)

7. Report circumstances to the physician, including orifices involved, trauma sustained, and other pertinent history.
8. The specimens for a pregnancy test and serology for syphilis may be obtained while the nurse prepares for the examination and evidence collection.

GENERAL PROCEDURAL STEPS

Specific information on each aspect of this procedure is found later in the chapter.

1. Collect clothing if the patient has not changed since the assault.
2. Collect head and pubic hair combings and controls. Only controls are collected if the patient has showered and shampooed since the assault. These may be used to compare to trace evidence found either on the assailant or at the scene.
3. Collect fingernail scrapings/clippings. This is indicated primarily if the patient scratched the assailant or clawed at anything in the environment, however, some jurisdictions routinely collect them on all victims.
4. Photograph injuries as indicated. If possible, arrange to have the photography done by a forensic photographer in conjunction with the law enforcement agency.
5. Collect bite mark evidence. See Ch. 180: Collection of Bite Mark Evidence.
6. *Examine the perineum with an ultraviolet or Wood's Lamp. Semen fluoresces yellow under ultraviolet light. Suspicious areas should be swabbed. (See specific information on swab collection later in this chapter.)
7. *Swab the perineum with toluidine blue. Fourchette lacerations visible only with toluidine blue may be the only evidence of forced penetration (Lauber, 1982).
8. *Perform pelvic/rectal/oral exams as indicated by assault history. Moisten speculum only with water as most lubricants contain bacteriostatic agents that may alter results. See Ch. 104: Pelvic Examination.
9. *Obtain swabs for the crime lab from each involved orifice.
10. *Obtain wet mounts for motile sperm from each involved orifice.
11. *Obtain baseline cultures for chlamydia and gonorrhea from each involved orifice.
   (**Note:** Some facilities still obtain aspirate from each involved orifice to be tested for the presence of acid phosphatase. Most crime labs can obtain this information from the dried swabs provided to them.)
12. *Obtain pap smear and gram stain.
   (**Note:** Some facilities continue to do this even though this is duplicated information obtained from other tests.)
13. *Provide prophylaxis for sexually transmitted diseases or pregnancy as indicated/ordered. Common prophylaxis protocols are

for STDs:	Cephtriaxone 250 mg IM, and
	Doxycycline 250 po bid ×7 days
for Pregnancy:	Ovral 2 stat and 2 in 12 hrs, and
	Antiemetic of choice

   (Note: AZT may be given for HIV prophylaxis by some practitioners.)

*Indicates portions of the procedure usually performed by a physician.

ADDITIONAL INFORMATION

1. Specimens commonly retained by the hospital include
   a. Tests for venereal diseases
   b. Swab or aspirate for acid phosphase

    c. Wet mount for sperm motility (performed within 30 min of obtaining sample)

    d. Gram stain

    e. Pap smear (permanent slide) (optional)

2. Specimens commonly released to law enforcement personnel include
   a. Clothing
   b. Fingernail and hair samples
   c. 2–3 air dried swabs from each involved orifice
   d. 1–2 air dried swabs from fluorescing areas
3. Samples must be taken from each involved area and labeled as such.
4. If law enforcement personnel are not present to take custody of the evidence, the chain of custody must be preserved and documented. This may require placing the evidence in a locked area with limited accessibility.

LABELING EVIDENCE

1. All specimens must be labeled with permanent ink.
2. Labels must be nonremovable.
3. Information must include
   a. Patient's name
   b. Contents of envelope or bag
   c. The name of the person collecting the specimen and the person labeling the specimen (only one signature needed if the same person collects and labels the specimen)
   d. Date and time of collection.
4. Swabs may be marked with a line on the wood so that the person doing the marking will be able to identify it at a later date (in court). After the swab has dried, place it in an envelope or tube and label the envelope or tube with the above information.
5. Signatures should appear across the seal of all envelopes and clothing bags.

CLOTHING COLLECTION

EQUIPMENT

Evidence inventory form (see example Figure 181.2) (optional)

Many small and large, new plastic bags

Many permanent labels

Butcher or stretcher paper

Stapler

Pen

PROCEDURAL STEPS

1. Place sufficient paper on floor to allow patient to undress standing on the paper. This is to gather any trace evidence that may fall off clothing or the patient while undressing.
2. Have the patient remove one piece of clothing at a time. Have the patient place the clothing into a bag.
3. Seal, initial, and label the bag.
4. Remove the contents of each bag on evidence inventory form and on the bag.
5. Carefully fold up the paper to collect any evidence that may have fallen onto it, place it in a bag, seal and label.

3. Seal, initial, and label the bag.
4. Remove the contents of each bag on evidence inventory form and on the bag.
5. Carefully fold up the paper to collect any evidence that may have fallen onto it, place it in a paper bag, seal and label.

HAIR COLLECTION

EQUIPMENT

2 Cotton stuffed combs (one for head hair and one for pubic hair)
Iris scissors

4 envelopes
4 pieces of paper
Labels

PROCEDURAL STEPS

1. Place paper on shoulders and under buttocks before combing.
2. Comb hair until no more hair comes out using the cotton stuffed comb. Comb the entire head with one comb and the entire pubic area with the other. (The patient may prefer to do this under supervision.)
3. Wrap the combs up in their respective papers. Place in separate envelopes, seal and label them as "combings."
4. Obtain control samples: Pluck at least 2 hairs from all areas of the head and clip at least 10 more hairs and place on piece of paper (minimum 72 hairs). Fold up paper and seal in envelope. Label as "controls."

    Areas of the scalp are

    Left temple
    Right temple
    Top front
    Top center
    Back of head
    Nape of neck (near hairline)

Repeat with the pubis. Only 3 additional hairs clipped from each area are required (minimum 20 hairs).

    Areas of the pubis are:

    Center
    Periphery (sides)
    Top near naval
    From labia or scrotum (clip only)

(C. Quicklick, personal communication, 1985).

COLLECTION OF FINGERNAIL SCRAPING

EQUIPMENT

Small disposable nail scraper (such as found in disposable scrub brushes), toothpick, or orange stick

Specimen tube or envelope
Label

EVIDENCE INVENTORY

CLOTHING: IDENTIFY TYPE AND COLOR

Coat/Jacket   _____

Sweater   _____

Shirt/Blouse   _____

T-Shirt   _____

Undershirt   _____

Bra/Camisole   _____

Slip   _____

Dress   _____

Pants   _____

Skirt   _____

Nylons   _____

Panties   _____

Socks   _____

Shoes   _____

Other   _____

Other   _____

Other   _____

SWABS: Vaginal _____   Oral _____

        Rectal _____   Other _____

COMBINGS: Head Hair _____   Control _____

          Pubic Hair _____   Control _____

          Other _____   Control _____

OTHER TRACE EVIDENCE   _____

                        _____

                        _____

                        _____

_____

R.N. SIGNATURE

_____

RECEIVED BY

Figure 181.2   Sample of a evidence inventory form.
(Courtesy of Valley Medical Center, Renton, WA.)

PROCEDURAL STEPS

1. Using nail scraper or toothpick, scape under the patient's fingernails.
2. Place all material collected and the scraper into the specimen tube/envelope.
3. Label the tube/envelope. The label should overlap the stopper or envelope flap.

(Note: Some jurisdictions require that scrapings be separated and labeled "right hand" and "left hand." Also, some jurisdictions require fingernail clippings instead of scrapings. The clippings are handled in the same manner.

COLLECTION OF SWABS

EQUIPMENT

3 cotton swabs per area sampled
1 envelope or dry specimen tube
    per area sampled
Labels
Swab holder (for air drying)

Hair dryer
(Note: Locking boxes for swab
    drying are commercially
    available.)

PROCEDURAL STEPS

1. *Insert the swabs into the orifice for 10–15 seconds (vaginal pool, rectum, or buccal area)
2. Dry the swabs with cool air only (**no** heat) per local crime lab recommendations.
3. Mark the swabs, place them in individual paper wraps, and then in an envelope. Use one envelope per area sampled. The swabs may also be placed in dry specimen tubes.
4. Seal and label the envelopes/tubes.
5. If areas of fluorescence are seen during the ultraviolet light exam, a saline moistened swab is swabbed over the area and dried as above. Controls are taken in the same manner from an adjacent nonfluroescing area.
6. Extreme care must be taken to label the swabs correctly with the site from which they were obtained and to label control swabs as such.

TOLUIDINE BLUE EXAM

EQUIPMENT

1% Solution of toluidine blue
Cotton swabs
Cotton (or rayon) balls
Lubricating jelly

PROCEDURAL STEPS

1. **Prior** to insertion of the speculum, apply toluidine blue to the fourchette using cotton swabs (very little dye is necessary).
2. Allow to dry 5–10 seconds

3. *Gently wipe the area using cotton balls moistened with lubricating jelly.
4. *Repeat wiping until no further recovery of dye occurs.
5. *Lacerations may be differentiated from dye trapped in crevices by finer stroking with a dry cotton swab. Areas retaining deep royal blue stain in linear marks are interpreted as positive. No dye uptake or diffuse dye uptake is interpreted as negative (Lauber, 1982).
6. Care must be taken to wipe the area completely dry and to avoid allowing dye or jelly to enter the vagina.

PATIENT TEACHING

1. The testing done for sexually transmitted diseases and pregnancy is for a baseline only. There must be follow up in 1 and 6 weeks for repeat testing.
2. If you have elected to use the "morning after pill" (Ovral) to prevent pregnancy, you should have vaginal bleeding within a week. If not, you must be retested for pregnancy.
3. You will be provided with telephone numbers for emotional support centers. It is not unusual to have delayed reactions, such as fear, uncontrollable crying, anxiety, sleep disturbances, and anger.
4. You will be given the telephone number for the appropriate law enforcement agency if you have not yet reported the assault.

REFERENCES

Gunson, K. 1992. *Preserving forensic evidence: What nurses need to know.* Lecture presented at Oregon Health Sciences University, Portland, OR, September 17, 1992.

Lauber, A.A., & Souma, M.L., 1982. Use of toluidine blue for documentation of traumatic intercourse. *American Journal of Obstetrics and Gynecology,* 60:644–648.

SUGGESTED READINGS

McCauley, J., & Gorman, R.L., 1986. Toluidine blue in the detection of perineal lacerations in pediatric and adolescent sexual abuse victims. *Pediatrics,* 78, 6:1039–1043.

Osborn, M., & Bryan, G., 1989. Evidentiary examination in sexual assault. *Journal of emergency nursing,* 15, 3:284–290.

182

Identifying and Caring for the Potential Organ and/or Tissue Donor

Linell M. Jones, RN, BSN, CEN, CCRN

INDICATIONS

1. To help patients waiting for transplantable organs and tissues.
2. To assure the viability of organs to be used for transplantation such as heart, heart-lung, liver, kidneys, and pancreas (Gill, 1988).
3. To assure the viability of tissues to be used such as bone, cartilage, tendons, dura mater, fascia lata, skin, corneas, heart valves, whole eyes, and middle ear ossicles.
4. To assist the family in decision making by presenting available options, answering questions, and allaying fears.
5. To comply with "required request" laws and federal legislation mandating hospitals to have policies and procedures for identifying potential donors and for providing next of kin the opportunity to donate (Hart, 1986).

CONTRAINDICATIONS AND CAUTIONS

The contraindications are relative and any question of suitability should be answered by the local organ procurement agency (Northwest Kidney Center, 1986).

1. Cancer (except primary brain tumor)
   (Note: This varies with organ and tissue to be donated.)
2. Sepsis
3. Active transmissible disease, such as hepatitis, AIDS, tuberculosis, or meningitis
4. History of alternative lifestyle, such as drug abuse or homosexuality
5. Pre-existing disease or trauma of the organ or organs under consideration for donation
6. Next of kin denies consent (even if patient had signed organ donor card)
7. Religious prohibition
   (Note: Very few religions have restrictions. The decision is usually left up to the individual. If there are any questions, it is recommended that the family consult with their own religious leader or teacher (American Council on Transplantation, 1988).
8. Prolonged hypotension (< 70 mm Hg for > 30 minutes)
9. Malignant hypertension
10. Prolonged use of vasopressors
11. Medical examiner refuses to consent.

EQUIPMENT

609

Ch. 182 Identifying and Caring for
the Potential Organ and/or Tissue
Donor

Equipment is identical to that which is required of any critically ill or injured patient who is maintained on life support equipment.

PATIENT PREPARATION AND PROCEDURE

1. Identify the potential organ donor. The donor is usually young (0 months to 70 years old), and arrived in the emergency department alive

Table 182.1 Organ donor checklist (Northwest Organ Procurement Agency)

1. Patient's name, age, sex, race
2. Patient's height and weight
3. Admission date and time
4. Current diagnosis, nature of illness or injury
5. Past medical history
6. Social history, i.e., IV drug abuse, homosexual lifestyle
7. Prehospital and emergency care
8. Invasive, operative, and arrest care
9. Blood type
10. Clinical status. Include duration and extent of hypotension and use of vasopressors.
11. Laboratory data
    All donors
    Blood type
    Chemistry profile
    Arterial blood gases
    HIV (Human immunodeficiency virus)
    Serology for syphilis
    Cultures of blood, urine, and sputum
    Complete blood count (CBC)
    Platelets
    HbSA (Hepatitis B surface antigen)
    HAA (Hepatitis Associated Antigen)
    Kidney donors
    Urinalysis
    Blood Urea Nitrogen (BUN)
    Creatinine
    Glucose
    Heart, Heart-Lung donors
    EKG
    Cardiac enzymes/isoenzymes
    Echocardiogram
    Chest x-ray
    Liver donors
    Prothrombin time (PT)
    Partial thromboplastin time (PTT)
    Bilirubin total, direct and indirect
    Liver enzymes
    Alkaline phosphatase
    Pancreas donors
    Amylase
12. Declaration of brain death, date and time
13. Consent status (next of kin, medical examiner)

610

Ch. 182 Identifying and Caring for
the Potential Organ and/or Tissue
Donor

but with total and irreversible brain damage. The admitting diagnosis is usually massive head trauma, intracerebral hemorrhage, primary brain tumor, cerebral hypoxia or anoxia from cardiac or respiratory arrest, drug overdose, or cerebral vascular accident.

2. Obtain the attending physician's consent.

3. Obtain information needed to determine donor suitability, see Table 182.1.

4. Contact the local organ procurement agency. If unknown call 1-800-24-DONOR, The United Network of Organ Sharing in Richmond, VA for referral to the local agency (Johnson, 1986). The procurement agency can assist with obtaining consents from next of kin and medical examiner as well as answer any questions that may arise. To find your local tissue bank contact the American Association of Tissue Banks, 703-827-9582 in McLean, VA.

5. Inquire of the next of kin if they have an interest in donating. Legal next of kin in order of preference are (1) spouse, (2) adult child, (3) parent, (4) sibling, (5) legal guardian, (6) any other legally authorized person.

†Needed for potential organ donors only

6. †*Declare the patient brain dead. See Table 182.2.

*Indicates portions of the procedure usually performed by a physician.

Table 182.2   Declaration of brain death

In 1981 the Uniform Determination of Death Act was adopted to establish standards to be used in the determination of death. "An individual who has sustained either (1) irreversible cessation of circulatory and respiratory functions, or (2) irreversible cessation of all functions of the entire brain, including the brain stem, is dead. A determination must be made in accordance with accepted medical standards."

Currently there is no uniform procedure used throughout the nation to determine brain death. Each institution must utilize its current policy and procedure to declare brain death. Criteria frequently include

1. Absence of all cerebral function. No movement or response to external stimulation.

2. Absence of all brain stem functions. Apnea, no movement or respiration when off the ventilator for three or more minutes after being on room air for ten minutes. Fixed, dilated pupils. Absent reflexes, totally flaccid, absent doll's eyes (oculocephalic reflex), negative cold caloric test (oculovestibular reflex), absent corneal reflex, and absent gag.

3. Electroencephalogram shows no activity (flat, isoelectric, electrocerebral silence).

4. Cerebral angiogram or radioisotope brain scan shows no blood flow to the brain.

5. All reversible causes have been ruled out including drug intoxication, hypothermia, metabolic coma, and shock.

7. Notify the medical examiner (ME) for consent. Almost all cases will fall under the ME's jurisdiction and his or her consent is required. Consent may be given over the phone or he or she may want to be present during the organ or tissue retrieval.

8. Obtain written consent from the next of kin. See Figure 182.1.

9. †Draw blood for tissue typing. Typically this consists of 50 ml in 1.000 U preservative-free heparin and 3–10 cc unheparinized tubes (red tops) (Northwest Kidney Center, 1986).

10. †Maintain adequate tissue oxygenation and organ perfusion. Prevent and treat complications.
Physiologic parameters (Brown, 1989) include
Systolic blood pressure > 90 mm Hg
Urinary output 50–100 ml/hr
Temperature > 32.2°C (36.6–37.5°C)
FiO_2 0.30–0.40, pH 7.35–7.45, pO_2 80–100, pCO_2 35–45, HCO_3 22–26 meg/l
CVP 5–12 cc H_2O
Normal electrolytes, blood chemistry

Consent for Organ and Tissue Donation

Out of consideration for those in need, and by reason of my relationship to the deceased, I hereby consent to the removal of the following organs or tissue for transplantation or the advancement of medical science and education.

I,_____, authorize the donation of the following

   (full legal name of next of kin)

organs/tissue from _____.

                (full legal name of donor)

Tissues		Organs	
_____	Eyes	_____	Kidneys
_____	Bone and connective tissue:	_____	Heart
_____	Skin grafts	_____	Lungs
_____	Heart for valves	_____	Liver
_____	Additional research tissues	_____	Pancreas

Limitations:_____ _____ Other (specify) _____

I understand that tissue samples may be tested and pertinent diagnostic and medical information will be reviewed to assure medical suitability and that all donors must be tested for transmissible diseases (AIDS, hepatitis, syphilis) before transplantation can occur.

I hereby acknowledge that this consent is voluntarily given and motivated by humanitarian instincts without expectation of reward or compensation. It implies no obligation on the part of the recipient, this facility or its designees. Distribution and determination of use of these gifts will be coordinated by the procurement program in accordance with medical and ethical standards.

I understand that any additional charges directly associated with the donation will be covered by the procurement agency. Disposition of the body after the removal of organs and tissue will remain the responsibility of the next of kin.

_____

Signature of next of kin   Date/time   Relationship

_____

Address   Phone

_____

City, State, Zip

_____

Signature of person obtaining consent   Date

_____

Witness   Date

_____

Facility   City/State

Figure 182.1   Sample consent form for anatomical gift.
(Northwest Organ Procurement Agency, 1990. Reprinted by permission.)

612

Ch. 182 Identifying and Caring for
the Potential Organ and/or Tissue
Donor

COMPLICATIONS

The nurse should be aware that many complications may arise secondary to the initial injury or current medical treatment. These complications may include

1. Neurogenic shock, treated with fluids or dopamine if necessary.
2. Diabetes insipidus from damage to hypothalamus, treated with vasopressin.
3. Electrolyte imbalance
4. Hypothermia from hypothalamic destruction, treated with gradual warming methods.
5. Hyperthermia from brain stem destruction, treated with cooling measures.
6. Nosocomial infections of respiratory and urinary tracts, prevented with aggressive pulmonary toilet and aseptic technique and treated with appropriate antibiotics.
7. Pulmonary edema from left ventricular failure
8. Adult Respiratory Distress Syndrome (ARDS)
9. Atelectasis
10. Barotrauma from mechanical ventilation
11. Skin breakdown

PATIENT TEACHING

Support must be given to the family of the potential organ/tissue donor. The option of organ/tissue donation may represent the final option available to the family.

1. Be honest. Do not give false hope of recovery.
2. Relay information early.
3. The initial approach of donation should be kept simple and unpressured. Allow the family time to think.
4. Reassure the family. The patient will feel no pain, care is taken to maintain a normal appearance after the donation, and funeral arrangements remain unchanged. Financial responsibility from the declaration of brain death through organ retrieval is that of the organ procurement agency. Financial responsibility for the funeral is that of the family.
5. Encourage inclusion of clergy.
6. It is important to remember that even if the patient does not meet the criteria for organ donation, tissue donation is accepted up to 24 hours after cessation of circulation (Howard, 1989).

REFERENCES

Brown, M. 1989. Clinical management of the organ donor. *Dimensions of Critical Care Nursing*, 8:134–142.

Gill, B. 1988. Cardiac transplantation: Issues of donor procurement and management. *Journal of Cardiovascular Nursing* 2, 2:31–38.

Hart, D. 1986. Helping the family of the potential organ donor: Crisis intervention and decision making. *Journal of Emergency Nursing*, 12, 4:210–212.

Howard, S. 1989. "How Do I Ask?" Requesting tissue or organ donations from bereaved families. *Nursing*, 19, 1:70–73.

Johnson, L. 1986. A case for organ donation. *Journal of Emergency Nursing*, 12, 4:196–198.

Kozlowski, L. 1988. Case study in identification and maintenance of an organ donor. *Heart Lung*, 17:366–371.

Northwest Organ Procurement Agency. 1986. *Organ Recovery Procedure Manual.* Seattle, WA.

President's commission for the study of ethical problems in medicine and biomedical and behavioral research: Guidelines for the determination of brain death. 1981. *Journal of the American Medical Association,* 246:2184–2186.

SUGGESTED READING

Bouressa, G., O'Mara, R. 1987. Ethical dilemmas in organ procurement and donation. *Critical Care Nursing Quarterly,* 10, 2:37–47.

Cox, J. 1986. Organ donation: The challenge for emergency nursing. *Journal of Emergency Nursing,* 12, 4:199–204.

Diggs, C. 1986. Recognition and nursing care of organ donors. *Journal of Emergency Nursing,* 12, 4:205–209.

Lenehan, G. 1986. The gift of life: Organ donation and the emergency nurse. *Journal of Emergency Nursing,* 12, 4:189–191.

Index